S A U N D E R S

PHARMACEUTICAL XREF BOOK

2002

RANDY DRAKE, BS
ELLEN DRAKE, CMT

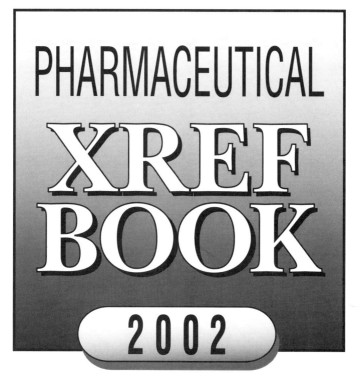

S A U N D E R S

PHARMACEUTICAL
XREF
BOOK
2002

W.B. SAUNDERS COMPANY
Philadelphia London New York St. Louis Sydney Toronto

W.B. SAUNDERS COMPANY

The Curtis Center
Independence Square West
Philadelphia, Pennsylvania 19106

www.wbsaunders.com

SAUNDERS PHARMACEUTICAL XREF BOOK 2002   ISBN 0–7216–9687–2

ISSN 1527–0696

Printed in the United States of America.

Last digit is the print number: 9   8   7   6   5   4   3   2   1

To the Lord Jesus

I saw the Holy City, the new Jerusalem,
    coming down out of heaven from God,
    prepared as a bride beautifully dressed for her husband.

And I heard a loud voice from the throne saying,
"Now the dwelling of God is with men,
    and He will live with them.
They will be His people, and God himself
    will be with them and be their God.

"He will wipe every tear from their eyes.
There will be no more death or mourning or crying or pain,
    for the old order of things has passed away."

                  — Revelation 21:2–4

Contents

Preface ix

Notes on Using the Text xi
    How the Book Is Arranged

Section 1: XRef Generic Names to ℞ Brand Name Drugs 1

Section 2: XRef Indications to Generic and ℞ Brand Name Drugs 97

Section 3: XRef Investigational Code Names to Generic Names 230
    4117 Manufacturer Drug Codes with Names

Section 4: XRef Street Drug Slang to Pharmaceutical Names 275
    1540 Slang Terms for Illegally Abused Drugs

Section 5: Hazardous Materials 301
    3156 HazMat Entries with Potential Adverse Effects

Preface

This book is intended to be a companion to our main drug reference, *Saunders* *Pharmaceutical Word Book*, and to provide new ways to access the information it contains. It has been written in response to numerous requests for a cross-reference between generic drugs and the brands that contain them, and a listing of drugs by indication (also known as the drug's "designated use," "approved use," or "therapeutic action"). This book, now in its third year of publication, contains both of these cross-referencing schemes.

The Investigational Codes and Street Drug Slang, which originally appeared as appendices to our main book, are also included. These specialized lists are of use to those in medical research, mental health, and emergency medicine.

We have also included a listing of over 3000 hazardous materials and their potential adverse effects. The correct names and spellings of such materials are exceedingly hard to locate; they have been collected here for quick reference.

We urge you to take a moment to study the contents page and to read "Notes on Using the Text" on the following pages. It will be well worth your time to help make the most of this valuable tool.

As you use the book, you may have suggestions for changes or additions that would make the book more complete or easier to use. In particular, you may find that Section 2 should have more, less, or different indications listed. The categorization of drugs by indications is not an exact science, and there are several different schemes to accomplish it. We have chosen a scheme and then modified it slightly, to present the information in a form we feel is most useful for our readers. The indications listing will be refined in future editions, and we welcome your input. We also welcome your comments regarding additions, inconsistencies, or inaccuracies in either book. Please send them to us via e-mail at the address below, or via regular mail to W.B. Saunders Company, The Curtis Center, Independence Square West, Philadelphia, PA 19106-3399.

Authors' e-mail address:
    spwb@saunders.net
Authors' web site:
    spwb.saunders.net

RANDY DRAKE, BS
ELLEN DRAKE, CMT
Atlanta, Georgia

Notes on Using the Text

The purpose of the *Saunders Pharmaceutical XRef Book* is to provide medical transcriptionists (as well as medical records administrators and technicians, coders, nurses, ward clerks, court reporters, legal secretaries, medical assistants, allied health students, physicians, and even pharmacists) with a quick, easy-to-use cross-reference to the information contained in our main reference book, *Saunders Pharmaceutical Word Book*. Specifically, *Saunders Pharmaceutical XRef Book 2002* is a cross-reference to the entries contained in *Saunders Pharmaceutical Word Book 2002*. As such, it is not intended to be used as a stand-alone reference book.

How the Book Is Arranged

This book is arranged in five sections. Section markings in the right margin make it easy to quickly turn to the needed section.

Section 1 is a cross-reference between generic drugs and the ℞ brand name drugs that contain those generics. The drug names in bold are the generic ingredients; the indented list that follows are the brands which contain that ingredient. *Every* generic contained in *every* ℞ brand name drug appearing in *Saunders Pharmaceutical Word Book* is included in the list of generics. A brand name drug with more than one active ingredient is listed under each ingredient, with an asterisk denoting it as a combination product. For example, Ser-Ap-Es* appears three times —under hydrochlorothiazide, under reserpine, and under hydralazine HCl.

Section 2 is a cross-reference between a drug's indication (also known as the drug's "designated use," "approved use," or "therapeutic action") and generic or ℞ brand name drugs. In effect, all drugs used for a particular indication are listed together under the indication heading. For example, all beta-blockers appear under the heading "Antihypertensives, β-Blockers."

Combination brands may be listed under multiple indications, according to the generic ingredients they contain. Hyzaar, for example, is listed under both "Antihypertensives, Angiotensin II Inhibitors" (because of its losartan content) and under "Antihypertensives, Diuretics" (because of its hydrochlorothiazide content). Not all combination brands are listed under multiple categories, however. The combination product Ortho-Novum appears only under "Gynecological Agents, Contraceptives, Oral" for example. Both generic drugs and single-ingredient brands may appear under more than one category, if they're used for multiple purposes. The generic bupropion HCl, for example, appears under "Psychotherapeutics, Antidepressants"(along with the Wellbutrin brand), and also under "Smoking Cessation Agents" (along with the Zyban brand). Valium (diazepam) appears in four categories, reflecting its use as an anticonvulsant, anxiolytic, sedative/hypnotic, and muscle relaxant.

Section 3 is a listing of investigational code names, cross-referenced to the subsequently assigned generic name, if any. A code name is a temporary identification assigned to a substance by its manufacturer. The number or letter-number combination is used while it is undergoing testing. The generic names shown in this section may be found in the main list of *Saunders Pharmaceutical Word Book*. If no name has been assigned, the code itself can be found in *Saunders Pharmaceutical Word Book*, along with its investigational use.

Section 4 has over 1500 "street slang" terms for illegally abused drugs. Each slang term is cross-referenced to the official name of the substance, which can be found in the main list of *Saunders Pharmaceutical Word Book*. For example, "magic mushroom" shows a cross-reference to psilocybin and psilocin, which can be found in the main list.

Section 5 lists over 3000 hazardous materials (HazMat) and their potential adverse effects. These industrial chemicals, poisons, flammable materials, radioactive substances, petroleum products, and biological agents produce a wide variety of adverse effects in the human body. Although this section has no cross-reference to the main book, the information can be of great use to people working in or with emergency departments and law enforcement agencies.

XRef Generic Names to ℞ Brand Name Drugs

Each brand name drug entry in the *Saunders Pharmaceutical Word Book* shows the generic name for each of the active ingredients it contains. It is often helpful, however, to cross-reference the generic ingredients back to the brand name drugs. Listed below is every active ingredient contained in every ℞ brand name entry in *Saunders Pharmaceutical Word Book 2002*. Following each generic name is a list of the ℞ brand name drugs which contain that generic. Brands with multiple active ingredients are listed under each ingredient and noted with an asterisk.

abacavir sulfate
  Trizivir*
  Ziagen
abciximab
  ReoPro
absorbable collagen
  Helistat
absorbable gelatin
  Gelfilm; Gelfilm Ophthalmic
  Gelfoam
acarbose
  Prandase ⒸⒶⓃ
  Precose
acebutolol HCl
  Gen-Acebutolol ⒸⒶⓃ
  Sectral
acecarbromal
  Paxarel
acemannan
  Carrisyn
acetaminophen
  Aceta with Codeine*
  Aclophen*
  Alumadrine*
  Amaphen*
  Anatuss*
  Anexsia 5/500; Anexsia 7.5/650;
    Anexsia 10/660*
  Anoquan*
  Axocet*
  Bancap HC*
  Bucet*

acetaminophen (cont.)
  Bupap*
  Butex Forte*
  Capital with Codeine*
  Ceta Plus*
  Co-Gesic*
  Darvocet-N 50; Darvocet-N 100*
  DHC Plus*
  Dolacet*
  Dolene*
  Dolgic*
  Duocet*
  Duradrin*
  Endocet*
  Endolor*
  Esgic*
  Esgic-Plus*
  Femcet*
  Fioricet*
  Fioricet with Codeine*
  Fiorpap*
  Flexaphen*
  Flextra-DS*
  Histex SR*
  Hy-Phen*
  Hycomine Compound*
  Hydrocet*
  Hydrogesic*
  Isocet*
  Isocom*

*This brand is a combination product.

acetaminophen (cont.)
  Isopap*
  Lobac*
  Lorcet*
  Lorcet-HD*
  Lorcet Plus; Lorcet 10/650*
  Lortab*
  Lortab 2.5/500; Lortab 5/500; Lortab 7.5/500; Lortab 10/500*
  Margesic*
  Margesic H*
  Marten-Tab*
  Maxidone*
  Medigesic*
  Medipain 5*
  Midchlor*
  Midrin*
  Migratine*
  Myapap
  Norco*
  Norel Plus*
  Oncet*
  Oxycocet ⓒ*
  Panacet 5/500*
  Panlor DC*
  Percocet*
  Phenaphen with Codeine No. 3 & No. 4*
  Phenate*
  Phrenilin*
  Phrenilin Forte*
  Prominol*
  Propacet 100*
  Repan*
  Repan CF*
  Roxicet*
  Roxicet 5/500*
  Roxilox*
  Sedapap*
  Stagesic*
  T-Gesic*
  Talacen*
  Tencet*
  Tencon*
  Triad*
  Triaprin*
  Two-Dyne*
  Tylenol with Codeine*
  Tylenol with Codeine No. 2, No. 3, and No. 4*

acetaminophen (cont.)
  Tylox*
  Ultracet*
  Vicodin; Vicodin ES; Vicodin HP*
  Wygesic*
  Zydone*
acetazolamide
  Dazamide
  Diamox
acetazolamide sodium
  Diamox
acetic acid
  AA-HC Otic*
  Acetasol
  Acetasol HC*
  Borofair Otic*
  Otic Domeboro*
  Otomycet-HC*
  VōSol HC Otic*
  VōSol Otic
  Vasotate HC*
acetohexamide
  Dymelor
acetohydroxamic acid
  Lithostat
acetylcholine chloride
  Miochol-E
acetylcysteine
  Fluimucil
  Mucomyst 10
acetylcysteine sodium
  Mucomyst
  Mucosil-10; Mucosil-20
acetylhydrolase
  Pafase
acidulated phosphate fluoride
  Minute-Gel
  Phos-Flur
acitretin
  Soriatane
acrivastine
  Semprex-D*
acyclovir
  Apo-Acyclovir ⓒ
  Genvir
  Zovirax
acyclovir sodium
  Zovirax

*This brand is a combination product.

adapalene
Differin
adefovir dipivoxil
Preveon
adenosine
Adenocard
Adenoscan
agalsidase alfa
Replagal
agalsidase beta
Fabrazyme
alatrofloxacin mesylate
Trovan
albendazole
Albenza
albuterol
Proventil
Ventolin
Ventolin HFA
albuterol sulfate
AccuNeb
Airet
Combivent*
DuoNeb*
Proventil
Proventil HFA
Ventolin
Ventolin ⓒᴬᴺ
Volmax
alclometasone dipropionate
Aclovate
alcohol
Accurbron*
Actifed with Codeine Cough*
5% Alcohol and 5% Dextrose in
    Water; 10% Alcohol and 5%
    Dextrose in Water*
Ambenyl Cough*
Ana-Kit*
Bromanate DC Cough*
Bromarest DX Cough*
Bromphen DX Cough*
Brompheniramine DC Cough*
Bronkotuss Expectorant*
Calcidrine*
Cheracol Cough*
Codehist DH*
Contuss*
Cophene XP*
Cresylate*

alcohol (cont.)
Cyclofed Pediatric*
Cycofed Pediatric*
Decohistine DH*
Decongestant Expectorant*
Deconsal Pediatric*
Deproist Expectorant with Codeine*
Detussin*
Detussin Expectorant*
Dexacort Phosphate*
Dihistine Expectorant*
Dilaudid Cough*
Dimetane-DC Cough*
Dimetane-DX Cough*
Endal Expectorant*
Entuss-D Jr.*
Erygel*
Gantrisin*
Gengraf*
Guiatuss AC*
Guiatuss DAC*
Guiatussin DAC*
Guiatussin with Codeine Expecto-
    rant*
Histor-D*
H-Tuss-D*
Hycotuss Expectorant*
Hydramyn*
Hyphed*
Isoclor Expectorant*
Kaochlor 10%; Kaochlor S-F*
Kaon-Cl 20%*
Kaylixir*
Levsin PB*
Liquid Pred*
Myphetane DC Cough*
Myphetane DX Cough*
Mytussin AC Cough*
Mytussin DAC*
Norisodrine with Calcium Iodide*
Novagest Expectorant with
    Codeine*
Novahistine DH*
Novahistine Expectorant*
Nucofed Expectorant; Nucofed
    Pediatric Expectorant*
P-V-Tussin*
Pancof-HC*

*This brand is a combination product.

Generic ◆ Brands

alcohol (cont.)
  Pediacof*
  Peridex*
  PerioGard*
  Phenameth DM*
  Phenergan Fortis*
  Phenergan VC*
  Phenergan VC with Codeine*
  Phenergan with Codeine*
  Phenergan with Dextromethorphan*
  Phenhist DH with Codeine*
  Phenhist Expectorant*
  Pherazine DM*
  Pherazine VC with Codeine*
  Pherazine with Codeine*
  Point-Two*
  Polaramine Expectorant*
  Potasalan*
  Prelone*
  Prometh VC with Codeine*
  Prometh with Dextromethorphan*
  Promethazine DM*
  Promethazine VC Plain*
  Promethazine VC with Codeine*
  Promethist with Codeine*
  Robafen AC Cough*
  Robafen DAC*
  Robitussin A-C*
  Robitussin-DAC*
  Rolatuss Expectorant*
  Ru-Tuss with Hydrocodone*
  SangCya*
  Septisol*
  Sil-Tex*
  SRC Expectorant*
  Statuss Expectorant*
  Statuss Green*
  Synophylate-GG*
  Theomax DF*
  Theostat 80*
  Tinver*
  Toposar*
  Triacin-C Cough*
  Triaminic Expectorant DH*
  Trifed-C Cough*
  Tusquelin*
  Tussafin Expectorant*
  Tussanil DH*
  Tussar SF; Tussar-2*
  Tussend*

alcohol (cont.)
  Tusstat*
  Tyrodone*
  Vanex Expectorant*
  Versiclear*
  Vetuss HC*
  Xerac AC*
aldesleukin
  Maxamine
  Proleukin
alemtuzumab
  Campath
alendronate sodium
  Fosamax
alfacalcidol
  One-Alpha (CAN)
alfentanil HCl
  Alfenta
alglucerase
  Ceredase
alitretinoin
  Panretin
allantoin
  Alasulf*
  D.I.T.I.-2*
  Deltavac*
allergenic extracts
  Allpyral
  Center-Al
allopurinol
  Purinol (CAN)
  Zyloprim
allopurinol sodium
  Aloprim
almotriptan malate
  Axert
alosetron HCl
  Lotronex
alpha-galactosidase A
  CC-Galactosidase
  FABRase
alpha lipoic acid
  Strovite Advance*
alpha$_1$-proteinase inhibitor
  Prolastin
dl-alpha tocopheryl acetate
  Aquavit-E

---

*This brand is a combination product.

alprazolam
Xanax
alprostadil
Alprox-TD
Caverject
Edex
Muse
Prostin VR Pediatric
Topiglan
Vasoprost
alteplase
Activase
altretamine
Hexalen
aluminum acetate
Borofair Otic*
Otic Domeboro*
aluminum chloride
Drysol
Xerac AC*
aluminum hydroxide gel
Dialume
amantadine HCl
Symmetrel
ambenonium chloride
Mytelase
amcinonide
Cyclocort
amifostine
Ethyol
amikacin
MiKasome
amikacin sulfate
Amikin
amiloride HCl
Midamor
Moduretic*
aminacrine HCl
Alasulf*
D.I.T.I.-2*
Deltavac*
Vagisec Plus
amino acids, multiple
Aminess 5.2%*
Aminosyn 3.5% (5%, 7%, 8.5%, 10%); Aminosyn (pH6) 10%; Aminosyn II 3.5% (5%, 7%, 8.5%, 10%, 15%); Aminosyn-PF 7% (10%)*

amino acids, multiple (cont.)
Aminosyn 3.5% M; Aminosyn II 3.5% M*
Aminosyn 7% (8.5%) with Electrolytes; Aminosyn II 7% (8.5%, 10%) with Electrolytes*
Aminosyn-HBC 7%*
Aminosyn II 3.5% in 5% (25%) Dextrose; Aminosyn II 4.25% in 10% (20%, 25%) Dextrose; Aminosyn II 5% in 25% Dextrose*
Aminosyn II 3.5% M in 5% Dextrose; Aminosyn II 4.25% M in 10% Dextrose*
Aminosyn-RF 5.2%*
BranchAmin 4%*
FreAmine HBC 6.9%*
FreAmine III 3% (8.5%) with Electrolytes*
FreAmine III 8.5%; FreAmine III 10%*
HepatAmine*
NephrAmine 5.4%*
Novamine; Novamine 15%*
ProcalAmine*
ProSol 20%*
RenAmin*
Travasol 2.75% in 5% (10%, 25%) Dextrose; Travasol 4.25% in 5% (10%, 25%) Dextrose*
Travasol 3.5% (5.5%, 8.5%) with Electrolytes*
Travasol 5.5% (8.5%, 10%)*
TrophAmine 6%; TrophAmine 10%*
aminobenzoate potassium
Potaba
aminocaproic acid
Amicar
Caprogel
aminoglutethimide
Cytadren
aminolevulinic acid HCl
Levulan Kerastick
aminophylline
Mudrane*
Phyllocontin
Truphylline

---

*This brand is a combination product.

5-aminosalicylic acid
FIV-ASA
Salofalk ⓒᴬᴺ
aminosalicylic acid
Pamisyl
Paser
Rezipas
aminosidine
Gabbromicina
Paromomycin
amiodarone HCl
Alti-Amiodarone ⓒᴬᴺ
Amio-Aqueous
Cordarone
Gen-Amiodarone ⓒᴬᴺ
Novo-Amiodarone ⓒᴬᴺ
Pacerone
Rhoxal-amiodarone ⓒᴬᴺ
amiprilose HCl
Therafectin
amitriptyline HCl
Apo-Amitriptylene ⓒᴬᴺ
Elavil
Etrafon; Etrafon 2–10; Etrafon-A;
    Etrafon-Forte*
Limbitrol DS 10-25*
Novo-Triptyn ⓒᴬᴺ
Triavil*
Triavil 4-50*
amlexanox
Aphthasol
OraDisc
amlodipine
Norvasc
amlodipine besylate
Lotrel*
ammoniated mercury
Emersal*
Unguentum Bossi*
ammonium chloride
Rolatuss Expectorant*
ammonium lactate
Lac-Hydrin
ammonium molybdate tetrahydrate
Molypen
amobarbital sodium
Amytal Sodium
Tuinal*
amoxapine
Asendin

amoxicillin
Alti-Amoxi Clav ⓒᴬᴺ*
Amoxil
Augmentin*
Augmentin ES*
Biomox
Losec 1-2-3 A ⓒᴬᴺ*
Polymox
Prevpac*
Trimox
Wymox
amoxicillin sodium
Augmentin*
amoxicillin trihydrate
Apo-Amoxi ⓒᴬᴺ
Gen-Amoxicillin ⓒᴬᴺ
Hp-PAC ⓒᴬᴺ*
Lin-Amox ⓒᴬᴺ
Novamoxin ⓒᴬᴺ
amphetamine aspartate
Adderall*
Adderall XR*
amphetamine sulfate
Adderall*
Adderall XR*
amphotericin B
Fungizone
amphotericin B cholesteryl
Amphotec
amphotericin B deoxycholate
Amphocin
Fungizone
amphotericin B lipid complex
Abelcet
AmBisome
ampicillin
D-Amp
Marcillin
Omnipen
Polycillin
Polycillin-PRB*
Principen
Probampacin*
Totacillin
ampicillin sodium
Omnipen-N
Polycillin-N
Totacillin-N

*This brand is a combination product.

Generic ▶ Brands

ampicillin sodium (cont.)
Unasyn*
amprenavir
Agenerase
amsacrine
Amsidyl
amyl nitrite inhalant
Cyanide Antidote Package*
amylase
Arco-Lase Plus*
Cotazym*
Cotazym-S*
Creon*
Creon 10*
Creon 20*
Donnazyme*
Gustase Plus*
Ilozyme*
Ku-Zyme*
Ku-Zyme HP*
Kutrase*
Lipram-CR20*
Lipram-PN10*
Lipram-PN16*
Lipram-UL12*
Lipram-UL18*
Lipram-UL20*
Pancrease; Pancrease MT 4; Pancrease MT 10; Pancrease MT 16; Pancrease MT 20*
Pancrecarb MS-8*
Protilase*
Ultrase; Ultrase MT 12; Ultrase MT 18; Ultrase MT 20*
Viokase*
Zymase*
anagrelide HCl
Agrylin
anakinra
Antril
Kineret
ananain
Vianain*
anastrozole
Arimidex
ancestim
Stemgen ⒸⒶ⒩
ancrod
Arvin

ancrod (cont.)
Viprinex ⒸⒶ⒩
anisindione
Miradon
anistreplase
Eminase
antazoline phosphate
Vasocon-A*
anthralin
Anthra-Derm
Drithocreme; Drithocreme HP 1%; Dritho-Scalp
Lasan
Lasan HP-1
Miconal
anti-B4-blocked ricin MAb
Oncolysin B
anti-inhibitor coagulant complex
Autoplex T
Feiba VH Immuno
antihemophilic factor VIII
Bioclate
Helixate
Hemofil M
Humate-P
Koāte-DVI
Koāte-HP
Kogenate
Kogenate FS*
Recombinate
antihemophilic factor VIII:C
Alphanate
Antihemophilic Factor (Porcine) Hyate:C
Monoclate P
Profilate HP
antipyrine
Allergen Ear Drops*
Auralgan Otic*
Auroto Otic*
Otocalm*
Tympagesic*
antithrombin III
ATnativ
Kybernin
Thrombate III
antithymocyte globulin
Thymoglobulin

*This brand is a combination product.

antivenin (Crotalidae) polyvalent immune Fab
  CroFab
apomorphine HCl
  Apokinon
  Uprima
  Zydis
apraclonidine HCl
  Iopidine
aprobarbital
  Alurate
aprotinin
  Trasylol
aptiganel HCl
  Cerestat
arbutamine HCl
  GenESA
arcitumomab
  CEA-Scan
ardeparin sodium
  Normiflo
argatroban
  Acova
arginine HCl
  R-gene 10
arsenic trioxide
  Trisenox
articaine HCl
  Astracaine; Astracaine Forte ⓒⒶⓃ*
  Septocaine*
ascorbic acid
  Anemagen*
  Cevalin
  Cevi-Fer*
  Chromagen*
  Contrin*
  Fero-Folic-500*
  Ferotrinsic*
  Foltrin*
  Fumatinic*
  Livitrinsic-f*
  Nephplex Rx*
  Nephro-Vite Rx + Fe*
  Nephron FA*
  Pronemia Hematinic*
  TriHemic 600*
  Trinsicon*
asparaginase
  Elspar

aspirin
  Aggrenox*
  Alor 5/500*
  Aspirin with Codeine No. 2, No. 3, and No. 4*
  Axotal*
  Azdone*
  Butalbital Compound*
  Damason-P*
  Darvon Compound-65*
  Easprin
  Empirin with Codeine No. 3 & No. 4*
  Equagesic*
  Fiorgen PF*
  Fiorinal*
  Fiorinal with Codeine*
  Fiorinal-C ¼; Fiorinal-C ½ ⓒⒶⓃ*
  Fiortal*
  Isollyl Improved*
  Lanorinal*
  Lortab ASA*
  Marnal*
  Micrainin*
  Norgesic; Norgesic Forte*
  Orphengesic; Orphengesic Forte*
  Panasal 5/500*
  Percodan; Percodan-Demi*
  Robaxisal*
  Roxiprin*
  Sodol Compound*
  Soma Compound*
  Soma Compound with Codeine*
  Synalgos-DC*
  Talwin Compound*
  ZORprin
astemizole
  Hismanal
atenolol
  Apo-Atenolol ⓒⒶⓃ
  Tenoretic 50; Tenoretic 100*
  Tenormin
atorvastatin calcium
  Lipitor
atovaquone
  Malarone; Malarone Pediatric*
  Mepron

---

*This brand is a combination product.

atracurium besylate
Tracrium
atropine sulfate
Antispasmodic*
Antrocol*
Arco-Lase Plus*
Atrohist Plus*
AtroPen
Atropine Care
Atropine-1
Atropisol
Atrosept*
Barbidonna; Barbidonna No. 2*
Bellacane*
Deconhist L.A.*
Dolsed*
Donna-Sed*
Donnatal*
Donnatal No. 2*
Enlon Plus*
Hyosophen*
Isopto Atropine
Logen*
Lomanate*
Lomotil*
Lonox*
Malatal*
Motofen*
Phenahist-TR*
Phenchlor S.H.A.*
Prosed/DS*
Sal-Tropine
Spasmolin*
Stahist*
Susano*
Trac Tabs 2X*
UAA*
Uridon Modified*
Urinary Antiseptic No. 2*
Urised*
Uritin*
auranofin
Ridaura
aurothioglucose
Solganal
autologous cell vaccine
O-Vax
azatadine maleate
Optimine
Rynatan*

azatadine maleate (cont.)
Trinalin*
azathioprine
Imuran
azathioprine sodium
Imuran
azelaic acid
Azelex
Finevin
azelastine HCl
Astelin
Optivar
azithromycin
Trovan/Zithromax Compliance Pak*
Zithromax
aztreonam
Azactam
bacampicillin HCl
Spectrobid
bacitracin
AK-Tracin
Baci-IM
bacitracin zinc
AK-Spore*
AK-Spore H.C.*
AK-Poly-Bac*
Cortisporin*
Neosporin*
Neotricin HC*
Ocutricin*
Triple Antibiotic*
baclofen
Lioresal
**bactericidal and permeability-
  increasing protein**
Neuprex
balsalazide disodium
Colazal
barium sulfate
Anatrast
Baricon
Baro-cat
Barobag
Baroflave
Barosperse
Barosperse, Liquid
Bear-E-Bag Pediatric
Bear-E-Yum CT

---

*This brand is a combination product.

barium sulfate (cont.)
Bear-E-Yum GI
Enecat
Enhancer
Entrobar*
Epi-C
Flo-Coat
HD 200 Plus
HD 85
Imager ac
Intropaste
Liqui-Coat HD
Liquipake
Medebar Plus
Medescan
Novopaque
Prepcat
Quick AC Enema Kit
Tomocat
Tonopaque
basic fuchsin
Castellani Paint Modified*
BCG vaccine
ImmuCyst ⒸⒶⓃ
OncoTICE ⒸⒶⓃ
Pacis
TheraCys
Tice BCG
becaplermin
Regranex
beclomethasone dipropionate
Apo-Beclomethasone ⒸⒶⓃ
Becloforte Inhaler ⒸⒶⓃ
Beclovent
Beclovent Inhaler ⒸⒶⓃ
Beconase
Beconase AQ
Nu-Beclomethasone ⒸⒶⓃ
QVAR
Vancenase
Vancenase AQ
Vanceril; Vanceril Double Strength
belladonna alkaloids
Bel-Phen-Ergot SR*
Bellacane SR*
Folergot-DF*
Phenerbel-S*
belladonna extract
B & O Supprettes No. 15A; B & O
Supprettes No. 16A*

belladonna extract (cont.)
Bellafoline
Bellergal-S*
Butibel*
Cafatine-PB*
Chardonna-2*
benazepril HCl
Lotensin
Lotensin HCT 5/6.25; Lotensin
HCT 10/12.5; Lotensin HCT
20/12.5; Lotensin HCT 20/25*
Lotrel*
bendroflumethiazide
Corzide 40/5; Corzide 80/5*
Naturetin
Rauzide*
benoxinate HCl
Flu-Oxinate*
Flurate*
Fluress*
bentiromide
Chymex
benzocaine
Allergen Ear Drops*
Americaine Anesthetic Lubricant
Americaine Otic
Auralgan Otic*
Auroto Otic*
Cetacaine*
Otocain
Otocalm*
T-Gen*
Tebamide*
Tigan*
Triban; Pediatric Triban*
Tympagesic*
benzoic acid
Atrosept*
Bensal HP*
Cystex*
Dolsed*
Prosed/DS*
Trac Tabs 2X*
UAA*
Uridon Modified*
Urinary Antiseptic No. 2*
Urised*
Uritin*

---

*This brand is a combination product.

benzonatate
  Tessalon
benzoyl peroxide
  Benzac AC 2½; Benzac W 2½; Benzac 5; Benzac AC 5; Benzac W 5; Benzac 10; Benzac AC 10; Benzac W 10
  Benzac AC Wash 2½; Benzac AC Wash 5; Benzac W Wash 5; Benzac AC Wash 10; Benzac W Wash 10
  Benzaclin*
  5 Benzagel; 10 Benzagel
  Benzagel Wash
  Benzamycin*
  Benzashave
  Benzox-10
  Brevoxyl
  Brevoxyl Cleansing
  Brevoxyl Creamy Wash
  Del Aqua-5; Del Aqua-10
  Desquam-E; Desquam-E 5; Desquam-E 10
  Desquam-X 5 Wash; Desquam-X 10 Wash
  Desquam-X 5; Desquam-X 10
  Panoxyl
  Panoxyl AQ 2½; Panoxyl 5; Panoxyl AQ 5; Panoxyl 10; Panoxyl AQ 10
  Peroxin A 5; Peroxin A 10
  Persa-Gel; Persa-Gel W 5%; Persa-Gel W 10%
  Sulfoxyl Regular; Sulfoxyl Strong*
  Triaz
  Vanoxide-HC*
benzphetamine HCl
  Didrex
benzthiazide
  Exna
benztropine mesylate
  Cogentin
benzydamine HCl
  Apo-Benzydamine ⒸⒶⓃ
  Tantrum
benzylpenicillin
  Pre-Pen/MDM
benzylpenicilloyl polylysine
  Pre-Pen
bepridil HCl
  Vascor

beractant
  Survanta
beta alethine
  Beta LT
betaine HCl
  Cystadane
betamethasone acetate
  Betaject ⒸⒶⓃ*
  Celestone Soluspan*
betamethasone dipropionate
  Alphatrex
  Diprolene
  Diprolene AF
  Diprosone
  Lotrisone*
  Maxivate
  Teladar
betamethasone sodium phosphate
  Betaject ⒸⒶⓃ*
  Cel-U-Jec
  Celestone Phosphate
  Celestone Soluspan*
betamethasone valerate
  Beta-Val
  Betatrex
  Celestoderm-V; Celestoderm-V/2 ⒸⒶⓃ
  Luxiq
  Valisone
  Valisone Reduced Strength
betaxolol HCl
  Betoptic; Betoptic S
  Kerlone
  Sab-Betaxolol ⒸⒶⓃ
bethanechol chloride
  Duvoid
  Myotonachol
  PMS-Bethanechol Chloride ⒸⒶⓃ
  Urecholine
bexarotene
  Targretin
bezafibrate
  PMS-Bezafibrate ⒸⒶⓃ
bicalutamide
  Casodex
bile salts
  Digepepsin*
bimatoprost
  Lumigan

*This brand is a combination product.

Generic ♠ Brands

biotin
  B-C with Folic Acid Plus*
  Bacmin*
  Berocca Parenteral Nutrition*
  Berocca Plus*
  Berplex Plus*
  Cernevit-12*
  Enfamil Natalins Rx*
  Formula B Plus*
  M.V.I. Pediatric*
  M.V.I.-12*
  Materna*
  Mynatal*
  Mynatal FC*
  Mynatal Rx*
  Natalins Rx*
  Natarex Prenatal*
  Nephplex Rx*
  Nephro-Vite Rx + Fe*
  Nephro-Vite Rx*
  Nephrocaps*
  Nephron FA*
  Prenatal Maternal*
  Prenatal Rx with Betacarotene*
  Strovite Advance*
  Strovite Plus; Strovite Forte*
  Zodeac-100*
biperiden HCl
  Akineton
biperiden lactate
  Akineton
biricodar dicitrate
  Incel
bisacodyl tannex
  Clysodrast
bismuth subsalicylate
  Helidac*
bisoprolol
  Probeta
bisoprolol fumarate
  Monocor ⒸⒶⓃ
  Zebeta
  Ziac*
bithionol
  Bitin
  Lorothidol
bitolterol mesylate
  Tornalate
bivalirudin
  Angiomax

bivalirudin (cont.)
  Hirulog
bleomycin sulfate
  Blenoxane
blood mononuclear cells
  CytoImplant
boric acid
  Succus Cineraria Maritima*
bosentan
  Tracleer
botulinum toxin
  Botox
  Dysport
  Myobloc
  Ortholinum
bovine cells
  CereCRIB
bovine myelin
  Myloral
bretylium tosylate
  Bretylol
brimonidine tartrate
  Alphagan; Alphagan P
brinzolamide
  Azopt
brofaromine
  Consonar
bromelains
  Vianain*
bromfenac sodium
  Duract
bromocriptine mesylate
  Ergoset
  Parlodel
  PMS-Bromocriptine ⒸⒶⓃ
bromodiphenhydramine HCl
  Ambenyl Cough*
  Amgenal Cough*
  Bromanyl*
  Bromotuss with Codeine*
brompheniramine maleate
  Allent*
  Anaplex DM Cough*
  Anaplex HD*
  Andehist*
  Andehist DM*
  Brofed*
  Bromadine-DM*

---

*This brand is a combination product.

brompheniramine maleate (cont.)
    Bromadine-DX*
    Bromanate DC Cough*
    Bromarest DX Cough*
    Bromatane DX Cough*
    Bromfed*
    Bromfed-DM Cough*
    Bromfed-PD*
    Bromfenex*
    Bromfenex PD*
    Bromophen T.D.*
    Bromphen DC with Codeine Cough*
    Bromphen DX Cough*
    Brompheniramine DC Cough*
    Coldec DM*
    Cophene-B
    Dallergy-JR*
    Dehist
    Diamine T.D.
    Dimetane-DC Cough*
    Dimetane-DX Cough*
    E.N.T.*
    Endafed*
    Histine DM; Histinex DM*
    Iofed*
    Iofed PD*
    Iohist DM*
    Liqui-Histine DM*
    Lodrane LD*
    Myphetane DC Cough*
    Myphetane DX Cough*
    Nasahist B
    ND Stat
    Oraminic II
    Poly-Histine CS*
    Poly-Histine DM*
    Respahist*
    Rondec*
    Siltapp with Dextromethorphan
        HBr Cold & Cough*
    Sinusol-B
    Tamine S.R.*
    Touro A & H; Touro Allergy*
    UltraBrom*
    UltraBrom PD*
    Veltane
broxuridine
    Broxine
    Neomark

budesonide
    Entocort Ⓒ
    Pulmicort
    Rhinocort
    Rhinocort Ⓒ
    Rhinocort Aqua
bumetanide
    Bumex
bupivacaine HCl
    Marcaine HCl
    Marcaine HCl*
    Marcaine Spinal
    Sensorcaine
    Sensorcaine*
    Sensorcaine MPF
    Sensorcaine MPF*
    Sensorcaine MPF Spinal
buprenorphine HCl
    Buprenex
bupropion HCl
    Wellbutrin
    Wellbutrin SR
    Zyban
buserelin acetate
    Suprefact Ⓒ
    Suprefact; Suprefact Depot Ⓒ
buspirone HCl
    BuSpar
    Lin-Buspirone Ⓒ
busulfan
    Busulfex
    Myleran
butabarbital
    Pyridium Plus*
butabarbital sodium
    Butibel*
    Butisol Sodium
butalbital
    Amaphen*
    Anoquan*
    Axocet*
    Axotal*
    Bucet*
    Bupap*
    Butalbital Compound*
    Butex Forte*
    Dolgic*
    Endolor*

*This brand is a combination product.

Generic ♦ Brands

butalbital (cont.)
  Esgic*
  Esgic-Plus*
  Femcet*
  Fiorgen PF*
  Fioricet*
  Fioricet with Codeine*
  Fiorinal*
  Fiorinal with Codeine*
  Fiorinal-C ¼; Fiorinal-C ½ ⓒᴬᴺ*
  Fiorpap*
  Fiortal*
  Isocet*
  Isollyl Improved*
  Lanorinal*
  Margesic*
  Marnal*
  Marten-Tab*
  Medigesic*
  Phrenilin*
  Phrenilin Forte*
  Prominol*
  Repan*
  Repan CF*
  Sedapap*
  Tencet*
  Tencon*
  Triad*
  Triaprin*
  Two-Dyne*
butamben
  Cetacaine*
butenafine HCl
  Mentax
butoconazole nitrate
  Gynazole-1
butorphanol tartrate
  Apo-Butorphanol ⓒᴬᴺ
  Stadol
  Stadol NS
C1-esterase-inhibitor
  Berinert-P
cabergoline
  Dostinex
caffeine
  Amaphen*
  Anoquan*
  Butalbital Compound*
  Cafatine*
  Cafatine-PB*

caffeine (cont.)
  Cafergot*
  Cafetrate*
  Darvon Compound-65*
  DHC Plus*
  Endolor*
  Ercaf*
  Esgic*
  Esgic-Plus*
  Femcet*
  Fiorgen PF*
  Fioricet*
  Fioricet with Codeine*
  Fiorinal*
  Fiorinal with Codeine*
  Fiorinal-C ¼; Fiorinal-C ½ ⓒᴬᴺ*
  Fiorpap*
  Fiortal*
  Hycomine Compound*
  Isocet*
  Isollyl Improved*
  Lanorinal*
  Margesic*
  Marnal*
  Medigesic*
  Neocaf
  Norgesic; Norgesic Forte*
  Orphengesic; Orphengesic Forte*
  Panlor DC*
  Repan*
  Synalgos-DC*
  Tencet*
  Triad*
  Two-Dyne*
  Wigraine*
caffeine citrate
  Cafcit
  Tussirex*
calcifediol
  Calderol
calcipotriene
  Dovonex
calcitonin (human)
  Cibacalcin
calcitonin (salmon)
  Calcimar
  Fortical
  Macritonin

*This brand is a combination product.

calcitonin (salmon) (cont.)
  Miacalcin
  Osteocalcin
  Salmonine
calcitriol
  Calcijex
  Rocaltrol
calcium
  Adeflor M*
  Enfamil Natalins Rx*
  Lactocal-F*
  Marnatal-F*
  Materna*
  Mission Prenatal Rx*
  Mynatal*
  Mynatal FC*
  Mynatal P.N.*
  Mynatal P.N. Forte*
  Mynatal Rx*
  Mynate 90 Plus*
  NatalCare Plus*
  Natalins Rx*
  Natarex Prenatal*
  Nestabs CFB; Nestabs FA*
  Niferex-PN Forte*
  O-Cal f.a.*
  Par-F*
  Par-Natal Plus 1 Improved*
  Pramilet FA*
  PreCare Conceive*
  PreCare Prenatal*
  Prenatal H.P.*
  Prenatal Maternal*
  Prenatal MR 90*
  Prenatal Plus Iron*
  Prenatal Plus with Betacarotene*
  Prenatal Plus; Prenatal Plus
    Improved*
  Prenatal Rx*
  Prenatal Rx with Betacarotene*
  Prenatal Z*
  Prenatal-1 + Iron*
  Prenate Advance; Prenate 90*
  Prenate Ultra*
  Strong Start*
  Stuartnatal Plus*
calcium acetate
  PhosLo
calcium carbonate
  Cotazym*

calcium carbonate (cont.)
  Didrocal ⓒ*
  MagneBind 400 Rx*
  PremesisRx*
  R & D Calcium Carbonate/600
calcium chloride
  Plegisol*
calcium citrate
  Citracal Prenatal*
calcium gluconate
  Calgonate
  H-F Gel
calcium glycerophosphate
  Calphosan*
calcium iodide
  Calcidrine*
  Norisodrine with Calcium Iodide*
calcium lactate
  Calphosan*
calfactant
  Infasurf
candesartan cilexetil
  Atacand
  Atacand HCT*
***Candida albicans* skin test antigen**
  Candin
cantharidin
  Verr-Canth
capecitabine
  Xeloda
capreomycin sulfate
  Capastat Sulfate
captopril
  Capoten
  Capozide 25/15; Capozide 25/25;
    Capozide 50/15; Capozide 50/25*
  PMS-Captopril ⓒ
caramiphen edisylate
  Ordrine AT*
  Rescaps-D S.R.*
  Tuss-Ornade*
  Tuss-Allergine Modified T.D.*
  Tussogest*
carbachol
  Carbastat
  Carboptic
  Isopto Carbachol
  Miostat

*This brand is a combination product.

Generic ◆ Brands

carbamazepine
Atretol
Carbatrol
Depitol
Epitol
Gen-Carbamazepine CR ⓒ
PMS-Carbamazepine CR ⓒ
Tegretol
Tegretol-XR
carbenicillin indanyl sodium
Geocillin
carbetapentane citrate
Cophene-X*
carbetapentane tannate
Rentamine Pediatric*
Rynatuss*
Tannic-12*
Tri-Tannate Plus Pediatric*
Tuss-Tan*
Tussi-12*
carbetocin
Duratocin ⓒ
carbidopa
Lodosyn
Sinemet 10/100; Sinemet 25/100;
    Sinemet 25/250*
Sinemet CR*
carbinoxamine maleate
Andehist*
Andehist DM*
Carbinoxamine Compound*
Carbiset*
Carbiset-TR*
Carbodec*
Carbodec DM*
Carbodec TR*
Cardec-DM*
Cardec-S*
Histex HC*
Histex PD
Palgic-D*
Palgic-DS*
Pseudo-Car DM*
Rondamine-DM*
Rondec*
Rondec-DM*
Rondec-TR*
Sildec-DM*
Tussafed*

carbohydrate polymer gel
Adcon-L
carbon C 13 urea
Helicosol
carbon-coated beads
Durasphere
carbonyl iron
Ultra-Natal*
carboplatin
Paraplatin
carboprost tromethamine
Hemabate
carisoprodol
Sodol Compound*
Soma
Soma Compound*
Soma Compound with Codeine*
carmustine
BiCNU
Gliadel
carprofen
Rimadyl
carteolol HCl
Ocupress
carvedilol
Coreg
caspofungin acetate
Cancidas
castor oil
Granulderm*
Granulex*
CD4
Receptin
cefaclor
Apo-Cefaclor ⓒ
Ceclor
Ceclor CD
Ceclor CDpak
Novo-Cefaclor ⓒ
cefadroxil
Apo-Cefadroxil ⓒ
Duricef
Novo-Cefadroxil ⓒ
cefamandole nafate
Mandol
cefazolin sodium
Ancef
Kefzol

*This brand is a combination product.

cefazolin sodium (cont.)
  Zolicef
cefdinir
  Omnicef
cefditoren pivoxil
  Spectracef
cefepime HCl
  Maxipime
cefixime
  Suprax
cefmetazole sodium
  Zefazone
cefodizime
  Modivid
cefonicid sodium
  Monocid
cefoperazone sodium
  Cefobid
cefotaxime sodium
  Claforan
cefotetan disodium
  Cefotan
cefoxitin sodium
  Mefoxin
cefpodoxime proxetil
  Vantin
cefprozil
  Cefzil
ceftazidime
  Fortaz
  Tazicef
  Tazidime
ceftazidime pentahydrate
  Ceptaz
ceftibuten
  Cedax
ceftizoxime sodium
  Cefizox
ceftriaxone sodium
  Rocephin
cefuroxime axetil
  Ceftin
cefuroxime sodium
  Kefurox
  Zinacef
celecoxib
  Celebrex
celiprolol HCl
  Selecor

cellulase
  Arco-Lase Plus*
  Gustase Plus*
cellulose, oxidized
  Oxycel
  Surgicel
cellulose sodium phosphate
  Calcibind
cephalexin
  Biocef
  Keflex
cephalexin HCl
  Keftab
cephapirin sodium
  Cefadyl
cephradine
  Velosef
cerivastatin sodium
  Baycol
cetirizine HCl
  Reactine ⒸⒶⒽ
  Zyrtec
  Zyrtec-D*
cetrorelix acetate
  Cetrotide
cevimeline HCl
  Evoxac
chenodiol
  Chenix
chimeric monoclonal antibody
  Cotara
chloral hydrate
  Aquachloral
chlorambucil
  Leukeran
chloramphenicol
  AK-Chlor
  Chloromycetin
  Chloromycetin Hydrocortisone*
  Chloromycetin Otic
  Chloroptic
  Chloroptic S.O.P.
  Elase-Chloromycetin*
chloramphenicol sodium succinate
  Chloromycetin Sodium Succinate
chlorazepate dipotassium
  Gen-Xene

*This brand is a combination product.

Generic ◆ Brands

chlorcyclizine HCl
  Mantadil*
chlordiazepoxide
  Libritabs
  Limbitrol DS 10-25*
  Menrium 5-2; Menrium 5-4; Menrium 10-4*
chlordiazepoxide HCl
  Clindex*
  Librax*
  Librium
  Mitran
  Reposans-10
chlorhexidine gluconate
  Apo-Chlorhexidine ⒸⒶⓃ
  Peridex*
  PerioChip
  PerioGard*
chlormezanone
  Trancopal
chlorobutanol
  Cresylate*
  Pontocaine HCl*
  Pred-G S.O.P.*
  TobraDex*
chloroguanide HCl
  Malarone; Malarone Pediatric*
chlorophyllin copper complex
  Panafil*
  Papain Urea Chlorophyllin*
chloroprocaine HCl
  Nesacaine; Nesacaine MPF
chloroquine HCl
  Aralen HCl
chloroquine phosphate
  Aralen Phosphate
chlorothiazide
  Aldoclor-150; Aldoclor-250*
  Diurigen
  Diuril
  Sodium Diuril
chlorotrianisene
  Tace
chloroxine
  Capitrol
chloroxylenol
  Cortic*
  Oti-Med*
  Otomar-HC*
  Tri-Otic*

chloroxylenol (cont.)
  Zoto-HC*
chlorphenesin carbamate
  Maolate
chlorpheniramine maleate
  Aclophen*
  AH-chew*
  AlleRx*
  Alumadrine*
  Ana-Kit*
  Anamine*
  Anamine T.D.*
  Anaplex*
  Atrohist Pediatric*
  Atrohist Plus*
  Atuss DM*
  Atuss HD*
  Biohist-LA*
  Brexin-L.A.*
  Bronkotuss Expectorant*
  Chlor-Pro
  Chlor-100
  Chlor-Trimeton
  Chlorafed; Chlorafed HS*
  Chlordrine S.R.*
  Chlorgest-HD*
  Chlorphedrine SR*
  Chlorspan-12
  Codehist DH*
  Codimal-L.A.; Codimal-L.A. Half*
  Colfed-A*
  Comhist*
  Comhist LA*
  Cophene No. 2*
  D.A.*
  D.A. II*
  Dallergy*
  Decohistine DH*
  Deconamine*
  Deconamine SR*
  Decongestabs*
  Decongestant*
  Deconhist L.A.*
  Deconomed SR*
  Dehistine*
  Donatussin*
  Drize*
  Dura-Tap/PD*

---

*This brand is a combination product.

chlorpheniramine maleate (cont.)
Dura-Vent/A*
Dura-Vent/DA*
Duralex*
Ed A-Hist*
ED-TLC; ED Tuss HC*
Endagen-HD*
Endal-HD; Endal-HD Plus*
Ex-Histine*
Extendryl*
Extendryl JR*
Extendryl SR*
Fedahist*
Hista-Vadrin*
Histade*
Histalet*
Histalet Forte*
Histex SR*
Histinex HC*
Histinex PV*
Histor-D*
Histussin HC*
Hycomine Compound*
Hydro-PC*
Hydrocodone CP; Hydrocodone HD*
Hyphed*
Iodal HD*
Iotussin HC*
Klerist-D*
Kronofed-A Jr.*
Kronofed-A*
Mescolor*
Naldecon*
Naldelate*
Nalgest*
ND Clear*
Nolamine*
Norel Plus*
Novafed A*
Novahistine DH*
OMNIhist L.A.*
Ornade*
P-V-Tussin*
Pancof-HC*
Pannaz*
Para-Hist HD*
Pediacof*
Pedituss Cough*
Phenahist-TR*
Phenate*

chlorpheniramine maleate (cont.)
Phenchlor S.H.A.*
Phenetron
Phenhist DH with Codeine*
Prehist*
Prehist D*
Pseudo-Chlor*
Resaid*
Rescon*
Rescon-ED*
Rescon JR*
Rhinolar-EX; Rhinolar-EX 12*
Rinade B.I.D.*
Rolatuss Expectorant*
Ryna-C*
S-T Forte 2*
Stahist*
T-Koff*
Telachlor
Time-Hist*
Tri-Phen-Chlor*
Tri-Phen-Chlor T.R.*
Tri-Phen-Mine*
Tri-Phen-Mine S.R.*
Tusquelin*
Tussanil DH*
Tussend*
Uni-Decon*
Unituss HC*
Vanex Forte*
Vanex Forte-R*
Vanex-HD*
Xiral*
chlorpheniramine polistirex
Tussionex Pennkinetic*
chlorpheniramine tannate
Atrohist Pediatric*
Gelhist*
R-Tannamine*
R-Tannate*
Rentamine Pediatric*
Rhinatate*
Rynatan*
Rynatan-S*
Rynatuss*
Tanafed*
Tannic-12*
Tanoral*

*This brand is a combination product.

Generic ♦ Brands

chlorpheniramine tannate (cont.)
Tri-Tannate*
Tri-Tannate Plus Pediatric*
Triotann*
Tritan*
Tuss-Tan*
Tussi-12*
chlorpromazine
Thorazine
chlorpromazine HCl
Ormazine
chlorpropamide
Diabinese
chlorthalidone
Clorpres*
Combipres 0.1; Combipres 0.2;
Combipres 0.3*
Demi-Regroton*
Hygroton
Regroton*
Tenoretic 50; Tenoretic 100*
Thalitone
chlorzoxazone
Flexaphen*
Paraflex
Parafon Forte DSC
Remular-S
cholestyramine resin
Cholestyramine Light
LoCholest; LoCholest Light
Prevalite
Questran; Questran Light
choline bitartrate
Ilopan-Choline*
choline chloride
Intrachol
choline magnesium trisalicylate
Tricosal
choline salicylate
Arthropan
Trilisate*
chondrocytes, cultured autologous
Carticel
chondroitan sulfate sodium
Uracyst-S; Uracyst-S Concentrate Ⓒᴬᴺ
chondroitin sulfate sodium
Viscoat*
choriogonadotropin alfa
Ovidrel

chorionic gonadotropin
A.P.L.
Chorex-5; Chorex-10
Choron-10
Gonic
Novarel
Pregnyl
Profasi
chromic chloride hexahydrate
Chroma-Pak
Chromium Chloride
chromic phosphate P 32
Phosphocol P 32
chymopapain
Chymodiactin
chymotrypsin
Catarase 1:5000
ciclopirox
Penlac
ciclopirox olamine
Loprox
cidofovir
Forvade
Vistide
cifenline succinate
Cipralan
cilastatin sodium
Primaxin I.M.*
Primaxin I.V.*
cilmostim
Macstim
cilostazol
Pletal
cimetidine
Apo-Cimetidine Ⓒᴬᴺ
Tagamet
cimetidine HCl
Tagamet
cinoxacin
Cinobac
cipemastat
Trocade
ciprofloxacin
Cipro
Cipro HC Otic*
ciprofloxacin HCl
Ciloxan

*This brand is a combination product.

cisapride
  Prepulsid ⒸⒶⓃ
  Propulsid
cisatracurium besylate
  Nimbex
cisplatin
  IntraDose*
  Platinol
  Platinol-AQ
citalopram hydrobromide
  Celexa
citicoline sodium
  CerAxon
citric acid
  Bicitra*
  Cytra-2*
  Cytra-3*
  Cytra-K*
  Cytra-LC*
  Oracit*
  PMS-Dicitrate ⒸⒶⓃ*
  Polycitra*
  Polycitra-K*
  Polycitra-LC*
  Renacidin*
  Renacidin Irrigation*
cladribine
  Leustatin
clarithromycin
  Biaxin
  Biaxin XL
  Hp-PAC ⒸⒶⓃ*
  Losec 1-2-3 A ⒸⒶⓃ*
  Losec 1-2-3 M ⒸⒶⓃ*
  Prevpac*
clavulanate potassium
  Augmentin*
  Augmentin ES*
  Timentin*
clavulanic acid
  Alti-Amoxi Clav ⒸⒶⓃ*
clemastine fumarate
  Tavist
clidinium bromide
  Clindex*
  Librax*
  Quarzan
clindamycin
  Clindets
  HyClinda

clindamycin HCl
  Alti-Clindamycin ⒸⒶⓃ
  Cleocin
  Dalacin C ⒸⒶⓃ
clindamycin palmitate HCl
  Cleocin Pediatric
  Dalacin C ⒸⒶⓃ
clindamycin phosphate
  Benzaclin*
  C/T/S
  Cleocin
  Cleocin Phosphate
  Cleocin T
  Clinda-Derm
  Dalacin ⒸⒶⓃ
  Dalacin C Phosphate ⒸⒶⓃ
  Dalacin T ⒸⒶⓃ
clioquinol
  Ala-Quin*
  Corque*
  1+1-F Creme*
  Pedi-Cort V Creme*
clobazam
  Alti-Clobazam ⒸⒶⓃ
  Frisium
clobetasol propionate
  Cormax
  Olux*
  Temovate
  Temovate Emollient
  ViaFoam
clocortolone pivalate
  Cloderm
clodronate disodium
  Ostac ⒸⒶⓃ
clodronate disodium tetrahydrate
  Bonefos ⒸⒶⓃ
clofazimine
  Lamprene
clofibrate
  Atromid-S
clomiphene citrate
  Clomid
  Milophene
  Serophene
clomipramine HCl
  Anafranil

*This brand is a combination product.

clonazepam
  Apo-Clonazepam (CAN)
  Klonopin
  Novo-Clonazepam (CAN)
clonidine HCl
  Catapres
  Catapres-TTS-1; Catapres-TTS-2;
    Catapres-TTS-3
  Clorpres*
  Combipres 0.1; Combipres 0.2;
    Combipres 0.3*
  Duraclon
clopidogrel bisulfate
  Plavix
clorazepate dipotassium
  Tranxene
  Tranxene-SD
clotrimazole
  Fungoid
  Lotrimin
  Lotrisone*
  Mycelex
  Mycelex-G
  Mycelex Twin Pack
cloxacillin sodium
  Cloxapen
  Tegopen
clozapine
  Clozaril
coagulation factor IX
  AlphaNine
  Mononine
coagulation factors II, VII, IX, and X
  AlphaNine SD
  Hemonyne
  Konyne 80
  Profilnine SD
  Proplex T
coal tar
  Sal-Oil-T*
  Unguentum Bossi*
  Zetar Emulsion
cocaine
  Cocaine Viscous
coccidioidin
  BioCox
  Spherulin
codeine phosphate
  Aceta with Codeine*

codeine phosphate (cont.)
  Actagen-C Cough*
  Actifed with Codeine Cough*
  Allerfrin with Codeine*
  Ambenyl Cough*
  Amgenal Cough*
  Aprodine with Codeine*
  Aspirin with Codeine No. 2, No. 3,
    and No. 4*
  Bromanate DC Cough*
  Bromanyl*
  Bromotuss with Codeine*
  Bromphen DC with Codeine Cough*
  Brompheniramine DC Cough*
  Brontex*
  Calcidrine*
  Calmylin with Codeine (CAN)*
  Capital with Codeine*
  Cheracol Cough*
  Codegest Expectorant*
  Codehist DH*
  Conex with Codeine*
  Cotridin (CAN)*
  Cotridin Expectorant (CAN)*
  Cyclofed Pediatric*
  Cycofed Pediatric*
  Decohistine DH*
  Decongestant Expectorant*
  Deconsal Pediatric*
  Deproist Expectorant with Codeine*
  Dihistine Expectorant*
  Dimetane-DC Cough*
  Empirin with Codeine No. 3 & No.
    4*
  Endal Expectorant*
  Fioricet with Codeine*
  Fiorinal with Codeine*
  Fiorinal-C ¼; Fiorinal-C ½ (CAN)*
  Guiatuss AC*
  Guiatuss DAC*
  Guiatussin DAC*
  Guiatussin with Codeine Expectorant*
  Iophen-C*
  Isoclor Expectorant*
  Myphetane DC Cough*
  Mytussin AC Cough*
  Mytussin DAC*

*This brand is a combination product.

codeine phosphate (cont.)
- Naldecon CX Adult*
- Novagest Expectorant with Codeine*
- Novahistine DH*
- Novahistine Expectorant*
- Nucofed*
- Nucofed Expectorant; Nucofed Pediatric Expectorant*
- Pediacof*
- Pedituss Cough*
- Pentazine VC with Codeine*
- Phenaphen with Codeine No. 3 & No. 4*
- Phenergan VC with Codeine*
- Phenergan with Codeine*
- Phenhist DH with Codeine*
- Phenhist Expectorant*
- Pherazine VC with Codeine*
- Pherazine with Codeine*
- Poly-Histine CS*
- Prometh VC with Codeine*
- Prometh with Codeine*
- Promethazine VC with Codeine*
- Promethist with Codeine*
- Robafen AC Cough*
- Robafen DAC*
- Robitussin A-C*
- Robitussin-DAC*
- Rolatuss Expectorant*
- Romilar AC*
- Ryna-C*
- Ryna-CX*
- Soma Compound with Codeine*
- Statuss Expectorant*
- T-Koff*
- Triacin-C Cough*
- Triafed with Codeine*
- Triaminic Expectorant with Codeine*
- Tricodene Cough and Cold*
- Trifed-C Cough*
- Tussar SF; Tussar-2*
- Tussi-Organidin NR; Tussi-Organidin-S NR*
- Tussirex*
- Tylenol with Codeine*
- Tylenol with Codeine No. 2, No. 3, and No. 4*

colchicine
- Col-Probenecid*
- ColBenemid*
- Proben-C*

colesevelam HCl
- Welchol

colestipol HCl
- Colestid

colfosceril palmitate
- Alec*
- Exosurf
- Exosurf Neonatal

colistimethate sodium
- Coly-Mycin M

colistin sulfate
- Coly-Mycin S Otic*
- Cortisporin-TC*

collagenase
- Cordase
- Plaquase
- Santyl

comosain
- Vianain*

conjugated estrogens
- C.E.S. (CAN)
- Cenestin
- PMB 200; PMB 400*
- PMS-Conjugated Estrogens (CAN)
- Premarin
- Premarin Intravenous
- Premarin with Methyltestosterone*
- Premphase*
- Prempro*

corticorelin ovine triflutate
- Acthrel

corticotropin
- ACTH
- ACTH-80
- Acthar
- H.P. Acthar Gel

cortisone acetate
- Cortone Acetate

cosyntropin
- Cortrosyn

coumarin
- Oncostate
- Onkolox

---

*This brand is a combination product.

m-cresyl acetate
  Cresylate*
crofelemer
  Provir
  Virend
cromolyn sodium
  Apo-Cromolyn ⓒⒶⓃ
  Crolom
  Gastrocrom
  Intal
  Opticrom 4%
crotamiton
  Eurax
***Cryptosporidium parvum* bovine colostrum IgG concentrate**
  Immuno-C
  Sporidin-G
cyanocobalamin
  Anemagen*
  Bedoz ⓒⒶⓃ
  Chromagen*
  Contrin*
  Crystamine
  Crysti 1000
  Cyanoject
  Cyomin
  Ferotrinsic*
  Foltrin*
  Fumatinic*
  Livitrinsic-f*
  Nascobal
  Niferex-150 Forte*
  Nu-Iron Plus*
  Pronemia Hematinic*
  Rubramin PC
  TriHemic 600*
  Trinsicon*
cyclandelate
  Cyclan
  Cyclospasmol
  Cyclospasmol ⓒⒶⓃ
cyclobenzaprine HCl
  Flexeril
cyclopentolate HCl
  AK-Pentolate
  Cyclogyl
  Cyclomydril*
  Pentolair
cyclophosphamide
  Cytoxan

cyclophosphamide (cont.)
  Neosar
cycloserine
  Seromycin
cyclosporine
  Gengraf*
  Neoral
  Optimmune
  Restasis
  Sandimmune
  SangCya*
cyproheptadine HCl
  Periactin
cyproterone acetate
  Diane-35 ⓒⒶⓃ*
  Gen-Cyproterone ⓒⒶⓃ
  Novo-Cyproterone ⓒⒶⓃ
cysteamine bitartrate
  Cystagon
cystine
  Amino-Cerv pH 5.5*
cytarabine
  Cytosar-U
  DepoCyt
  Tarabine PFS
cytomegalovirus immune globulin
  CytoGam
dacarbazine
  DTIC-Dome
daclizumab
  Zenapax
dactinomycin
  Cosmegen
dalfopristin
  Synercid*
dalteparin sodium
  Fragmin
danaparoid sodium
  Orgaran
danazol
  Danocrine
dantrolene sodium
  Dantrium
dapiprazole HCl
  Rēv-Eyes
daptomycin
  Cidecin

*This brand is a combination product.

darbepoetin alfa
  Aranesp
daunorubicin citrate
  DaunoXome
daunorubicin HCl
  Cerubidine
deferoxamine
  Bio-Rescue*
deferoxamine mesylate
  Desferal
  PMS-Desferoxamine ⒸⒶⓃ
dehydrocholic acid
  Digestozyme*
dehydroemetine
  Mebadin
delavirdine mesylate
  Rescriptor
demecarium bromide
  Humorsol
demeclocycline HCl
  Declomycin
denileukin diftitox
  Ontak
depreotide
  NeoTect
deserpidine
  Enduronyl; Enduronyl Forte*
desflurane
  Suprane
desipramine HCl
  Norpramin
desirudin
  Revasc
desloratadine
  Aerius ⒸⒶⓃ
deslorelin
  Somagard
desmopressin acetate
  Apo-Desmopressin ⒸⒶⓃ
  DDAVP
  Stimate
desogestrel
  Apri*
  Cyclessa*
  Desogen*
  Marvelon ⒸⒶⓃ*
  Mircette*
  Ortho-Cept*
desonide
  DesOwen

desonide (cont.)
  Tridesilon
desoximetasone
  Desoxi ⒸⒶⓃ
  Topicort
  Topicort LP
desoxyribonuclease
  Elase*
  Elase-Chloromycetin*
dessicated stomach substance
  Anemagen*
dexamethasone
  AK-Trol*
  Aeroseb-Dex
  Alti-Dexamethasone ⒸⒶⓃ
  Decadron
  Dexacidin*
  Dexameth
  Dexasporin*
  Dexone
  Hexadrol
  Maxidex
  Maxitrol*
  PMS-Dexamethasone ⒸⒶⓃ
  Storz-N-P-D*
  Surodex
  TobraDex*
dexamethasone acetate
  Dalalone D.P.
  Dalalone L.A.
  Decadron-LA
  Decaject-L.A.
  Dexasone L.A.
  Dexone LA
  Solurex LA
dexamethasone sodium phosphate
  AK-Dex
  AK-Neo-Dex*
  Dalalone
  Decadron Phosphate
  Decadron with Xylocaine*
  Decaject
  Dexacort Phosphate
  Dexacort Phosphate*
  Dexasone
  Dexone
  Diodex ⒸⒶⓃ
  Hexadrol Phosphate

*This brand is a combination product.

dexamethasone sodium phosphate (cont.)
  Neo-Dexair*
  Neo-Dexameth*
  NeoDecadron*
  PMS-Dexamethasone ⓒ️ᴬᴺ
  R.O.-Dexsone ⓒ️ᴬᴺ
  Solurex
  Spersadex ⓒ️ᴬᴺ
  Storz-N-D*
dexbrompheniramine maleate
  Dexaphen S.A.*
  Disobrom*
  Drixomed*
dexchlorpheniramine maleate
  Dexchlor
  Poladex
  Polaramine
  Polaramine Expectorant*
dexfenfluramine HCl
  Redux
dexmedetomidine HCl
  Precedex
dexmethylphenidate HCl
  Ritadex
dexpanthenol
  Ilopan
  Ilopan-Choline*
dexrazoxane
  Zinecard
dextran
  Bio-Rescue*
  Gendex 75
  Gentran 40
  Gentran 70
  Hyskon*
  10% LMD
  Macrodex
  Promit
  Rheomacrodex
dextran sulfate
  Uendex
dextranomer
  Debrisan
dextroamphetamine saccharate
  Adderall*
  Adderall XR*
dextroamphetamine sulfate
  Adderall*
  Adderall XR*

dextroamphetamine sulfate (cont.)
  Dexedrine
  Dextrostat
  Oxydess II
  Spancap No. 1
dextromethorphan
  MorphiDex*
dextromethorphan hydrobromide
  Anaplex DM Cough*
  Anatuss*
  Andehist DM*
  Aquatab C*
  Aquatab DM*
  Atuss DM*
  Bromadine-DM*
  Bromadine-DX*
  Bromarest DX Cough*
  Bromatane DX Cough*
  Bromfed-DM Cough*
  Bromphen DX Cough*
  Carbinoxamine Compound*
  Carbodec DM*
  Cardec-DM*
  Coldec DM*
  Dimetane-DX Cough*
  Donatussin*
  Duratuss DM*
  Fenesin DM*
  Guaifenex DM*
  Histine DM; Histinex DM*
  Humibid DM*
  Humibid DM Sprinkle*
  Iobid DM*
  Iohist DM*
  Iophen-DM*
  Liqui-Histine DM*
  MED-Rx DM*
  Monafed DM*
  Muco-Fen-DM*
  Myphetane DX Cough*
  PanMist-DM*
  Phenameth DM*
  Phenergan with Dextromethorphan*
  Pherazine DM*
  Poly-Histine DM*
  Profen Forte DM*
  Profen II DM*
  Prometh with Dextromethorphan*

*This brand is a combination product.

dextromethorphan hydrobromide (cont.)
  Promethazine DM*
  Protuss DM*
  Pseudo-Car DM*
  Respa-DM*
  Rondamine-DM*
  Rondec-DM*
  Sildec-DM*
  Siltapp with Dextromethorphan HBr Cold & Cough*
  Touro CC*
  Touro DM*
  Tusquelin*
  Tussafed*
  Tussafed-LA*
  Tussi-Organidin DM NR; Tussi-Organidin DM-S NR*
  Tusso-DM*

dextrose
  5% Alcohol and 5% Dextrose in Water; 10% Alcohol and 5% Dextrose in Water*
  Aminosyn II 3.5% in 5% (25%) Dextrose; Aminosyn II 4.25% in 10% (20%, 25%) Dextrose; Aminosyn II 5% in 25% Dextrose*
  Aminosyn II 3.5% M in 5% Dextrose; Aminosyn II 4.25% M in 10% Dextrose*
  D-2.5-W; D-5-W; D-10-W; D-20-W; D-25-W; D-30-W; D-40-W; D-50-W; D-60-W; D-70-W
  5% Dextrose and Electrolyte #48; 5% Dextrose and Electrolyte #75; 10% Dextrose and Electrolyte #48*
  50% Dextrose with Electrolyte Pattern A (or N)*
  Dialyte Pattern LM*
  Hyskon*
  Isolyte E (G; H; M; P; R; S) with 5% Dextrose*
  Normosol-M and 5% Dextrose; Normosol-R and 5% Dextrose*
  Plasma-Lyte M (R; 56; 148) and 5% Dextrose*
  Primacor in 5% Dextrose*
  Travasol 2.75% in 5% (10%, 25%) Dextrose; Travasol 4.25% in 5% (10%, 25%) Dextrose*

dextrose (cont.)
  5% Travert and Electrolyte No. 2; 10% Travert and Electrolyte No. 2*
  Xylocaine HCl*

dextrothyroxine sodium
  Choloxin

dezocine
  Dalgan

diatrizoate meglumine
  Angiovist 282
  Angiovist 292; Angiovist 370*
  Cystografin; Cystografin Dilute
  Gastrografin*
  Hypaque-76*
  Hypaque-Cysto
  Hypaque-M 75; Hypaque-M 90*
  Hypaque Meglumine 30%; Hypaque Meglumine 60%
  MD-60; MD-76*
  MD-76 R*
  MD-Gastroview*
  Reno-30
  Reno-Dip; Reno-60
  RenoCal-76*
  Renografin-60*
  Renografin-76*
  Renovist; Renovist II*
  Sinografin*
  Urovist Cysto
  Urovist Meglumine DIU/CT

diatrizoate sodium
  Angiovist 292; Angiovist 370*
  Gastrografin*
  Hypaque-76*
  Hypaque-M 75; Hypaque-M 90*
  Hypaque Sodium
  Hypaque Sodium 20%
  Hypaque Sodium 25%; Hypaque Sodium 50%
  MD-60; MD-76*
  MD-76 R*
  MD-Gastroview*
  RenoCal-76*
  Renografin-60*
  Renografin-76*
  Renovist; Renovist II*
  Urovist Sodium 300

*This brand is a combination product.

diazepam
  Apo-Diazepam (CAN)
  Diastat
  Diazemuls (CAN)
  Dizac
  Valium
  Valium Roche Oral (CAN)
diazoxide
  Hyperstat
  Proglycem
dichloralphenazone
  Duradrin*
  Isocom*
  Isopap*
  Midchlor*
  Midrin*
  Migratine*
dichloroacetic acid
  Bichloracetic Acid
dichlorodifluoromethane
  Fluori-Methane*
dichlorotetrafluoroethane
  Fluro-Ethyl*
dichlorphenamide
  Daranide
diclofenac potassium
  Apo-Diclo Rapide (CAN)
  Cataflam
  Novo-Difenac-K (CAN)
  Pennsaid
  Riva-Diclofenac-K (CAN)
  Solaraze
  Voltaren Rapide (CAN)
diclofenac sodium
  Arthrotec*
  Diclotec (CAN)
  PMS-Diclofenac (CAN)
  PMS-Diclofenac SR (CAN)
  Riva-Diclofenac (CAN)
  Vofenal (CAN)
  Voltaren
  Voltaren (CAN)
  Voltaren Ophtha (CAN)
  Voltaren Ophthalmic
  Voltaren SR (CAN)
  Voltaren XR
dicloxacillin sodium
  Dycill
  Dynapen
  Pathocil

dicyclomine HCl
  Antispas
  Bentyl
  Byclomine
  Di-Spaz
  Dibent
didanosine
  Scriptene*
  Videx
  Videx EC
dienestrol
  Ortho Dienestrol
diethylcarbamazine citrate
  Hetrazan
diethyldithiocarbamate
  Imuthiol
diethylpropion HCl
  Tenuate
diethylstilbestrol diphosphate
  Stilphostrol
difenoxin HCl
  Motofen*
diflorasone diacetate
  Florone
  Florone E
  Maxiflor
  Psorcon E
diflunisal
  Dolobid
digitoxin
  Crystodigin
digoxin
  Digitek
  Digoxin Injection C.S.D. (CAN)
  Digoxin Pediatric Injection C.S.D. (CAN)
  Lanoxicaps
  Lanoxin
digoxin immune Fab
  Digibind
  Digidote
dihydrocodeine bitartrate
  DHC Plus*
  Panlor DC*
  Synalgos-DC*
dihydroergotamine mesylate
  D.H.E. 45
  Migranal

---

*This brand is a combination product.

dihydrotachysterol
DHT
Hytakerol
dihydrotestosterone
Androgel-DHT
diloxanide furoate
Furamide
diltiazem HCl
Apo-Diltiaz (CAN)
Apo-Diltiaz CD (CAN)
Apo-Diltiaz SR (CAN)
Cardizem
Cardizem CD
Cardizem SR
Cardizem XL
Cartia XT
Dilacor XR
Diltia XT
Novo-Diltiazem CD (CAN)
Nu-Diltiaz-CD (CAN)
Rhoxal-diltiazem CD (CAN)
Tiazac
diltiazem maleate
Teczem*
Tiamate
dimenhydrinate
Dimetabs
Dinate
Dramamine
Dramanate
Dramilin
Dymenate
Hydrate
Marmine
dimercaprol
BAL in Oil
dimethyl sulfoxide
Kemsol (CAN)
Rimso-50
dinoprostone
Cervidil
Prepidil
Prostin E2
dioxybenzone
Nuquin HP*
Solaquin Forte*
Viquin Forte*
diphenhydramine HCl
Ben-Allergin-50
Benadryl

diphenhydramine HCl (cont.)
Benadryl Allergy
Genahist
Hydramyn*
Hyrexin-50
Tusstat*
diphenidol HCl
Vontrol
diphenoxylate HCl
Logen*
Lomanate*
Lomotil*
Lonox*
diphtheria & tetanus toxoids & acellular pertussis (DTaP) vaccine
Adacel (CAN)
Acel-Imune
ActHIB/Tripedia*
Certiva
Infanrix
TriHIBit*
Tripedia
diphtheria & tetanus toxoids & whole-cell pertussis (DTwP) vaccine
Tetramune*
Tri-Immunol
dipivefrin HCl
AKPro
Apo-Dipivefrin (CAN)
PMS-Dipivefrin (CAN)
Propine
dipyridamole
Aggrenox*
Persantinc
Persantine IV
dirithromycin
Dynabac
disaccharide tripeptide glycerol dipalmitoyl
ImmTher
disopyramide phosphate
Norpace
Norpace CR
disulfiram
Antabuse
divalproex sodium
Apo-Divalproex (CAN)

*This brand is a combination product.

divalproex sodium (cont.)
  Depakote
  Depakote ER
  Epival (CAN)
  Epival ER (CAN)
  Novo-Divalproex (CAN)
  Nu-Divalproex (CAN)
dobutamine HCl
  Dobutrex
docetaxel
  Taxotere
docosanol
  Lidakol
docusate sodium
  Citracal Prenatal*
  Nephron FA*
  TriHemic 600*
dofetilide
  Tikosyn
dolasetron mesylate
  Anzemet
domperidone maleate
  Apo-Domperidone (CAN)
  Motilium (CAN)
  Novo-Domperidone (CAN)
donepezil HCl
  Aricept
dopamine HCl
  Intropin
dopaminergic cells
  NeuroCell-PD
dornase alfa
  Pulmozyme
dorzolamide HCl
  Cosopt*
  Trusopt
dothiepin HCl
  Prothiaden
doxacurium chloride
  Nuromax
doxapram HCl
  Dopram
doxazosin mesylate
  Alti-Doxazosin (CAN)
  Apo-Doxazosin (CAN)
  Cardura
  Gen-Doxazosin (CAN)
doxepin HCl
  Sinequan
  Zonalon

doxercalciferol
  Hectorol
doxorubicin
  Evacet
doxorubicin HCl
  Adriamycin PFS
  Adriamycin RDF
  Caelyx (CAN)
  Doxil
  Rubex
doxycycline
  Monodox
  Vibramycin
doxycycline calcium
  Vibramycin
doxycycline hyclate
  Atridox
  Bio-Tab
  Doryx
  Doxy 100; Doxy 200
  Doxy Caps
  Doxychel Hyclate
  Periostat
  Vibra-Tabs
  Vibramycin
doxycycline monohydrate
  Adoxa
dronabinol
  Marinol
droperidol
  Inapsine
  Innovar*
drospirenone
  Yasmin*
drotrecogin alfa
  Xigris
dyclonine HCl
  Dyclone
dyphylline
  Dilor
  Dilor 400
  Dilor-G*
  Dy-G*
  Dyflex-G*
  Dyline-GG*
  Lufyllin
  Lufyllin 400
  Lufyllin-EPG*

---

*This brand is a combination product.

Generic ◆ Brands

dyphylline (cont.)
Lufyllin-GG*
Panfil G*
echothiophate iodide
Phospholine Iodide
econazole nitrate
Spectazole
edetate calcium disodium
Calcium Disodium Versenate
edetate disodium
Disotate
Endrate
edrecolomab
Panorex
edrophonium chloride
Enlon
Enlon Plus*
Reversol
Tensilon
efavirenz
Sustiva
eflornithine HCl
Ornidyl
Vaniqa
electrolytes
Aminosyn 3.5% M; Aminosyn II
3.5% M*
Aminosyn 7% (8.5%) with Electro-
lytes; Aminosyn II 7% (8.5%,
10%) with Electrolytes*
Aminosyn-HBC 7%*
Aminosyn II 3.5% M in 5% Dex-
trose; Aminosyn II 4.25% M in
10% Dextrose*
Co-Lav*
5% Dextrose and Electrolyte #48; 5%
Dextrose and Electrolyte #75; 10%
Dextrose and Electrolyte #48*
50% Dextrose with Electrolyte Pat-
tern A (or N)*
FreAmine HBC 6.9%*
FreAmine III 3% (8.5%) with Elec-
trolytes*
Go-Evac*
HepatAmine*
Hyperlyte; Hyperlyte CR; Hyperlyte R
Isolyte E (G; H; M; P; R; S) with
5% Dextrose*
Isolyte E; Isolyte S; Isolyte S pH 7.4
Isolyte S pH 7.4

electrolytes (cont.)
Lypholyte; Lypholyte II
Multilyte-20; Multilyte-40
NephrAmine 5.4%*
Normosol-M and 5% Dextrose; Nor-
mosol-R and 5% Dextrose*
Normosol-R; Normosol-R pH 7.4
Nutrilyte; Nutrilyte II
Plasma-Lyte A pH 7.4; Plasma-Lyte
R; Plasma-Lyte 56; Plasma-Lyte 148
Plasma-Lyte M (R; 56; 148) and 5%
Dextrose*
ProcalAmine*
RenAmin*
TPN Electrolytes; TPN Electrolytes
II; TPN Electrolytes III
Tracelyte; Tracelyte II; Tracelyte
with Double Electrolytes; Trace-
lyte II with Double Electrolytes*
Travasol 3.5% (5.5%, 8.5%) with
Electrolytes*
5% Travert and Electrolyte No. 2;
10% Travert and Electrolyte No. 2*
eletriptan hydrobromide
Relpax
emedastine difumarate
Emadine
emivirine
Coactinon
emtricitabine
Coviracil
enalapril maleate
Lexxel*
Nu-Enalapril ⓒ
Teczem*
Vaseretic 5-12.5; Vaseretic 10-25*
Vasotec
enalaprilat
Vasotec I.V.
encapsulated bovine cells
CereCRIB
enflurane
Ethrane
enoxacin
Penetrex
enoxaparin sodium
Lovenox

*This brand is a combination product.

enprostil
  Gardrin
entacapone
  Comtan
ephedrine HCl
  Broncholate*
  KIE*
  Lufyllin-EPG*
  Mudrane*
  Mudrane GG*
  Quadrinal*
ephedrine sulfate
  Bronkotuss Expectorant*
  Hydrophed*
  Marax*
  Marax-DF*
  Theomax DF*
ephedrine tannate
  Rentamine Pediatric*
  Rynatuss*
  Tri-Tannate Plus Pediatric*
  Tuss-Tan*
epinephrine
  AccuSite*
  Ana-Guard
  Ana-Kit*
  Astracaine; Astracaine Forte ⒸⒶⓃ*
  Citanest Forte*
  Duranest; Duranest MPF*
  EpiPen; EpiPen Jr.
  IntraDose*
  Octocaine HCl*
  Sensorcaine*
  Sensorcaine MPF*
  Septocaine*
  Sus-Phrine
  Xylocaine HCl*
  Xylocaine MPF*
epinephrine bitartrate
  E-Pilo-1; E-Pilo-2; E-Pilo-4; E-Pilo-6*
  Marcaine HCl*
  P_1E_1; P_2E_1; P_4E_1; P_6E_1*
  P_3E_1*
epinephrine HCl
  Adrenalin Chloride
  Epifrin
  Epinephrine Pediatric
  Glaucon
epinephryl borate
  Epinal

epirubicin HCl
  Ellence
  Pharmorubicin PFS; Pharmorubicin
    RDF ⒸⒶⓃ
epoetin alfa
  Epogen
  Procrit
epoetin beta
  Marogen
epoprostenol
  Cyclo-Prostin
  Flolan
eptacog alfa
  NiaStase ⒸⒶⓃ
eptifibatide
  Integrilin
ergocalciferol (vitamin D$_2$)
  Calciferol
  Drisdol
ergoloid mesylates
  Gerimal
  Hydergine
  Hydergine LC
ergonovine maleate
  Ergotrate Maleate
ergotamine tartrate
  Bel-Phen-Ergot SR*
  Bellacane SR*
  Bellergal-S*
  Cafatine*
  Cafatine-PB*
  Cafergot*
  Cafetrate*
  Ercaf*
  Ergomar
  Folergot-DF*
  Phenerbel-S*
  Wigraine*
ersofermin
  Ossigel*
erwinia ʟ-asparaginase
  Erwinase
erythromycin
  A/T/S
  Akne-mycin
  Benzamycin*
  Del-Mycin
  E-Base

---

*This brand is a combination product.

erythromycin (cont.)
  E-Mycin
  Emgel
  Ery-Tab
  ERYC
  Erycette
  EryDerm 2%
  Erygel*
  Erymax
  Erythra-Derm
  Ilotycin
  PCE
  Robimycin
  Staticin
  T-Stat
  Theramycin Z
erythromycin estolate
  Ilosone
erythromycin ethylsuccinate
  E.E.S.
  E.E.S. 200
  E.E.S. 400
  EryPed
  EryPed 200; EryPed 400
  Eryzole*
  Pediazole*
erythromycin gluceptate
  Ilotycin Gluceptate
erythromycin lactobionate
  Erythrocin
erythromycin stearate
  Eramycin
  Erythrocin Stearate
erythropoietin
  Dynepo
escitalopram oxalate
  Cipralex
esmolol HCl
  Brevibloc
esomeprazole magnesium
  Nexium
esopiclone
  Estorra
estazolam
  ProSom
esterified estrogens
  Estratab
  Estratest; Estratest H.S.*
  Menest
  Menogen; Menogen H.S.*

esterified estrogens (cont.)
  Menrium 5-2; Menrium 5-4; Menrium 10-4*
estradiol
  Activella*
  Alora
  Climara
  CombiPatch*
  E2II
  Esclim
  Estrace
  Estraderm
  Estradiol Transdermal System
  Estring
  FemPatch
  Gynodiol
  Menorest
  TheraDerm-MTX*
  Vivelle; Vivelle-Dot
estradiol cypionate
  depAndrogyn*
  depGynogen
  Depo-Estradiol Cypionate
  Depo-Testadiol*
  DepoGen
  Depotestogen*
  Duo-Cyp*
  Duratestrin*
  Estro-Cyp
  Lunelle*
  Test-Estro Cypionates*
estradiol hemihydrate
  Vagifem
estradiol valerate
  Delestrogen
  Dioval XX; Dioval 40
  Estra-L 20
  Estra-L 40
  Gynogen L.A. 20
  Valergen 20; Valergen 40
  Valertest No. 1*
estradiol-17β
  Estalis 140/50; Estalis 250/50 ⓒᴬᴺ*
  Estrasorb
  Ortho-Prefest*
estradiol-17β hemihydrate
  Oesclim ⓒᴬᴺ

---

*This brand is a combination product.

estramustine phosphate sodium
  Emcyt
estrogen
  E2III
estrogen-17β
  Estrogel ⓒ
estrone
  Aquest
  Estrogenic Substance Aqueous
  Estrone 5
  Estrone Aqueous
  Kestrone 5
  Ogen
  Ortho-Est
estropipate
  Ogen
etanercept
  Enbrel
ethacrynate sodium
  Edecrin Sodium
ethacrynic acid
  Edecrin
ethambutol HCl
  Myambutol
ethanol
  Olux*
ethanolamine oleate
  Ethamolin
ethchlorvynol
  Placidyl
ethinyl estradiol
  Alesse*
  Apri*
  Aviane-28*
  Brevicon*
  Cyclessa*
  Demulen 1/35; Demulen 1/50*
  Desogen*
  Diane-35 ⓒ*
  Enpresse*
  Estinyl
  Estrostep 21*
  Estrostep Fe*
  femhrt 1/5*
  Genora 0.5/35; Genora 1/35*
  Jenest-28*
  Levlen*
  Levlite*
  Levora 0.15/30*
  Lo/Ovral*

ethinyl estradiol (cont.)
  Loestrin 21 1/20; Loestrin 21 1.5/30*
  Loestrin Fe 1/20; Loestrin Fe 1.5/30*
  Low-Ogestrel*
  Marvelon ⓒ*
  Microgestin Fe 1/20; Microgestin Fe 1.5/30*
  Minesse*
  Mircette*
  Modicon*
  N.E.E. 1/35*
  Necon 0.5/35; Necon 1/35*
  Necon 10/11*
  Nelova 0.5/35E; Nelova 1/35E*
  Nelova 10/11*
  Nordette*
  Norethin 1/35E*
  Norinyl 1 + 35*
  Nortrel*
  Ogestrel*
  Ortho 0.5/35; Ortho 1/35 ⓒ*
  Ortho 7/7/7 ⓒ*
  Ortho-Cept*
  Ortho-Cyclen*
  Ortho-Novum 1/35*
  Ortho-Novum 10/11*
  Ortho-Novum 7/7/7*
  Ortho Tri-Cyclen*
  Ovcon-35*
  Ovcon-50*
  Ovral*
  Preven*
  Tri-Levlen*
  Tri-Norinyl*
  Triphasil*
  Trivora-28*
  Yasmin*
  Zovia 1/35E; Zovia 1/50E*
ethiodized oil
  Ethiodol
ethionamide
  Trecator-SC
ethopropazine HCl
  Parsidol
ethosuximide
  Zarontin
ethotoin
  Peganone

*This brand is a combination product.

ethyl chloride
Fluro-Ethyl*
ethyl dihydroxypropyl PABA
Solaquin Forte*
ethynodiol diacetate
Demulen 1/35; Demulen 1/50*
Zovia 1/35E; Zovia 1/50E*
etidocaine
Duranest; Duranest MPF*
etidocaine HCl
Duranest; Duranest MPF
etidronate disodium
Didrocal ⓒ*
Didronel
etodolac
Apo-Etodolac ⓒ
Gen-Etodolac ⓒ
Lodine
Lodine XL
etomidate
Amidate
etoposide
Toposar*
VePesid
etoposide phosphate diethanolate
Etopophos
etretinate
Tegison
evernimicin
Ziracin
everolimus
Certican
exemestane
Aromasin
exisulind
Aptosyn
Prevatac
extended-release niacin
Advicor*
extracts of honeybee, yellow jacket, yellow hornet, white-faced hornet, mixed vespid, and wasp venom
Albay
Pharmalgen
Venomil
factor IX complex
Bebulin VH
factor VIIa
NovoSeven

factor XIII
Fibrogammin P
famciclovir
Famvir
famotidine
Alti-Famotidine ⓒ
Pepcid
Pepcid RPD
Rhoxal-famotidine ⓒ
fat emulsion
Intralipid 10%; Intralipid 20%
Liposyn II 20%; Liposyn III 20%
felbamate
Felbatol
felodipine
Lexxel*
Plendil
fenfluramine HCl
Pondimin
fenofibrate
Gen-Fenofibrate Micro ⓒ
Lipidil Supra ⓒ
PMS-Fenofibrate Micro ⓒ
Tricor
fenoldopam mesylate
Corlopam
fenoprofen calcium
Nalfon
fenoterol hydrobromide
Berotec
fentanyl
Duragesic-25; Duragesic-50; Duragesic-75; Duragesic-100
fentanyl citrate
Actiq
Fentanyl Oralet
Innovar*
Sublimaze
ferric pyrophosphate
Senilezol*
Vitafōl*
ferrous fumarate
Anemagen*
B-C with Folic Acid Plus*
Berocca Plus*
Berplex Plus*
Chromagen*
Contrin*

---

*This brand is a combination product.

Generic ◆ Brands

ferrous fumarate (cont.)
Estrostep Fe*
Feocyte*
Ferotrinsic*
Foltrin*   ,
Formula B Plus*
Fumatinic*
Hemocyte-F*
Hemocyte Plus*
Livitrinsic-f*
Loestrin Fe 1/20; Loestrin Fe 1.5/30*
Microgestin Fe 1/20; Microgestin Fe
    1.5/30*
NataChew*
Nephro-Fer Rx*
Nephro-Vite Rx + Fe*
Nephron FA*
Pronemia Hematinic*
Theragran Hematinic*
TriHemic 600*
Trinsicon*
Vitafōl; Vitafōl-PN*
Zodeac-100*
ferrous gluconate
Feocyte*
Hytinic*
ferrous sulfate
Feocyte*
Fero-Folic-500*
Florvite + Iron*
Florvite + Iron; Half Strength
    Florvite + Iron*
Iberet-Folic-500*
NataFort*
Vi-Daylin/F ADC + Iron*
Vi-Daylin/F Multivitamin + Iron*
ferucarbotran
Resovist
ferumoxides
Feridex
ferumoxsil
GastroMARK
ferumoxtran-10
Combidex
fexofenadine HCl
Allegra
Allegra-D*
fibrinolysin
Elase*
Elase-Chloromycetin*

filgrastim
Neupogen
finasteride
Propecia
Proscar
flavoxate HCl
Urispas
flecainide acetate
Tambocor
floxuridine
FUDR
fluconazole
Apo-Fluconazole ⊛
Diflucan
flucytosine
Ancobon
fludarabine phosphate
Fludara
fludrocortisone acetate
Florinef Acetate
flumazenil
Romazicon
flumecinol
Zixoryn
flunarizine HCl
Sibelium
flunisolide
AeroBid; AeroBid-M
Alti-Flunisolide ⊛
Apo-Flunisolide ⊛
Bronalide ⊛
Nasalide
Nasarel
flunitrazepam
Rohypnol
fluocinolone acetonide
Capex
Derma-Smoothe/FS
Fluonid
Flurosyn
Synalar
Synalar-HP
Synemol
fluocinonide
Fluonex
Lidex
Lidex-E
Lyderm ⊛

---

*This brand is a combination product.

Generic ♦ Brands

fluorescein
  AK-Fluor
fluorescein sodium
  Flu-Oxinate*
  Fluor-I-Strip; Fluor-I-Strip A.T.
  Fluoracaine*
  Fluorescite
  Flurate*
  Fluress*
  Ful-Glo
  Funduscein-10; Funduscein-25
  Healon Yellow*
  Ophthifluor
fluorexon
  Fluoresoft
fluoride
  ADC with Fluoride*
  Adeflor M*
  Apatate with Fluoride*
  Chewable Multivitamins with Fluoride*
  Chewable Triple Vitamins with Fluoride*
  Multivitamin with Fluoride*
  Mulvidren-F*
  Polytabs-F*
  Polyvitamin Fluoride*
  Polyvitamin Fluoride with Iron*
  Polyvitamin with Iron and Fluoride*
  Polyvitamins with Fluoride and Iron*
  Soluvite C.T.*
  Soluvite-f*
  Tri-Flor-Vite with Fluoride*
  Tri Vit with Fluoride*
  Tri-Vitamin with Fluoride*
  Tri-A-Vite F*
  Triple Vitamin ADC with Fluoride*
  Trivitamin Fluoride*
fluorometholone
  Fluor-Op
  FML S.O.P.
  FML; FML Forte
  FML-S*
  PMS-Fluorometholone ⓒⓐⓝ
fluorometholone acetate
  Eflone
  Flarex
fluorouracil
  AccuSite*
  Adrucil

fluorouracil (cont.)
  Carac
  Efudex
  Fluoroplex
fluoxetine HCl
  Alti-Fluoxetine ⓒⓐⓝ
  CO Fluoxetine ⓒⓐⓝ
  Gen-Fluoxetine ⓒⓐⓝ
  Prozac
  Prozac Weekly
  Rhoxal-fluoxetine ⓒⓐⓝ
  Sarafem
fluoxymesterone
  Halotestin
fluphenazine decanoate
  Modecate; Modecate Concentrate ⓒⓐⓝ
  PMS-Fluphenazine ⓒⓐⓝ
  PMS-Fluphenazine Decanoate ⓒⓐⓝ
  Prolixin Decanoate
  Rho-Fluphenazine Decanoate ⓒⓐⓝ
fluphenazine enanthate
  Moditen Enanthate ⓒⓐⓝ
  Prolixin Enanthate
fluphenazine HCl
  Apo-Fluphenazine ⓒⓐⓝ
  Moditen HCl ⓒⓐⓝ
  Permitil
  Prolixin
flurandrenolide
  Cordran
  Cordran SP
flurazepam HCl
  Dalmane
flurbiprofen
  Ansaid
flurbiprofen sodium
  Ocufen
flutamide
  Apo-Flutamide ⓒⓐⓝ
  Euflex ⓒⓐⓝ
  Eulexin
fluticasone propionate
  Advair*
  Cutivate
  Flonase
  Flovent
fluvastatin sodium
  Lescol

*This brand is a combination product.

fluvastatin sodium (cont.)
Lescol XL
fluvestrant
Faslodex
fluvoxamine maleate
Gen-Fluvoxamine ⒸⒶⓃ
Luvox
Novo-Fluvoxamine ⒸⒶⓃ
Nu-Fluvoxamine ⒸⒶⓃ
PMS-Fluvoxamine ⒸⒶⓃ
folic acid
B-C with Folic Acid*
B-C with Folic Acid Plus*
B-Plex*
Bacmin*
Berocca*
Berocca Parenteral Nutrition*
Berocca Plus*
Berplex Plus*
Cefol*
Cernevit-12*
Cevi-Fer*
Cezin-S*
Chewable Multivitamins with Fluoride*
Citracal Prenatal*
Contrin*
Eldercaps*
Enfamil Natalins Rx*
Fe-Tinic 150 Forte*
Feocyte*
Fero-Folic-500*
Ferotrinsic*
Ferrex 150 Forte*
Ferrex PC; Ferrex PC Forte*
Florvite + Iron; Half Strength Florvite + Iron*
Florvite; Florvite Half Strength*
Foltrin*
Foltx*
Folvite
Formula B*
Formula B Plus*
Hemocyte-F*
Hemocyte Plus*
Iberet-Folic-500*
Lactocal-F*
Liver Combo No. 5*
Livitrinsic-f*
M.V.I. Pediatric*

folic acid (cont.)
M.V.I.-12*
MagneBind 400 Rx*
Marnatal-F*
Materna*
May-Vita*
Megaton*
Mission Prenatal Rx*
Mynatal*
Mynatal FC*
Mynatal P.N.*
Mynatal P.N. Forte*
Mynatal Rx*
Mynate 90 Plus*
NataChew*
NataFort*
NatalCare Plus*
Natalins Rx*
Natarex Prenatal*
Nephplex Rx*
Nephro-Fer Rx*
Nephro-Vite Rx + Fe*
Nephro-Vite Rx*
Nephrocaps*
Nephron FA*
Nestabs CFB; Nestabs FA*
Niferex-PN*
Niferex-PN Forte*
Niferex-150 Forte*
Nu-Iron Plus*
Nu-Iron V*
O-Cal f.a.*
Par-F*
Par-Natal Plus 1 Improved*
Poly-Vi-Flor*
Poly-Vi-Flor with Iron*
Polytabs-F*
Polyvitamin Fluoride*
Polyvitamin Fluoride with Iron*
Polyvitamins with Fluoride and Iron*
Pramilet FA*
PreCare Conceive*
PreCare Prenatal*
PremesisRx*
Prenatal H.P.*
Prenatal Maternal*
Prenatal MR 90*
Prenatal Plus Iron*

---

*This brand is a combination product.

folic acid (cont.)
  Prenatal Plus with Betacarotene*
  Prenatal Plus; Prenatal Plus
    Improved*
  Prenatal Rx*
  Prenatal Rx with Betacarotene*
  Prenatal Z*
  Prenatal-1 + Iron*
  Prenate Advance; Prenate 90*
  Prenate Ultra*
  Pronemia Hematinic*
  Soluvite C.T.*
  Strong Start*
  Strovite*
  Strovite Advance*
  Strovite Plus; Strovite Forte*
  Stuartnatal Plus*
  Theragran Hematinic*
  TriHemic 600*
  Trinsicon*
  Ultra-Natal*
  Vi-Daylin/F Multivitamin*
  Vi-Daylin/F Multivitamin + Iron*
  Vicon Forte*
  Vitafōl*
  Vitafōl; Vitafōl-PN*
  Zenate, Advanced Formula*
  Zincvit*
  Zodeac-100*
follitropin alfa
  Gonal-F
follitropin beta
  Follistim
  Puregon ⓒⒶⓃ
fomepizole
  Antizol
fomivirsen sodium
  Vitravene
fondaparinux sodium
  Arixtra
formaldehyde
  Formalyde-10
  Lazer Formalyde
formoterol fumarate
  Foradil
  Oxeze ⓒⒶⓃ
foscarnet sodium
  Foscavir
fosfomycin tromethamine
  Monurol

fosinopril sodium
  Monopril
  Monopril-HCT*
fosphenytoin sodium
  Cerebyx
frovatriptan succinate
  Miguard, Migard
fructose
  5% Travert and Electrolyte No. 2;
    10% Travert and Electrolyte No. 2*
fructose-1,6-diphosphate
  Cordox
furazolidone
  Furoxone
furosemide
  Apo-Furosemide ⓒⒶⓃ
  Lasix
  Novo-Semide ⓒⒶⓃ
fusidic acid
  Fucidin ⓒⒶⓃ
gabaergic cells
  NeuroCell-HD
gabapentin
  Neurontin
  PMS-Gabapentin ⓒⒶⓃ
gadodiamide
  Omniscan
gadopentetate dimeglumine
  Magnevist
gadoteridol
  ProHance
gadoversetamide
  Optimark
galactose
  Echovist ⓒⒶⓃ
  Levovist ⓒⒶⓃ*
galantamine hydrobromide
  Reminyl
gallium nitrate
  Ganite
gamma hydroxybutyrate
  Gamma-OH
ganciclovir
  Cytovene
  Vitrasert
ganciclovir sodium
  Cytovene

*This brand is a combination product.

Generic ◆ Brands

ganirelix acetate
Antagon
gatifloxacin
Tequin
gemcitabine HCl
Gemzar
gemfibrozil
Apo-Gemfibrozil ⒸⒶⓃ
Gemcor
Lopid
Novo-Gemfibrozil ⒸⒶⓃ
gemifloxacin mesylate
Factive
gemtuzumab ozogamicin
Mylotarg
gentamicin sulfate
G-myticin
Garamycin
Garamycin Pediatric
Genoptic
Genoptic S.O.P.
Gentacidin
Gentak
Jenamicin
Maitec
Pred-G*
Pred-G S.O.P.*
Septopal
gestodene
Minesse*
glatiramer acetate
Copaxone
gliclazide
Gen-Gliclazide ⒸⒶⓃ
glimepiride
Amaryl
glipizide
Glucotrol
Glucotrol XL
glucagon
GlucaGen Diagnostic Kit
GlucaGen Emergency Kit
Glucagon Diagnostic Kit
Glucagon Emergency Kit
D-gluconic acid lactone
Renacidin*
glucono-delta-lactone
Renacidin Irrigation*
glucose
Glucose-40

glucose (cont.)
Iveegam*
Xylocaine MPF*
L-glutathione
Cachexon
glyburide
Apo-Glyburide ⒸⒶⓃ
Diaβeta (or DiaBeta)
Euglucon ⒸⒶⓃ
Gen-Glybe ⒸⒶⓃ
Glucovance*
Glynase
Micronase
Micronized Glyburide
Novo-Glyburide ⒸⒶⓃ
glycerin
Ophthalgan
Osmoglyn
glycopyrrolate
Robinul
Robinul Forte
gold sodium thiomalate
Aurolate
gonadorelin acetate
Lutrepulse
gonadorelin HCl
Factrel
goserelin acetate
Zoladex
Zoladex LA ⒸⒶⓃ
gp120 antigens
AIDSVax
gp160 antigens
VaxSyn HIV-1
graftskin
Apligraf
gramicidin
AK-Spore*
Neosporin*
granisetron HCl
Kytril
grepafloxacin HCl
Raxar
griseofulvin
Fulvicin P/G
Fulvicin U/F
Grifulvin V
Gris-PEG

*This brand is a combination product.

griseofulvin (cont.)
  Grisactin 250
  Grisactin 500
  Grisactin Ultra
guaifenesin
  Ami-Tex LA*
  Anatuss*
  Anatuss LA*
  Aquatab C*
  Aquatab D*
  Aquatab DM*
  Atuss G*
  Bronchial*
  Broncholate*
  Brondelate*
  Bronkotuss Expectorant*
  Brontex*
  Calmylin with Codeine ⒸⒶⓃ*
  Cheracol Cough*
  Co-Tuss V*
  Codegest Expectorant*
  Codiclear DH*
  Coldloc*
  Coldloc-LA*
  Conex with Codeine*
  Congess JR*
  Congess SR*
  Contuss*
  Cophene XP*
  Cotridin Expectorant ⒸⒶⓃ*
  Cyclofed Pediatric*
  Cycofed Pediatric*
  Deconamine CX*
  Decongestant Expectorant*
  Deconsal II*
  Deconsal Pediatric*
  Deconsal Sprinkle*
  Defen-LA*
  Deproist Expectorant with Codeine*
  Despec*
  Detussin Expectorant*
  Dihistine Expectorant*
  Dilaudid Cough*
  Dilor-G*
  Donatussin*
  Donatussin DC*
  Dura-Gest*
  Dura-Vent*
  Duratuss DM*
  Duratuss-G

guaifenesin (cont.)
  Duratuss; Duratuss-GP*
  Dy-G*
  Dyflex-G*
  Dyline-GG*
  Elixophyllin GG*
  Endal*
  Endal Expectorant*
  Enomine*
  Entex*
  Entex LA*
  Entex PSE*
  Entuss-D*
  Entuss-D Jr.*
  Entuss Expectorant*
  Eudal-SR*
  Exgest LA*
  Fenesin
  Fenesin DM*
  GFN/PSE*
  Glyceryl-T*
  GP-500*
  Guai-Vent/PSE*
  Guaifed*
  Guaifed-PD*
  Guaifenex*
  Guaifenex DM*
  Guaifenex LA
  Guaifenex PPA 75*
  Guaifenex PSE 60; Guaifenex PSE 120; Guaifenex Rx DM*
  Guaifenex Rx*
  GuaiMAX-D*
  Guaipax*
  Guaitex*
  Guaitex LA*
  Guaitex PSE*
  Guaivent*
  Guaivent PD*
  Guiatex LA*
  Guiatex PSE*
  Guiatuss AC*
  Guiatuss DAC*
  Guiatussin DAC*
  Guiatussin with Codeine Expectorant*
  Histalet X*
  Humibid DM*

*This brand is a combination product.

Generic ♦ Brands

guaifenesin (cont.)
    Humibid DM Sprinkle*
    Humibid L.A.
    Humibid Sprinkle
    HycoClear Tuss*
    Hycotuss Expectorant*
    Hydrocodone GF*
    Iobid DM*
    Iosal II*
    Isoclor Expectorant*
    Kwelcof*
    Levall 5.0*
    Liquibid-D*
    Liquibid; Liquibid-1200
    Lufyllin-EPG*
    Lufyllin-GG*
    MED-Rx*
    MED-Rx DM*
    Monafed
    Monafed DM*
    Muco-Fen-DM*
    Muco-Fen-LA
    Mudrane GG*
    Mudrane GG-2*
    Mytussin AC Cough*
    Mytussin DAC*
    Naldecon CX Adult*
    Nasabid*
    Nasabid SR*
    Nasatab LA*
    Norel*
    Novagest Expectorant with
        Codeine*
    Novahistine Expectorant*
    Nucofed Expectorant; Nucofed
        Pediatric Expectorant*
    Organidin NR
    P-V-Tussin*
    Pancof-XL; Pancof XP*
    Panfil G*
    Panmist JR*
    PanMist-DM*
    Partuss LA*
    Phenhist Expectorant*
    Phenylfenesin L.A.*
    Pneumomist
    Pneumotussin*
    Pneumotussin HC*
    Polaramine Expectorant*
    Profen Forte DM*

guaifenesin (cont.)
    Profen II DM*
    Profen II; Profen LA*
    Protuss DM*
    Quibron; Quibron-300*
    Respa-DM*
    Respa-GF
    Respa-1st*
    Respaire-60; Respaire-120*
    Robafen AC Cough*
    Robafen DAC*
    Robitussin A-C*
    Robitussin-DAC*
    Romilar AC*
    Ru-Tuss DE*
    Rymed*
    Rymed-TR*
    Ryna-CX*
    Sil-Tex*
    Sinufed*
    Sinumist-SR
    Sinupan*
    SinuVent*
    Slo-phyllin GG*
    SRC Expectorant*
    Stamoist E*
    Stamoist LA*
    Statuss Expectorant*
    Sudal 120/600*
    Sudal 60/500*
    Syn-Rx*
    Synophylate-GG*
    Theolate*
    Touro CC*
    Touro DM*
    Touro Ex
    Touro LA*
    Triaminic Expectorant DH*
    Triaminic Expectorant with
        Codeine*
    Tuss-LA*
    Tussafed HC*
    Tussafed-LA*
    Tussafin Expectorant*
    Tussanil DH*
    Tussar SF; Tussar-2*
    Tussi-Organidin DM NR; Tussi-
        Organidin DM-S NR*

---

*This brand is a combination product.

guaifenesin (cont.)
  Tussi-Organidin NR; Tussi-Organi-
    din-S NR*
  ULR-LA*
  V-Dec-M*
  Vanex Expectorant*
  Versacaps*
  Vicodin Tuss*
  Zephrex*
  Zephrex LA*
guanabenz acetate
  Wytensin
guanadrel sulfate
  Hylorel
guanethidine monosulfate
  Esimil*
  Ismelin
guanfacine HCl
  Tenex
halcinonide
  Halog
  Halog-E
halobetasol propionate
  Ultravate
halofantrine HCl
  Halfan
haloperidol
  Haldol
haloperidol decanoate
  Apo-Haloperidol LA ⒸⒶⓃ
  Haldol Decanoate 50; Haldol Deca-
    noate 100
  Haloperidol LA ⒸⒶⓃ
  PMS-Haloperidol LA ⒸⒶⓃ
haloperidol lactate
  Haldol
  PMS-Haloperidol ⒸⒶⓃ
haloprogin
  Halotex
halothane
  Fluothane
hamamelis water
  Succus Cineraria Maritima*
heme arginate
  Normosang
hemin
  Hemex*
  Panhematin
hemoglobin glutamer 250 bovine
  Hemopure

Hemophilus b conjugate vaccine
  ActHIB*
  ActHIB/Tripedia*
  HibTITER
  OmniHIB*
  PedvaxHIB*
  ProHIBiT
  Tetramune*
  TriHIBit*
**Hemophilus b purified capsular
  polysaccharide**
  Comvax*
heparin
  Aeropin
heparin sodium
  Hep-Lock; Hep-Lock U/P
  Heparin Lock Flush
  Hepflush-10
  Liquaemin Sodium
hepatitis A vaccine
  Avaxim; Avaxim Pediatric ⒸⒶⓃ
  Havrix
  Twinrix*
  Vaqta
hepatitis B immune globulin
  BayHep B
  H-BIG
  Nabi-HB
hepatitis B virus vaccine
  Comvax*
  Engerix-B
  Recombivax HB
  Twinrix*
hetastarch
  Hespan
hexachlorophene
  pHisoHex
  Septisol*
hexoprenaline sulfate
  Delaprem
histoplasmin
  Histolyn-CYL
histrelin acetate
  Supprelin
HIV immune globulin
  HIV-IG
  Remune

*This brand is a combination product.

Generic ♦ Brands

homatropine hydrobromide
  AK-Homatropine
  Hydrocodone Compound*
  Isopto Homatropine
homatropine methylbromide
  Gustase Plus*
  Hycodan*
  Hydromet*
  Tussigon*
human albumin
  Albuminar-5; Albuminar-25
  Albunex
  Albutein 5%; Albutein 25%
  Buminate 5%; Buminate 25%
  Plasbumin-5; Plasbumin-25
human hemoglobin
  Optro
  PolyHeme
hyaluronate sodium
  AMO Vitrax
  Amvisc; Amvisc Plus
  Healon Yellow*
  Healon; Healon GV
  Hyalgan
  Ossigel*
  Staarvisc
  Supartz
  Viscoat*
hyaluronate sodium 5000
  Healon5 ⓒⒶⓝ
hyaluronidase
  Wydase
hydralazine
  Bidil*
hydralazine HCl
  Apresazide 25/25; Apresazide 50/50;
    Apresazide 100/50*
  Apresoline
  Hydrap-ES*
  Marpres*
  Ser-Ap-Es*
  Tri-Hydroserpine*
hydriodic acid
  Bronkotuss Expectorant*
hydrochlorothiazide
  Accuretic*
  Aldactazide*
  Aldoril 15; Aldoril 25; Aldoril D30;
    Aldoril D50*

hydrochlorothiazide (cont.)
  Apo-Hydro ⓒⒶⓝ
  Apresazide 25/25; Apresazide 50/50;
    Apresazide 100/50*
  Atacand HCT*
  Avalide*
  Capozide 25/15; Capozide 25/25;
    Capozide 50/15; Capozide 50/25*
  Diovan HCT*
  Dyazide*
  Esidrix
  Esimil*
  Ezide
  Hydrap-ES*
  Hydro-Par
  Hydro-Serp*
  HydroDIURIL
  Hydropres-50*
  Hydroserpine #1; Hydroserpine #2*
  Hyzaar*
  Inderide 40/25; Inderide 80/25*
  Inderide LA 80/50; Inderide LA
    120/50; Inderide LA 160/50*
  Lopressor HCT 50/25; Lopressor HCT
    100/25; Lopressor HCT 100/50*
  Lotensin HCT 5/6.25; Lotensin
    HCT 10/12.5; Lotensin HCT
    20/12.5; Lotensin HCT 20/25*
  Marpres*
  Maxzide*
  Micardis HCT*
  Micardis Plus ⓒⒶⓝ*
  Microzide
  Moduretic*
  Monopril-HCT*
  Novo-Hydrazide ⓒⒶⓝ
  Oretic
  Prinzide*
  Prinzide 12.5; Prinzide 25*
  Ser-Ap-Es*
  Timolide 10-25*
  Tri-Hydroserpine*
  Uniretic*
  Vaseretic 5-12.5; Vaseretic 10-25*
  Zestoretic*
  Ziac*
hydrocodone bitartrate
  Alor 5/500*

*This brand is a combination product.

hydrocodone bitartrate (cont.)
  Anaplex HD*
  Anexsia 5/500; Anexsia 7.5/650;
    Anexsia 10/660*
  Atuss EX*
  Atuss G*
  Atuss HD*
  Azdone*
  Bancap HC*
  Ceta Plus*
  Chlorgest-HD*
  Co-Gesic*
  Co-Tuss V*
  Codamine*
  Codiclear DH*
  Codimal DH*
  Cophene XP*
  Damason-P*
  Deconamine CX*
  Detussin*
  Detussin Expectorant*
  Dolacet*
  Donatussin DC*
  Duocet*
  ED-TLC; ED Tuss HC*
  Endagen-HD*
  Endal-HD; Endal-HD Plus*
  Entuss-D*
  Entuss-D Jr.*
  Entuss Expectorant*
  H-Tuss-D*
  Histex HC*
  Histinex HC*
  Histinex PV*
  Histussin D*
  Histussin HC*
  Hy-Phen*
  HycoClear Tuss*
  Hycodan*
  Hycomine*
  Hycomine Compound*
  Hycotuss Expectorant*
  Hydro-PC*
  Hydrocet*
  Hydrocodone Compound*
  Hydrocodone CP; Hydrocodone HD*
  Hydrocodone GF*
  Hydrocodone PA*
  Hydrogesic*
  Hydromet*

hydrocodone bitartrate (cont.)
  Hyphed*
  Iodal HD*
  Iotussin HC*
  Kwelcof*
  Levall 5.0*
  Lorcet*
  Lorcet-HD*
  Lorcet Plus; Lorcet 10/650*
  Lortab*
  Lortab 2.5/500; Lortab 5/500; Lortab
    7.5/500; Lortab 10/500*
  Lortab ASA*
  Marcof Expectorant*
  Margesic H*
  Maxidone*
  Medipain 5*
  Norco*
  Oncet*
  P-V-Tussin*
  Panacet 5/500*
  Panasal 5/500*
  Pancof-HC*
  Pancof-XL; Pancof XP*
  Para-Hist HD*
  Pneumotussin*
  Pneumotussin HC*
  Protuss*
  Protuss-D*
  Rolatuss with Hydrocodone*
  Ru-Tuss with Hydrocodone*
  S-T Forte 2*
  SRC Expectorant*
  Stagesic*
  Status Green*
  T-Gesic*
  Triaminic Expectorant DH*
  Tussafed HC*
  Tussafin Expectorant*
  Tussanil DH*
  Tussend*
  Tussigon*
  Unituss HC*
  Vanex Expectorant*
  Vanex-HD*
  Vetuss HC*
  Vicodin Tuss*
  Vicodin; Vicodin ES; Vicodin HP*

*This brand is a combination product.

Generic ▶ Brands

hydrocodone bitartrate (cont.)
  Vicoprofen*
  Zydone*
hydrocodone polistirex
  Tussionex Pennkinetic*
hydrocortisone
  AK-Spore H.C.*
  AA-HC Otic*
  Acetasol HC*
  Acticort 100
  Aeroseb-HC
  Ala-Cort
  Ala-Quin*
  Ala-Scalp
  AntibiŌtic*
  Antibiotic Ear Solution*
  Antibiotic Ear Suspension*
  Anusol-HC
  Cetacort
  Cipro HC Otic*
  Corque*
  Cort-Dome
  Cortatrigen Modified*
  Cortef
  Cortenema
  Cortic*
  Cortisporin*
  Cortisporin Otic*
  Dermacort
  Dermol HC
  Drotic*
  Ear-Eze*
  1+1-F Creme*
  Fungoid-HC*
  1% HC
  Hi-Cor 1.0; Hi-Cor 2.5
  Hycort
  HydroTex
  Hydrocort
  Hydrocortisone Iodoquinol 1%*
  Hydrocortone
  Hytone
  Hytone 1%
  LactiCare-HC
  LazerSporin-C*
  Neo-Cortef*
  Nutracort
  Octicare*
  Oti-Med*
  Otic-Care*

hydrocortisone (cont.)
  OtiTricin*
  Otobiotic Otic*
  Otocort*
  Otomar-HC*
  Otomycet-HC*
  Otomycin-HPN Otic*
  Otosporin*
  Pedi-Cort V Creme*
  Pediotic*
  Pedotic*
  Penecort
  Proctocort
  S-T Cort
  Sab-Cortimyxin ⒸⒶⓃ*
  Synacort
  Texacort
  Tri-Otic*
  UAD Otic*
  VōSol HC Otic*
  Vanoxide-HC*
  Vasotate HC*
  Vytone*
  Zoto-HC*
hydrocortisone acetate
  Analpram-HC*
  Anucort HC
  Anumed HC
  Anusol-HC
  Anusol-HC 1
  Carmol HC*
  Chloromycetin Hydrocortisone*
  Coly-Mycin S Otic*
  Cort-Dome High Potency
  Cortate ⒸⒶⓃ
  Cortifoam
  Cortisporin*
  Cortisporin-TC*
  Enzone*
  Epifoam*
  Hemorrhoidal HC
  Hemril-HC
  Hydrocortone Acetate
  Lida-Mantle-HC*
  Mantadil*
  Neotricin HC*
  Orabase HCA
  Pramosone*

*This brand is a combination product.

hydrocortisone acetate (cont.)
Pramoxine HC*
ProctoCream-HC*
ProctoCream-HC 2.5%
Proctodan-HC ⒸⒶⓃ*
Proctofoam-HC*
Rectacort
Terra-Cortril*
U-Cort
Zone-A Forte*
hydrocortisone butyrate
Locoid
hydrocortisone probutate
Pandel
hydrocortisone sodium phosphate
Hydrocortone Phosphate
hydrocortisone sodium succinate
A-Hydrocort
Solu-Cortef
hydrocortisone valerate
Westcort
hydrodocone bitartrate
Tyrodone*
hydroflumethiazide
Diucardin
Saluron
Salutensin; Salutensin-Demi*
hydromorphone HCl
Dilaudid
Dilaudid Cough*
Dilaudid-HP
HydroStat IR
hydroquinone
Alustra*
Glyquin
Lustra
Lustra-AF
Melanex
Melpaque HP
Melquin HP
Nuquin HP*
Solaquin Forte*
Viquin Forte*
hydroxocobalamin
Hydro Cobex
Hydro-Crysti 12
LA-12
hydroxyamphetamine hydrobromide
Paredrine

hydroxyamphetamine hydrobromide (cont.)
Paremyd*
hydroxychloroquine sulfate
Plaquenil Sulfate
hydroxyprogesterone caproate
Hylutin
Hyprogest 250
hydroxypropyl methylcellulose
Occucoat
hydroxyurea
Droxia
Hydrea
Mylocel
hydroxyzine HCl
Anxanil
Atarax
Atarax 100
E-Vista
Hydrophed*
Hyzine-50
Marax-DF*
Quiess
Theomax DF*
Vistacon
Vistaquel 50
Vistaril
Vistazine 50
hydroxyzine pamoate
Vistaril
hylan G-F 20
Synvisc
hyoscyamine
Urisedamine*
hyoscyamine hydrobromide
Barbidonna; Barbidonna No. 2*
Donna-Sed*
Hyosophen*
Malatal*
Pyridium Plus*
Spasmolin*
Susano*
hyoscyamine sulfate
A-Spas S/L
Anaspaz
Antispasmodic*
Arco-Lase Plus*
Atrohist Plus*

*This brand is a combination product.

Generic ♦ Brands

hyoscyamine sulfate (cont.)
  Atrosept*
  Bellacane*
  Cystospaz
  Cystospaz-M
  Deconhist L.A.*
  Dolsed*
  Donnamar
  Donnatal*
  Donnatal No. 2*
  Ed-Spaz
  Gastrosed
  Levbid
  Levsin
  Levsin PB*
  Levsin with Phenobarbital*
  Levsin/SL
  Levsinex
  NuLev
  Phenahist-TR*
  Phenchlor S.H.A.*
  Prosed/DS*
  Stahist*
  Symax-SR
  Trac Tabs 2X*
  UAA*
  Uridon Modified*
  Urimar-T*
  Urimax*
  Urinary Antiseptic No. 2*
  Urised*
  Uritin*
  Urogesic Blue*
hypericin
  VIMRxyn
ibandronate sodium
  Bondronat
  Bonviva
ibritumomab tiuxetan
  Zevalin
ibuprofen
  Ibu
  Ibuprohm
  Motrin
  Saleto-400; Saleto-600; Saleto-800
  Salprofen
  Vicoprofen*
ibutilide fumarate
  Corvert

icodextrin
  Extraneal Peritoneal Dialysis Solution
idarubicin HCl
  Idamycin
  Idamycin PFS
idoxuridine
  Herplex
ifosfamide
  Ifex
IGF-BP3 complex
  SomatoKine
ilomastat
  Galardin
iloperidone
  Zomaril
imatinib mesylate
  Gleevec
imiglucerase
  Cerezyme
imipenem
  Primaxin I.M.*
  Primaxin I.V.*
imipramine HCl
  Tofranil
imipramine pamoate
  Tofranil-PM
imiquimod
  Aldara
immune globulin
  BayGam
  Gamimune N
  Gammagard S/D
  Gammar-P I.V.
  Iveegam*
  Panglobulin
  Polygam
  Polygam S/D
  Sandoglobulin
  Venoglobulin-I
  Venoglobulin-S
inamrinone lactate
  Inocor
indapamide
  Lozol
  PMS-Indapamide Ⓒ
indinavir sulfate
  Crixivan

*This brand is a combination product.

indium In 111 IGIV pentetate
Macroscint
indium In 111 pentetreotide
OctreoScan 111
indium In 111 satumomab pentetide
OncoScint CR/OV
indocyanine green
Cardio-Green (CG)
indomethacin
Indochron E-R
Indocin
Indocin SR
indomethacin sodium trihydrate
Indocin I.V.
infliximab
Remicade
influenza vaccine
Fluogen
FluShield
Fluvirin
Fluzone
Vaxigrip ⓒⒶⓃ
inosine pranobex
Isoprinosine
inositol
Amino-Cerv pH 5.5*
insulin, human
Humulin R Regular U-500 (concentrated)
insulin, pork
Regular Iletin II U-500 (concentrated)
insulin aspart
NovoLog
insulin glargine
Lantus
insulin lispro
Humalog
Humalog Mix 50/50*
Humalog Mix 75/25*
Humalog Mix25 ⓒⒶⓃ*
insulin lispro protamine
Humalog Mix 50/50*
Humalog Mix 75/25*
Humalog Mix25 ⓒⒶⓃ*
interferon alfa
Omniferon
Veldona

interferon alfa-2a
Roferon-A
interferon alfa-2b
Intron A
Rebetron*
interferon alfa-n1
Wellferon
Wellferon ⓒⒶⓃ
interferon alfa-n3
Alferon LDO
Alferon N
interferon alfacon-1
Infergen
interferon beta
rIFN-beta
interferon beta-1a
Avonex
R-Frone
Rebif ⓒⒶⓃ
interferon beta-1b
Betaseron
interferon gamma-1b
Actimmune
interleukin-4 receptor
Nuvance
interleukin-10
Tenovil
intrinsic factor concentrate
Chromagen*
Contrin*
Ferotrinsic*
Foltrin*
Livitrinsic-f*
Pronemia Hematinic*
TriHemic 600*
Trinsicon*
invert sugar
5% Travert and Electrolyte No. 2;
10% Travert and Electrolyte No. 2*
iocetamic acid
Cholebrine
iodamide meglumine
Renovue-Dip; Renovue-65
iodinated glycerol
Iophen
Iophen-C*
Iophen-DM*
Iophylline*

*This brand is a combination product.

iodinated glycerol (cont.)
Par Glycerol
R-Gen
Tusso-DM*
iodine
Lugol*
Strong Iodine*
iodine I 131 Lym-1 MAb
Oncolym
iodine I 131 murine MAb IgG$_2$a to B cell
ImmuRAIT-LL2
iodine I 131 tositumomab
Bexxar
iodipamide meglumine
Cholografin Meglumine
Sinografin*
iodixanol
Visipaque
iodoquinol
Hydrocortisone Iodoquinol 1%*
Vytone*
Yodoxin
iohexol
Omnipaque
iopamidol
Isovue-M 200; Isovue-M 300
Isovue-128; Isovue-200; Isovue-250; Isovue-300; Isovue-370
iopanoic acid
Telepaque
iopromide
Ultravist
iothalamate meglumine
Conray; Conray 30; Conray 43
Cysto-Conray; Cysto-Conray II
Vascoray*
iothalamate sodium
Angio-Conray
Conray 325
Conray 400
Vascoray*
ioversol
Optiray 160; Optiray 240; Optiray 300; Optiray 320; Optiray 350
ioxaglate meglumine
Hexabrix*
ioxaglate sodium
Hexabrix*

ipodate calcium
Oragrafin Calcium
ipodate sodium
Bilivist
Oragrafin Sodium
ipratropium bromide
Alti-Ipratropium Ⓒ
Apo-Ipravent Ⓒ
Atrovent
Combivent*
DuoNeb*
Gen-Ipratropium Ⓒ
irbesartan
Avalide*
Avapro
irinotecan HCl
Camptosar
iron
Adeflor M*
Bacmin*
Cevi-Fer*
Citracal Prenatal*
Enfamil Natalins Rx*
Lactocal-F*
Marnatal-F*
Materna*
Mission Prenatal Rx*
Mynatal*
Mynatal FC*
Mynatal P.N.*
Mynatal P.N. Forte*
Mynatal Rx*
Mynate 90 Plus*
NatalCare Plus*
Natalins Rx*
Natarex Prenatal*
Nestabs CFB; Nestabs FA*
O-Cal f.a.*
Par-F*
Par-Natal Plus 1 Improved*
Poly-Vi-Flor with Iron*
Polyvitamin Fluoride with Iron*
Polyvitamin with Iron and Fluoride*
Polyvitamins with Fluoride and Iron*
Pramilet FA*
PreCare Conceive*
PreCare Prenatal*
Prenatal H.P.*

---

*This brand is a combination product.

iron (cont.)
  Prenatal Maternal*
  Prenatal MR 90*
  Prenatal Plus Iron*
  Prenatal Plus with Betacarotene*
  Prenatal Plus; Prenatal Plus
    Improved*
  Prenatal Rx*
  Prenatal Rx with Betacarotene*
  Prenatal Z*
  Prenatal-1 + Iron*
  Prenate Advance; Prenate 90*
  Prenate Ultra*
  Strong Start*
  Stuartnatal Plus*
  Tri-Vi-Flor with Iron*
  Zenate, Advanced Formula*
iron dextran
  DexFerrum
  Dexiron ⒸⒶⓃ
  InFeD
  Infurfer ⒸⒶⓃ
iron sucrose
  Venofer
isocarboxazid
  Marplan
isoetharine HCl
  Beta-2
  Bronkosol
isoetharine mesylate
  Bronkometer
isoflurane
  Forane
isoleucine
  VIL*
isometheptene mucate
  Duradrin*
  Isocom*
  Isopap*
  Midchlor*
  Midrin*
  Migratine*
isoniazid
  Laniazid
  Laniazid C.T.
  Nydrazid
  Rifamate*
  Rifater*
isopropyl alcohol
  Ovide*

isoproterenol HCl
  Duo-Medihaler*
  Isuprel
isoproterenol sulfate
  Medihaler-Iso
  Norisodrine with Calcium Iodide*
isosorbide
  Ismotic
isosorbide dinitrate
  Bidil*
  Dilatrate-SR
  Isordil
  Isotrate ER
  Sorbitrate
isosorbide mononitrate
  Imdur
  Ismo
  Monoket
isosulfan blue
  Lymphazurin 1%
isotretinoin
  Accutane
isoxicam
  Maxicam
isoxsuprine HCl
  Vasodilan
  Voxsuprine
isradipine
  DynaCirc
  DynaCirc CR
itraconazole
  Sporanox
ivermectin
  Stromectol
Japanese encephalitis virus vaccine
  JE-VAX
kanamycin sulfate
  Kantrex
ketamine HCl
  Ketalar
ketoconazole
  Apo-Ketoconazole ⒸⒶⓃ
  Nizoral
  Novo-Ketoconazole ⒸⒶⓃ
ketoprofen
  Orudis
  Oruvail

Generic ◆ Brands

*This brand is a combination product.

ketorolac tromethamine
  Acular; Acular PF
  Apo-Ketorolac ⒸⒶⓃ
  Toradol
ketotifen fumarate
  Zaditor
labetalol HCl
  Normodyne
  Trandate
lacidipine
  Lacipil
lactic acid
  Lactinol
  Lactinol-E*
lactulose
  Apo-Lactulose ⒸⒶⓃ
  Cephulac
  Cholac
  Chronulac
  Constilac
  Constulose
  Duphalac
  Enulose
  Evalose
  Heptalac
  Kristalose
lamivudine
  Combivir*
  Epivir
  Epivir-HBV
  Heptovir ⒸⒶⓃ
  Trizivir*
  Zeffix
lamotrigine
  Lamictal
lansoprazole
  Hp-PAC ⒸⒶⓃ*
  Prevacid
  Prevpac*
lanthanum carbonate
  Lambda
laronidase
  Aldurazyme
latanoprost
  Xalatan
  Xalcom*
lazabemide HCl
  Tempium
leflunomide
  Arava

leteprinim potassium
  Neotrofin
letrozole
  Femara
leucine
  VIL*
ʟ-leucovorin
  Isovorin
leucovorin calcium
  Orzel*
  Wellcovorin
leuprolide acetate
  Leuprogel
  Lupron Depot
  Lupron Depot-Ped
  Lupron Depot−3 month; Lupron
    Depot−4 month
  Lupron; Lupron Pediatric
  Viadur
levacecarnine
  Alcar
levalbuterol
  Contramid
levalbuterol HCl
  Xopenex
levamisole HCl
  Ergamisol
levetiracetam
  Keppra
levobetaxolol HCl
  Betaxon
levobunolol
  BetaSite
levobunolol HCl
  AKBeta
  Apo-Levobunolol ⒸⒶⓃ
  Betagan Liquifilm
  PMS-Levobunolol ⒸⒶⓃ
levobupivacaine HCl
  Chirocaine
levocabastine HCl
  Livostin
  Livostin ⒸⒶⓃ
levocarnitine
  Carnitor
  VitaCarn
levodopa
  Dopar

*This brand is a combination product.

Generic ◆ Brands

levodopa (cont.)
  Larodopa
  Sinemet 10/100; Sinemet 25/100;
    Sinemet 25/250*
  Sinemet CR*
levofloxacin
  Levaquin
  Quixin
levomethadyl acetate HCl
  Orlaam
levonordefrin
  Carbocaine with Neo-Cobefrin*
  Isocaine HCl*
  Polocaine*
levonorgestrel
  Alesse*
  Aviane-28*
  Enpresse*
  Levlen*
  Levlite*
  Levora 0.15/30*
  Mirena
  Nordette*
  Norplant
  Plan B
  Preven*
  Tri-Levlen*
  Triphasil*
  Trivora-28*
levorphanol tartrate
  Levo-Dromoran
levothyroxine sodium
  Eltroxin
  Levo-T
  Levothroid
  Levothroid ⒸⒶⓃ
  Levoxyl
  Synthroid
  Triacana*
  Unithroid
lexipafant
  Zacutex
lidocaine
  EMLA*
  Lida-Mantle-HC*
  Lidoderm
  Terramycin IM*
lidocaine HCl
  Anestacon
  Decadron with Xylocaine*

lidocaine HCl (cont.)
  Dentipatch
  Dilocaine
  Duo-Trach Kit
  Lidoject-1; Lidoject-2
  LidoPen
  Nervocaine 1%
  Octocaine HCl*
  Xylocaine
  Xylocaine 10% Oral
  Xylocaine HCl*
  Xylocaine HCl IV for Cardiac
    Arrhythmias
  Xylocaine MPF
  Xylocaine MPF*
  Xylocaine Viscous
lincomycin HCl
  Lincocin
  Lincorex
lindane
  G-Well
  Scabene
linezolid
  Zyvox
  Zyvoxam ⒸⒶⓃ
liothyronine sodium
  Cytomel
  Triostat
liotrix
  Thyrolar-0.25; -0.5; -1; -2; -3
lipase
  Arco-Lase Plus*
  Cotazym*
  Cotazym-S*
  Donnazyme*
  Ilozyme*
  Ku-Zyme*
  Ku-Zyme HP*
  Kutrase*
  Lipram-CR20*
  Lipram-PN10*
  Lipram-PN16*
  Lipram-UL12*
  Lipram-UL18*
  Lipram-UL20*
  Pancrease; Pancrease MT 4; Pan-
    crease MT 10; Pancrease MT 16;
    Pancrease MT 20*

*This brand is a combination product.

lipase (cont.)
   Pancrecarb MS-8*
   Protilase*
   Ultrase; Ultrase MT 12; Ultrase MT
     18; Ultrase MT 20*
   Viokase*
   Zymase*
lipoprotein OspA
   LYMErix
lisinopril
   Prinivil
   Prinzide*
   Prinzide 12.5; Prinzide 25*
   Zestoretic*
   Zestril
lithium carbonate
   Apo-Lithium (CAN)
   Carbolith (CAN)
   Duralith (CAN)
   Eskalith
   Eskalith CR
   Lithane (CAN)
   Lithobid
   Lithonate
   Lithotabs
   PMS-Lithium Carbonate (CAN)
lithium citrate
   PMS-Lithium Citrate (CAN)
liver derivative complex
   Kutapressin
liver, desiccated
   Feocyte*
liver extracts
   Liver Combo No. 5*
lobeline sulfate
   NicErase-SL
lodoxamide tromethamine
   Alomide
lomefloxacin HCl
   Maxaquin
lomustine
   CeeNu
loperamide HCl
   Imodium
lopinavir
   Kaletra*
loracarbef
   Lorabid
loratadine
   Claritin

loratadine (cont.)
   Claritin-D; Claritin-D 12 Hour;
     Claritin-D 24 Hour*
lorazepam
   Apo-Lorazepam (CAN)
   Ativan
   Novo-Lorazem (CAN)
   Riva-Lorazepam (CAN)
losartan potassium
   Cozaar
   Hyzaar*
loteprednol etabonate
   Alrex
   Lotemax
lovastatin
   Advicor*
   Mevacor
loxapine
   Loxapac (CAN)
loxapine HCl
   Loxapac (CAN)
   Loxitane C
   Loxitane IM
loxapine succinate
   Apo-Loxapine (CAN)
   Loxitane
lucinactant
   Surfaxin
lutein
   Strovite Advance*
lymphocyte immune globulin
   Atgam
   Nashville Rabbit Antithymocyte
     Serum
lypressin
   Diapid
mafenide acetate
   Sulfamylon
magnesium carbonate
   MagneBind 400 Rx*
   Renacidin Irrigation*
magnesium chloride
   Plegisol*
magnesium hydroxycarbonate
   Renacidin*
magnesium salicylate
   Magan
   Magsal*

*This brand is a combination product.

Generic ◆ Brands

magnesium salicylate (cont.)
Mobidin
Trilisate*
malathion
Ovide*
mangofodipir trisodium
Teslascan
mannitol
Osmitrol
Resectisol
maprotiline HCl
Ludiomil
masoprocol
Actinex
maxacalcitol
Prezios
mazindol
Mazanor
Sanorex
measles and rubella virus vaccine
M-R-Vax II
measles, mumps, and rubella virus vaccine
M-M-R II
Priorix (CAN)
measles virus vaccine
Attenuvax
mebendazole
Vermox
mecamylamine HCl
Inversine
mecasermin
Myotrophin
mechlorethamine HCl
Mustargen
meclizine HCl
Antivert; Antivert/25; Antivert/50
Antrizine
Meni-D
Ru-Vert-M
meclocycline sulfosalicylate
Meclan
medroxyprogesterone acetate
Alti-MPA (CAN)
Amen
Curretab
Cycrin
Depo-Provera
Lunelle*

medroxyprogesterone acetate (cont.)
Novo-Medrone (CAN)
Premphase*
Prempro*
Proclim (CAN)
Provera
medrysone
HMS
mefenamic acid
Ponstel
mefloquine HCl
Lariam
Mephaquin
megakaryocyte growth and development factor
Megagen
megestrol acetate
Lin-Megestrol (CAN)
Megace
melanoma vaccine
Melacine
melarsoprol
Arsobal
meloxicam
Mobic
Mobicox (CAN)
melphalan
Alkeran
meningococcal polysaccharide vaccine
Menomune-A/C/Y/W-135
menotropins
Humegon
Pergonal
Repronex
menthol
Tussafed*
mepenzolate bromide
Cantil
meperidine HCl
Demerol HCl
Mepergan*
Mepergan Fortis*
mephentermine sulfate
Wyamine Sulfate
mephenytoin
Mesantoin

*This brand is a combination product.

mephobarbital
  Mebaral
mepivacaine HCl
  Carbocaine
  Carbocaine with Neo-Cobefrin*
  Isocaine HCl
  Isocaine HCl*
  Polocaine
  Polocaine*
  Polocaine MPF
meprobamate
  Equagesic*
  Equanil
  Meprospan
  Micrainin*
  Miltown
  Miltown-600
  Neuramate
  PMB 200; PMB 400*
mequinol
  Solage*
mercaptopurine
  Purinethol
meropenem
  Merrem
mesalamine
  Asacol
  Canasa
  FIV-ASA
  Pentasa
  Rowasa
  Salofalk Ⓒᴬᴺ
mesna
  Mesnex
mesoridazine besylate
  Serentil
mestranol
  Enovid*
  Genora 1/50*
  Necon 1/50*
  Nelova 1/50M*
  Norethin 1/50M*
  Norinyl 1 + 50*
  Ortho-Novum 1/50*
metaproterenol sulfate
  Alupent
  Metaprel
metaraminol bitartrate
  Aramine

metaxalone
  Skelaxin
metformin HCl
  Alti-Metformin HCl Ⓒᴬᴺ
  Gen-Metformin Ⓒᴬᴺ
  Glucophage
  Glucophage XR
  Glucovance*
  Metformin XT
  Novo-Metformin Ⓒᴬᴺ
methacholine chloride
  Provocholine
methadone HCl
  Dolophine HCl
  Metadol Ⓒᴬᴺ
  Methadose
methamphetamine HCl
  Desoxyn
methandrostenolone
  Dianabol
methantheline bromide
  Banthīne
methazolamide
  GlaucTabs
  MZM
  Neptazane
methdilazine HCl
  Tacaryl
methenamine
  Atrosept*
  Cystex*
  Dolsed*
  Prosed/DS*
  Trac Tabs 2X*
  UAA*
  Uridon Modified*
  Urimar-T*
  Urimax*
  Urinary Antiseptic No. 2*
  Urised*
  Uritin*
  Uro-Phosphate*
  Urogesic Blue*
methenamine hippurate
  Hiprex
  Urex
methenamine mandelate
  Mandameth

---

*This brand is a combination product.

methenamine mandelate (cont.)
Mandelamine
Urisedamine*
Uroqid-Acid No. 2*
methenamine sulfosalicylate
Unguentum Bossi*
methicillin sodium
Staphcillin
methimazole
Tapazole
methionine
Amino-Cerv pH 5.5*
methocarbamol
Robaxin
Robaxisal*
methohexital sodium
Brevital Sodium
Brietal Sodium CAN
methotrexate
Trexall
methotrexate sodium
Folex PFS
Rheumatrex
methotrimeprazine HCl
Levoprome
methotrimeprazine maleate
Apo-Methoprazine CAN
methoxamine HCl
Vasoxyl
methoxsalen
8-MOP
Oxsoralen
Oxsoralen-Ultra
Uvadex
8-methoxycarbonyloctyl oligosaccharides
Synsorb-Pk
methoxyflurane
Penthrane
methscopolamine bromide
Ex-Histine*
Pamine
methscopolamine nitrate
AH-chew*
AlleRx*
D.A.*
D.A. II*
Dallergy*
Dehistine*
Dura-Vent/DA*

methscopolamine nitrate (cont.)
Extendryl*
Extendryl JR*
Extendryl SR*
Mescolor*
OMNIhist L.A.*
Pannaz*
Prehist D*
Xiral*
methsuximide
Celontin
methyclothiazide
Aquatensen
Diutensen-R*
Enduron
Enduronyl; Enduronyl Forte*
methyldopa
Aldoclor-150; Aldoclor-250*
Aldomet
Aldoril 15; Aldoril 25; Aldoril D30; Aldoril D50*
Amodopa
methyldopate HCl
Aldomet; Aldomet Ester HCl
methylene blue
Atrosept*
Dolsed*
Methblue 65
Prosed/DS*
Trac Tabs 2X*
UAA*
Uridon Modified*
Urimar-T*
Urimax*
Urinary Antiseptic No. 2*
Urised*
Uritin*
Urogesic Blue*
Urolene Blue
methylergonovine maleate
Methergine
methylphenidate HCl
Concerta
Metadate CD
Metadate ER
Methylin
Methylin ER
Ritalin

*This brand is a combination product.

methylphenidate HCl (cont.)
Ritalin-SR
methylprednisolone
Medrol
methylprednisolone acetate
Adlone
depMedalone 40; depMedalone 80
Depo-Medrol
Depoject
Depopred-40; Depopred-80
Duralone-40; Duralone-80
M-Prednisol-40; M-Prednisol-80
Medralone 40; Medralone 80
methylprednisolone sodium succinate
A-Methapred
Solu-Medrol
methyltestosterone
Android
Android-10; Android-25
Estratest; Estratest H.S.*
Menogen; Menogen H.S.*
Methitest
Oreton Methyl
Premarin with Methyltestosterone*
Testred
Virilon
methysergide maleate
Sansert
metipranolol HCl
OptiPranolol
metoclopramide HCl
Clopra
Emitasol
Maxolon
Octamide PFS
Pramidin
Reclomide
Reglan
Sensamide
metocurine iodide
Metubine Iodide
metolazone
Mykrox
Zaroxolyn
metoprolol succinate
Toprol-XL
metoprolol tartrate
Apo-Metoprolol Ⓒ🅐🅝

metoprolol tartrate (cont.)
Apo-Metoprolol L Ⓒ🅐🅝
Gen-Metoprolol Ⓒ🅐🅝
Lopressor
Lopressor HCT 50/25; Lopressor HCT 100/25; Lopressor HCT 100/50*
Novo-Metoprol Ⓒ🅐🅝
metrifonate
ProMem
metrizamide
Amipaque
metronidazole
Flagyl
Flagyl ER
Flagyl IV RTU
Helidac*
Losec 1-2-3 M Ⓒ🅐🅝*
Metro I.V.
MetroCream
MetroGel Vaginal
MetroGel; MetroLotion
Nidagel Ⓒ🅐🅝
Noritate
Protostat
metronidazole HCl
Flagyl IV
metyrapone
Metopirone
metyrosine
Demser
mexiletine HCl
Mexitil
mezlocillin sodium
Mezlin
mibefradil dihydrochloride
Posicor
miconazole
Monistat i.v.
miconazole nitrate
Fungoid-HC*
Monistat-Derm
Monistat Dual-Pak
microbubble contrast agent
Filmix
microfibrillar collagen hemostat
Avitene Hemostat
Hemopad
Hemotene

---

*This brand is a combination product.

midazolam HCl
  Versed
midodrine HCl
  ProAmatine
mifepristone
  Mifeprex
miglitol
  Glyset
milodistim
  Pixykine
milrinone lactate
  Primacor
  Primacor in 5% Dextrose*
minerals, multiple
  B-C with Folic Acid Plus*
  Bacmin*
  Berocca Plus*
  Berplex Plus*
  Cezin-S*
  Eldercaps*
  Enfamil Natalins Rx*
  Ferrex PC; Ferrex PC Forte*
  Florvite + Iron*
  Florvite + Iron; Half Strength
    Florvite + Iron*
  Formula B Plus*
  Hemocyte Plus*
  Lactocal-F*
  Marnatal-F*
  Materna*
  Megaton*
  Mynatal*
  Mynatal FC*
  Mynatal P.N. Forte*
  Mynatal Rx*
  NataTab CFe; NataTab FA*
  NataChew*
  NatalCare Plus*
  Niferex-PN*
  Niferex-PN Forte*
  O-Cal f.a.*
  Par-F*
  Poly-Vi-Flor with Iron*
  Polyvitamin Fluoride with Iron*
  Pramilet FA*
  PreCare Conceive*
  PreCare Prenatal*
  Prenatal Maternal*
  Strovite Advance*
  Strovite Plus; Strovite Forte*

minerals, multiple (cont.)
  Theragran Hematinic*
  Ultra-Natal*
  Vicon Forte*
  Zincvit*
  Zodeac-100*
minocycline
  MPTS (minocycline periodontal
    therapeutic system)
minocycline HCl
  Arestin
  Dynacin
  Minocin
  PMS-Minocycline ⓒ
  Rhoxal-minocycline ⓒ
  Vectrin
minoxidil
  Loniten
mirtazapine
  Remeron
misoprostol
  Arthrotec*
  Cytotec
mitomycin
  Mutamycin
mitotane
  Lysodren
mitoxantrone HCl
  Novantrone
mivacurium chloride
  Mivacron
mixed respiratory vaccine
  MRV
moclobemide
  Apo-Moclobemide ⓒ
  Manerix ⓒ
  Novo-Moclobemide ⓒ
  Nu-Moclobemide ⓒ
  PMS-Moclobemide ⓒ
modafinil
  Alertec ⓒ
  Provigil
moexipril HCl
  Uniretic*
  Univasc
molgramostim
  Leucomax

*This brand is a combination product.

molindone HCl
Moban
mometasone furoate
Elocom Ⓒ
Elocon
Nasonex
monobenzone
Benoquin
monochloroacetic acid
Mono-Chlor
monoclonal antibodies
Ceprate SC
monoclonal antibody B43.13
BrevaRex
OvaRex
monoclonal antibody CD22 antigen on B-cells
LymphoCide
monoclonal antibody to CEA, humanized
CEA-Cide
monoctanoin
Moctanin
monolaurin
Glylorin
montelukast sodium
Singulair
moricizine HCl
Ethmozine
morphine
Morphelan
morphine sulfate
AERx
Astramorph PF
DepoMorphine
Duramorph
Infumorph
Kadian
M-Eslon Ⓒ
MorphiDex*
MS Contin
MS/L; MS/L Concentrate
MS/S
MSIR
OMS Concentrate
Oramorph SR
RMS
Roxanol
Roxanol; Roxanol 100; Roxanol Rescudose; Roxanol T; Roxanol UD

morphine sulfate (cont.)
UltraJect
morrhuate sodium
Scleromate
motexafin gadolinium
Gd-Tex
Xcytrin
motexafin lutetium
Antrin
Lu-Tex
Lutrin
Optrin
moxifloxacin HCl
Avelox
moxonidine
Physiotens
multiple amino acids
Aminess 5.2%*
Aminosyn 3.5% (5%, 7%, 8.5%, 10%); Aminosyn (pH6) 10%; Aminosyn II 3.5% (5%, 7%, 8.5%, 10%, 15%); Aminosyn-PF 7% (10%)*
Aminosyn 3.5% M; Aminosyn II 3.5% M*
Aminosyn 7% (8.5%) with Electrolytes; Aminosyn II 7% (8.5%, 10%) with Electrolytes*
Aminosyn-HBC 7%*
Aminosyn II 3.5% in 5% (25%) Dextrose; Aminosyn II 4.25% in 10% (20%, 25%) Dextrose; Aminosyn II 5% in 25% Dextrose*
Aminosyn II 3.5% M in 5% Dextrose; Aminosyn II 4.25% M in 10% Dextrose*
Aminosyn-RF 5.2%*
BranchAmin 4%*
FreAmine HBC 6.9%*
FreAmine III 3% (8.5%) with Electrolytes*
FreAmine III 8.5%; FreAmine III 10%*
HepatAmine*
NephrAmine 5.4%*
Novamine; Novamine 15%*
ProcalAmine*
ProSol 20%*

---

*This brand is a combination product.

multiple amino acids (cont.)
RenAmin*
Travasol 2.75% in 5% (10%, 25%)
   Dextrose; Travasol 4.25% in 5%
   (10%, 25%) Dextrose*
Travasol 3.5% (5.5%, 8.5%) with
   Electrolytes*
Travasol 5.5% (8.5%, 10%)*
TrophAmine 6%; TrophAmine 10%*
multiple B vitamins
B-C with Folic Acid*
B-Ject-100*
B-Plex*
Berocca*
Formula B*
Hemocyte Plus*
Hytinic*
Iberet-Folic-500*
Key-Plex*
Lypholized Vitamin B Complex &
   Vitamin C with B_{12}*
May-Vita*
Megaton*
Nephplex Rx*
Nephro-Vite Rx + Fe*
Nephro-Vite Rx*
Nephrocaps*
Nephron FA*
Neurodep*
Senilezol*
Strovite*
Vicam*
Vitafōl*
Vitamin B Complex 100*
multiple electrolytes
Dialyte Pattern LM*
multiple leukocytes and interleukins
MultiKine
multiple minerals
B-C with Folic Acid Plus*
Bacmin*
Berocca Plus*
Berplex Plus*
Cezin-S*
Eldercaps*
Enfamil Natalins Rx*
Ferrex PC; Ferrex PC Forte*
Florvite + Iron*
Florvite + Iron; Half Strength
   Florvite + Iron*

multiple minerals (cont.)
Formula B Plus*
Hemocyte Plus*
Lactocal-F*
Marnatal-F*
Materna*
Megaton*
Mynatal*
Mynatal FC*
Mynatal P.N. Forte*
Mynatal Rx*
NataTab CFe; NataTab FA*
NataChew*
NatalCare Plus*
Niferex-PN*
Niferex-PN Forte*
O-Cal f.a.*
Par-F*
Poly-Vi-Flor with Iron*
Polyvitamin Fluoride with Iron*
Pramilet FA*
PreCare Conceive*
PreCare Prenatal*
Prenatal Maternal*
Strovite Advance*
Strovite Plus; Strovite Forte*
Theragran Hematinic*
Ultra-Natal*
Vicon Forte*
Zincvit*
Zodeac-100*
multiple trace elements (metals)
ConTE-Pak-4
M.T.E.-4; M.T.E.-5; M.T.E.-6;
   M.T.E.-7; M.T.E.-4 Concentrated;
   M.T.E.-5 Concentrated; M.T.E.-6
   Concentrated
MulTE-Pak-4; MulTE-Pak-5
Multiple Trace Element with Sele-
   nium; Multiple Trace Element
   with Selenium Concentrated
Multiple Trace Element; Multiple
   Trace Element Concentrated;
   Multiple Trace Element Neonatal;
   Multiple Trace Element Pediatric
Multitrace-5 Concentrate
Neotrace-4
P.T.E.-4; P.T.E.-5

*This brand is a combination product.

multiple trace elements (metals) (cont.)
PedTE-Pak-4
Pedtrace-4
Trace Metals Additive in 0.9% NaCl
Tracelyte; Tracelyte II; Tracelyte with Double Electrolytes; Trace-lyte II with Double Electrolytes*

multiple vitamins
Adeflor M*
B Complex with C and B-12*
B-C with Folic Acid Plus*
Bacmin*
Berocca Parenteral Nutrition*
Berocca Plus*
Berplex Plus*
Cefol*
Cernevit-12*
Cezin-S*
Chewable Multivitamins with Fluoride*
Eldercaps*
Enfamil Natalins Rx*
Ferrex PC; Ferrex PC Forte*
Florvite + Iron*
Florvite + Iron; Half Strength Florvite + Iron*
Florvite*
Florvite; Florvite Half Strength*
Formula B Plus*
Infuvite Pediatric*
Lactocal-F*
M.V.I. Neonatal*
M.V.I. Pediatric*
M.V.I.-12*
Marnatal-F*
Materna*
Mission Prenatal Rx*
Multi-12; Multi-12 Pediatric ⓒⓐⓝ*
Multi Vitamin Concentrate*
Multivitamin with Fluoride*
Mulvidren-F*
Mynatal*
Mynatal FC*
Mynatal P.N.*
Mynatal P.N. Forte*
Mynatal Rx*
Mynate 90 Plus*
NataTab CFe; NataTab FA*
NataChew*

multiple vitamins (cont.)
NataFort*
NatalCare Plus*
Natalins Rx*
Natarex Prenatal*
Nestabs CFB; Nestabs FA*
Niferex-PN*
Niferex-PN Forte*
Nu-Iron V*
O-Cal f.a.*
Par-F*
Par-Natal Plus 1 Improved*
Poly-Vi-Flor*
Poly-Vi-Flor with Iron*
Polytabs-F*
Polyvitamin Fluoride*
Polyvitamin Fluoride with Iron*
Polyvitamin with Iron and Fluoride*
Polyvitamins with Fluoride and Iron*
Pramilet FA*
PreCare Conceive*
PreCare Prenatal*
Prenatal H.P.*
Prenatal Maternal*
Prenatal MR 90*
Prenatal Plus Iron*
Prenatal Plus with Betacarotene*
Prenatal Plus; Prenatal Plus Improved*
Prenatal Rx*
Prenatal Rx with Betacarotene*
Prenatal Z*
Prenatal-1 + Iron*
Prenate Advance; Prenate 90*
Prenate Ultra*
Soluvite C.T.*
Strong Start*
Strovite Advance*
Strovite Plus; Strovite Forte*
Stuartnatal Plus*
Theragran Hematinic*
Ultra-Natal*
Vi-Daylin/F Multivitamin*
Vi-Daylin/F Multivitamin + Iron*
Vicon Forte*
Vitafōl; Vitafōl-PN*
Zenate, Advanced Formula*
Zincvit*

*This brand is a combination product.

Generic ♦ Brands

multiple vitamins (cont.)
Zodeac-100*
mumps and rubella virus vaccine
Biavax II
mumps skin test antigen
MSTA (Mumps Skin Test Antigen)
mumps virus vaccine
Mumpsvax
mupirocin
Bactroban
mupirocin calcium
Bactroban
Bactroban Nasal
muromonab-CD3
Orthoclone OKT3
mycophenolate mofetil
CellCept
mycophenolate mofetil HCl
CellCept
nabumetone
Apo-Nabumetone ⒸⒶⓃ
Relafen
nadolol
Corgard
Corzide 40/5; Corzide 80/5*
nadroparin calcium
Fraxiparine ⒸⒶⓃ
Fraxiparine Forte ⒸⒶⓃ
nafarelin acetate
Synarel
nafcillin sodium
Nafcil
Nallpen
Unipen
naftifine HCl
Naftin
nalbuphine HCl
Nubain
nalidixic acid
NegGram
nalmefene
Revex
naloxone HCl
Narcan
Talwin NX*
naltrexone HCl
Depade
ReVia
nandrolone decanoate (in oil)
Androlone-D 200

Deca-Durabolin
Hybolin Decanoate-50; Hybolin
   Decanoate-100
Neo-Durabolic
nandrolone phenpropionate (in oil)
Durabolin
Hybolin Improved
naphazoline HCl
AK-Con
Albalon*
Nafazair
Naphcon Forte
Naphoptic-A*
Vasocon Regular
Vasocon-A*
naproxen
Anaprox; Anaprox DS
Apo-Naproxen ⒸⒶⓃ
Apo-Naproxen SR ⒸⒶⓃ
EC-Naprosyn
Gen-Naproxen EC ⒸⒶⓃ
Naprelan
Napron X
Naprosyn
Novo-Naprox ⒸⒶⓃ
Novo-Naprox-EC ⒸⒶⓃ
Novo-Naprox SR ⒸⒶⓃ
Riva-Naproxen ⒸⒶⓃ
naratriptan HCl
Amerge
natalizumab
Antegren
natamycin
Natacyn
nateglinide
Starlix
nebacumab
Centoxin
nedocromil sodium
Alocril
Tilade
nefazodone HCl
Apo-Nefazodone ⒸⒶⓃ
Serzone
Serzone-5HT$_2$ ⒸⒶⓃ
Neisseria meningitidis **OMPC**
Comvax*
PedvaxHIB*

---

*This brand is a combination product.

nelfinavir mesylate
Viracept
neomycin sulfate
AK-Spore*
AK-Spore H.C.*
AK-Trol*
AK-Neo-Dex*
AntibiÕtic*
Antibiotic Ear Solution*
Antibiotic Ear Suspension*
Coly-Mycin S Otic*
Cortatrigen Modified*
Cortisporin*
Cortisporin Otic*
Cortisporin-TC*
Dexacidin*
Dexasporin*
Drotic*
Ear-Eze*
LazerSporin-C*
Maxitrol*
Mycifradin Sulfate
Myco-Biotic II*
Neo-Cortef*
Neo-Dexair*
Neo-Dexameth*
Neo-fradin
Neo-Tabs
NeoDecadron*
Neosporin*
Neosporin G.U. Irrigant*
Neotricin HC*
Octicare*
Ocutricin*
Otic-Care*
OtiTricin*
Otocort*
Otomycin-HPN Otic*
Otosporin*
Pediotic*
Pedotic*
Poly-Pred*
Sab-Cortimyxin ⒸⒶⓃ*
Storz-N-D*
Storz-N-P-D*
Triple Antibiotic*
UAD Otic*
neostigmine bromide
Prostigmin

neostigmine methylsulfate
Prostigmin
nesiritide citrate
Natrecor
netilmicin sulfate
Netromycin
neural dopaminergic cells
NeuroCell-PD
neural gabaergic cells
NeuroCell-HD
nevirapine
Viramune
niacin
Niacor
Niaspan
Nicolar
nicardipine HCl
Cardene
Cardene I.V.
Cardene SR
nicotine
Habitrol
Nicotrol
Nicotrol NS
ProStep
nicotine polacrilex
Nicorette DS
nifedipine
Adalat
Adalat CC; Adalat Oros
Adalat XL ⒸⒶⓃ
Nifedical XL
Procardia
Procardia XL
nifurtimox
Lampit
nilutamide
Anandron ⒸⒶⓃ
Nilandron
nisoldipine
Sular
nitazoxanide
Cryptaz
nitrazepam
Mogadon
nitrendipine
Baypress

---

*This brand is a combination product.

nitric oxide
  INOmax
nitrofurantoin
  Furadantin
  Furalan
  Macrobid*
  Macrodantin
nitrofurantoin monohydrate
  Macrobid*
nitrofurazone
  Furacin
  Furacin Soluble Dressing
nitroglycerin
  Anogesic
  Deponit
  Minitran
  NitroTab
  Nitrek
  Nitro-Bid
  Nitro-Bid IV
  Nitro-Derm
  Nitro-Dur
  Nitro-Time
  Nitrodisc
  Nitrogard
  Nitroglyn
  Nitrol
  Nitrolingual Pumpspray
  Nitrong
  NitroQuick
  Nitrostat
  Transderm-Nitro
  Tridil
  Trinipatch (CAN)
nizatidine
  Axid
  Novo-Nizatidine (CAN)
  PMS-Nizatidine (CAN)
nofetumomab merpentan
  Verluma
nolatrexed dihydrochloride
  Thymitaq
nonacog alfa
  Benefix
norelgestromin
  Ortho Evra
norepinephrine bitartrate
  Levophed
  Ravocaine & Novocaine with
    Levophed*

norethindrone
  Brevicon*
  Genora 0.5/35; Genora 1/35*
  Genora 1/50*
  Jenest-28*
  Micronor
  Modicon*
  N.E.E. 1/35*
  Necon 0.5/35; Necon 1/35*
  Necon 1/50*
  Necon 10/11*
  Nelova 0.5/35E; Nelova 1/35E*
  Nelova 1/50M*
  Nelova 10/11*
  Nor-Q.D.
  Norethin 1/35E*
  Norethin 1/50M*
  Norinyl 1 + 35*
  Norinyl 1 + 50*
  Nortrel*
  Ortho 0.5/35; Ortho 1/35 (CAN)*
  Ortho 7/7/7 (CAN)*
  Ortho-Novum 1/35*
  Ortho-Novum 1/50*
  Ortho-Novum 10/11*
  Ortho-Novum 7/7/7*
  Ovcon-35*
  Ovcon-50*
  Tri-Norinyl*
norethindrone acetate
  Activella*
  Aygestin
  CombiPatch*
  Estalis 140/50; Estalis 250/50 (CAN)*
  Estrostep 21*
  Estrostep Fe*
  femhrt 1/5*
  Loestrin 21 1/20; Loestrin 21 1.5/30*
  Loestrin Fe 1/20; Loestrin Fe 1.5/30*
  Microgestin Fe 1/20; Microgestin Fe
    1.5/30*
norethynodrel
  Enovid*
norfloxacin
  Apo-Norflox (CAN)
  Chibroxin
  Noroxin
  Novo-Norfloxacin (CAN)

---

*This brand is a combination product.

Generic ♦ Brands

norfloxacin (cont.)
Riva-Norfloxacin ⓒᴬᴺ
norgestimate
Ortho-Cyclen*
Ortho-Prefest*
Ortho Tri-Cyclen*
norgestrel
Lo/Ovral*
Low-Ogestrel*
Ogestrel*
Ovral*
Ovrette
nortriptyline HCl
Alti-Nortriptylene Hydrochloride ⓒᴬᴺ
Aventyl HCl
Pamelor
novobiocin sodium
Albamycin
nystatin
Myco-Biotic II*
Myco-Triacet II*
Mycogen II*
Mycolog-II*
Myconel*
Mycostatin
Mytrex*
N.G.T.*
Nilstat
Nyotran
Nystatin-LF
Nystex
Pedi-Dri
Tri-Statin II*
octreotide acetate
Sandostatin
Sandostatin LAR Depot
ofloxacin
Apo-Oflox ⓒᴬᴺ
Floxin
Floxin Otic
Ocuflox
olanzapine
Zyprexa
Zyprexa IntraMuscular
olopatadine HCl
Patanol
olsalazine sodium
Dipentum
omalizumab
Xolair

omapatrilat
Vanlev
omeprazole
Prilosec
omeprazole magnesium
Losec ⓒᴬᴺ
ondansetron HCl
Zofran
Zofran ODT
opium
B & O Supprettes No. 15A; B & O
Supprettes No. 16A*
oprelvekin
Neumega
orciprenaline sulfate
Apo-Orciprenaline ⓒᴬᴺ
orgotein
OxSODrol
orlistat
Xenical
orphenadrine citrate
Banflex
Flexoject
Flexon
Myolin
Norflex
Norgesic; Norgesic Forte*
Orphengesic; Orphengesic Forte*
Rhoxal-orphenadrine ⓒᴬᴺ
orphenadrine HCl
Disipal ⓒᴬᴺ
oseltamivir phosphate
Tamiflu
oxacillin sodium
Bactocill
Prostaphlin
oxaliplatin
Dacplat
Eloxatin
Foloxatine
Transplatin
oxamniquine
Vansil
oxandrolone
Hepandrin
Oxandrin
oxaprozin
Daypro

*This brand is a combination product.

oxaprozin (cont.)
Rhoxal-oxaprozin (CAN)
oxazepam
Apo-Oxazepam (CAN)
Novoxapam (CAN)
Serax
oxcarbazepine
Trileptal
oxiconazole nitrate
Oxistat
Oxizole (CAN)
oxidronate sodium
OctreoScan
oxothiazolidine carboxylate
Procysteine
oxtriphylline
Choledyl SA
oxybenzone
Solaquin Forte*
Viquin Forte*
oxybutynin chloride
Ditropan
Ditropan XL
PMS-Oxybutynin (CAN)
oxycodone HCl
Endocet*
Endocodone
M-oxy
Oxycocet (CAN)*
OxyContin
OxyFast
OxyIR
Percocet*
Percodan; Percodan-Demi*
Percolone
Roxicet*
Roxicet 5/500*
Roxicodone
Roxilox*
Roxiprin*
Tylox*
oxycodone terephthalate
Percodan; Percodan-Demi*
Roxiprin*
oxymetholone
Anadrol-50
oxymorphone HCl
Numorphan
oxyphencyclimine HCl
Daricon

oxytetracycline
Terramycin IM*
oxytetracycline HCl
Terak with Polymyxin B Sulfate*
Terra-Cortril*
Terramycin
Terramycin with Polymyxin B*
Uri-Tet
Urobiotic-250*
oxytocin
Pitocin
Syntocinon
p30 protein
Onconase
paclitaxel
Onxol
Paxene
Taxol
padimate O
Viquin Forte*
paflufocon A
Fluoroperm 92
paflufocon B
Fluoroperm 62
paflufocon C
Fluoroperm 32
paflufocon D
Fluoroperm 151
paflufocon E
PVS Basics
palivizumab
Synagis
palladium Pd 103
Theraseed
palmitic acid
Levovist (CAN)*
pamidronate disodium
Aredia
pancreatin
Creon*
Creon 10*
Creon 20*
Digepepsin*
Digestozyme*
Donnazyme*
pancuronium bromide
Pavulon

*This brand is a combination product.

pantoprazole
Pantozol
pantoprazole sodium
Panto IV ⓒᴬᴺ
Pantoloc ⓒᴬᴺ
Protonix
Protonix I.V.
papain
Accuzyme*
Panafil*
Panafil White*
Papain Urea Chlorophyllin*
Papain Urea Debriding*
papaverine HCl
Genabid
Pavabid
Pavagen TD
Pavarine
Pavatine
Paverolan
paraldehyde
Paral
parathyroid hormone
Allelix
Fortéo
paricalcitol
Zemplar
paromomycin sulfate
Humatin
paroxetine HCl
Paxil
Paxil CR
PEG-camptothecin
Prothecan
PEG-glucocerebrosidase
Lysodase
PEG-interferon alfa-2a
Pegasys
pegademase bovine
Adagen
pegaspargase
Oncaspar
pegvisomant
Somavert
pemetrexed disodium
Rolazar
Tifolar
pemirolast potassium
Alamast

pemoline
Cylert
PemADD
PemADD CT
penbutolol sulfate
Levatol
penciclovir
Denavir
penicillamine
Cuprimine
Depen
penicillin G benzathine
Bicillin C-R; Bicillin C-R 900/300*
Bicillin L-A
Permapen
penicillin G potassium
Pfizerpen
penicillin G procaine
Bicillin C-R; Bicillin C-R 900/300*
Crysticillin 300 A.S.; Crysticillin 600 A.S.
Pfizerpen-AS
Wycillin
penicillin V potassium
Apo-Pen VK ⓒᴬᴺ
Beepen-VK
Betapen-VK
Ledercillin VK
Pen-V
Pen-Vee K
Penicillin VK
Robicillin VK
V-Cillin K
Veetids
Veetids '125'; Veetids '250'
pentagastrin
Peptavlon
pentamidine isethionate
NebuPent
Pentacarinat
Pentam 300
Pneumopent
pentastarch
Pentaspan
pentazocine HCl
Talacen*
Talwin Compound*
Talwin NX*

*This brand is a combination product.

pentazocine lactate
Talwin
pentobarbital
Nembutal
pentobarbital sodium
Cafatine-PB*
Nembutal Sodium
pentosan polysulfate sodium
Elmiron
pentostatin
Nipent
pentoxifylline
Trental
pepsin
Digepepsin*
Digestozyme*
perflenapent
EchoGen*
perflexane
Imagent US
perflisopent
EchoGen*
perflubron
LiquiVent
Oxygent
perfluoroalkylpolyether
SERPACWA (Skin Exposure
   Reduction Paste Against Chemi-
   cal Warfare Agents)*
perflutren microspheres
Definity
pergolide mesylate
Permax
perindopril erbumine
Aceon
permethrin
Acticin
Elimite
perphenazine
Apo-Perphenazine (CAN)
Etrafon; Etrafon 2–10; Etrafon-A;
   Etrafon-Forte*
Triavil*
Triavil 4-50*
Trilafon
pertussis vaccine
Acel-P (CAN)
peruvian balsam
Dermuspray*
Granulderm*

peruvian balsam (cont.)
Granulex*
GranuMed*
pexiganan acetate
Cytolex
Locilex
PGG glucan
Betafectin
phenacemide
Phenurone
phenazopyridine HCl
Azo-Sulfisoxazole*
Baridium
Geridium
Phenazo (CAN)
Pyridiate; Pyridate No. 2
Pyridium
Pyridium Plus*
Uristat
Urobiotic-250*
Urodine
Urogesic
phendimetrazine tartrate
Adipost
Bontril
Bontril PDM
Dital
Dyrexan-OD
Melfiat-105
Prelu-2
Rexigen Forte
phenelzine sulfate
Nardil
phenindamine tartrate
Nolamine*
P-V-Tussin*
pheniramine maleate
Iohist D*
Liqui-Histine-D*
Naphoptic-A*
Poly-Histine*
Poly-Histine-D*
Poly-Histine-D Ped Caps*
Rolatuss with Hydrocodone*
Ru-Tuss with Hydrocodone*
Statuss Green*
Tri-P*
Triaminic*

---

*This brand is a combination product.

pheniramine maleate (cont.)
    Triaminic Expectorant DH*
    Tussirex*
    Vetuss HC*
phenobarbital
    Antispasmodic*
    Antrocol*
    Arco-Lase Plus*
    Barbidonna; Barbidonna No. 2*
    Bel-Phen-Ergot SR*
    Bellacane*
    Bellacane SR*
    Bellatal
    Bellergal-S*
    Chardonna-2*
    Donna-Sed*
    Donnatal*
    Donnatal No. 2*
    Folergot-DF*
    Gustase Plus*
    Hyosophen*
    Levsin PB*
    Levsin with Phenobarbital*
    Lufyllin-EPG*
    Malatal*
    Mudrane*
    Mudrane GG*
    Phenerbel-S*
    Quadrinal*
    Solfoton
    Spasmolin*
    Susano*
phenobarbital sodium
    Luminal Sodium
phenol
    Castellani Paint Modified*
phenoxybenzamine HCl
    Dibenzyline
phensuximide
    Milontin
phentermine HCl
    Adipex-P
    Fastin
    Ionamin
    Obenix
    Obephen
    Oby-Cap
    Phentrol 2; Phentrol 4; Phentrol 5
    Zantryl

phentolamine mesylate
    Invicorp*
    Regitine
    Vasofem
    Vasomax
phenyl salicylate
    Atrosept*
    Dolsed*
    Prosed/DS*
    Trac Tabs 2X*
    UAA*
    Uridon Modified*
    Urimar-T*
    Urimax*
    Urinary Antiseptic No. 2*
    Urised*
    Uritin*
    Urogesic Blue*
phenylephrine bitartrate
    Duo-Medihaler*
phenylephrine HCl
    AK-Dilate
    Aclophen*
    AH-chew*
    AH-chew D
    Atrohist Plus*
    Atuss DM*
    Atuss G*
    Atuss HD*
    Bromophen T.D.*
    Chlorgest-HD*
    Codimal DH*
    Coldloc*
    Comhist*
    Comhist LA*
    Contuss*
    Cophene-X*
    Cyclomydril*
    D.A.*
    D.A. II*
    Dallergy*
    Decongestabs*
    Decongestant*
    Deconhist L.A.*
    Deconsal Sprinkle*
    Dehistine*
    Despec*
    Donatussin*

---

*This brand is a combination product.

Generic ♦ Brands

phenylephrine HCl (cont.)
Donatussin DC*
Dura-Gest*
Dura-Vent/DA*
Ed A-Hist*
ED-TLC; ED Tuss HC*
Endagen-HD*
Endal*
Endal-HD; Endal-HD Plus*
Enomine*
Entex*
Ex-Histine*
Extendryl*
Extendryl JR*
Extendryl SR*
Guaifenex*
Guaitex*
Hista-Vadrin*
Histalet Forte*
Histex SR*
Histinex HC*
Histor-D*
Histussin HC*
Hycomine Compound*
Hydro-PC*
Hydrocodone CP; Hydrocodone HD*
Iodal HD*
Iotussin HC*
Levall 5.0*
Liquibid-D*
Murocoll-2*
Mydfrin 2.5%
Naldecon*
Naldelate*
Nalgest*
Neo-Synephrine
No-Hist*
Norel*
OMNIhist L.A.*
Para-Hist HD*
Pediacof*
Pedituss Cough*
Phenahist-TR*
Phenchlor S.H.A.*
Phenergan VC*
Phenergan VC with Codeine*
Phenoptic
Pherazine VC with Codeine*
Prehist*
Prehist D*

phenylephrine HCl (cont.)
Prometh VC Plain*
Prometh VC with Codeine*
Promethazine VC*
Promethazine VC Plain*
Promethazine VC with Codeine*
Promethist with Codeine*
Rolatuss Expectorant*
Rolatuss with Hydrocodone*
Ru-Tuss with Hydrocodone*
Sil-Tex*
Sinupan*
Stahist*
Statuss Green*
Storzfen
T-Koff*
Tamine S.R.*
Tri-Phen-Chlor*
Tri-Phen-Chlor T.R.*
Tri-Phen-Mine*
Tri-Phen-Mine S.R.*
Tusquelin*
Tussafed HC*
Tussanil DH*
Tussirex*
Tympagesic*
Uni-Decon*
Unituss HC*
Vanex Forte*
Vanex-HD*
Vasosulf*
Vetuss HC*

phenylephrine tannate
Atrohist Pediatric*
Gelhist*
R-Tanna 12*
R-Tannamine*
R-Tannate*
R-Tannic-S A/D*
Rentamine Pediatric*
Rhinatate*
Rynatan*
Rynatan-12 S*
Rynatan-S*
Rynatuss*
Tannic-12*
Tanoral*
Tri-Tannate*

*This brand is a combination product.

phenylephrine tannate (cont.)
    Tri-Tannate Plus Pediatric*
    Triotann*
    Tritan*
    Tuss-Tan*
    Tussi-12*
phenylpropanolamine HCl
    Alumadrine*
    Ami-Tex LA*
    Anatuss*
    Aquatab C*
    Aquatab D*
    Atrohist Plus*
    Bromanate DC Cough*
    Bromophen T.D.*
    Bromphen DC with Codeine Cough*
    Brompheniramine DC Cough*
    Codamine*
    Codegest Expectorant*
    Coldloc*
    Coldloc-LA*
    Conex with Codeine*
    Contuss*
    Cophene-X*
    Decongestabs*
    Decongestant*
    Deconhist L.A.*
    Despec*
    Dimetane-DC Cough*
    Drize*
    Dura-Gest*
    Dura-Vent*
    Dura-Vent/A*
    E.N.T.*
    Endal Expectorant*
    Enomine*
    Entex*
    Entex LA*
    Exgest LA*
    Guaifenex*
    Guaifenex PPA 75*
    Guaipax*
    Guaitex*
    Guaitex LA*
    Guiatex LA*
    Hista-Vadrin*
    Histade*
    Histalet Forte*
    Histine DM; Histinex DM*
    Hycomine*

phenylpropanolamine HCl (cont.)
    Hydrocodone PA*
    Iohist D*
    Iohist DM*
    Liqui-Histine-D*
    Liqui-Histine DM*
    Myphetane DC Cough*
    Naldecon*
    Naldecon CX Adult*
    Naldelate*
    Nalgest*
    No-Hist*
    Nolamine*
    Norel*
    Norel Plus*
    Ordrine AT*
    Ornade*
    Partuss LA*
    Phenahist-TR*
    Phenate*
    Phenchlor S.H.A.*
    Phenylfenesin L.A.*
    Poly-Histine CS*
    Poly-Histine-D*
    Poly-Histine-D Ped Caps*
    Poly-Histine DM*
    Profen II; Profen LA*
    Resaid*
    Rescaps-D S.R.*
    Rhinolar-EX; Rhinolar-EX 12*
    Rolatuss with Hydrocodone*
    Ru-Tuss with Hydrocodone*
    Rymed-TR*
    Sil-Tex*
    Siltapp with Dextromethorphan
        HBr Cold & Cough*
    SinuVent*
    Stamoist LA*
    Statuss Expectorant*
    Statuss Green*
    T-Koff*
    Tamine S.R.*
    Tri-P*
    Tri-Phen-Chlor*
    Tri-Phen-Chlor T.R.*
    Tri-Phen-Mine*
    Tri-Phen-Mine S.R.*
    Triaminic*

*This brand is a combination product.

phenylpropanolamine HCl (cont.)
    Triaminic Expectorant DH*
    Triaminic Expectorant with
        Codeine*
    Tusquelin*
    Tuss-Ornade*
    Tuss-Allergine Modified T.D.*
    Tussanil DH*
    Tussogest*
    ULR-LA*
    Uni-Decon*
    Vanex Forte*
    Vanex Forte-R*
    Vetuss HC*
phenyltoloxamine
    Lobac*
phenyltoloxamine citrate
    Comhist*
    Comhist LA*
    Decongestabs*
    Decongestant*
    Flextra-DS*
    Iohist D*
    Liqui-Histine-D*
    Magsal*
    Naldecon*
    Naldelate*
    Nalgest*
    Poly-Histine*
    Poly-Histine-D*
    Poly-Histine-D Ped Caps*
    Tri-Phen-Chlor*
    Tri-Phen-Chlor T.R.*
    Tri-Phen-Mine*
    Tri-Phen-Mine S.R.*
    Uni-Decon*
phenyltoloxamine dihydrogen citrate
    Norel Plus*
phenytoin
    Dilantin
    Dilantin-125
phenytoin sodium
    Dilantin
    Diphenylan Sodium
phosphatidylglycerol
    Alec*
physiological irrigating solution
    Cytosol
    Physiolyte

physiological irrigating solution (cont.)
    PhysioSol
    Tis-U-Sol
physostigmine
    Synapton SR
physostigmine salicylate
    Antilirium
physostigmine sulfate
    Eserine Sulfate
phytonadione
    AquaMEPHYTON
    Konakion
    Mephyton
pilocarpine
    Ocusert Pilo-20; Ocusert Pilo-40
pilocarpine HCl
    Adsorbocarpine
    Akarpine
    E-Pilo-1; E-Pilo-2; E-Pilo-4; E-Pilo-6*
    Isopto Carpine
    P_1E_1; P_2E_1; P_4E_1; P_6E_1*
    P_3E_1*
    Pilocar
    Pilopine HS
    Piloptic-½; Piloptic-1; Piloptic-2;
        Piloptic-3; Piloptic-4; Piloptic-6
    Pilopto-Carpine
    Pilostat
    Salagen
    Storzine 2
pilocarpine nitrate
    Pilagan
pimozide
    Orap
pinacidil
    Pindac
pindolol
    PMS-Pindolol ⓒⒶⓃ
    Visken
pioglitazone HCl
    Actos
pipecuronium bromide
    Arduan
piperacillin sodium
    Pipracil
    Zosyn*

*This brand is a combination product.

piracetam
Nootropil
pirbuterol acetate
Maxair
pirenzepine HCl
Gastrozepine
piroxicam
Feldene
Fexicam (CAN)
piroxicam betadex
Brexidol 20 (CAN)
plasma protein fraction
Plasma-Plex
Plasmanate
Plasmatein
Protenate
pleconaril
Picovir
plicamycin
Mithracin
pneumococcal vaccine
Pneumo 23 (CAN)
Pneumovax 23
Pnu-Imune 23
Prevnar
podofilox
Condylox
Wartec (CAN)
podophyllum
Podocon-25
Podofin
Verrex*
poliovirus vaccine
IPOL
Orimune
poloxamer 188
Flocor
poloxamer 331
Protox
poly I: poly C12U
Ampligen
polydimethylsiloxane
AdatoSil 5000
**polyethylene glycol–electrolyte
solution**
Co-Lav*
Colovage
CoLyte
Go-Evac*
GoLYTELY

**polyethylene glycol–electrolyte
solution (cont.)**
MiraLax
NuLytely
OCL
polymyxin B sulfate
AK-Spore*
AK-Spore H.C.*
AK-Trol*
AK-Poly-Bac*
AntibiOtic*
Antibiotic Ear Solution*
Antibiotic Ear Suspension*
Cortatrigen Modified*
Cortisporin*
Cortisporin Otic*
Dexacidin*
Dexasporin*
Drotic*
Ear-Eze*
LazerSporin-C*
Maxitrol*
Neosporin*
Neosporin G.U. Irrigant*
Neotricin HC*
Octicare*
Ocutricin*
Otic-Care*
OtiTricin*
Otobiotic Otic*
Otocort*
Otomycin-HPN Otic*
Otosporin*
Pediotic*
Pedotic*
PMS-Polytrimethoprim (CAN)*
Poly-Pred*
Polytrim*
Sab-Cortimyxin (CAN)*
Storz-N-P-D*
Terak with Polymyxin B Sulfate*
Terramycin with Polymyxin B*
Triple Antibiotic*
UAD Otic*
polysaccharide-iron complex
Fe-Tinic 150 Forte*
Ferrex 150 Forte*
Ferrex PC; Ferrex PC Forte*

---

*This brand is a combination product.

polysaccharide-iron complex (cont.)
Hemocyte Plus*
Niferex-PN*
Niferex-PN Forte*
Niferex-150 Forte*
Nu-Iron Plus*
Nu-Iron V*

polytef
SERPACWA (Skin Exposure Reduction Paste Against Chemical Warfare Agents)*

polythiazide
Minizide 1; Minizide 2; Minizide 5*
Renese
Renese-R*

polyvinyl alcohol
Albalon*

polyvinyl chloride
Sitzmarks

poractant alfa
Curosurf

porfimer sodium
Photofrin

potassium acetate
Tri-K*

potassium acid phosphate
K-Phos M.F.*
K-Phos No. 2*
K-Phos Original

potassium bicarbonate
Effer-K*
Effervescent Potassium*
K+ Care ET
K-Lyte; K-Lyte DS*
Klor-Con/EF*
Tri-K*

potassium chloride
Cena-K
Gen-K
K+ 8; K+ 10
K+ Care
K-Tab
K-vescent
K-Dur 10; K-Dur 20
K-Lease
K-Lor
K-Lyte/Cl
K-Lyte/Cl; K-Lyte/Cl 50
K-Norm

potassium chloride (cont.)
Kaochlor 10%; Kaochlor S-F*
Kaon-Cl 20%*
Kaon-Cl; Kaon-Cl 10
Kay Ciel
Klor-Con 8; Klor-Con 10; Klor-Con M10; Klor-Con M20
Klor-Con; Klor-Con/25
Klorvess
Klotrix
Kolyum*
Micro-K LS
Micro-K; Micro-K 10
Plegisol*
Potasalan*
Rum-K
Slow-K
Ten-K

potassium citrate
Citrolith*
Cytra-3*
Cytra-K*
Cytra-LC*
Effer-K*
Effervescent Potassium*
K-Lyte ⓒⓐⓝ
K-Lyte; K-Lyte DS*
Klor-Con/EF*
Polycitra*
Polycitra-K*
Polycitra-LC*
Tri-K*
Twin-K*
Urocit-K

potassium gluconate
K-G Elixir
Kaon
Kaylixir*
Kolyum*
Twin-K*

potassium guaiacolsulfonate
Atuss EX*
Cophene-X*
Entuss Expectorant*
Marcof Expectorant*
Protuss*
Protuss-D*

Generic ♦ Brands

---

*This brand is a combination product.

potassium iodide
  Elixophyllin-KI*
  KIE*
  Lugol*
  Mudrane*
  Pediacof*
  Pedituss Cough*
  Pima
  Quadrinal*
  SSKI
  Strong Iodine*
  Theophyllin KI*
  Thyro-Block
potassium perchlorate
  Perchloracap
potassium phosphate
  K-Phos Neutral*
  Uro-KP-Neutral*
povidone-iodine
  Betadine 5% Sterile Ophthalmic Prep
pralidoxime chloride
  Protopam Chloride
pramipexole dihydrochloride
  Mirapex
pramlintide acetate
  Symlin
pramoxine
  Analpram-HC*
  Epifoam*
  1+1-F Creme*
  Pramosone*
  Zone-A Forte*
pramoxine HCl
  Cortic*
  Enzone*
  Oti-Med*
  Otomar-HC*
  Pramoxine HC*
  ProctoCream-HC*
  Proctodan-HC ⒸⒶⓃ*
  Proctofoam-HC*
  Tri-Otic*
  Zoto-HC*
pravastatin sodium
  Apo-Pravastatin ⒸⒶⓃ
  Lin-Pravastatin ⒸⒶⓃ
  Pravachol
praziquantel
  Biltricide

prazosin HCl
  Minipress
  Minizide 1; Minizide 2; Minizide 5*
prednicarbate
  Dermatop
prednimustine
  Sterecyt
prednisolone
  Delta-Cortef
  Prelone*
prednisolone acetate
  Articulose-50
  Blephamide*
  Cetapred*
  Econopred; Econopred Plus
  Isopto Cetapred*
  Key-Pred 25; Key-Pred 50
  Metimyd*
  Poly-Pred*
  Pred-G*
  Pred-G S.O.P.*
  Pred Mild; Pred Forte
  Predalone 50
  Predcor-50
  Vasocidin*
  Vasocine*
prednisolone sodium phosphate
  AK-Pred
  Hydeltrasol
  Inflamase Mild; Inflamase Forte
  Key-Pred-SP
  Orapred
  Pediapred
  Sulster*
  Vasocidin*
prednisolone tebutate
  Hydeltra-T.B.A.
  Prednisol TBA
prednisone
  Apo-Prednisone ⒸⒶⓃ
  Deltasone
  Liquid Pred*
  Meticorten
  Orasone
  Panasol-S
  Prednicen-M
  Sterapred; Sterapred DS

*This brand is a combination product.

Generic ♦ Brands

prezatide copper acetate
  Iamin
priliximab
  Centara
prilocaine
  EMLA*
prilocaine HCl
  Citanest Forte*
  Citanest Plain
primidone
  Mysoline
probenecid
  Benemid ⓒⒶⓃ
  Benuryl ⓒⒶⓃ
  Col-Probenecid*
  ColBenemid*
  Polycillin-PRB*
  Probalan
  Probampacin*
  Proben-C*
probucol
  Panavir
procainamide HCl
  Procanbid
  Pronestyl
  Pronestyl-SR
procaine
  Ravocaine & Novocaine with
    Levophed*
procaine HCl
  Anticort
  Hytinic*
  Novocain
procarbazine HCl
  Matulane
prochlorperazine
  Compazine
  Stemetil ⓒⒶⓃ
prochlorperazine bimaleate
  Nu-Prochlor ⓒⒶⓃ
  Stemetil ⓒⒶⓃ
prochlorperazine edisylate
  Compazine
prochlorperazine maleate
  Apo-Prochlorazine ⓒⒶⓃ
  Compazine
prochlorperazine mesylate
  Stemetil ⓒⒶⓃ
procyclidine HCl
  Kemadrin

progesterone
  Crinone
  Progestasert
  Prometrium
proguanil HCl
  Malarone; Malarone Pediatric*
promazine HCl
  Prozine-50
  Sparine
promethazine HCl
  Anergan 50
  K-Phen-50
  Mepergan*
  Mepergan Fortis*
  Pentazine
  Pentazine VC with Codeine*
  Phenameth
  Phenameth DM*
  Phenazine 50
  Phenergan
  Phenergan Fortis*
  Phenergan Plain
  Phenergan VC*
  Phenergan VC with Codeine*
  Phenergan with Codeine*
  Phenergan with Dextromethorphan*
  Phenoject-50
  Pherazine DM*
  Pherazine VC with Codeine*
  Pherazine with Codeine*
  Pro-50
  Prometh-50
  Prometh VC Plain*
  Prometh VC with Codeine*
  Prometh with Codeine*
  Prometh with Dextromethorphan*
  Promethazine DM*
  Promethazine VC*
  Promethazine VC Plain*
  Promethazine VC with Codeine*
  Promethist with Codeine*
  Prorex-25; Prorex-50
  Prothazine
  Prothazine Plain
propafenone HCl
  Apo-Propafenone ⓒⒶⓃ
  Rythmol

*This brand is a combination product.

propantheline bromide
  Pro-Banthīne
proparacaine HCl
  Alcaine
  Fluoracaine*
  Ophthaine
  Ophthetic
propiomazine HCl
  Largon
propiram fumarate
  Dirame
propofol
  Diprivan
propoxycaine HCl
  Ravocaine & Novocaine with
    Levophed*
propoxyphene HCl
  Darvon
  Darvon Compound-65*
  Dolene*
  Wygesic*
propoxyphene napsylate
  Darvocet-N 50; Darvocet-N 100*
  Darvon-N
  Propacet 100*
propranolol HCl
  Betachron E-R
  Inderal
  Inderal LA
  Inderide 40/25; Inderide 80/25*
  Inderide LA 80/50; Inderide LA
    120/50; Inderide LA 160/50*
propylhexedrine
  Benzedrex
propyliodone
  Dionosil Oily
protease
  Arco-Lase Plus*
  Cotazym*
  Cotazym-S*
  Creon*
  Creon 10*
  Creon 20*
  Donnazyme*
  Gustase Plus*
  Ilozyme*
  Ku-Zyme*
  Ku-Zyme HP*
  Kutrase*
  Lipram-CR20*

protease (cont.)
  Lipram-PN10*
  Lipram-PN16*
  Lipram-UL12*
  Lipram-UL18*
  Lipram-UL20*
  Pancrease; Pancrease MT 4; Pan-
    crease MT 10; Pancrease MT 16;
    Pancrease MT 20*
  Pancrecarb MS-8*
  Protilase*
  Ultrase; Ultrase MT 12; Ultrase MT
    18; Ultrase MT 20*
  Viokase*
  Zymase*
protein A
  Prosorba Column
protirelin
  Thymone
  Thypinone
  Thyrel-TRH
protriptyline HCl
  Vivactil
pseudoephedrine HCl
  Actagen-C Cough*
  Actifed with Codeine Cough*
  Allegra-D*
  Allent*
  Allerfrin with Codeine*
  AlleRx*
  Anamine*
  Anamine T.D.*
  Anaplex*
  Anaplex DM Cough*
  Anaplex HD*
  Anatuss LA*
  Andehist*
  Andehist DM*
  Aprodine with Codeine*
  Atrohist Pediatric*
  Biohist-LA*
  Brexin-L.A.*
  Brofed*
  Bromadine-DM*
  Bromadine-DX*
  Bromarest DX Cough*
  Bromatane DX Cough*
  Bromfed*

*This brand is a combination product.

pseudoephedrine HCl (cont.)
  Bromfed-DM Cough*
  Bromfed-PD*
  Bromfenex*
  Bromfenex PD*
  Bromphen DX Cough*
  Calmylin with Codeine ⓒⒶⓃ*
  Carbinoxamine Compound*
  Carbiset*
  Carbiset-TR*
  Carbodec*
  Carbodec DM*
  Carbodec TR*
  Cardec-DM*
  Cardec-S*
  Chlorafed; Chlorafed HS*
  Chlordrine S.R.*
  Chlorphedrine SR*
  Codehist DH*
  Codimal-L.A.; Codimal-L.A. Half*
  Coldec DM*
  Colfed-A*
  Congess JR*
  Congess SR*
  Cophene No. 2*
  Cophene XP*
  Cotridin ⓒⒶⓃ*
  Cotridin Expectorant ⓒⒶⓃ*
  Cyclofed Pediatric*
  Cycofed Pediatric*
  Dallergy-JR*
  Decohistine DH*
  Deconamine*
  Deconamine CX*
  Deconamine SR*
  Decongestant Expectorant*
  Deconomed SR*
  Deconsal II*
  Deconsal Pediatric*
  Defen-LA*
  Deproist Expectorant with Codeine*
  Detussin*
  Detussin Expectorant*
  Dihistine Expectorant*
  Dimetane-DX Cough*
  Dura-Tap/PD*
  Duralex*
  Duratuss; Duratuss-GP*
  Endafed*
  Entex PSE*

pseudoephedrine HCl (cont.)
  Entuss-D*
  Entuss-D Jr.*
  Eudal-SR*
  Fedahist*
  GFN/PSE*
  GP-500*
  Guai-Vent/PSE*
  Guaifed*
  Guaifed-PD*
  Guaifenex PSE 60; Guaifenex PSE
    120; Guaifenex Rx DM*
  Guaifenex Rx*
  GuaiMAX-D*
  Guaitex PSE*
  Guaivent*
  Guaivent PD*
  Guiatex PSE*
  Guiatuss DAC*
  Guiatussin DAC*
  H-Tuss-D*
  Histalet*
  Histalet X*
  Histinex PV*
  Histussin D*
  Hyphed*
  Iofed*
  Iofed PD*
  Iosal II*
  Isoclor Expectorant*
  Klerist-D*
  Kronofed-A Jr.*
  Kronofed-A*
  Lodrane LD*
  MED-Rx*
  MED-Rx DM*
  Mescolor*
  Myphetane DX Cough*
  Mytussin DAC*
  Nasabid*
  Nasabid SR*
  Nasatab LA*
  ND Clear*
  No-Hist*
  Novafed A*
  Novagest Expectorant with
    Codeine*
  Novahistine DH*

*This brand is a combination product.

pseudoephedrine HCl (cont.)
Novahistine Expectorant*
Nucofed*
Nucofed Expectorant; Nucofed
    Pediatric Expectorant*
P-V-Tussin*
Palgic-D*
Palgic-DS*
Pancof-HC*
Pancof-XL; Pancof XP*
Panmist JR*
PanMist-DM*
Pannaz*
Phenhist DH with Codeine*
Phenhist Expectorant*
Profen Forte DM*
Profen II DM*
Protuss-D*
Protuss DM*
Pseudo-Car DM*
Pseudo-Chlor*
Rescon*
Rescon-ED*
Rescon JR*
Respa-1st*
Respahist*
Respaire-60; Respaire-120*
Rinade B.I.D.*
Robafen DAC*
Robitussin-DAC*
Rondamine-DM*
Rondec*
Rondec-DM*
Rondec-TR*
Ru-Tuss DE*
Rymed*
Ryna-C*
Ryna-CX*
Seldane-D*
Semprex-D*
Sildec-DM*
Sinufed*
SRC Expectorant*
Stahist*
Stamoist E*
Sudal 120/600*
Sudal 60/500*
Syn-Rx*
Time-Hist*
Touro A & H; Touro Allergy*

pseudoephedrine HCl (cont.)
Touro CC*
Touro LA*
Triacin-C Cough*
Triafed with Codeine*
Trifed-C Cough*
Tuss-LA*
Tussafed*
Tussafed-LA*
Tussafin Expectorant*
Tussar SF; Tussar-2*
Tussend*
Tyrodone*
UltraBrom*
UltraBrom PD*
V-Dec-M*
Vanex Expectorant*
Versacaps*
Xiral*
Zephrex*
Zephrex LA*
Zyrtec-D*
pseudoephedrine maleate
Histex HC*
pseudoephedrine sulfate
Claritin-D; Claritin-D 12 Hour;
    Claritin-D 24 Hour*
Dexaphen S.A.*
Disobrom*
Drixomed*
Polaramine Expectorant*
Rynatan*
Trinalin*
pseudoephedrine tannate
Tanafed*
pyrazinamide
Rifater*
pyridostigmine bromide
Mestinon
Regonol
pyrilamine maleate
Codimal DH*
Histalet Forte*
Iohist D*
Liqui-Histine-D*
Poly-Histine*
Poly-Histine-D*
Poly-Histine-D Ped Caps*

*This brand is a combination product.

pyrilamine maleate (cont.)
Rolatuss with Hydrocodone*
Ru-Tuss with Hydrocodone*
Statuss Green*
Tri-P*
Triaminic*
Triaminic Expectorant DH*
Tricodene Cough and Cold*
Vanex Forte*
Vetuss HC*

pyrilamine tannate
Atrohist Pediatric*
Gelhist*
R-Tanna 12*
R-Tannamine*
R-Tannate*
R-Tannic-S A/D*
Rhinatate*
Rynatan*
Rynatan-12 S*
Rynatan-S*
Tanoral*
Tri-Tannate*
Triotann*
Tritan*

pyrimethamine
Daraprim
Fansidar*

quazepam
Doral

quetiapine fumarate
Seroquel

quinapril HCl
Accupril
Accuretic*

quinethazone
Hydromox

quinidine gluconate
Quinaglute
Quinalan

quinidine polygalacturonate
Cardioquin

quinidine sulfate
Quinidex
Quinora

quinupristin
Synercid*

rabeprazole sodium
Aciphex

rabies immune globulin
BayRab
Imogam
Imogam Rabies-HT

rabies vaccine
Imovax
RabAvert

racemethionine
M-Caps
Pedameth
Uracid

raloxifene HCl
Evista

raltitrexed
Tomudex

ramipril
Altace

ranitidine bismuth citrate
Pylorid ⓒⒶⓃ
Tritec

ranitidine HCl
Apo-Ranitidine ⓒⒶⓃ
Gen-Ranitidine ⓒⒶⓃ
Novo-Ranidine ⓒⒶⓃ
PMS-Ranitidine ⓒⒶⓃ
Rhoxal-ranitidine ⓒⒶⓃ
Zantac
Zantac EFFERdose
Zantac GELdose

rapacuronium bromide
Raplon

rauwolfia serpentina
Rauzide*

reboxetine mesylate
Edronax
Vestra

regramostim
Leucotropin

remifentanil HCl
Ultiva

reovirus
Reosyn

repaglinide
GlucoNorm ⓒⒶⓃ
Prandin

reserpine
Demi-Regroton*
Diutensen-R*

*This brand is a combination product.

Generic ♠ Brands

reserpine (cont.)
Hydrap-ES*
Hydro-Serp*
Hydropres-50*
Hydroserpine #1; Hydroserpine #2*
Marpres*
Metatensin #2; Metatensin #4*
Regroton*
Renese-R*
Salutensin; Salutensin-Demi*
Ser-Ap-Es*
Tri-Hydroserpine*
resorcinol
Castellani Paint Modified*
respiratory syncytial virus immune globulin
Hypermune RSV
RespiGam
reteplase
Retavase
Rh_0(D) immune globulin
BayRho-D Full Dose; BayRho-D Mini-Dose
Gamulin Rh
MICRhoGAM
Mini-Gamulin Rh
RhoGAM
WinRho SD
WinRho SDF
ribavirin
Rebetol
Rebetron*
Virazole
rifabutin
Mycobutin
rifampin
Rifadin
Rifamate*
Rifater*
Rimactane
rifapentine
Priftin
rifaximin
Normix
riluzole
Rilutek
rimantadine HCl
Flumadine
rimexolone
Vexol

risedronate sodium
Actonel
risperidone
Risperdal
ritamycin
Rifaximin
ritodrine HCl
Yutopar
ritonavir
Kaletra*
Norvir
rituximab
Rituxan
rivastigmine tartrate
Exelon
rizatriptan benzoate
Maxalt
Maxalt-MLT
Maxalt-RPD ⓒᴬᴺ
rocuronium bromide
Zemuron
rofecoxib
Vioxx
ropinirole HCl
Requip
ropivacaine HCl
Naropin
roquinimex
Linomide
rosiglitazone maleate
Avandia
rostaporfin
PhotoPoint
rosuvastatin calcium
Crestor
rotavirus vaccine
RotaShield
rovelizumab
LeukArrest
roxatidine acetate HCl
Roxin
rubella virus vaccine
Meruvax II
sacrosidase
Sucraid
salbutamol
Apo-Salvent ⓒᴬᴺ

*This brand is a combination product.

salbutamol sulfate
  Airomir ⓒᴬᴺ
  Apo-Salvent ⓒᴬᴺ
  Novo-Salmol ⓒᴬᴺ
  Salbutamol Nebuamp ⓒᴬᴺ
salicylamide
  Lobac*
  Tussanil DH*
salicylic acid
  Bensal HP*
  DuoPlant
  Emersal*
  Gordofilm
  Paplex Ultra
  PROPApH Foaming Face Wash
  Sal-Oil-T*
  Tinver*
  Verrex*
  Versiclear*
salmeterol xinafoate
  Advair*
  Serevent
salsalate
  Amigesic
  Argesic-SA
  Disalcid
  Marthritic
  Mono-Gesic
  Salsitab
samarium Sm 153 lexidronam
  Quadramet
saquinavir
  Fortovase
saquinavir mesylate
  Invirase
sargramostim
  Leukine
saruplase
  r-ProUK
scarlet red
  Scarlet Red Ointment Dressings
scopolamine hydrobromide
  Antispasmodic*
  Atrohist Plus*
  Barbidonna; Barbidonna No. 2*
  Bellacane*
  Deconhist L.A.*
  Donna-Sed*
  Donnatal*
  Donnatal No. 2*

scopolamine hydrobromide (cont.)
  Hyosophen*
  Isopto Hyoscine
  Malatal*
  Murocoll-2*
  Phenahist-TR*
  Phenchlor S.H.A.*
  Spasmolin*
  Stahist*
  Susano*
  Transderm Scōp
scopolamine hydrobromine
  Scopace
secalciferol
  Osteo-D
secobarbital sodium
  Seconal Sodium
  Tuinal*
secretin
  Secretin Ferring
selegiline HCl
  Carbex
  Eldepryl
selenious acid
  Sele-Pak
  Selepen
selenium sulfide
  Exsel
  Selsun
senecio compositae
  Succus Cineraria Maritima*
sermorelin acetate
  Geref
Serratia marcescens **extract**
  Imuvert
Sertoli cells
  N-Graft
sertraline HCl
  Apo-Sertraline ⓒᴬᴺ
  Novo-Sertraline ⓒᴬᴺ
  Zoloft
  Zoloft ⓒᴬᴺ
sevelamer HCl
  Renagel
sevirumab
  Protovir
sevoflurane
  Ultane

*This brand is a combination product.

shark cartilage
 BeneFin
short chain fatty acids
 Colomed
sibutramine HCl
 Meridia
sildenafil citrate
 Viagra
silicone plug
 Herrick Lacrimal Plug
 Punctum Plug
 TearSaver Punctum Plugs
silver sulfadiazine
 Silvadene
 SSD; SSD AF
 Thermazene
simethicone
 Baros*
simethicone-coated cellulose
 SonoRx
simvastatin
 Zocor
sincalide
 Kinevac
sirolimus
 Rapamune
sodium acid phosphate
 K-Phos M.F.*
 K-Phos No. 2*
 Uroqid-Acid No. 2*
sodium ascorbate
 Cenolate
 Hemocyte Plus*
 Iberet-Folic-500*
sodium benzoate
 Ucephan*
sodium bicarbonate
 Baros*
 Neut
sodium biphosphate
 Urimar-T*
 Urimax*
 Uro-Phosphate*
 Urogesic Blue*
sodium chloride
 AMO Endosol; AMO Endosol Extra
 B-Salt Forte
 Bacteriostatic Sodium Chloride
  Injection
 BSS; BSS Plus

sodium chloride (cont.)
 Dey-Pak Sodium Chloride 3% & 10%
 Plegisol*
sodium citrate
 Bicitra*
 Citrolith*
 Cytra-2*
 Cytra-3*
 Cytra-LC*
 Oracit*
 PMS-Dicitrate CAN*
 Polycitra*
 Polycitra-LC*
 Tussirex*
sodium cromoglycate
 Apo-Cromolyn CAN
sodium dichloroacetate
 Ceresine
sodium ferric gluconate
 Ferrlecit
sodium fluoride
 Florvite + Iron*
 Florvite + Iron; Half Strength
  Florvite + Iron*
 Florvite*
 Florvite; Florvite Half Strength*
 Fluoride Loz
 Fluorinse
 Fluoritab
 Flura
 Flura-Drops
 Flura-Loz
 Karidium
 Karigel; Karigel-N
 Luride
 Luride SF
 Neosten
 O-Cal f.a.*
 Pediaflor
 Pharmaflur; Pharmaflur df; Phar-
  maflur 1.1
 Point-Two*
 Poly-Vi-Flor*
 Poly-Vi-Flor with Iron*
 PreviDent
 PreviDent 5000 Plus
 PreviDent Rinse
 Slow Fluoride

---

*This brand is a combination product.

sodium fluoride (cont.)
Thera-Flur; Thera-Flur-N
Tri-Vi-Flor*
Tri-Vi-Flor with Iron*
Vi-Daylin/F ADC*
Vi-Daylin/F ADC + Iron*
Vi-Daylin/F Multivitamin*
Vi-Daylin/F Multivitamin + Iron*
sodium hypochlorite
Carisolv ⒸⒶⓃ
sodium iodide
Iodopen
sodium iodide I 131
Iodotope
sodium monomercaptoundecahydro-closo-dodecaborate
Borocell
sodium nitrite
Cyanide Antidote Package*
sodium nitroprusside
Nitropress
sodium oxybate
Xyrem
sodium phenylacetate
Ucephan*
sodium phenylbutyrate
Buphenyl
sodium phosphate
K-Phos Neutral*
Uro-KP-Neutral*
Visicol
sodium polystyrene sulfonate
Kayexalate
SPS
sodium propionate
Amino-Cerv pH 5.5*
sodium salicylate
Cystex*
Tussirex*
sodium stibogluconate
Pentostam
sodium tetradecyl sulfate
Sotradecol
sodium thiosalicylate
Rexolate
sodium thiosulfate
Cyanide Antidote Package*
Tinver*
Versiclear*

somatostatin
Reducin
Zecnil
somatrem
Protropin
somatropin
Genotropin
Genotropin MiniQuick
Humatrope
Norditropin
Norditropin SimpleXx
Nutropin
Nutropin AQ
Nutropin Depot
Protropin II
Saizen
Serostim
Umatrope
sorivudine
Bravavir
sotalol HCl
Betapace
Betapace AF
PMS-Sotalol ⒸⒶⓃ
sparfloxacin
Zagam
spectinomycin HCl
Trobicin
spironolactone
Aldactazide*
Aldactone
squalamine
BeneFin
stannous fluoride
Gel-Kam
Stop
stanozolol
Winstrol
staphage lysate
SPL-Serologic types I and III*
***Staphylococcus aureus* vaccine**
SPL-Serologic types I and III*
Staphylococcus bacteriophage plaque-forming units
SPL-Serologic types I and III*
stavudine
Zerit

*This brand is a combination product.

streptokinase
  Kabikinase
  Streptase
streptozocin
  Zanosar
strontium chloride Sr 89
  Metastron
succimer
  Chemet
succinylcholine chloride
  Anectine
  Quelicin
sucralfate
  Carafate
  PMS-Sucralfate Ⓒᴬᴺ
sucrose
  Kogenate FS*
sufentanil citrate
  Sufenta
sulbactam sodium
  Unasyn*
sulconazole nitrate
  Exelderm
sulfabenzamide
  Dayto Sulf*
  Gyne-Sulf*
  Sultrin Triple Sulfa*
  Triple Sulfa*
  Trysul*
  V.V.S.*
sulfacetamide
  Dayto Sulf*
  Gyne-Sulf*
  Sultrin Triple Sulfa*
  Triple Sulfa*
  Trysul*
  V.V.S.*
sulfacetamide sodium
  AK-Sulf
  Bleph-10
  Blephamide*
  Cetamide
  Cetapred*
  FML-S*
  Isopto Cetamide
  Isopto Cetapred*
  Klaron
  Metimyd*
  Novacet*
  Ocusulf-10

sulfacetamide sodium (cont.)
  Sebizon
  Sodium Sulamyd
  Storz-Sulf
  Sulf-10
  Sulfacet-R*
  Sulster*
  Vanocin*
  Vasocidin*
  Vasocine*
  Vasosulf*
sulfacytine
  Renoquid
sulfadoxine
  Fansidar*
sulfamethizole
  Thiosulfil Forte
  Urobiotic-250*
sulfamethoxazole
  Bactrim IV*
  Bactrim Pediatric*
  Bactrim; Bactrim DS*
  Cotrim Pediatric*
  Cotrim; Cotrim D.S.*
  Gantanol
  Septra*
  Septra DS*
  Septra IV*
  Sulfatrim*
  Urobak
sulfanilamide
  Alasulf*
  AVC
  D.I.T.I.-2*
  Deltavac*
sulfasalazine
  Azulfidine
  Azulfidine EN-tabs
sulfathiazole
  Dayto Sulf*
  Gyne-Sulf*
  Sultrin Triple Sulfa*
  Triple Sulfa*
  Trysul*
  V.V.S.*
sulfinpyrazone
  Anturane

---

*This brand is a combination product.

sulfisoxazole
Azo-Sulfisoxazole*
sulfisoxazole acetyl
Eryzole*
Gantrisin*
Pediazole*
sulfur
Novacet*
Sulfacet-R*
Sulfoxyl Regular; Sulfoxyl Strong*
Vanocin*
sulindac
Clinoril
sumatriptan succinate
Imitrex
superoxide dismutase
OxSODrol
suprofen
Profenal
suramin hexasodium
Metaret
suramin sodium
Antrypol
Belganyl
Fourneau 309
Germanin
Moranyl
Naganol
Naphuride
tacrine HCl
Cognex
tacrolimus
Prograf
Protopic
tadalafil
Cialis
talc, sterile
Sclerosol
tamoxifen citrate
Nolvadex
PMS-Tamoxifen Ⓒ
tamsulosin HCl
Flomax
tartaric acid
Baros*
Wigraine*
tasosartan
Verdia
tazarotene
Tazorac

tazobactam sodium
Zosyn*
technetium Tc 99m
Fibrimage
technetium Tc 99m antimelanoma murine MAb
OncoTrac
technetium Tc 99m apcitide
AcuTect
technetium Tc 99m bectumomab
LymphoScan
technetium Tc 99m bicisate
Neurolite
technetium Tc 99m murine MAb to human alpha-fetoprotein (AFP)
ImmuRAID-AFP
technetium Tc 99m murine MAb to human chorionic gonadotropin (hCG)
ImmuRAID-hCG
technetium Tc 99m sestamibi
Cardiolite
Miraluma
technetium Tc 99m tetrofosmin
Myoview
tegafur
Orzel*
UFT*
tegaserod
Zelmac
teicoplanin
Targocid
telmisartan
Micardis
Micardis HCT*
Micardis Plus Ⓒ*
temazepam
Apo-Temazepam Ⓒ
Restoril
temoporfin
Foscan
temozolomide
Temodal Ⓒ
Temodar
tenecteplase
TNKase
tenidap
Enable

---

*This brand is a combination product.

Generic ◆ Brands

teniposide
Vumon
tenofovir disoproxil fumarate
Viread
terazosin HCl
Apo-Terazosin ⒸⒶⓃ
Hytrin
Hytrin ⒸⒶⓃ
Novo-Terazosin ⒸⒶⓃ
PMS-Terazosin ⒸⒶⓃ
terbinafine HCl
Apo-Terbinafine ⒸⒶⓃ
Lamisil
Lamisil DermGel
PMS-Terbinafine ⒸⒶⓃ
terbutaline sulfate
Brethaire
Brethine
Bricanyl
terconazole
Terazol 3
Terazol 7
terfenadine
Seldane
Seldane-D*
teriparatide acetate
Parathar
terlipressin
Glypressin
testolactone
Teslac
testosterone
Androderm
AndroGel
Androtest-SL
Histerone 100
Tesamone
Testandro
Testoderm TTS
Testoderm; Testoderm with Adhesive
Testopel
Testosterone Aqueous
TheraDerm
TheraDerm-MTX*
Tostrex
testosterone cypionate
depAndro 100; depAndro 200
depAndrogyn*
Depo-Testadiol*
Depo-Testosterone

testosterone cypionate (cont.)
Depotest 100; Depotest 200
Depotestogen*
Duo-Cyp*
Duratest 100; Duratest 200
Duratestrin*
Test-Estro Cypionates*
testosterone enanthate
Andro L.A. 200
Andropository-200
Delatestryl
Durathate-200
Everone 200
Valertest No. 1*
tetanus immune globulin
BayTet
tetanus toxoid
ActHIB*
OmniHIB*
tetracaine HCl
Cetacaine*
Pontocaine HCl
Pontocaine HCl*
tetracycline
Actisite
tetracycline HCl
Achromycin V
Helidac*
Nor-Tet
Panmycin
Robitet
Sumycin
Sumycin '250'; Sumycin '500'
Teline; Teline-500
Tetracap
Tetralan
Tetralan "250"; Tetralan-500
Topicycline
tetrahydrozoline HCl
Tyzine
thalidomide
Thalomid
theophylline
Accurbron*
Aerolate Sr.; Aerolate Jr.; Aerolate III
Aquaphyllin
Asmalix
Bronchial*

---

*This brand is a combination product.

theophylline (cont.)
Brondelate*
Bronkodyl
Elixomin
Elixophyllin
Elixophyllin GG*
Elixophyllin-KI*
Glyceryl-T*
Hydrophed*
Iophylline*
Lanophyllin
Marax*
Marax-DF*
Mudrane GG*
Mudrane GG-2*
Quadrinal*
Quibron; Quibron-300*
Quibron-T
Quibron-T/SR
Respbid
Slo-bid
Slo-phyllin
Slo-phyllin GG*
Sustaire
Synophylate-GG*
T-Phyl
Theo-24
Theo-Dur
Theo-Sav
Theo-X
Theobid
Theochron
Theoclear-80
Theoclear L.A.
Theolair
Theolair-SR
Theolate*
Theomax DF*
Theophyllin KI*
Theospan-SR
Theostat 80*
Theovent
Uni-Dur
Uniphyl
thiabendazole
Mintezol
thiethylperazine maleate
Norzine
Torecan

thiopental sodium
Pentothal
thioridazine HCl ℞
Apo-Thioridazine ⒸⒶⓃ
Mellaril
Mellaril-S
thiotepa
Thioplex
thiothixene
Navane
thiothixene HCl
Navane
thonzonium bromide
Cortisporin-TC*
L-threonine
Threostat
thrombin
Thrombin-JMI
Thrombinar
Thrombogen
Thrombostat
thymalfasin
Zadaxin
thymopentin
Timunox
thyroid, desiccated
Armour Thyroid
S-P-T
Thyrar
Thyroid Strong
thyrotropin
Thytropar
thyrotropin alfa
Thyrogen
tiagabine HCl
Gabitril
tiazofurin
Tiazole
tibolone
Livial
Xyvion
ticarcillin disodium
Ticar
Timentin*
ticlodipine HCl
Gen-Ticlodipine ⒸⒶⓃ
ticlopidine HCl
Alti-Ticlopidine ⒸⒶⓃ

*This brand is a combination product.

Generic ◆ Brands

ticlopidine HCl (cont.)
   Apo-Ticlopidine Ⓒⓐⓝ
   PMS-Ticlopidine Ⓒⓐⓝ
   Rhoxal-ticlopidine Ⓒⓐⓝ
   Ticlid
tiludronate disodium
   Skelid
timolol
   Xalcom*
timolol hemihydrate
   Betimol
timolol maleate
   Alti-Timolol Ⓒⓐⓝ
   Beta-Tim Ⓒⓐⓝ
   Blocadren
   Cosopt*
   Med Timolol Ⓒⓐⓝ
   Novo-Timol Ⓒⓐⓝ
   Nu-Timolol Ⓒⓐⓝ
   Rhoxal-timolol Ⓒⓐⓝ
   Timodal Ⓒⓐⓝ
   Timolide 10-25*
   Timoptic
   Timoptic-XE
tinzaparin sodium
   Innohep
tiopronin
   Thiola
tiotropium
   Spiriva
tiratricol
   Triacana*
tirilazad mesylate
   Freedox
tirofiban HCl
   Aggrastat
tizanidine HCl
   Zanaflex
tobramycin
   AKTob
   Defy
   PMS-Tobramycin Ⓒⓐⓝ
   TOBI
   TobraDex*
   Tobrex
   Tomycine Ⓒⓐⓝ
tobramycin sulfate
   Nebcin
   Scheinpharm Tobramycin Ⓒⓐⓝ

tocainide HCl
   Tonocard
tolazamide
   Tolinase
tolazoline HCl
   Priscoline HCl
tolbutamide
   Orinase
tolbutamide sodium
   Orinase Diagnostic
tolcapone
   Tasmar
tolmetin sodium
   Tolectin 200; Tolectin 600
   Tolectin DS
tolrestat
   Alredase
tolterodine tartrate
   Detrol
   Detrol LA
topiramate
   Topamax
topotecan HCl
   Hycamtin
toremifene citrate
   Fareston
torsemide
   Demadex
tourniquet
   Ana-Kit*
trafermin
   Fiblast
tramadol HCl
   Ultracet*
   Ultram
   Ultram XL
trandolapril
   Mavik
   Mavik Ⓒⓐⓝ
   Tarka*
tranexamic acid
   Cyklokapron
tranylcypromine sulfate
   Parnate
trastuzumab
   Herceptin
travoprost
   Travatan

*This brand is a combination product.

trazodone HCl
Desyrel
treosulfan
Ovastat
treprostinil sodium
Remodulin
tretinoin
Altinac
Alustra*
Atragen
Avita
Rejuva-A (CAN)
Renova
Retin-A
Retin-A Micro
Solage*
Vesanoid
Vitinoin (CAN)
triamcinolone
Aristocort
Atolone
Kenacort
triamcinolone acetonide
Aristocort
Aristocort A
Azmacort
Delta-Tritex
Flutex
Kenaject-40
Kenalog
Kenalog-H
Kenalog in Orabase
Kenalog-10; Kenalog-40
Kenonel
Myco-Biotic II*
Myco-Triacet II*
Mycogen II*
Mycolog-II*
Myconel*
Mytrex*
N.G.T.*
Nasacort
Nasacort AQ
Oralone Dental
Tac-3
Tac-40
Tri-Kort
Tri-Nasal
Tri-Statin II*
Triacet

triamcinolone acetonide (cont.)
Triam-A
Triamonide 40
Triderm
Trilog
triamcinolone diacetate
Amcort
Aristocort Forte
Aristocort Intralesional
Articulose L.A.
Triam Forte
Triamolone 40
Trilone
Tristoject
triamcinolone hexacetonide
Aristospan Intra-articular
Aristospan Intralesional
triamterene
Dyazide*
Dyrenium
Maxzide*
triazolam
Halcion
trichlormethiazide
Diurese
Metahydrin
Metatensin #2; Metatensin #4*
Naqua
trichloroacetic acid
Tri-Chlor
trichloromonofluoromethane
Fluori-Methane*
triclosan
Septi-Soft
Septisol
tridihexethyl chloride
Pathilon
trientine HCl
Syprine
trifluoperazine HCl
Apo-Trifluoperazine (CAN)
Stelazine
triflupromazine HCl
Vesprin
trifluridine
Viroptic
trihexyphenidyl HCl
Artane

*This brand is a combination product.

trihexyphenidyl HCl (cont.)
Trihexy-2; Trihexy-5
trimethadione
Tridione
trimethobenzamide HCl
Arrestin
T-Gen*
Tebamide*
Ticon
Tigan
Tigan*
Triban; Pediatric Triban*
Trimazide
trimethoprim
Bactrim IV*
Bactrim Pediatric*
Bactrim; Bactrim DS*
Cotrim Pediatric*
Cotrim; Cotrim D.S.*
Polytrim*
Proloprim
Septra*
Septra DS*
Septra IV*
Sulfatrim*
Trimpex
trimethoprim HCl
Primsol
trimethoprim sulfate
PMS-Polytrimethoprim ⓒⒶⓃ*
trimetrexate glucuronate
NeuTrexin
trimipramine maleate
Surmontil
trioxsalen
Trisoralen
tripelennamine HCl
PBZ
PBZ-SR
Pelamine
triprolidine HCl
Actagen-C Cough*
Actifed with Codeine Cough*
Allerfrin with Codeine*
Aprodine with Codeine*
Cotridin ⓒⒶⓃ*
Cotridin Expectorant ⓒⒶⓃ*
Myidyl
Triacin-C Cough*
Triafed with Codeine*

triprolidine HCl (cont.)
Trifed-C Cough*
triptorelin pamoate
Trelstar Depot
trisaccharides A and B
Biosynject
troglitazone
Rezulin
trolamine polypeptide oleate-condensate
Cerumenex
troleandomycin
Tao
tromethamine
Tham
tropicamide
Mydriacyl
Opticyl
Paremyd*
Tropi-Storz
Tropicacyl
trospectomycin
Spexil
trovafloxacin mesylate
Trovan
Trovan/Zithromax Compliance Pak*
trypsin
Dermuspray*
Granulderm*
Granulex*
GranuMed*
tuberculin purified protein derivative
Tubersol
tuvirumab
Ostavir
typhoid vaccine
Typherix ⓒⒶⓃ
Typhim Vi
Typhoid Vaccine (AKD)
Typhoid Vaccine (H-P)
Vivotif Berna
tyropanoate sodium
Bilopaque
undecylenic acid
Fungoid
unoprostone isopropyl
Rescula

*This brand is a combination product.

Generic ♦ Brands

uracil
  Orzel*
  UFT*
urea
  Accuzyme*
  Amino-Cerv pH 5.5*
  Carmol HC*
  Gordon's Urea 40%
  Panafil*
  Panafil White*
  Papain Urea Chlorophyllin*
  Papain Urea Debriding*
  Ureaphil
urofollitropin
  Fertinex
  Metrodin
urokinase
  Abbokinase
  Abbokinase Open-Cath
ursodiol
  Actigall
  Urso
vaccinia virus vaccine for human papillomavirus
  TA-HPV
valacyclovir HCl
  Valtrex
valganciclovir HCl
  Valcyte
valine
  VIL*
valproate sodium
  Depacon
  Depakene
  Epiject (CAN)
valproic acid
  Apo-Valproic (CAN)
  Depakene
  Deproic (CAN)
  Nu-Valproic (CAN)
  Rhoxal-valproic (CAN)
valrubicin
  Valstar
  Valtaxin (CAN)
valsartan
  Diovan
  Diovan HCT*
valspodar
  Amdray

vancomycin HCl
  Lyphocin
  Vancocin
  Vancoled
varicella virus vaccine
  Varivax
vascular endothelial growth factor
  Trinam
vasoactive intestinal polypeptide
  Invicorp*
vasopressin
  Pitressin
vecuronium bromide
  Norcuron
venlafaxine HCl
  Effexor
  Effexor XR
verapamil HCl
  Calan
  Calan SR
  Chronovera (CAN)
  Covera-HS
  Gen-Verapamil (CAN)
  Isoptin
  Isoptin SR
  Tarka*
  Verelan
  Verelan PM
verteporfin
  Visudyne
vidarabine
  Vira-A
vigabatrin
  Sabril
viloxazine
  Catatrol
vinblastine sulfate
  Velban
vincristine sulfate
  Oncovin
  Vincasar PFS
vindesine sulfate
  Eldisine
vinorelbine tartrate
  Navelbine
visilizumab
  Nuvion

*This brand is a combination product.

vitamin A
  ADC with Fluoride*
  Aquasol A
  Chewable Triple Vitamins with Fluoride*
  Del-Vi-A
  Soluvite-f*
  Tri-Flor-Vite with Fluoride*
  Tri-Vi-Flor*
  Tri-Vi-Flor with Iron*
  Tri Vit with Fluoride*
  Tri-Vitamin with Fluoride*
  Tri-A-Vite F*
  Triple Vitamin ADC with Fluoride*
  Trivitamin Fluoride*
  Vi-Daylin/F ADC*
  Vi-Daylin/F ADC + Iron*

vitamin B$_1$
  Apatate with Fluoride*

vitamin B$_6$
  Apatate with Fluoride*
  Feocyte*
  Foltx*
  PremesisRx*

vitamin B$_{12}$
  Apatate with Fluoride*
  Fe-Tinic 150 Forte*
  Feocyte*
  Ferrex 150 Forte*
  Foltx*
  Liver Combo No. 5*
  PremesisRx*

vitamin B complex
  B-C with Folic Acid*
  B-Ject-100*
  B-Plex*
  Berocca*
  Formula B*
  Hemocyte Plus*
  Hytinic*
  Iberet-Folic-500*
  Key-Plex*
  Lypholized Vitamin B Complex & Vitamin C with B$_{12}$*
  May-Vita*
  Megaton*
  Nephplex Rx*
  Nephro-Vite Rx + Fe*
  Nephro-Vite Rx*
  Nephrocaps*

vitamin B complex (cont.)
  Nephron FA*
  Neurodep*
  Senilezol*
  Strovite*
  Vicam*
  Vitafōl*
  Vitamin B Complex 100*

vitamin C
  ADC with Fluoride*
  B-C with Folic Acid*
  B-Plex*
  Berocca*
  Chewable Triple Vitamins with Fluoride*
  Feocyte*
  Formula B*
  Key-Plex*
  Lypholized Vitamin B Complex & Vitamin C with B$_{12}$*
  Nephro-Vite Rx*
  Nephrocaps*
  Neurodep*
  Soluvite-f*
  Strovite*
  Tri-Flor-Vite with Fluoride*
  Tri-Vi-Flor*
  Tri-Vi-Flor with Iron*
  Tri Vit with Fluoride*
  Tri-Vitamin with Fluoride*
  Tri-A-Vite F*
  Triple Vitamin ADC with Fluoride*
  Trivitamin Fluoride*
  Vi-Daylin/F ADC*
  Vi-Daylin/F ADC + Iron*
  Vicam*

vitamin D
  ADC with Fluoride*
  Chewable Triple Vitamins with Fluoride*
  Soluvite-f*
  Tri-Flor-Vite with Fluoride*
  Tri-Vi-Flor*
  Tri-Vi-Flor with Iron*
  Tri Vit with Fluoride*
  Tri-Vitamin with Fluoride*
  Tri-A-Vite F*
  Triple Vitamin ADC with Fluoride*

*This brand is a combination product.

Generic ♦ Brands

vitamin D (cont.)
   Trivitamin Fluoride*
   Vi-Daylin/F ADC*
   Vi-Daylin/F ADC + Iron*
vitamin E
   Aquavit-E
   Lactinol-E*
   TriHemic 600*
vitamins, multiple
   Adeflor M*
   B Complex with C and B-12*
   B-C with Folic Acid Plus*
   Bacmin*
   Berocca Parenteral Nutrition*
   Berocca Plus*
   Berplex Plus*
   Cefol*
   Cernevit-12*
   Cezin-S*
   Chewable Multivitamins with Fluo-
      ride*
   Eldercaps*
   Enfamil Natalins Rx*
   Ferrex PC; Ferrex PC Forte*
   Florvite + Iron*
   Florvite + Iron; Half Strength
      Florvite + Iron*
   Florvite*
   Florvite; Florvite Half Strength*
   Formula B Plus*
   Infuvite Pediatric*
   Lactocal-F*
   M.V.I. Neonatal*
   M.V.I. Pediatric*
   M.V.I.-12*
   Marnatal-F*
   Materna*
   Mission Prenatal Rx*
   Multi-12; Multi-12 Pediatric ⓒ*
   Multi Vitamin Concentrate*
   Multivitamin with Fluoride*
   Mulvidren-F*
   Mynatal*
   Mynatal FC*
   Mynatal P.N.*
   Mynatal P.N. Forte*
   Mynatal Rx*
   Mynate 90 Plus*
   NataTab CFe; NataTab FA*
   NataChew*

vitamins, multiple (cont.)
   NataFort*
   NatalCare Plus*
   Natalins Rx*
   Natarex Prenatal*
   Nestabs CFB; Nestabs FA*
   Niferex-PN*
   Niferex-PN Forte*
   Nu-Iron V*
   O-Cal f.a.*
   Par-F*
   Par-Natal Plus 1 Improved*
   Poly-Vi-Flor*
   Poly-Vi-Flor with Iron*
   Polytabs-F*
   Polyvitamin Fluoride*
   Polyvitamin Fluoride with Iron*
   Polyvitamin with Iron and Fluoride*
   Polyvitamins with Fluoride and Iron*
   Pramilet FA*
   PreCare Conceive*
   PreCare Prenatal*
   Prenatal H.P.*
   Prenatal Maternal*
   Prenatal MR 90*
   Prenatal Plus Iron*
   Prenatal Plus with Betacarotene*
   Prenatal Plus; Prenatal Plus
      Improved*
   Prenatal Rx*
   Prenatal Rx with Betacarotene*
   Prenatal Z*
   Prenatal-1 + Iron*
   Prenate Advance; Prenate 90*
   Prenate Ultra*
   Soluvite C.T.*
   Strong Start*
   Strovite Advance*
   Strovite Plus; Strovite Forte*
   Stuartnatal Plus*
   Theragran Hematinic*
   Ultra-Natal*
   Vi-Daylin/F Multivitamin*
   Vi-Daylin/F Multivitamin + Iron*
   Vicon Forte*
   Vitafōl; Vitafōl-PN*
   Zenate, Advanced Formula*
   Zincvit*

*This brand is a combination product.

vitamins, multiple (cont.)
  Zodeac-100*
voglibose
  Basen
  Glustat
warfarin sodium
  Apo-Warfarin ⓒⒶⓃ
  Coumadin
  Taro-Warfarin ⓒⒶⓃ
yellow fever vaccine
  YF-Vax
yohimbine HCl
  Aphrodyne
  Dayto Himbin
  Yocon
  Yohimex
zafirlukast
  Accolate
zalcitabine
  Hivid
zaleplon
  Sonata
  Starnoc ⓒⒶⓃ
zidovudine
  Aztec
  Combivir*
  Retrovir
  Scriptene*
  Trizivir*

zileuton
  Zyflo
zinc acetate
  Galzin
zinc mesoporphyrin
  Hemex*
zinc sulfate
  Anuzinc ⓒⒶⓃ
  Proctodan-HC ⓒⒶⓃ*
  Zinca-Pak
  Zincate
ziprasidone HCl
  Geodon
ziprasidone mesylate
  Geodon
zoledronic acid
  Zometa
zolmitriptan
  Zomig
  Zomig ⓒⒶⓃ
  Zomig-ZMT
zolpidem tartrate
  Ambien
zonisamide
  Zonegran
zopiclone
  Alti-Zopiclone ⓒⒶⓃ
  Gen-Zopiclone ⓒⒶⓃ
  Imovane ⓒⒶⓃ

---

*This brand is a combination product.

XRef Indications to Generic and ℞ Brand Name Drugs

The "indications" for a drug—also called its "designated use," "approved use," or "therapeutic action"—is the reason a drug is prescribed. We can categorize drugs by their indications, grouping together drugs used for a similar purpose. The indications shown below are broad categories of therapeutic action. Individual drugs may be placed in subcategories or have specifically targeted diseases beyond the scope of this listing. Such nuances of use are shown in each individual drug's entry in *Saunders Pharmaceutical Word Book*.

Indications

Abortifacients [*see: Gynecological Agents, Abortifacients*]

Acne Preparations [*see: Dermatological Preparations, Acne Products*]

Adhesion Prevention Agents [*see: Wound Treatment*]

AIDS [*see: HIV Infections*]

Alcoholism Agents
[*see also: Psychotherapeutics, Antidepressants*]
Antabuse
Depade
disulfiram
naltrexone HCl
ReVia

Allergy and Anaphylaxis Agents
[*see also: Corticosteroids, Systemic; Dermatological Preparations, Antiinflammatory Agents; Nasal Preparations; Ophthalmologicals*]
Albay
allergenic extracts (aqueous, glycerinated, or alum-precipitated)
Allpyral
Ana-Guard
Ana-Kit

Allergy and Anaphylaxis Agents (cont.)
Center-Al
cromolyn sodium
dextran 1
epinephrine
EpiPen; EpiPen Jr.
Gastrocrom
Intal
omalizumab
Pharmalgen
Promit
Sus-Phrine
Venomil
Xolair

Alzheimer Disease Agents
AD7C
Aricept
Cognex
donepezil HCl
ergoloid mesylates
Exelon
galantamine hydrobromide
Gerimal
Hydergine
Hydergine LC
lazabemide HCl
lecithin
leteprinim potassium
memantine

Alzheimer Disease Agents (cont.)
metrifonate
Neotrofin
nimodipine
Nootropil
physostigmine
piracetam
ProMem
Reminyl
rivastigmine tartrate
Synapton SR
tacrine HCl
Tempium
velnacrine maleate
Anabolic Steroids [*see: Hormones, Anabolic/Androgenic*]

Analgesics
[*see also: Gout Agents; Rheumatic Disease Agents*]
Analgesics, Antimigraine
acetaminophen & butalbital & caffeine
almotriptan malate
Amaphen
Amerge
Anoquan
aspirin & butalbital & caffeine
Axert
Axocet
Axotal
Bucet
Bupap
butalbital & acetaminophen & caffeine
butalbital & aspirin & caffeine
Butalbital Compound
Butex Forte
Cafatine
Cafatine-PB
Cafergot
Cafetrate
D.H.E. 45
dihydroergotamine mesylate
Dolgic
Duradrin
eletriptan hydrobromide
Endolor
Ercaf

Analgesics, Antimigraine (cont.)
Ergomar
ergotamine tartrate
Esgic
Esgic-Plus
Femcet
feverfew (*Chrysanthemum parthenium; Leucanthemum parthenium; Pyrethrum parthenium; Tanacetum parthenium*)
Fiorgen PF
Fioricet
Fioricet with Codeine
Fiorinal
Fiorinal with Codeine
Fiorinal-C ¼; Fiorinal-C ½ Ⓐ
Fiorpap
Fiortal
frovatriptan succinate
Imitrex
Isocet
Isocom
Isollyl Improved
isometheptene mucate
Isopap
Lanorinal
Margesic
Marnal
Marten-Tab
Maxalt
Maxalt-MLT
Maxalt-RPD Ⓐ
Medigesic
methysergide maleate
Midchlor
Midrin
Migranal
Migratine
Miguard, Migard
naratriptan HCl
Phrenilin
Phrenilin Forte
Prominol
Relpax
Repan
Repan CF
rizatriptan benzoate
Sansert
Sedapap
sumatriptan succinate

Analgesics, Antimigraine (cont.)

Tencet
Tencon
Triad
Triaprin
Two-Dyne
Wigraine
zolmitriptan
Zomig
Zomig Ⓒ
Zomig-ZMT

Analgesics, Narcotic

Aceta with Codeine
acetaminophen & codeine
acetaminophen & hydrocodone
  bitartrate
acetaminophen & pentazocine HCl
Actiq
AERx
Alfenta
alfentanil HCl
Alor 5/500
Anexsia 5/500; Anexsia 7.5/650;
  Anexsia 10/660
Apo-Butorphanol Ⓒ
Aspirin with Codeine No. 2, No. 3,
  and No. 4
Astramorph PF
Azdone
B & O Supprettes No. 15A; B & O
  Supprettes No. 16A
Bancap HC
Buprenex
buprenorphine HCl
butorphanol tartrate
Capital with Codeine
Ceta Plus
Co-Gesic
codeine phosphate
Dalgan
Damason-P
Darvocet-N 50; Darvocet-N 100
Darvon
Darvon Compound-65
Darvon-N
Demerol HCl
DepoMorphine
dezocine
DHC Plus
dihydrocodeine bitartrate

Analgesics, Narcotic (cont.)

Dilaudid
Dilaudid Cough
Dilaudid-HP
Dirame
Dolacet
Dolene
Dolophine HCl
Duocet
Duragesic-25; Duragesic-50; Dura-
  gesic-75; Duragesic-100
Duramorph
Empirin with Codeine No. 3 & No. 4
Endocet
Endocodone
fentanyl
fentanyl citrate
Fentanyl Oralet
Fioricet with Codeine
Fiorinal with Codeine
Fiorinal-C ¼; Fiorinal-C ½ Ⓒ
Hy-Phen
Hydrocet
hydrocodone bitartrate
hydrocodone bitartrate & acetamin-
  ophen
Hydrogesic
hydromorphone HCl
HydroStat IR
Infumorph
Innovar
Kadian
Levo-Dromoran
levomethadyl acetate
levorphanol tartrate
Lorcet
Lorcet-HD
Lorcet Plus; Lorcet 10/650
Lortab
Lortab 2.5/500; Lortab 5/500; Lortab
  7.5/500; Lortab 10/500
Lortab ASA
M-oxy
M-Eslon Ⓒ
Margesic H
Maxidone
Medipain 5
Mepergan
Mepergan Fortis
meperidine HCl

Analgesics, Narcotic (cont.)

Metadol ⒸⒶⓃ
methadone HCl
Methadose
MorphiDex
morphine HCl
morphine sulfate (MS)
MS Contin
MS/L; MS/L Concentrate
MS/S
MSIR
nalbuphine HCl
Norco
Nubain
Numorphan
OMS Concentrate
opium
Oramorph SR
Orlaam
Oxycocet ⒸⒶⓃ
oxycodone HCl
oxycodone terephthalate
OxyContin
OxyFast
OxyIR
oxymorphone HCl
Panacet 5/500
Panasal 5/500
Panlor DC
paregoric (PG)
pentazocine HCl
pentazocine HCl & acetaminophen
pentazocine lactate
Percocet
Percodan; Percodan-Demi
Percolone
Phenaphen with Codeine No. 3 & No. 4
Propacet 100
propiram fumarate
propoxyphene HCl
propoxyphene napsylate
RMS
Roxanol
Roxanol; Roxanol 100; Roxanol Rescudose; Roxanol T; Roxanol UD
Roxicet
Roxicet 5/500
Roxicodone
Roxilox

Analgesics, Narcotic (cont.)

Roxiprin
Soma Compound with Codeine
Stadol
Stadol NS
Stagesic
Sublimaze
Sufenta
sufentanil citrate
Synalgos-DC
T-Gesic
Talacen
Talwin
Talwin Compound
Talwin NX
Tylenol with Codeine
Tylenol with Codeine No. 2, No. 3, and No. 4
Tylox
UltraJect
Vicodin; Vicodin ES; Vicodin HP
Vicoprofen
Wygesic
Zydone

Analgesics, Neuralgia

Atretol
carbamazepine
Carbatrol
Depitol
Epitol
Gen-Carbamazepine CR ⒸⒶⓃ
PMS-Carbamazepine CR ⒸⒶⓃ
Tegretol

Analgesics, Nonsteroidal (NSAIDs)

[see also: Antiarthritics, Nonsteroidal (NSAIDs)]
acetaminophen
acetaminophen & butalbital & caffeine
Aclophen
Alumadrine
Amaphen
Amigesic
Anaprox; Anaprox DS
Anatuss
Anoquan
Apo-Diclo Rapide ⒸⒶⓃ
Apo-Etodolac ⒸⒶⓃ
Apo-Ketorolac ⒸⒶⓃ

Analgesics, Nonsteroidal (NSAIDs) (cont.)

Apo-Naproxen (CAN)
Apo-Naproxen SR (CAN)
Argesic-SA
Arthropan
Arthrotec
aspirin
aspirin & butalbital & caffeine
aspirin, buffered
Axocet
Axotal
Brexidol 20 (CAN)
bromfenac sodium
Bucet
Bupap
butalbital & acetaminophen & caffeine
butalbital & aspirin & caffeine
Butalbital Compound
Butex Forte
carprofen
Cataflam
choline magnesium trisalicylate
    (choline salicylate + magnesium
    salicylate)
choline salicylate
diclofenac potassium
diclofenac sodium
Diclotec (CAN)
diflunisal
Disalcid
Dolgic
Dolobid
Duract
Duradrin
Easprin
Enable
Endolor
Equagesic
Esgic
Esgic-Plus
etodolac
Femcet
fenoprofen calcium
Fexicam (CAN)
Fiorgen PF
Fioricet
Fiorinal
Fiorpap

Analgesics, Nonsteroidal (NSAIDs) (cont.)

Fiortal
Flexaphen
Flextra-DS
Gen-Etodolac (CAN)
Histex SR
Hycomine Compound
Ibu
ibuprofen
Ibuprohm
Indochron E-R
Isocet
Isocom
Isollyl Improved
Isopap
isoxicam
ketoprofen
ketorolac tromethamine
Lanorinal
Lobac
Lodine
Lodine XL
Magan
magnesium salicylate
Magsal
Margesic
Marnal
Marten-Tab
Marthritic
Maxicam
meclofenamate sodium
Medigesic
mefenamic acid
meloxicam
Micrainin
Midchlor
Midrin
Migratine
Mobic
Mobicox (CAN)
Mobidin
Mono-Gesic
Motrin
Myapap
Nalfon
Naprelan
Napron X
Naprosyn
naproxen

Analgesics, Nonsteroidal (NSAIDs) (cont.)

naproxen sodium
Norel Plus
Norgesic; Norgesic Forte
Novo-Difenac-K ⓒⒶⓃ
Novo-Naprox ⓒⒶⓃ
Novo-Naprox-EC ⓒⒶⓃ
Novo-Naprox SR ⓒⒶⓃ
Orphengesic; Orphengesic Forte
Orudis
Pennsaid
Phenate
Phrenilin
Phrenilin Forte
piroxicam betadex
PMS-Diclofenac ⓒⒶⓃ
PMS-Diclofenac SR ⓒⒶⓃ
Ponstel
Prominol
Repan
Repan CF
Rexolate
Rimadyl
Riva-Diclofenac ⓒⒶⓃ
Riva-Diclofenac-K ⓒⒶⓃ
Riva-Naproxen ⓒⒶⓃ
Robaxisal
rofecoxib
Saleto-400; Saleto-600; Saleto-800
salicylamide
Salprofen
salsalate
Salsitab
Sedapap
sodium salicylate (SS)
sodium thiosalicylate
Sodol Compound
Soma Compound
Soma Compound with Codeine
Tencet
Tencon
tenidap
Toradol
Triad
Triaprin
Tricosal
Trilisate
Tussanil DH
Tussirex

Analgesics, Nonsteroidal (NSAIDs) (cont.)

Two-Dyne
Ultracet
Vioxx
Voltaren
Voltaren ⓒⒶⓃ
Voltaren Rapide ⓒⒶⓃ
ZORprin

Analgesics, Topical
[see also: Dermatological Preparations]
capsaicin
diclofenac potassium
menthol
Pennsaid

Analgesics, Other
CereCRIB
clonidine
Duraclon
Levoprome
Metastron
methotrimeprazine
methotrimeprazine maleate
Oralease
Quadramet
samarium Sm 153 lexidronam
strontium chloride Sr 89
tramadol HCl
Ultracet
Ultram
Ultram XL
ziconotide

Anemia Agents
Anemia Agents, B Vitamins
[see also: Vitamin Replacement, B
    Vitamins]
Anemagen
B Complex with C and B-12
B-Ject-100
Bedoz ⓒⒶⓃ
Cevi-Fer
Chromagen
Contrin
Crystamine
Crysti 1000
cyanocobalamin (vitamin B_{12})
Cyanoject
Cyomin

Anemia Agents, B Vitamins (cont.)
  Fe-Tinic 150 Forte
  Feocyte
  Fero-Folic-500
  Ferotrinsic
  Ferrex 150 Forte
  folic acid
  Foltrin
  Folvite
  Fumatinic
  Hemocyte-F
  Hemocyte Plus
  Hydro Cobex
  Hydro-Crysti 12
  hydroxocobalamin
  Hytinic
  Iberet-Folic-500
  intrinsic factor concentrate
  Key-Plex
  LA-12
  Liver Combo No. 5
  Livitrinsic-f
  Lypholized Vitamin B Complex &
    Vitamin C with B_{12}
  May-Vita
  Megaton
  Nascobal
  Nephplex Rx
  Nephro-Fer Rx
  Nephro-Vite Rx
  Nephro-Vite Rx + Fe
  Nephrocaps
  Nephron FA
  Neurodep
  niacin (vitamin B_3)
  Niacor
  Niaspan
  Niferex-150 Forte
  Nu-Iron Plus
  Pronemia Hematinic
  Rubramin PC
  Senilezol
  Strovite
  Theragran Hematinic
  TriHemic 600
  Trinsicon
  Vicam
  Vitafōl
  Vitafōl; Vitafōl-PN
  Vitamin B Complex 100

Anemia Agents, B Vitamins (cont.)
  Zodeac-100
Anemia Agents, Iron
  [see also: Mineral Replacement, Iron]
  Anemagen
  carbonyl iron
  Cevi-Fer
  Chromagen
  Contrin
  DexFerrum
  Dexiron Ⓒ🅰🅽
  Fe-Tinic 150 Forte
  Feocyte
  Fero-Folic-500
  Ferotrinsic
  Ferrex 150 Forte
  Ferrlecit
  ferrous fumarate
  ferrous gluconate
  ferrous sulfate
  ferrous sulfate, dried
  Foltrin
  Fumatinic
  Hemocyte-F
  Hemocyte Plus
  Hytinic
  Iberet-Folic-500
  InFeD
  Infurfer Ⓒ🅰🅽
  iron
  iron dextran
  iron sucrose
  Livitrinsic-f
  Nephro-Fer Rx
  Nephro-Vite Rx + Fe
  Nephron FA
  Niferex-150 Forte
  Nu-Iron Plus
  polysaccharide-iron complex
  Pronemia Hematinic
  Senilezol
  Theragran Hematinic
  TriHemic 600
  Trinsicon
  Venofer
  Vitafōl
  Vitafōl; Vitafōl-PN
  Zodeac-100
Anemia Agents, Other
  Androlone-D 200

Indications

Anemia Agents, Other (cont.)
antithymocyte globulin (ATG)
Aranesp
Atgam
darbepoetin alfa
Deca-Durabolin
Droxia
epoetin alfa (EPO)
epoetin beta
Epogen
hemoglobin, recombinant human (rHb1.1)
Hybolin Decanoate-50; Hybolin Decanoate-100
Hydrea
hydroxyurea
lymphocyte immune globulin (LIG)
Marogen
nandrolone decanoate
Neo-Durabolic
Optro
Procrit

Anesthetics
Anesthetics, General
Alfenta
alfentanil HCl
Amidate
Brevital Sodium
Brietal Sodium ⒸⒶⓃ
desflurane
Diprivan
droperidol
enflurane
Ethrane
etomidate
fentanyl citrate
Fluothane
Forane
halothane
Inapsine
Innovar
isoflurane
Ketalar
ketamine HCl
methohexital sodium
methoxyflurane
midazolam HCl
Penthrane

Anesthetics, General (cont.)
Pentothal
propofol
rapacuronium bromide
Raplon
remifentanil HCl
sevoflurane
Sublimaze
Sufenta
sufentanil citrate
Suprane
thiopental sodium
Ultane
Ultiva
Versed

Anesthetics, Local
[see also: Hemorrhoidal Agents; Ophthalmologicals, Local Anesthetics]
articaine HCl
Astracaine; Astracaine Forte ⒸⒶⓃ
benzocaine
bupivacaine HCl
butamben
butamben picrate
Carbocaine
Carbocaine with Neo-Cobefrin
Cetacaine
Chirocaine
chloroprocaine HCl
Citanest Plain
cocaine
cocaine HCl
Cocaine Viscous
Decadron with Xylocaine
Dentipatch
dibucaine
dibucaine HCl
dichlorodifluoromethane
dichlorotetrafluoroethane
Dilocaine
diperodon
Duranest; Duranest MPF
Dyclone
dyclonine HCl
EMLA
Enzone
Epifoam
ethyl chloride
etidocaine
1+1-F Creme

Anesthetics, Local (cont.)
Fluori-Methane
Fluro-Ethyl
Isocaine HCl
levobupivacaine HCl
Lida-Mantle-HC
lidocaine
lidocaine HCl
Lidoderm
Lidoject-1; Lidoject-2
Marcaine HCl
Marcaine Spinal
mepivacaine HCl
Naropin
Nervocaine 1%
Nesacaine; Nesacaine MPF
Novocain
Octocaine HCl
Polocaine
Polocaine MPF
Pontocaine HCl
Pramosone
pramoxine
pramoxine HCl
prilocaine
prilocaine HCl
procaine HCl
propoxycaine HCl
ropivacaine HCl
RSD-921
Sensorcaine
Sensorcaine MPF
Sensorcaine MPF Spinal
Septocaine
tetracaine HCl
Triban; Pediatric Triban
trichloromonofluoromethane
Xylocaine
Xylocaine HCl
Xylocaine MPF
Zone-A Forte
Angina [see: Cardiac Agents, Antianginals]
Anorexiants [see: Weight Reduction Agents, CNS Modifiers]

Antacids
[see also: Antisecretories, Gastrointestinal; Peptic Ulcer and Gastric Reflux Agents]
aluminum hydroxide gel
calcium carbonate
Cotazym
Dialume
magaldrate
magnesia, milk of
magnesium carbonate
magnesium hydroxide
magnesium oxide
sodium bicarbonate
sodium citrate

Anthelmintics
albendazole
Albenza
Biltricide
bithionol
Bitin
diethylcarbamazine citrate
Hetrazan
ivermectin
Lorothidol
mebendazole
Mintezol
niclosamide
oxamniquine
piperazine citrate
praziquantel
pyrantel pamoate
Stromectol
thiabendazole (TBZ)
Vansil
Vermox
Antiarrhythmics [see: Cardiac Agents, Antiarrhythmics]

Antiarthritics
[see also: Analgesics; Rheumatic Disease Agents]
Antiarthritics, Nonsteroidal (NSAIDs)
[see also: Analgesics, Nonsteroidal (NSAIDs)]

Indications

Antiarthritics, Nonsteroidal (NSAIDs) (cont.)
Anaprox; Anaprox DS
Ansaid
Apo-Diclo Rapide ⓒᴬᴺ
Apo-Nabumetone ⓒᴬᴺ
Apo-Naproxen ⓒᴬᴺ
Apo-Naproxen SR ⓒᴬᴺ
Brexidol 20 ⓒᴬᴺ
Cataflam
Celebrex
celecoxib
Clinoril
Daypro
diclofenac potassium
diclofenac sodium
EC-Naprosyn
etodolac
Feldene
fenoprofen calcium
flurbiprofen
Gen-Etodolac ⓒᴬᴺ
Gen-Naproxen EC ⓒᴬᴺ
ibuprofen
Indocin
Indocin SR
indomethacin
ketoprofen
Lodine
Lodine XL
meclofenamate sodium
meloxicam
Mobic
Mobicox ⓒᴬᴺ
Motrin
nabumetone
Nalfon
Naprelan
Naprosyn
naproxen
naproxen sodium
Novo-Difenac-K ⓒᴬᴺ
Novo-Naprox ⓒᴬᴺ
Novo-Naprox-EC ⓒᴬᴺ
Novo-Naprox SR ⓒᴬᴺ
Orudis
Oruvail
oxaprozin
piroxicam
piroxicam betadex

Antiarthritics, Nonsteroidal (NSAIDs) (cont.)
PMS-Diclofenac ⓒᴬᴺ
PMS-Diclofenac SR ⓒᴬᴺ
Relafen
Rhoxal-oxaprozin ⓒᴬᴺ
Riva-Diclofenac ⓒᴬᴺ
Riva-Diclofenac-K ⓒᴬᴺ
Riva-Naproxen ⓒᴬᴺ
rofecoxib
sulindac
Tolectin 200; Tolectin 600
Tolectin DS
tolmetin sodium
Vioxx
Voltaren
Voltaren ⓒᴬᴺ
Voltaren Rapide ⓒᴬᴺ
Voltaren SR ⓒᴬᴺ
Voltaren XR
Antiarthritics, Other
Colloral
Hyalgan
hyaluronate sodium
hylan G-F 20
Supartz
Synvisc
trinecol (pullus)

Antibiotics
[see also: Antidiarrheal Agents, Intestinal Antibacterials; Antiprotozoals; Antituberculosis Agents; Dermatological Preparations, Acne Products; Ophthalmologicals, Antibiotics; Otologicals; Urinary Tract Agents, Antibacterials; Vaginal Preparations, Antibacterial; Wound Treatment, Medicated Dressings]
Antibiotics, Aminoglycosides
amikacin
amikacin sulfate
Amikin
Garamycin
Garamycin Pediatric
gentamicin sulfate
Humatin
Jenamicin
kanamycin sulfate

Antibiotics, Aminoglycosides (cont.)
Kantrex
MiKasome
Mycifradin Sulfate
Nebcin
Neo-fradin
Neo-Tabs
neomycin sulfate
netilmicin sulfate
Netromycin
paromomycin sulfate
Scheinpharm Tobramycin ⒸⒶ⒩
Septopal
streptomycin sulfate
TOBI
tobramycin
tobramycin sulfate
Antibiotics, Carbapenems
imipenem
Ivanaz
Lorabid
loracarbef
meropenem
Merrem
Primaxin I.M.
Primaxin I.V.
Antibiotics, Cephalosporins
Ancef
Apo-Cefaclor ⒸⒶ⒩
Apo-Cefadroxil ⒸⒶ⒩
Biocef
Ceclor
Ceclor CD
Ceclor CDpak
Cedax
cefaclor
cefadroxil
Cefadyl
cefamandole nafate
cefazolin sodium
cefdinir
cefditoren pivoxil
cefepime HCl
cefixime
Cefizox
cefmetazole sodium
Cefobid
cefodizime
cefonicid sodium
cefoperazone sodium

Antibiotics, Cephalosporins (cont.)
Cefotan
cefotaxime sodium
cefotetan disodium
cefoxitin sodium
cefpodoxime proxetil
cefprozil
ceftazidime
ceftibuten
Ceftin
ceftizoxime sodium
ceftriaxone sodium
cefuroxime axetil
cefuroxime sodium
Cefzil
cephalexin
cephalexin HCl
cephalothin sodium
cephapirin sodium
cephradine
Ceptaz
Claforan
Duricef
Fortaz
Keflex
Keftab
Kefurox
Kefzol
Mandol
Maxipime
Mefoxin
Modivid
Monocid
Novo-Cefaclor ⒸⒶ⒩
Novo-Cefadroxil ⒸⒶ⒩
Omnicef
Rocephin
Spectracef
Suprax
Tazicef
Tazidime
Vantin
Velosef
Zefazone
Zinacef
Zolicef
Antibiotics, Fluoroquinolones
alatrofloxacin mesylate
Apo-Norflox ⒸⒶ⒩

Indications

Antibiotics, Fluoroquinolones (cont.)
Apo-Oflox Ⓒ
Avelox
Chibroxin
Ciloxan
Cipro
Cipro HC Otic
ciprofloxacin
ciprofloxacin HCl
enoxacin
Floxin
Floxin Otic
gatifloxacin
grepafloxacin HCl
Levaquin
levofloxacin
lomefloxacin HCl
Maxaquin
moxifloxacin HCl
norfloxacin
Noroxin
Novo-Norfloxacin Ⓒ
Ocuflox
ofloxacin
Penetrex
Quixin
Raxar
Riva-Norfloxacin Ⓒ
sparfloxacin
Tequin
trovafloxacin mesylate
Trovan
Trovan/Zithromax Compliance Pak
Zagam

Antibiotics, Glycopeptides
Lyphocin
Targocid
teicoplanin
Vancocin
Vancoled
vancomycin HCl

Antibiotics, Lincosamides
Alti-Clindamycin Ⓒ
Cleocin; Cleocin Pediatric
Cleocin Phosphate
clindamycin
clindamycin HCl
clindamycin palmitate HCl
clindamycin phosphate

Antibiotics, Lincosamides (cont.)
Dalacin C Ⓒ
Dalacin C Phosphate Ⓒ
HyClinda
Lincocin
lincomycin HCl
Lincorex

Antibiotics, Macrolides
azithromycin
Biaxin
Biaxin XL
clarithromycin
dirithromycin
Dynabac
E.E.S.
E.E.S. 200
E.E.S. 400
Eramycin
Ery-Tab
EryPed
EryPed 200; EryPed 400
Erythrocin
Erythrocin Stearate
erythromycin
erythromycin estolate
erythromycin ethylsuccinate (EES)
erythromycin gluceptate
erythromycin lactobionate
erythromycin stearate
Eryzole
Ilosone
Ilotycin Gluceptate
PCE
Pediazole
Prevpac
Robimycin
Tao
troleandomycin
Trovan/Zithromax Compliance Pak
Zithromax

Antibiotics, Penicillins
Alti-Amoxi Clav Ⓒ
amoxicillin
amoxicillin sodium
Amoxil
ampicillin
ampicillin sodium
Apo-Pen VK Ⓒ
Apo-Amoxi Ⓒ
Augmentin

Antibiotics, Penicillins (cont.)
Augmentin ES
bacampicillin HCl
Bactocill
Beepen-VK
Betapen-VK
Bicillin C-R; Bicillin C-R 900/300
Bicillin L-A
Biomox
carbenicillin indanyl sodium
cloxacillin sodium
Cloxapen
Crysticillin 300 A.S.; Crysticillin 600 A.S.
D-Amp
dicloxacillin sodium
Dycill
Dynapen
Gen-Amoxicillin ⒸⒶⓃ
Geocillin
Ledercillin VK
Lin-Amox ⒸⒶⓃ
Marcillin
methicillin sodium
Mezlin
mezlocillin sodium
Nafcil
nafcillin sodium
Nallpen
Novamoxin ⒸⒶⓃ
Omnipen
Omnipen-N
oxacillin sodium
Pathocil
Pen-V
Pen-Vee K
penicillin G benzathine
penicillin G potassium
penicillin G procaine
penicillin G sodium
penicillin V potassium
Penicillin VK
Permapen
Pfizerpen
Pfizerpen-AS
piperacillin sodium
Pipracil
Polycillin
Polycillin-N
Polycillin-PRB

Antibiotics, Penicillins (cont.)
Polymox
Principen
Probampacin
Prostaphlin
Robicillin VK
Spectrobid
Staphcillin
Tegopen
Ticar
ticarcillin disodium
Timentin
Totacillin
Totacillin-N
Trimox
Unasyn
Unipen
V-Cillin K
Veetids
Veetids '125'; Veetids '250'
Wycillin
Wymox
Zosyn
Antibiotics, Sulfonamides
Bactrim IV
Bactrim Pediatric
Bactrim; Bactrim DS
Cotrim Pediatric
Cotrim; Cotrim D.S.
Eryzole
Gantanol
Gantrisin
Pediazole
Septra
Septra DS
Septra IV
sulfacytine
sulfadoxine
sulfamethizole
sulfamethoxazole (SMX; SMZ)
Sulfatrim
sulfisoxazole
sulfisoxazole acetyl
Thiosulfil Forte
trisulfapyrimidines
Antibiotics, Tetracyclines
Achromycin V
Actisite
Adoxa
Arestin

Indications

Antibiotics, Tetracyclines (cont.)
Bio-Tab
Declomycin
demeclocycline HCl
Doryx
Doxy 100; Doxy 200
Doxy Caps
Doxychel Hyclate
doxycycline
doxycycline calcium
doxycycline hyclate
doxycycline monohydrate
Dynacin
Helidac
Minocin
minocycline HCl
Monodox
Nor-Tet
oxytetracycline
oxytetracycline HCl
Panmycin
Periostat
PMS-Minocycline ⒸⒶⓃ
Rhoxal-minocycline ⒸⒶⓃ
Robitet
Sumycin
Sumycin '250'; Sumycin '500'
Teline; Teline-500
Terramycin
Terramycin IM
Tetracap
tetracycline HCl
Tetralan
Tetralan "250"; Tetralan-500
Uri-Tet
Vectrin
Vibra-Tabs
Vibramycin

Antibiotics, Topical
[see also: Dermatological Preparations, Acne Products]
A/T/S
AK-Neo-Dex
Akne-mycin
AK-Tracin
Ala-Quin
Atridox
bacitracin
bacitracin zinc
Bactroban

Antibiotics, Topical (cont.)
Bactroban Nasal
Benzaclin
Benzamycin
C/T/S
Castellani Paint Modified
chloramphenicol
chloramphenicol palmitate
chlorhexidine gluconate
chlortetracycline HCl
Cleocin T
Clinda-Derm
clindamycin phosphate
Clindets
clioquinol
Corque
Cortisporin
Cytolex
Dalacin T ⒸⒶⓃ
Del-Mycin
doxycycline hyclate
Elase-Chloromycetin
Emgel
Erycette
EryDerm 2%
Erygel
Erymax
Erythra-Derm
erythromycin
1+1-F Creme
fuchsin, basic
Fucidin ⒸⒶⓃ
Furacin
fusidate sodium
fusidic acid
G-myticin
Garamycin
gentamicin sulfate
Klaron
Locilex
mafenide
mafenide acetate
MetroCream
MetroGel; MetroLotion
mupirocin
mupirocin calcium
Myco-Biotic II
Neo-Cortef
Neo-Dexair
Neo-Dexameth

Antibiotics, Topical (cont.)
NeoDecadron
neomycin sulfate
Neosporin G.U. Irrigant
nitrofurazone
Noritate
Novacet
oxytetracycline HCl
Pedi-Cort V Creme
pexiganan acetate
polymyxin B sulfate
Protegrin
Sebizon
Silvadene
silver sulfadiazine (SSD)
SSD; SSD AF
Staticin
Storz-N-D
Sulfacet-R
sulfacetamide sodium
Sulfamylon
T-Stat
tetracycline HCl
Theramycin Z
Thermazene
Topicycline
Vanocin

Antibiotics, Other (including Synergists)
Albamycin
Altracin
Azactam
aztreonam
Baci-IM
bacitracin
bactericidal and permeability-increasing (BPI) protein, recombinant
Bactrim IV
Bactrim Pediatric
Bactrim; Bactrim DS
Centoxin
chloramphenicol
chloramphenicol sodium succinate
Chloromycetin Sodium Succinate
Cidecin
clavulanate potassium
clavulanic acid
clofazimine
colistimethate sodium
colistin sulfate

Antibiotics, Other (including Synergists) (cont.)
Coly-Mycin M
Cotrim Pediatric
Cotrim; Cotrim D.S.
dalfopristin
dapsone
daptomycin
drotrecogin alfa
evernimicin
Factive
Flagyl
Flagyl ER
Flagyl IV
Flagyl IV RTU
furazolidone
Furoxone
gemifloxacin mesylate
Helidac
Ketek
Lamprene
linezolid
Metaret
Metro I.V.
metronidazole
metronidazole HCl
Mycobutin
nebacumab
Neuprex
Normix
novobiocin calcium
oritavancin diphosphate
polymyxin B sulfate
Primsol
Proloprim
Protostat
quinupristin
Renoquid
rifabutin
rifaximin
Rifaximin
ritamycin
Rituxan
rituximab
Septra
Septra DS
Septra IV
spectinomycin HCl
Spexil
sulbactam sodium

Indications

Antibiotics, Other (including Synergists) (cont.)
Sulfatrim
suramin hexasodium
Synercid
telithromycin
trimethoprim (TMP)
Trimpex
Trobicin
trospectomycin sulfate
Unasyn
Xigris
Ziracin
Zovant
Zyvox
Zyvoxam Ⓒⓐⓝ

Anticoagulants
ATnativ
Acova
ancrod
Angiomax
anisindione
antithrombin III (AT-III)
Apo-Warfarin Ⓒⓐⓝ
ardeparin sodium
argatroban
Arvin
bivalirudin
Coumadin
coumarin
dalteparin sodium
danaparoid sodium
desirudin
dicumarol
enoxaparin sodium
Flocor
Fragmin
Fraxiparine Ⓒⓐⓝ
Fraxiparine Forte Ⓒⓐⓝ
Hep-Lock; Hep-Lock U/P
heparin calcium
heparin sodium
Heparin Lock Flush
Hepflush-10
Hirulog
Innohep
Kybernin
lepirudin

Anticoagulants (cont.)
Liquaemin Sodium
Lovenox
Miradon
nadroparin calcium
Normiflo
Novastan
Orgaran
Refludan
Revasc
Taro-Warfarin Ⓒⓐⓝ
Thrombate III
tifacogin
tinzaparin sodium
Vasoflux
Viprinex Ⓒⓐⓝ
warfarin
warfarin sodium

Anticonvulsants
[see also: Psychotherapeutics, Anxiolytics; Sedatives and Hypnotics]
acetazolamide
acetazolamide sodium
Apo-Clonazepam Ⓒⓐⓝ
Apo-Diazepam Ⓒⓐⓝ
Apo-Divalproex Ⓒⓐⓝ
Apo-Valproic Ⓒⓐⓝ
Ativan
Atretol
Bellatal
carbamazepine
Carbatrol
Celontin
Cerebyx
clonazepam
Depacon
Depakene
Depakote
Depakote ER
Depitol
Deproic Ⓒⓐⓝ
Diamox
Diastat
Diazemuls Ⓒⓐⓝ
diazepam
Dilantin
Dilantin-125
Diphenylan Sodium

Anticonvulsants (cont.)
divalproex sodium
Dizac
Epiject (CAN)
Epitol
Epival (CAN)
Epival ER (CAN)
ethosuximide
ethotoin
felbamate
Felbatol
fosphenytoin sodium
gabapentin
Gabitril
Gen-Carbamazepine CR (CAN)
Keppra
Klonopin
Lamictal
lamotrigine
levetiracetam
lorazepam
Luminal Sodium
magnesium sulfate
Mebaral
mephenytoin
mephobarbital
Mesantoin
methsuximide
Milontin
Mogadon
Mysoline
neural gabaergic cells (or precursors), porcine fetal
NeuroCell-HD
Neurontin
nitrazepam
Novo-Clonazepam (CAN)
Novo-Divalproex (CAN)
Nu-Divalproex (CAN)
Nu-Valproic (CAN)
oxcarbazepine
Paral
paraldehyde
Peganone
phenacemide
phenobarbital
phenobarbital sodium
phensuximide
Phenurone
phenytoin

Anticonvulsants (cont.)
phenytoin sodium
PMS-Carbamazepine CR (CAN)
PMS-Gabapentin (CAN)
primidone
Rhoxal-valproic (CAN)
Sabril
Solfoton
Tegretol
Tegretol-XR
tiagabine HCl
Topamax
topiramate
Tridione
Trileptal
trimethadione
Valium
Valium Roche Oral (CAN)
valproate sodium
valproic acid
vigabatrin
Zarontin
Zonegran
zonisamide
Antidepressants [see: Psychotherapeutics, Antidepressants]

Antidiarrheal Agents
Antidiarrheal Agents, Antiflatulents
charcoal
simethicone
Antidiarrheal Agents, Antiperistaltics
Antispasmodic
Antrocol
Arco-Lase Plus
Barbidonna; Barbidonna No. 2
Bellacane
difenoxin HCl
diphenoxylate HCl
Donna-Sed
Donnatal
Donnatal No. 2
Hyosophen
Imodium
Logen
Lomanate
Lomotil
Lonox
loperamide HCl

Indications

Antidiarrheal Agents, Antiperistaltics (cont.)
Malatal
Motofen
Spasmolin
Susano

Antidiarrheal Agents, Intestinal Antibacterials
[see also: Antibiotics; Antifungals, Systemic]
Adoxa
Bactrim Pediatric
Bactrim; Bactrim DS
Bio-Tab
Cipro
ciprofloxacin
Cotrim Pediatric
Cotrim; Cotrim D.S.
Cryptosporidium parvum bovine colostrum IgG concentrate
Doryx
Doxy Caps
Doxychel Hyclate
doxycycline hyclate
Flagyl
Helidac
Immuno-C
metronidazole
Monodox
Mycostatin
Neo-fradin
neomycin sulfate
Nilstat
nystatin
Nystex
Protostat
Septra
Septra DS
Sporidin-G
Sulfatrim
Synsorb-Pk
Vancocin
vancomycin HCl
Vibra-Tabs
Vibramycin

Antidiarrheal Agents, Other
attapulgite, activated
bismuth subsalicylate (BSS)
calcium polycarbophil
dehydroemetine

Antidiarrheal Agents, Other (cont.)
Lactobacillus acidophilus
Mebadin
8-methoxycarbonyloctyl oligosaccharides
polycarbophil

Antidotes
Antidotes, Acetaminophen
acetylcysteine (N-acetylcysteine)
acetylcysteine sodium
Mucomyst
Mucomyst 10

Antidotes, Benzodiazepine
flumazenil
Romazicon

Antidotes, Chelating Agents
BAL in Oil
Bio-Rescue
Calcium Disodium Versenate
Chemet
deferoxamine
deferoxamine mesylate
Desferal
dimercaprol
Disotate
edetate calcium disodium
edetate disodium
Endrate
PMS-Desferoxamine ⒸⒶⓃ
succimer
Syprine
trientine HCl

Antidotes, Cyanide
amyl nitrite
Cyanide Antidote Package
Methblue 65
methylene blue (MB)
sodium nitrite
sodium thiosulfate
Urolene Blue

Antidotes, Digoxin
Digibind
Digidote
digoxin immune Fab (ovine)

Antidotes, Heparin
protamine sulfate

Antidotes, Insecticide
AtroPen

Antidotes, Insecticide (cont.)
atropine sulfate
pralidoxime chloride
Protopam Chloride
Sal-Tropine
Antidotes, Narcotic
buprenorphine HCl
Depade
nalmefene
naloxone HCl
naltrexone HCl
Narcan
ReVia
Revex
Antidotes, Other
Antilirium
Antizol
charcoal, activated
cupric sulfate
edrophonium chloride
Enlon
fomepizole
ipecac
physostigmine salicylate
Reversol
Tensilon

Antiemetics and Antinauseants

[see also: Antisecretories, Gastrointestinal; Peptic Ulcer and Gastric Reflux Agents]
alosetron HCl
Anergan 50
Antivert; Antivert/25; Antivert/50
Antrizine
Anzemet
Apo-Domperidone ⒸⒶⓃ
Apo-Perphenazine ⒸⒶⓃ
Apo-Prochlorazine ⒸⒶⓃ
Apo-Trifluoperazine ⒸⒶⓃ
Arrestin
chlorpromazine
chlorpromazine HCl
Clopra
Compazine
dimenhydrinate
Dimetabs
Dinate
diphenidol HCl

Antiemetics and Antinauseants (cont.)
dolasetron mesylate
domperidone
Dramamine
Dramanate
Dramilin
dronabinol
droperidol
Dymenate
E-Vista
Emitasol
granisetron HCl
Hydrate
hydroxyzine HCl
Hyzine-50
Inapsine
K-Phen-50
Kytril
Marinol
Marmine
Maxolon
meclizine HCl
Meni-D
metoclopramide HCl
metoclopramide monohydrochloride monohydrate
MK-869
Motilium ⒸⒶⓃ
Norzine
Novo-Domperidone ⒸⒶⓃ
Nu-Prochlor ⒸⒶⓃ
Octamide PFS
ondansetron HCl
Ormazine
Pentazine
perphenazine
Phenameth
Phenazine 50
Phenergan
Phenergan Fortis
Phenergan Plain
Phenoject-50
phosphorated carbohydrate solution (hyperosmolar solution with phosphoric acid)
Pramidin
Pro-50
prochlorperazine
prochlorperazine bimaleate

Antiemetics and Antinauseants (cont.)

prochlorperazine edisylate
prochlorperazine maleate
prochlorperazine mesylate
Prometh-50
promethazine HCl
Prorex-25; Prorex-50
Prothazine
Prothazine Plain
Quiess
Reclomide
Reglan
Ru-Vert-M
Scopace
scopolamine hydrobromide
Stelazine
Stemetil Ⓒ
T-Gen
Tebamide
thiethylperazine
thiethylperazine malate
Thorazine
Ticon
Tigan
Torecan
Transderm Scōp
Triban; Pediatric Triban
trifluoperazine HCl
Trilafon
Trimazide
trimethobenzamide HCl
Vistacon
Vistaril
Vistazine 50
Vontrol
Zofran
Zofran ODT

Antifungals
Antifungals, Systemic
[see also: Antidiarrheal Agents]
Abelcet
AmBisome
Amphocin
Amphotec
amphotericin B
amphotericin B cholesteryl
Ancobon

Antifungals, Systemic (cont.)

Apo-Fluconazole Ⓒ
Apo-Ketoconazole Ⓒ
Apo-Terbinafine Ⓒ
Cancidas
caspofungin acetate
Diflucan
fluconazole
flucytosine
Fulvicin P/G
Fulvicin U/F
Fungizone
Grifulvin V
Gris-PEG
Grisactin 250
Grisactin 500
Grisactin Ultra
griseofulvin
itraconazole
ketoconazole
Lamisil
miconazole
Monistat i.v.
Mycostatin
Nilstat
Nizoral
Novo-Ketoconazole Ⓒ
Nyotran
nystatin
Nystatin-LF
Nystex
PMS-Terbinafine Ⓒ
Sporanox
terbinafine HCl
Antifungals, Topical
[see also: Dermatological Preparations;
   Mouth and Throat Preparations;
   Vaginal Preparations, Antifungal]
Ala-Quin
amphotericin B
amphotericin B deoxycholate
amphotericin B lipid complex
   (ABLC)
Bensal HP
benzoic acid
betamethasone dipropionate & clo-
   trimazole
butenafine HCl
Castellani Paint Modified
ciclopirox

Antifungals, Topical (cont.)
ciclopirox olamine
clioquinol
clotrimazole (CLT)
clotrimazole & betamethasone
   dipropionate
Corque
econazole nitrate
Exelderm
Exsel
1+1-F Creme
fuchsin, basic
Fungizone
Fungoid
Fungoid-HC
gentian violet
haloprogin
Halotex
ketoconazole
Lamisil DermGel
Loprox
Lotrimin
Lotrisone
Mentax
miconazole nitrate
Monistat-Derm
Mycelex
Myco-Biotic II
Myco-Triacet II
Mycogen II
Mycolog-II
Myconel
Mycostatin
Mytrex
N.G.T.
naftifine HCl
Naftin
Nilstat
Nizoral
nystatin
Nystex
oxiconazole nitrate
Oxistat
Oxizole Ⓝ
Pedi-Cort V Creme
Pedi-Dri
Penlac
resorcinol
selenium sulfide
Selsun

Antifungals, Topical (cont.)
Spectazole
sulconazole nitrate
terbinafine HCl
tolnaftate
Tri-Statin II
undecylenic acid

Antihistamines
Antihistamines, Systemic
[*see also: Allergy and Anaphylaxis
   Agents*]
Aclophen
acrivastine
Actagen-C Cough
Actifed with Codeine Cough
Aerius Ⓝ
AH-chew
Allegra
Allegra-D
Allent
Allerfrin with Codeine
AlleRx
Alumadrine
Ambenyl Cough
Amgenal Cough
Ana-Kit
Anamine
Anamine T.D.
Anaplex
Anaplex DM Cough
Anaplex HD
Andehist
Andehist DM
Anergan 50
Aprodine with Codeine
astemizole
Atarax
Atarax 100
Atrohist Pediatric
Atrohist Plus
Atuss DM
Atuss HD
azatadine maleate
Ben-Allergin-50
Benadryl
Benadryl Allergy
Biohist-LA
Brexin-L.A.

Indications

Antihistamines, Systemic (cont.)

Brofed
Bromadine-DM
Bromadine-DX
Bromanate DC Cough
Bromanyl
Bromarest DX Cough
Bromatane DX Cough
Bromfed
Bromfed-DM Cough
Bromfed-PD
Bromfenex
Bromfenex PD
Bromophen T.D.
Bromotuss with Codeine
Bromphen DC with Codeine Cough
Bromphen DX Cough
brompheniramine maleate
brompheniramine maleate & pseu-
    doephedrine HCl & dextrometh-
    orphan hydrobromide
Brompheniramine DC Cough
Bronkotuss Expectorant
carbinoxamine maleate
Carbinoxamine Compound
Carbiset
Carbiset-TR
Carbodec
Carbodec DM
Carbodec TR
Cardec-DM
Cardec-S
cetirizine HCl
Chlor-Pro
Chlor-100
Chlor-Trimeton
Chlorafed; Chlorafed HS
Chlordrine S.R.
Chlorgest-HD
Chlorphedrine SR
chlorphenamine maleate
chlorpheniramine maleate
chlorpheniramine maleate & phen-
    ylpropanolamine HCl
chlorpheniramine polistirex
Chlorspan-12
Claritin
Claritin-D; Claritin-D 12 Hour;
    Claritin-D 24 Hour
clemastine fumarate

Antihistamines, Systemic (cont.)

Codehist DH
Codimal DH
Codimal-L.A.; Codimal-L.A. Half
Coldec DM
Colfed-A
Comhist
Comhist LA
Cophene-B
Cophene No. 2
Cotridin ⒸⒶⒺ
Cotridin Expectorant ⒸⒶⒺ
cyproheptadine HCl
D.A.
D.A. II
Dallergy
Dallergy-JR
Decohistine DH
Deconamine
Deconamine SR
Decongestabs
Decongestant
Deconhist L.A.
Deconomed SR
Dehist
Dehistine
Dexaphen S.A.
dexbrompheniramine maleate
Dexchlor
dexchlorpheniramine maleate
dextromethorphan hydrobromide &
    brompheniramine maleate &
    pseudoephedrine HCl
Diamine T.D.
Dimetane-DC Cough
Dimetane-DX Cough
diphenhydramine HCl
Disobrom
Donatussin
Drixomed
Drize
Dura-Tap/PD
Dura-Vent/A
Dura-Vent/DA
Duralex
E.N.T.
Ed A-Hist
ED-TLC; ED Tuss HC
Endafed
Endagen-HD

Antihistamines, Systemic (cont.)
Endal-HD; Endal-HD Plus
Ex-Histine
Extendryl
Extendryl JR
Extendryl SR
Fedahist
fexofenadine HCl
Gelhist
Genahist
Hismanal
Hista-Vadrin
Histade
Histalet
Histalet Forte
Histex HC
Histex PD
Histex SR
Histine DM; Histinex DM
Histinex HC
Histinex PV
Histor-D
Histussin HC
Hycomine Compound
Hydramyn
Hydro-PC
Hydrocodone CP; Hydrocodone HD
Hydrophed
hydroxyzine HCl
hydroxyzine pamoate
Hyphed
Hyrexin-50
Iodal HD
Iofed
Iofed PD
Iohist D
Iohist DM
Iotussin HC
K-Phen-50
ketotifen fumarate
Klerist-D
Kronofed-A Jr.
Kronofed-A
Kutrase
Liqui-Histine-D
Liqui-Histine DM
Lodrane LD
loratadine
Marax-DF
Mescolor

Antihistamines, Systemic (cont.)
methdilazine HCl
Myidyl
Myphetane DC Cough
Myphetane DX Cough
Naldecon
Naldelate
Nalgest
Nasahist B
ND Clear
ND Stat
Nolamine
Norel Plus
Novafed A
Novahistine DH
OMNIhist L.A.
Optimine
Oraminic II
Ornade
P-V-Tussin
Palgic-D
Palgic-DS
Pancof-HC
Pannaz
Para-Hist HD
PBZ
PBZ-SR
Pediacof
Pedituss Cough
Pelamine
Pentazine
Pentazine VC with Codeine
Periactin
Phenahist-TR
Phenameth
Phenameth DM
Phenate
Phenazine 50
Phenchlor S.H.A.
Phenergan
Phenergan Fortis
Phenergan Plain
Phenergan VC
Phenergan VC with Codeine
Phenergan with Codeine
Phenergan with Dextromethorphan
Phenetron
Phenhist DH with Codeine
phenindamine tartrate
pheniramine maleate

Antihistamines, Systemic (cont.)
Phenoject-50
phenylpropanolamine HCl & chlor-
    pheniramine maleate
phenyltoloxamine citrate
Pherazine DM
Pherazine VC with Codeine
Pherazine with Codeine
Poladex
Polaramine
Polaramine Expectorant
Poly-Histine
Poly-Histine CS
Poly-Histine-D
Poly-Histine-D Ped Caps
Poly-Histine DM
Prehist
Prehist D
Pro-50
Prometh-50
Prometh VC Plain
Prometh VC with Codeine
Prometh with Codeine
Prometh with Dextromethorphan
promethazine HCl
Promethazine DM
Promethazine VC
Promethazine VC Plain
Promethazine VC with Codeine
Promethist with Codeine
Prorex-25; Prorex-50
Prothazine
Prothazine Plain
Pseudo-Car DM
Pseudo-Chlor
pseudoephedrine HCl & dextro-
    methorphan hydrobromide &
    brompheniramine maleate
pyrilamine maleate
R-Tanna 12
R-Tannamine
R-Tannate
R-Tannic-S A/D
Reactine Ⓒᴬᴺ
Rentamine Pediatric
Resaid
Rescon
Rescon-ED
Rescon JR
Respahist

Antihistamines, Systemic (cont.)
Rhinatate
Rhinolar-EX; Rhinolar-EX 12
Rinade B.I.D.
Rolatuss Expectorant
Rolatuss with Hydrocodone
Rondamine-DM
Rondec
Rondec-DM
Rondec-TR
Ru-Tuss with Hydrocodone
Ryna-C
Rynatan
Rynatan-12 S
Rynatan-S
Rynatuss
S-T Forte 2
Seldane
Seldane-D
Semprex-D
Sildec-DM
Siltapp with Dextromethorphan
    HBr Cold & Cough
Sinusol-B
Stahist
Statuss Green
T-Koff
Tacaryl
Tamine S.R.
Tanafed
Tannic-12
Tanoral
Tavist
Telachlor
terfenadine
Theomax DF
Time-Hist
Touro A & H; Touro Allergy
Tri-P
Tri-Phen-Chlor
Tri-Phen-Chlor T.R.
Tri-Phen-Mine
Tri-Phen-Mine S.R.
Tri-Tannate
Tri-Tannate Plus Pediatric
Triacin-C Cough
Triafed with Codeine
Triaminic
Triaminic Expectorant DH
Tricodene Cough and Cold

Antihistamines, Systemic (cont.)
  Trifed-C Cough
  trimeprazine tartrate
  Trinalin
  Triotann
  tripelennamine HCl
  triprolidine HCl
  Tritan
  Tusquelin
  Tuss-Tan
  Tussafed
  Tussanil DH
  Tussend
  Tussi-12
  Tussionex Pennkinetic
  Tussirex
  Tusstat
  UltraBrom
  UltraBrom PD
  Uni-Decon
  Unituss HC
  Vanex Forte
  Vanex Forte-R
  Vanex-HD
  Veltane
  Vetuss HC
  Vistaril
  Vistazine 50
  Xiral
  Zyrtec
  Zyrtec-D
Antihistamines, Topical
  [see also: Dermatological Preparations;
    Nasal Preparations, Antiallergic;
    Ophthalmologicals, Antiallergic]
  chlorcyclizine HCl
  diphenhydramine HCl
  doxepin HCl
  Mantadil
  phenyltoloxamine citrate
  pyrilamine maleate
  tripelennamine HCl
  Zonalon

Antihypertensives
  [see also: Cardiac Agents]
Antihypertensives, α-Blockers
  Alti-Doxazosin ⓒⒶⓃ

Antihypertensives, α-Blockers (cont.)
  Apo-Doxazosin ⓒⒶⓃ
  Apo-Terazosin ⓒⒶⓃ
  Cardura
  doxazosin mesylate
  Gen-Doxazosin ⓒⒶⓃ
  Hytrin
  Hytrin ⓒⒶⓃ
  labetalol HCl
  Minipress
  Minizide 1; Minizide 2; Minizide 5
  Normodyne
  Novo-Terazosin ⓒⒶⓃ
  phentolamine mesylate
  PMS-Terazosin ⓒⒶⓃ
  prazosin HCl
  Regitine
  terazosin HCl
  Trandate
Antihypertensives, ACE Inhibitors
  Accupril
  Accuretic
  Aceon
  Altace
  benazepril HCl
  Capoten
  Capozide 25/15; Capozide 25/25;
    Capozide 50/15; Capozide 50/25
  captopril
  captopril & hydrochlorothiazide
  cilazapril
  enalapril maleate
  enalapril maleate & hydrochlorothi-
    azide
  enalaprilat
  fosinopril sodium
  gemopatrilat
  hydrochlorothiazide & captopril
  hydrochlorothiazide & enalapril
    maleate
  Lexxel
  lisinopril
  Lotensin
  Lotensin HCT 5/6.25; Lotensin
    HCT 10/12.5; Lotensin HCT
    20/12.5; Lotensin HCT 20/25
  Lotrel
  Mavik

Indications

Antihypertensives, ACE Inhibitors (cont.)

Mavik (CAN)
moexipril HCl
Monopril
Monopril-HCT
Nu-Enalapril (CAN)
omapatrilat
perindopril erbumine
PMS-Captopril (CAN)
Prinivil
Prinzide
Prinzide 12.5; Prinzide 25
quinapril HCl
ramipril
spirapril HCl
Tarka
Teczem
trandolapril
Uniretic
Univasc
Vanlev
Vaseretic 5-12.5; Vaseretic 10-25
Vasotec
Vasotec I.V.
Zestoretic
Zestril

Antihypertensives, Angiotensin II Inhibitors

Atacand
Atacand HCT
Avalide
Avapro
candesartan cilexetil
Cozaar
Diovan
Diovan HCT
eprosartan mesylate
Hyzaar
irbesartan
losartan potassium
Micardis
Micardis HCT
Micardis Plus (CAN)
olmesartan
tasosartan
telmisartan
Teveten
valsartan
Verdia

Antihypertensives, β-Blockers

acebutolol HCl
Apo-Metoprolol (CAN)
Apo-Metoprolol L (CAN)
Apo-Atenolol (CAN)
atenolol
Betachron E-R
betaxolol HCl
bisoprolol fumarate
bisoprolol fumarate & hydrochloro-thiazide
Blocadren
carteolol HCl
celiprolol HCl
Corgard
Corzide 40/5; Corzide 80/5
Gen-Metoprolol (CAN)
Gen-Acebutolol (CAN)
hydrochlorothiazide & bisoprolol fumarate
Inderal
Inderal LA
Inderide 40/25; Inderide 80/25
Inderide LA 80/50; Inderide LA 120/50; Inderide LA 160/50
Kerlone
labetalol HCl
Levatol
Lopressor
Lopressor HCT 50/25; Lopressor HCT 100/25; Lopressor HCT 100/50
metoprolol succinate
metoprolol tartrate
Monocor (CAN)
nadolol
Normodyne
Novo-Metoprol (CAN)
Nu-Timolol (CAN)
penbutolol sulfate
pindolol
PMS-Pindolol (CAN)
Probeta
propranolol HCl
Sectral
Selecor
Tenoretic 50; Tenoretic 100
Tenormin
Timolide 10-25
timolol maleate
Toprol-XL

Antihypertensives, β-Blockers (cont.)
Trandate
Visken
Zebeta
Ziac

Antihypertensives, Calcium Channel Blockers
Adalat
Adalat CC; Adalat Oros
Adalat XL (CAN)
amlodipine
amlodipine besylate
Apo-Diltiaz (CAN)
Apo-Diltiaz CD (CAN)
Apo-Diltiaz SR (CAN)
Baypress
Calan
Calan SR
Cardene
Cardene I.V.
Cardene SR
Cardizem
Cardizem CD
Cardizem SR
Cardizem XL
Cartia XT
Chronovera (CAN)
Covera-HS
Dilacor XR
Diltia XT
diltiazem HCl
diltiazem malate
DynaCirc
DynaCirc CR
felodipine
Gen-Verapamil (CAN)
Isoptin
Isoptin SR
isradipine
lacidipine
Lacipil
Lexxel
Lotrel
mibefradil dihydrochloride
nicardipine HCl
Nifedical XL
nifedipine
nimodipine
nisoldipine

Antihypertensives, Calcium Channel Blockers (cont.)
nitrendipine
Norvasc
Novo-Diltiazem CD (CAN)
Nu-Diltiaz-CD (CAN)
Plendil
Posicor
Procardia
Procardia XL
Rhoxal-diltiazem CD (CAN)
Sular
Tarka
Teczem
Tiamate
Tiazac
verapamil HCl
Verelan
Verelan PM

Antihypertensives, Diuretics
[see also: Diuretics]
Accuretic
Aldactazide
Aldactone
Aldoclor-150; Aldoclor-250
Aldoril 15; Aldoril 25; Aldoril D30; Aldoril D50
amiloride HCl
Apo-Furosemide (CAN)
Apo-Hydro (CAN)
Apresazide 25/25; Apresazide 50/50; Apresazide 100/50
Aquatensen
Atacand HCT
Avalide
bendroflumethiazide
benzthiazide
bisoprolol fumarate & hydrochlorothiazide
bumetanide
Bumex
Capozide 25/15; Capozide 25/25; Capozide 50/15; Capozide 50/25
captopril & hydrochlorothiazide
chlorothiazide
chlorthalidone
Clorpres
Combipres 0.1; Combipres 0.2; Combipres 0.3
Corzide 40/5; Corzide 80/5

Indications

Antihypertensives, Diuretics (cont.)

Demadex
Demi-Regroton
Diovan HCT
Diucardin
Diurese
Diurigen
Diuril
Diutensen-R
Dyazide
Dyrenium
Edecrin
Edecrin Sodium
enalapril maleate & hydrochlorothi-
    azide
Enduron
Enduronyl; Enduronyl Forte
Esidrix
Esimil
ethacrynate sodium
ethacrynic acid
Exna
Ezide
furosemide
Hydrap-ES
Hydro-Par
Hydro-Serp
hydrochlorothiazide (HCT; HCTZ)
hydrochlorothiazide & bisoprolol
    fumarate
hydrochlorothiazide & captopril
hydrochlorothiazide & enalapril
    maleate
hydrochlorothiazide & triamterene
HydroDIURIL
hydroflumethiazide
Hydromox
Hydropres-50
Hydroserpine #1; Hydroserpine #2
Hygroton
Hyzaar
indapamide
Inderide 40/25; Inderide 80/25
Inderide LA 80/50; Inderide LA
    120/50; Inderide LA 160/50
Lasix
Lopressor HCT 50/25; Lopressor HCT
    100/25; Lopressor HCT 100/50

Antihypertensives, Diuretics (cont.)

Lotensin HCT 5/6.25; Lotensin
    HCT 10/12.5; Lotensin HCT
    20/12.5; Lotensin HCT 20/25
Lozol
mannitol (D-mannitol)
Marpres
Maxzide
Metahydrin
Metatensin #2; Metatensin #4
methyclothiazide
metolazone
Micardis HCT
Micardis Plus (CAN)
Microzide
Midamor
Minizide 1; Minizide 2; Minizide 5
Moduretic
Monopril-HCT
Mykrox
Naqua
Naturetin
Novo-Hydrazide (CAN)
Novo-Semide (CAN)
Oretic
Osmitrol
PMS-Indapamide (CAN)
polythiazide
Prinzide
Prinzide 12.5; Prinzide 25
quinethazone
Rauzide
Regroton
Renese
Renese-R
Saluron
Salutensin; Salutensin-Demi
Ser-Ap-Es
Sodium Diuril
spironolactone
Tenoretic 50; Tenoretic 100
Thalitone
Timolide 10-25
torsemide
Tri-Hydroserpine
triamterene
triamterene & hydrochlorothiazide
trichlormethiazide
Uniretic
Vaseretic 5-12.5; Vaseretic 10-25

Antihypertensives, Diuretics (cont.)
Zaroxolyn
Zestoretic
Ziac
Antihypertensives, Vasodilators
Apresazide 25/25; Apresazide 50/50;
    Apresazide 100/50
Apresoline
Bidil
Corlopam
Cyclo-Prostin
diazoxide
epoprostenol
fenoldopam mesylate
Flolan
hydralazine HCl
Hydrap-ES
Hyperstat
Loniten
Marpres
minoxidil
Nitro-Bid IV
nitroglycerin
Nitropress
Proglycem
Ser-Ap-Es
sodium nitroprusside
Tri-Hydroserpine
Tridil
trimethaphan camsylate
Antihypertensives, Other
Aldomet
Aldomet; Aldomet Ester HCl
Amodopa
Catapres
Catapres-TTS-1; Catapres-TTS-2;
    Catapres-TTS-3
clonidine HCl
Demser
deserpidine
Dibenzyline
guanabenz acetate
guanadrel sulfate
guanethidine monosulfate
guanfacine HCl
Hylorel
Inversine
Ismelin
mecamylamine HCl
methyldopa

Antihypertensives, Other (cont.)
methyldopate HCl
metyrosine
moxonidine
phenoxybenzamine HCl
Physiotens
pinacidil
Pindac
rauwolfia serpentina
rescinnamine
reserpine
Tenex
Wytensin

Antineoplastics
[see also: Immunostimulants; Immuno-
    suppressants; Urinary Tract Agents,
    Antineoplastics]
Antineoplastics, Alkylating
Alkeran
BiCNU
busulfan
Busulfex
carboplatin
carmustine
CeeNu
chlorambucil
cisplatin
cyclophosphamide
Cytoxan
dacarbazine
Dacplat
DTIC-Dome
Eloxatin
Emcyt
estramustine phosphate sodium
Foloxatine
Gliadel
Ifex
ifosfamide
IntraDose
Leukeran
lomustine
mechlorethamine HCl
melphalan (MPL)
Mustargen
Myleran
Neosar
oxaliplatin

Indications

Antineoplastics, Alkylating (cont.)
Paraplatin
Platinol
Platinol-AQ
streptozocin
Temodal ⒸⒶⓃ
Temodar
temozolomide
Thioplex
thiotepa
Transplatin
Triapine
Zanosar

Antineoplastics, Angiogenesis Inhibitors
AE-941
BeneFin
Neovastat
squalamine
SU-5416
Vitaxin

Antineoplastics, Antibiotics
Adriamycin PFS
Adriamycin RDF
Blenoxane
bleomycin sulfate
Caelyx ⒸⒶⓃ
Cerubidine
Cosmegen
dactinomycin
DaunoXome
daunorubicin citrate, liposomal
daunorubicin HCl
Doxil
doxorubicin HCl
doxorubicin HCl, liposome-encapsulated (LED)
Ellence
epirubicin HCl
Evacet
Idamycin
Idamycin PFS
idarubicin HCl
Lysodren
Mithracin
mitomycin
mitotane
mitoxantrone HCl
MTC-DOX (magnetically targeted carrier with doxorubicin)

Antineoplastics, Antibiotics (cont.)
Mutamycin
Nipent
Novantrone
pentostatin
Pharmorubicin PFS; Pharmorubicin RDF ⒸⒶⓃ
plicamycin
Rubex
valrubicin
Valstar
Valtaxin ⒸⒶⓃ

Antineoplastics, Antimetabolites
Adrucil
alemtuzumab
allopurinol
allopurinol sodium
Aloprim
Campath
capecitabine
Carac
cladribine
cytarabine
cytarabine, liposomal
Cytosar-U
denileukin diftitox
DepoCyt
Efudex
floxuridine
Fludara
fludarabine phosphate
Fluoroplex
fluorouracil (5-FU)
Folex PFS
FUDR
gemcitabine
Gemzar
Hydrea
hydroxyurea
Leustatin
mercaptopurine (6-MP)
methotrexate (MTX)
methotrexate sodium
Mylocel
Ontak
prinomastat
Purinethol
raltitrexed
Rheumatrex
Tarabine PFS

Antineoplastics, Antimetabolites (cont.)
tegafur
thioguanine (6-TG)
Tomudex
Trexall
UFT
Xeloda
Zyloprim

Antineoplastics, DNA Synthesis Inhibitors
Camptosar
gemtuzumab ozogamicin
Hycamtin
irinotecan HCl
Mylotarg
topotecan HCl

Antineoplastics, Hormones
Andro L.A. 200
Android
Android-10; Android-25
Andropository-200
Aquest
buserelin acetate
chlorotrianisene
Delatestryl
Delestrogen
depAndro 100; depAndro 200
Depo-Provera
Depo-Testosterone
Depotest 100; Depotest 200
diethylstilbestrol (DES)
diethylstilbestrol diphosphate
Dioval XX; Dioval 40
Durabolin
Duratest 100; Duratest 200
Durathate-200
Emcyt
Estinyl
Estra-L 20
Estra-L 40
Estrace
estradiol
estradiol valerate
estramustine phosphate sodium
Estratab
Estrogenic Substance Aqueous
estrogens, conjugated
estrogens, esterified
estrone

Antineoplastics, Hormones (cont.)
Estrone 5
Estrone Aqueous
ethinyl estradiol
Everone 200
fluoxymesterone
goserelin acetate
Gynogen L.A. 20
Halotestin
Histerone 100
Hybolin Improved
Kestrone 5
Lin-Megestrol ⒸⒶⓃ
Lupron Depot
Lupron Depot–3 month; Lupron Depot–4 month
Lupron; Lupron Pediatric
medroxyprogesterone acetate (MPA)
Megace
megestrol acetate
Menest
Methitest
methyltestosterone
nandrolone phenpropionate
Oreton Methyl
PEG-camptothecin
Premarin
ProMaxx-100
Prothecan
Stilphostrol
Suprefact; Suprefact Depot ⒸⒶⓃ
Tace
Tesamone
Teslac
Testandro
testolactone
testosterone
testosterone cypionate
testosterone enanthate
Testosterone Aqueous
Testred
Trelstar Depot
triptorelin pamoate
Valergen 20; Valergen 40
Virilon
Zoladex
Zoladex LA ⒸⒶⓃ

Antineoplastics, Hormone Antagonists
aminoglutethimide

Indications

Antineoplastics, Hormone Antagonists (cont.)
Anandron ⒸⒶⓃ
anastrozole
Arimidex
Aromasin
bicalutamide
Casodex
cyproterone acetate
Cytadren
Euflex ⒸⒶⓃ
Eulexin
exemestane
Fareston
Faslodex
Femara
flutamide
fluvestrant
Gen-Cyproterone ⒸⒶⓃ
letrozole
Leuprogel
leuprolide acetate
Nilandron
nilutamide
Nolvadex
Novo-Cyproterone ⒸⒶⓃ
PMS-Tamoxifen ⒸⒶⓃ
tamoxifen citrate
toremifene citrate
trilostane
Viadur

Antineoplastics, Plant Alkaloids and Other Natural Products
docetaxel
Eldisine
Etopophos
etoposide
etoposide phosphate
Navelbine
Oncovin
Onxol
paclitaxel
Paxene
Taxol
Taxotere
teniposide
Toposar
triptolide
Velban
VePesid

Antineoplastics, Plant Alkaloids and Other Natural Products (cont.)
vinblastine sulfate
Vincasar PFS
vincristine sulfate
vindesine sulfate
vinorelbine tartrate
Vumon

Antineoplastics, Protective and Rescue Agents
amifostine
dexrazoxane
Ethyol
Isovorin
Leucotropin
L-leucovorin
leucovorin calcium
mesna
Mesnex
pilocarpine HCl
regramostim
Salagen
sucralfate
Wellcovorin
Zinecard

Antineoplastics, Therapeutic Vaccines (Theraccines)
AdjuVax-100a
autologous cell (AC) vaccine
Avicine
BCG vaccine (bacillus Calmette-Guérin)
BrevaRex
Gastrimmune
GVAX
M-Vax
Melacine
melanoma vaccine
monoclonal antibody B43.13
NovoVac
O-Vax
OncoVax-CL
OncoVax-Pr
OvaRex
Pacis
TA-HPV
TheraCys
Theratope-STn
Tice BCG

Antineoplastics, Therapeutic Vaccines (Theraccines) (cont.)

vaccinia virus vaccine for human papillomavirus (HPV)

Antineoplastics, Unclassified and Adjuncts

Abarelix-Depot-M

AdjuVax-100a

aldesleukin

Allovectin-7

altretamine

Amdray

9-aminocamptothecin (9-AC)

amsacrine

Amsidyl

Anticort

Apra

Aptosyn

Armour Thyroid

Aroplatin

arsenic trioxide (AsO_3)

asparaginase (L-asparaginase)

Atragen

Avicidin

azacitidine (5-AZA; 5-AZC)

beta alethine

Beta LT

Betathine

bexarotene

Bexxar

biricodar dicitrate

blood mononuclear cells, allogenic peripheral

Bondronat

Bonefos (CAN)

Bonviva

Broxine

broxuridine

calcifediol (25-hydroxycholecalciferol; 25-hydroxyvitamin D_3)

Calderol

CEA-Cide

Ceprate SC

chromic phosphate P 32

clodronate disodium

coumarin

CYT-103-Y-90

CytoImplant

Detox-B

Antineoplastics, Unclassified and Adjuncts (cont.)

disaccharide tripeptide glycerol dipalmitoyl

disodium clodronate tetrahydrate

edodekin alfa

edrecolomab

Elspar

EpiLeukin

Ergamisol

Erwinase

erwinia L-asparaginase

exisulind

Foscan

Gd-Tex

Genasense

Gleevec

Herceptin

Hexalen

ibandronate sodium

ibritumomab tiuxetan

ImmTher

imatinib mesylate

ImmuRAIT-LL2

Imuvert

Incel

interleukin-4 (IL-4) Pseudomonas toxin fusion protein

iodine I 131 Lym-1 MAb

iodine I 131 murine MAb IgG_2a to B cell

iodine I 131 murine MAb to alpha-fetoprotein (AFP)

iodine I 131 murine MAb to human chorionic gonadotropin (hCG)

iodine I 131 radiolabeled B1 MAb

iodine I 131 tositumomab

Iodotope

Leuvectin

levamisole HCl

lobradimil

Lu-Tex

Lutrin

LymphoCide

Matulane

methoxsalen (8-methoxsalen)

metoclopramide HCl

mitumomab

monoclonal antibody to CD22 antigen on B-cells, radiolabeled

Antineoplastics, Unclassified and Adjuncts (cont.)

monoclonal antibody to CEA, humanized
motexafin gadolinium
motexafin lutetium
MultiKine
MX-6
Neomark
nolatrexed dihydrochloride
Oncaspar
Onco-TCS
Oncocine-HspE7
Oncolym
Oncolysin B
Onconase
OncoPhage
OncoRad OV103
Oncostate
Onkolox
ONYX-015
Orzel
Ovastat
p30 protein
Panorex
pegaspargase (PEG-L-asparaginase)
pemetrexed disodium
perfosfamide
perillyl alcohol (POH)
Phosphocol P 32
Photofrin
Pivanex
porfimer sodium
prednimustine
Prevatac
procarbazine HCl
Purlytin
Regressin
Reosyn
reovirus
ricin (blocked) conjugated murine MAb (anti-B4)
Rolazar
rostaporfin
rubitecan
S-P-T
Sensamide
Serratia marcescens extract (polyribosomes)
sodium iodide (^{131}I)

Antineoplastics, Unclassified and Adjuncts (cont.)

sodium iodide I 131
sodium phosphate P 32
Sterecyt
Targretin
temoporfin
Theragyn
Thymitaq
Thyrar
Thyrogen
thyroid
thyrotropin alfa
tiazofurin
Tiazole
Tifolar
trastuzumab
treosulfan
tretinoin
Triacana
Trisenox
uracil
Uvadex
valspodar
Vesanoid
Virulizin
Xcytrin
Zevalin
zoledronic acid
Zometa

Antineoplastics, Chemotherapy Protocols

5 + 2 protocol (cytarabine, daunorubicin)
5 + 2 protocol (cytarabine, mitoxantrone)
7 + 3 protocol (cytarabine, daunorubicin)
7 + 3 protocol (cytarabine, idarubicin)
7 + 3 protocol (cytarabine, mitoxantrone)
8 in 1 (methylprednisolone, vincristine, lomustine, procarbazine, hydroxyurea, cisplatin, cytarabine, dacarbazine)
8 in 1 (methylprednisolone, vincristine, lomustine, procarbazine, hydroxyurea, cisplatin, cytarabine, cyclophosphamide)
A + D (ara-C, daunorubicin)

Antineoplastics, Chemotherapy Protocols (cont.)

A-DIC (Adriamycin, dacarbazine)

AA (ara-C, Adriamycin)

ABC (Adriamycin, BCNU, cyclophosphamide)

ABCM (Adriamycin, bleomycin, cyclophosphamide, mitomycin)

ABD (Adriamycin, bleomycin, DTIC)

ABDIC (Adriamycin, bleomycin, DIC, [CCNU, prednisone])

ABDV (Adriamycin, bleomycin, DTIC, vinblastine)

ABP (Adriamycin, bleomycin, prednisone)

ABV (actimomycin D, bleomycin, vincristine)

ABV (Adriamycin, bleomycin, vinblastine)

ABV (Adriamycin, bleomycin, vincristine)

ABVD (Adriamycin, bleomycin, vinblastine, dacarbazine)

ABVD/MOPP (alternating cycles of ABVD and MOPP)

AC (Adriamycin, carmustine)

AC (Adriamycin, CCNU)

AC (Adriamycin, cisplatin)

AC; A-C (Adriamycin, cyclophosphamide)

ACe (Adriamycin, cyclophosphamide)

ACE (Adriamycin, cyclophosphamide, etoposide)

ACFUCY (actinomycin D, fluorouracil, cyclophosphamide)

ACM (Adriamycin, cyclophosphamide, methotrexate)

ACOP (Adriamycin, cyclophosphamide, Oncovin, prednisone)

ACOPP; A-COPP (Adriamycin, cyclophosphamide, Oncovin, procarbazine, prednisone)

AD (Adriamycin, dacarbazine)

ADBC (Adriamycin, DTIC, bleomycin, CCNU)

ADE (ara-C, daunorubicin, etoposide)

ADOAP (Adriamycin, Oncovin, ara-C, prednisone)

Antineoplastics, Chemotherapy Protocols (cont.)

ADOP (Adriamycin, Oncovin, prednisone)

Adria + BCNU (Adriamycin, BCNU)

Adria-L-PAM (Adriamycin, L-phenylalanine mustard)

AFM (Adriamycin, fluorouracil, methotrexate [with leucovorin rescue])

ALOMAD (Adriamycin, Leukeran, Oncovin, methotrexate, actinomycin D, dacarbazine)

AOPA (ara-C, Oncovin, prednisone, asparaginase)

AOPE (Adriamycin, Oncovin, prednisone, etoposide)

AP (Adriamycin, Platinol)

APC (AMSA, prednisone, chlorambucil)

APE (Adriamycin, Platinol, etoposide)

APE (ara-C, Platinol, etoposide)

APO (Adriamycin, prednisone, Oncovin)

ara-C + 6-TG (ara-C, thioguanine)

ara-C + ADR (ara-C, Adriamycin)

ara-C + DNR + PRED + MP (ara-C, daunorubicin, prednisolone, mercaptopurine)

ara-C-HU (ara-C, hydroxyurea)

ARAC-DNR (ara-C, daunorubicin)

ASHAP; A-SHAP (Adriamycin, Solu-Medrol, high-dose ara-C, Platinol)

AV (Adriamycin, vincristine)

AVP (actinomycin D, vincristine, Platinol)

B-CHOP (bleomycin, Cytoxin, hydroxydaunomycin, Oncovin, prednisone)

B-DOPA (bleomycin, DTIC, Oncovin, prednisone, Adriamycin)

B-MOPP (bleomycin, nitrogen mustard, Oncovin, procarbazine, prednisone)

baby brain I

BAC (BCNU, ara-C, cyclophosphamide)

Antineoplastics, Chemotherapy Protocols (cont.)

BACOD (bleomycin, Adriamycin, CCNU, Oncovin, dexamethasone)

BACON (bleomycin, Adriamycin, CCNU, Oncovin, nitrogen mustard)

BACOP (bleomycin, Adriamycin, cyclophosphamide, Oncovin, prednisone)

BACT (BCNU, ara-C, cyclophosphamide, thioguanine)

Bagshawe protocol, modified

BAMON (bleomycin, Adriamycin, methotrexate, Oncovin, nitrogen mustard)

BAVIP (bleomycin, Adriamycin, vinblastine, imidazole carboxamide, prednisone)

BBVP-M (BCNU, bleomycin, VePesid, prednisone, methotrexate)

BCAP (BCNU, cyclophosphamide, Adriamycin, prednisone)

BCAVe; B-CAVe (bleomycin, CCNU, Adriamycin, Velban)

BCD (bleomycin, cyclophosphamide, dactinomycin)

BCMF (bleomycin, cyclophosphamide, methotrexate, fluorouracil)

BCOP (BCNU, cyclophosphamide, Oncovin, prednisone)

BCP (BCNU, cyclophosphamide, prednisone)

BCVP (BCNU, cyclophosphamide, vincristine, prednisone)

BCVPP (BCNU, cyclophosphamide, vinblastine, procarbazine, prednisone)

BEAC (BCNU, etoposide, ara-C, cyclophosphamide)

BEACOPP (bleomycin, etoposide, Adriamycin, cyclophosphamide, Oncovin, procarbazine, prednisone, [filgrastim])

BEAM (BCNU, etoposide, ara-C, melphalan)

BEMP (bleomycin, Eldisine, mitomycin, Platinol)

BEP (bleomycin, etoposide, Platinol)

Antineoplastics, Chemotherapy Protocols (cont.)

BHD (BCNU, hydroxyurea, dacarbazine)

BHDV; BHD-V (BCNU, hydroxyurea, dacarbazine, vincristine)

BIP (bleomycin, ifosfamide [with mesna rescue], Platinol)

BLEO-COMF (bleomycin, cyclophosphamide, Oncovin, methotrexate, fluorouracil)

BMP (BCNU, methotrexate, procarbazine)

BOAP (bleomycin, Oncovin, Adriamycin, prednisone)

BOLD (bleomycin, Oncovin, lomustine, dacarbazine)

BOMP (bleomycin, Oncovin, Matulane, prednisone)

BOMP; CLD-BOMP (bleomycin, Oncovin, mitomycin, Platinol)

BOP (BCNU, Oncovin, prednisone)

BOPAM (bleomycin, Oncovin, prednisone, Adriamycin, mechlorethamine, methotrexate)

BOPP (BCNU, Oncovin, procarbazine, prednisone)

BVAP (BCNU, vincristine, Adriamycin, prednisone)

BVCPP (BCNU, vinblastine, cyclophosphamide, procarbazine, prednisone)

BVDS (bleomycin, Velban, doxorubicin, streptozocin)

BVPP (BCNU, vincristine, procarbazine, prednisone)

CA-VP16; CAVP16 (cyclophosphamide, Adriamycin, VP-16)

CY-VA-DACT (Cytoxin, vincristine, Adriamycin, dactinomycin)

CaT (carboplatin, Taxol)

C-MOPP (cyclophosphamide, mechlorethamine, Oncovin, procarbazine, prednisone)

CA (cyclophosphamide, Adriamycin)

CA (cytarabine, asparaginase)

CABO (cisplatin, Abitrexate, bleomycin, Oncovin)

Antineoplastics, Chemotherapy Protocols (cont.)

CABOP; CA-BOP (Cytoxin, Adriamycin, bleomycin, Oncovin, prednisone)

CABS (CCNU, Adriamycin bleomycin, streptozocin)

CAC (cisplatin, ara-C, caffeine)

CAD (cyclophosphamide, Adriamycin, dacarbazine)

CAD (cytarabine [and] daunorubicin)

CAE (cyclophosphamide, Adriamycin, etoposide)

CAF (cyclophosphamide, Adriamycin, fluorouracil)

CAFP (cyclophosphamide, Adriamycin, fluorouracil, prednisone)

CAFTH (cyclophosphamide, Adriamycin, fluorouracil, tamoxifen, Halotestin)

CAFVP (cyclophosphamide, Adriamycin, fluorouracil, vincristine, prednisone)

CAL-G (cyclophosphamide, asparaginase, leurocristine, daunorubicin, prednisone)

CALF (cyclophosphamide, Adriamycin, leucovorin [rescue], fluorouracil)

CALF-E (cyclophosphamide, Adriamycin, leucovorin [rescue], fluorouracil, ethinyl estradiol)

CAM (cyclophosphamide, Adriamycin, methotrexate)

CAMB (Cytoxin, Adriamycin, methotrexate, bleomycin)

CAMELEON (cytosine arabinoside, methotrexate, Leukovorin, Oncovin)

CAMEO (cyclophosphamide, Adriamycin, methotrexate, etoposide, Oncovin)

CAMF (cyclophosphamide, Adriamycin, methotrexate, folinic acid)

CAMP (cyclophosphamide, Adriamycin, methotrexate, procarbazine HCl)

CAO (cyclophosphamide, Adriamycin, Oncovin)

Antineoplastics, Chemotherapy Protocols (cont.)

CAP (cyclophosphamide, Adriamycin, Platinol)

CAP (cyclophosphamide, Adriamycin, prednisone)

CAP; CAP-I (cyclophosphamide, Adriamycin, Platinol)

CAP-BOP (cyclophosphamide, Adriamycin, procarbazine, bleomycin, Oncovin, prednisone)

CAP-II (cyclophosphamide, Adriamycin, high-dose Platinol)

CAPPr (cyclophosphamide, Adriamycin, Platinol, prednisone)

carboplatin & etoposide & paclitaxel

CAT (cytarabine, Adriamycin, thioguanine)

CAV (cyclophosphamide, Adriamycin, vinblastine)

CAV (cyclophosphamide, Adriamycin, vincristine)

CAVE (cyclophosphamide, Adriamycin, vincristine, etoposide)

CAVe; CA-Ve (CCNU, Adriamycin, vinblastine)

CBV (cyclophosphamide, BCNU, VePesid)

CBV (cyclophosphamide, BCNU, VP-16-213)

CC (carboplatin, cyclophosphamide)

CCV-AV (CCNU, cyclophosphamide, vincristine [alternates with] Adriamycin, vincristine)

CCM (cyclophosphamide, CCNU, methotrexate)

CCVPP (CCNU, cyclophosphamide, Velban, procarbazine, prednisone)

CD (cytarabine, daunorubicin)

CDC (carboplatin, doxorubicin, cyclophosphamide)

CDDP/VP; CDDP/VP-16 (CDDP, VP-16)

CDE (cyclophosphamide, doxorubicin, etoposide)

CEB (carboplatin, etoposide, bleomycin)

CECA (cisplatin, etoposide, cyclophosphamide, Adriamycin)

Antineoplastics, Chemotherapy Protocols (cont.)

CEF (cyclophosphamide, epirubicin, fluorouracil, [co-trimoxazole])

CEM (cytosine arabinoside, etoposide, methotrexate)

CEP (CCNU, etoposide, prednimustine)

CEPP (cyclophosphamide, etoposide, prednisone)

CEPPB (cyclophosphamide, etoposide, prednisone, bleomycin)

CEV (cyclophosphamide, etoposide, vincristine)

CF (carboplatin, fluorouracil)

CF (cisplatin, fluorouracil)

CFL (cisplatin, fluorouracil, leucovorin [rescue])

CFM (cyclophosphamide, fluorouracil, mitoxantrone)

CFP (cyclophosphamide, fluorouracil, prednisone)

CFPT (cyclophosphamide, fluorouracil, prednisone, tamoxifen)

CH1VPP; Ch1VPP (chlorambucil, vinblastine, procarbazine, prednisone)

CHAD (cyclophosphamide, hexamethylmelamine, Adriamycin, DDP)

CHAMOCA (cyclophosphamide, hydroxyurea, actinomycin D, methotrexate, Oncovin, calcium folinate, Adriamycin)

CHAP (cyclophosphamide, Hexalen, Adriamycin, Platinol)

CHAP (cyclophosphamide, hexamethylmelamine, Adriamycin, Platinol)

ChexUP; Chex-Up; CHEX-UP (cyclophosphamide, hexamethylmelamine, fluorouracil, Platinol)

CHF (cyclophosphamide, hexamethylmelamine, fluorouracil)

CHL + PRED (chlorambucil, prednisone)

ChlVPP (chlorambucil, vinblastine, procarbazine, prednisone/prednisolone)

Antineoplastics, Chemotherapy Protocols (cont.)

ChlVPP/EVA (chlorambucil, vinblastine, procarbazine, prednisone/prednisolone, etoposide, vincristine, Adriamycin)

CHO (cyclophosphamide, hydroxydaunomycin, Oncovin)

CHOB (cyclophosphamide, hydroxydaunomycin, Oncovin, bleomycin)

CHOD (cyclophosphamide, hydroxydaunomycin, Oncovin, dexamethasone)

CHOP (cyclophosphamide, hydroxydaunomycin, Oncovin, prednisone)

CHOP-BLEO (cyclophosphamide, hydroxydaunomycin, Oncovin, prednisone, bleomycin)

CHOPE (cyclophosphamide, hydroxydaunomycin, Oncovin, prednisone, etoposide)

CHOR (cyclophosphamide, hydroxydaunomycin, Oncovin, radiation therapy)

CHVP (cyclophosphamide, hydroxydaunomycin, VM-26, prednisone)

CISCA; CisCA (cisplatin, cyclophosphamide, Adriamycin)

$CISCA_{II}/VB_{IV}$ (cisplatin, cyclophosphamide, Adriamycin, vinblastine, bleomycin)

cisplatin & docetaxel

cisplatin & vinorelbine tartrate

CIVPP (chlorambucil, vinblastine, procarbazine, prednisone)

CLD-BOMP

CMC (cyclophosphamide, methotrexate, CCNU)

CMC-VAP (cyclophosphamide, methotrexate, CCNU, vincristine, Adriamycin, procarbazine)

CMF/AV (cyclophosphamide, methotrexate, fluorouracil, Adriamycin, Oncovin)

CMF; CMF-IV (cyclophosphamide, methotrexate, fluorouracil)

Antineoplastics, Chemotherapy Protocols (cont.)

CMFAVP (cyclophosphamide, methotrexate, fluorouracil, Adriamycin, vincristine, prednisone)

CMFP; CMF-P (cyclophosphamide, methotrexate, fluorouracil, prednisone)

CMFPT (cyclophosphamide, methotrexate, fluorouracil, prednisone, tamoxifen)

CMFPTH (cyclophosphamide, methotrexate, fluorouracil, prednisone, tamoxifen, Halotestin)

CMFT (cyclophosphamide, methotrexate, fluorouracil, tamoxifen)

CMFVAT (cyclophosphamide, methotrexate, fluorouracil, vincristine, Adriamycin, testosterone)

CMFVP (cyclophosphamide, methotrexate, fluorouracil, vincristine, prednisone)

CMH (cyclophosphamide, m-AMSA, hydroxyurea)

CMV (cisplatin, methotrexate, vinblastine)

CNF (cyclophosphamide, Novantrone, fluorouracil)

CNOP (cyclophosphamide, Novantrone, Oncovin, prednisone)

COAP (cyclophosphamide, Oncovin, ara-C, prednisone)

COAP-BLEO (cyclophosphamide, Oncovin, ara-C, prednisone, bleomycin)

COB (cisplatin, Oncovin, bleomycin)

CODE (cisplatin, Oncovin, doxorubicin, etoposide)

COF/COM (cyclophosphamide, Oncovin, fluorouracil + cyclophosphamide, Oncovin, methotrexate)

COM (cyclophosphamide, Oncovin, MeCCNU)

COM (cyclophosphamide, Oncovin, methotrexate)

COMA-A (cyclophosphamide, Oncovin, methotrexate/citrovorum factor, Adriamycin, ara-C)

COMB (cyclophosphamide, Oncovin, MeCCNU, bleomycin)

Antineoplastics, Chemotherapy Protocols (cont.)

COMB (Cytoxin, Oncovin, methotrexate, bleomycin)

COMe (Cytoxin, Oncovin, methotrexate)

COMF (cyclophosphamide, Oncovin, methotrexate, fluorouracil)

COMLA (cyclophosphamide, Oncovin, methotrexate, leucovorin [rescue], ara-C)

COMP (CCNU, Oncovin, methotrexate, procarbazine)

COMP (cyclophosphamide, Oncovin, methotrexate, prednisone)

CONPADRI; CONPADRI-I (cyclophosphamide, Oncovin, L-phenylalanine mustard, Adriamycin)

Cooper regimen

COP (cyclophosphamide, Oncovin, prednisone)

COPA-BLEO (cyclophosphamide, Oncovin, prednisone, Adriamycin, bleomycin)

COP-BLAM (cyclophosphamide, Oncovin, prednisone, bleomycin, Adriamycin, Matulane)

COP-BLEO (cyclophosphamide, Oncovin, prednisone, bleomycin)

COPA (Cytoxin, Oncovin, prednisone, Adriamycin)

COPAC (CCNU, Oncovin, prednisone, Adriamycin, cyclophosphamide)

COPB (cyclophosphamide, Oncovin, prednisone, bleomycin)

COPE (cyclophosphamide, Oncovin, Platinol, etoposide)

COPP (CCNU, Oncovin, procarbazine, prednisone)

COPP (cyclophosphamide, Oncovin, procarbazine, prednisone)

CP (chlorambucil, prednisone)

CP (cyclophosphamide, Platinol)

CP (cyclophosphamide, prednisone)

CPB (cyclophosphamide, Platinol, BCNU)

CPC (cyclophosphamide, Platinol, carboplatin)

Indications

Antineoplastics, Chemotherapy Protocols (cont.)

CPM (CCNU, procarbazine, methotrexate)

CPOB (cyclophosphamide, prednisone, Oncovin, bleomycin)

CT (cisplatin, Taxol)

CT (cytarabine, thioguanine)

CTCb (cyclophosphamide, thiotepa, carboplatin)

Ctx-Plat (cyclophosphamide, Platinol)

CV (cisplatin, VePesid)

CVA-BMP; CVA + BMP (cyclophosphamide, vincristine, Adriamycin, BCNU, methotrexate, procarbazine)

CVA (cyclophosphamide, vincristine, Adriamycin)

CVAD; C-VAD (cyclophosphamide, vincristine, Adriamycin, dexamethasone)

CVB (CCNU, vinblastine, bleomycin)

CVBD (CCNU, bleomycin, vinblastine, dexamethasone)

CVD (cisplatin, vinblastine, dacarbazine)

CVD+IL-2I (cisplatin, vinblastine, dacarbazine, interleukin-2, interferon alfa)

CVEB (cisplatin, vinblastine, etoposide, bleomycin)

CVI (carboplatin, VePesid, ifosfamide [with mesna rescue])

CVM (cyclophosphamide, vincristine, methotrexate)

CVP (cyclophosphamide, vincristine, prednisone)

CVPP (CCNU, vinblastine, procarbazine, prednisone)

CVPP (cyclophosphamide, Velban, procarbazine, prednisone)

CVPP-CCNU (cyclophosphamide, vinblastine, procarbazine, prednisone, CCNU)

CyADIC (cyclophosphamide, Adriamycin, DIC)

CyHOP (cyclophosphamide, Halotestin, Oncovin, prednisone)

Antineoplastics, Chemotherapy Protocols (cont.)

CYTABOM (cytarabine, bleomycin, Oncovin, mechlorethamine)

CYVADIC; CY-VA-DIC; CyVADIC (cyclophosphamide, vincristine, Adriamycin, DIC)

CYVMAD (cyclophosphamide, vincristine, methotrexate, Adriamycin, DTIC)

DA (daunorubicin, ara-C)

DAL (daunorubicin, ara-C, L-asparaginase)

DAT (daunorubicin, ara-C, thioguanine)

DATVP (daunorubicin, ara-C, thioguanine, vincristine, prednisone)

DAV (daunorubicin, ara-C, VePesid)

DAVH (dibromodulcitol, Adriamycin, vincristine, Halotestin)

DC (daunorubicin, cytarabine)

DCMP (daunorubicin, cytarabine, mercaptopurine, prednisone)

DCPM (daunorubicin, cytarabine, prednisone, mercaptopurine)

DCT (daunorubicin, cytarabine, thioguanine)

DCV (DTIC, CCNU, vincristine)

DECAL (dexamethasone, etoposide, cisplatin, ara-C, L-asparaginase)

DFMO-MGBG (eflornithine, mitoguazone)

DFV (DDP, fluorouracil, VePesid)

DHAP (dexamethasone, high-dose ara-C, Platinol)

DI (doxorubicin, ifosfamide [with mesna rescue])

DMC (dactinomycin, methotrexate, cyclophosphamide)

1DMTX/6-MP (methotrexate [with leucovorin rescue], mercaptopurine)

DOAP (daunorubicin, Oncovin, ara-C, prednisone)

docetaxel & cisplatin

DTIC & tamoxifen citrate

DTIC-ACTD; DTIC-ACT-D (DTIC, actinomycin D)

DVB (DDP, vindesine, bleomycin)

Antineoplastics, Chemotherapy Protocols (cont.)

DVP (daunorubicin, vincristine, prednisone)

DVPL-ASP (daunorubicin, vincristine, prednisone, L-asparaginase)

DZAPO (daunorubicin, azacitidine, ara-C, prednisone, Oncovin)

E-VMAC (escalated methotrexate, vinblastine, Adriamycin, cisplatin)

E-VMAC (escalated methotrexate, vinblastine, Adriamycin, cyclophosphamide)

EAP (etoposide, Adriamycin, Platinol)

EC (etoposide, carboplatin)

ECHO (etoposide, cyclophosphamide, hydroxydaunomycin, Oncovin)

EDAP (etoposide, dexamethasone, ara-C, Platinol)

EFP (etoposide, fluorouracil, Platinol)

ELF (etoposide, leucovorin [rescue], fluorouracil)

EMA 86 (etoposide, mitoxantrone, ara-C)

EMACO (etoposide, methotrexate, actinomycin D, cyclophosphamide, Oncovin)

EP (etoposide, Platinol)

EPOCH (etoposide, prednisone, Oncovin, cyclophosphamide, Halotestin)

ESHAP (etoposide, Solu-Medrol, high-dose ara-C, Platinol)

ESHAP-MINE (alternating cycles of ESHAP and MINE)

estramustine & vinblastine sulfate

etoposide & paclitaxel & carboplatin

EVA (etoposide, vinblastine, Adriamycin)

F-CL (fluorouracil, leucovorin calcium [rescue])

FAC (fluorouracil, Adriamycin, cyclophosphamide)

FAC-LEV (fluorouracil, Adriamycin, Cytoxin, levamisole)

FAC-M (fluorouracil, Adriamycin, cyclophosphamide, methotrexate)

FAM (fluorouracil, Adriamycin, mitomycin)

Antineoplastics, Chemotherapy Protocols (cont.)

FAM-CF (fluorouracil, Adriamycin, mitomycin, citrovorum factor)

FAM-S (fluorouracil, Adriamycin, mitomycin, streptozocin)

FAME; FAMe (fluorouracil, Adriamycin, MeCCNU)

FAMMe (fluorouracil, Adriamycin, mitomycin, MeCCNU)

FAMTX (fluorouracil, Adriamycin, methotrexate [with leucovorin rescue])

FAP (fluorouracil, Adriamycin, Platinol)

FCAP (fluorouracil, cyclophosphamide, Adriamycin, Platinol)

FCE (fluorouracil, cisplatin, etoposide)

FCP (fluorouracil, cyclophosphamide, prednisone)

FEC (fluorouracil, epirubicin, cyclophosphamide)

FED (fluorouracil, etoposide, DDP)

FIME (fluorouracil, ICRF-159, MeCCNU)

FL (flutamide, leuprolide acetate)

FLAC (fluorouracil, leucovorin [rescue], Adriamycin, cyclophosphamide)

FLAP (fluorouracil, leucovorin [rescue], Adriamycin, Platinol)

FLe (fluorouracil, levamisole)

FLEP (fluorouracil, leucovorin, etoposide, Platinol)

FMS (fluorouracil, mitomycin, streptozocin)

FMV (fluorouracil, MeCCNU, vincristine)

FNC (fluorouracil, Novantrone, cyclophosphamide)

FNM (fluorouracil, Novantrone, methotrexate)

FOAM (fluorouracil, Oncovin, Adriamycin, mitomycin)

FOMI; FOMi (fluorouracil, Oncovin, mitomycin)

FU/LV (fluorouracil, leucovorin calcium [rescue])

FUM (fluorouracil, methotrexate)

Indications

Antineoplastics, Chemotherapy Protocols (cont.)

FUVAC (5-FU, vinblastine, Adriamycin, cyclophosphamide)

FZ (flutamide, Zoladex)

gemcitabine-cis (gemcitabine, cisplatin)

H-CAP (hexamethylmelamine, cyclophosphamide, Adriamycin, Platinol)

HAD (hexamethylmelamine, Adriamycin, DDP)

HAM (hexamethylmelamine, Adriamycin, melphalan)

HAM (hexamethylmelamine, Adriamycin, methotrexate)

HD-VAC (high-dose [methotrexate], vinblastine, Adriamycin, cisplatin)

HDMTX (high-dose methotrexate [with leucovorin rescue])

HDMTX/LV (high-dose methotrexate, leucovorin [rescue])

HDMTX-CF (high-dose methotrexate, citrovorum factor)

HDPEB (high-dose PEB protocol)

HexaCAF; Hexa-CAF (hexamethylmelamine, cyclophosphamide, amethopterin, fluorouracil)

HiDAC (high-dose ara-C)

HOAP-BLEO (hydroxydaunomycin, Oncovin, ara-C, prednisone, bleomycin)

HOP (hydroxydaunomycin, Oncovin, prednisone)

ICE (ifosfamide [with mesna rescue], carboplatin, etoposide)

ICE-T (ifosfamide [with mesna rescue], carboplatin, etoposide, Taxol)

IE (ifosfamide [with mesna rescue], etoposide)

IfoVP (ifosfamide [with mesna rescue], VePesid)

IMF (ifosfamide [with mesna rescue], methotrexate, fluorouracil)

Indiana protocol

IPA (ifosfamide, Platinol, Adriamycin)

L-VAM (leuprolide acetate, vinblastine, Adriamycin, mitomycin)

Antineoplastics, Chemotherapy Protocols (cont.)

LAPOCA (L-asparaginase, Oncovin, cytarabine, Adriamycin)

Linker protocol (daunorubicin, vincristine, prednisone, asparaginase, teniposide, cytarabine, methotrexate [with leucovorin rescue])

LMF (Leukeran, methotrexate, fluorouracil)

LOMAC (leucovorin, Oncovin, methotrexate, Adriamycin, cyclophosphamide)

m-BACOD; M-BACOD (methotrexate, bleomycin, Adriamycin, cyclophosphamide, Oncovin, dexamethasone)

m-PFL (methotrexate, Platinol, fluorouracil, leucovorin [rescue])

M-2 protocol (vincristine, carmustine, cyclophosphamide, prednisone, melphalan)

M-BACOS (methotrexate, bleomycin, Adriamycin, cyclophosphamide, Oncovin, Solu-Medrol)

MABOP (Mustargen, Adriamycin, bleomycin, Oncovin, prednisone)

MAC (methotrexate, actinomycin D, chlorambucil)

MAC (mitomycin, Adriamycin, cyclophosphamide)

MAC; MAC III (methotrexate, actinomycin D, cyclophosphamide)

MACC (methotrexate, Adriamycin, cyclophosphamide, CCNU)

MACHO (methotrexate, asparaginase, cyclophosphamide, hydroxydaunomycin, Oncovin)

MACOP-B (methotrexate, Adriamycin, cyclophosphamide, Oncovin, prednisone, bleomycin)

MAD (MeCCNU, Adriamycin)

MADDOC (mechlorethamine, Adriamycin, dacarbazine, DDP, Oncovin, cyclophosphamide)

MAID (mesna [rescue], Adriamycin, ifosfamide, dacarbazine)

MAP (mitomycin, Adriamycin, Platinol)

Antineoplastics, Chemotherapy Protocols (cont.)

MAZE (m-AMSA, azacitidine, etoposide)

MBC (methotrexate, bleomycin, cisplatin)

MBD (methotrexate, bleomycin, DDP)

MC (mitoxantrone, cytarabine)

MCBP (melphalan, cyclophosphamide, BCNU, prednisone)

MCP (melphalan, cyclophosphamide, prednisone)

MCV (methotrexate, cisplatin, vinblastine)

MECY (methotrexate, cyclophosphamide)

MF (methotrexate [with leucovorin rescue], fluorouracil)

MF (mitomycin, fluorouracil)

MFP (melphalan, fluorouracil, medroxyprogesterone acetate)

MICE (mesna [rescue], ifosfamide, carboplatin, etoposide)

MIFA (mitomycin, fluorouracil, Adriamycin)

MINE (mesna [rescue], ifosfamide, Novantrone, etoposide)

MINE-ESHAP (alternating cycles of MINE and ESHAP)

mini-BEAM (BCNU, etoposide, ara-C, melphalan)

mini-COAP (cyclophosphamide, Oncovin, ara-C, prednisone)

MIV (mitoxantrone, ifosfamide, VePesid)

MM (mercaptopurine, methotrexate)

MMOPP (methotrexate, mechlorethamine, Oncovin, procarbazine, prednisone)

MOB (mechlorethamine, Oncovin, bleomycin)

MOB-III (mitomycin, Oncovin, bleomycin, cisplatin)

MOBP (mitomycin, Oncovin, bleomycin, Platinol)

modified Bagshawe protocol

MOF (MeCCNU, Oncovin, fluorouracil)

Antineoplastics, Chemotherapy Protocols (cont.)

MOF-STREP; MOF-Strep (MeCCNU, Oncovin, fluorouracil, streptozocin)

MOMP (mechlorethamine, Oncovin, methotrexate, prednisone)

MOP (mechlorethamine, Oncovin, prednisone)

MOP (mechlorethamine, Oncovin, procarbazine)

MOP-BAP (mechlorethamine, Oncovin, procarbazine, bleomycin, Adriamycin, prednisone)

MOPP (mechlorethamine, Oncovin, procarbazine, prednisone)

MOPP (mustine HCl, Oncovin, procarbazine, prednisone)

MOPP/ABVD (alternating cycles of MOPP and ABVD)

MOPP-BLEO; MOPP-Bleo (mechlorethamine, Oncovin, procarbazine, prednisone, bleomycin)

MOPP/ABV (mechlorethamine, Oncovin, procarbazine, prednisone, Adriamycin, bleomycin, vinblastine)

MOPPHDB (mechlorethamine, Oncovin, procarbazine, prednisone, high-dose bleomycin)

MOPPLDB (mechlorethamine, Oncovin, procarbazine, prednisone, low-dose bleomycin)

MOPr (mechlorethamine, Oncovin, procarbazine)

MP (melphalan, prednisone)

MP (mitoxantrone, prednisone)

MPL + PRED (melphalan, prednisone)

MTX + MP + CTX (methotrexate, mercaptopurine, cyclophosphamide)

MTX-CDDPAdr (methotrexate [with leucovorin rescue], CDDP, Adriamycin)

MTX/6-MP (methotrexate, mercaptopurine)

MTX/6-MP/VP (methotrexate, mercaptopurine, vincristine, prednisone)

Antineoplastics, Chemotherapy Protocols (cont.)

MV (mitomycin, vinblastine)

MV (mitoxantrone, VePesid)

MVAC; M-VAC (methotrexate, vinblastine, Adriamycin, cisplatin)

MVF (mitoxantrone, vincristine, fluorouracil)

MVP (mitomycin, vinblastine, Platinol)

MVPP (mechlorethamine, vinblastine, procarbazine, prednisone)

MVT (mitoxantrone, VePesid, thiotepa)

MVVPP (mechlorethamine, vincristine, vinblastine, procarbazine, prednisone)

NAC (nitrogen mustard, Adriamycin, CCNU)

NFL (Novantrone, fluorouracil, leucovorin [rescue])

NOVP (Novantrone, Oncovin, vinblastine, prednisone)

OAP (Oncovin, ara-C, prednisone)

OMAD (Oncovin, methotrexate/citrovorum factor, Adriamycin, dactinomycin)

OPA (Oncovin, prednisone, Adriamycin)

OPAL (Oncovin, prednisone, L-asparaginase)

OPEN (Oncovin, prednisone, etoposide, Novantrone)

OPP (Oncovin, procarbazine, prednisone)

OPPA (Oncovin, prednisone, procarbazine, Adriamycin)

P-MVAC (Platinol, methotrexate, vinblastine, Adriamycin, carboplatin)

PA-CI (Adriamycin, cisplatin)

PAB-Esc-C (Platinol, Adriamycin, bleomycin, escalating doses of cyclophosphamide)

PAC; PAC-I (Platinol, Adriamycin, cyclophosphamide)

PACE (Platinol, Adriamycin, cyclophosphamide, etoposide)

paclitaxel & carboplatin & etoposide

paclitaxel & trastuzumab

Antineoplastics, Chemotherapy Protocols (cont.)

paclitaxel & vinorelbine tartrate

PATCO (prednisone, ara-C, thioguanine, cyclophosphamide, Oncovin)

PAVe (procarbazine, Alkeran, Velban)

PBV (Platinol, bleomycin, vinblastine)

PC (paclitaxel, carboplatin)

PC (paclitaxel, cisplatin)

PCE (Platinol, cyclophosphamide, etoposide)

PCV (procarbazine, CCNU, vincristine)

PE (paclitaxel, estramustine)

PEB (Platinol, etoposide, bleomycin)

PFL (Platinol, fluorouracil, leucovorin [rescue])

PFT (L-phenylalanine mustard, fluorouracil, tamoxifen)

PHRT (procarbazine, hydroxyurea, radiotherapy)

PIA (Platinol, ifosfamide, Adriamycin)

POC (procarbazine, Oncovin, CCNU)

POCA (prednisone, Oncovin, cytarabine, Adriamycin)

POCC (procarbazine, Oncovin, cyclophosphamide, CCNU)

POMP (prednisone, Oncovin, methotrexate, Purinethol)

ProMACE (prednisone, methotrexate [with leucovorin rescue], Adriamycin, cyclophosphamide, etoposide)

ProMACE/cytaBOM (ProMACE [above], cytarabine, bleomycin, Oncovin, mitoxantrone)

ProMACE/MOPP (full course of ProMACE, followed by MOPP)

Pt/VM (Platinol, VM-26)

pulse VAC

pulse VAC (vincristine, Adriamycin, cyclophosphamide)

PVA (prednisone, vincristine, asparaginase)

PVB (Platinol, vinblastine, bleomycin)

Antineoplastics, Chemotherapy Protocols (cont.)

PVDA (prednisone, vincristine, daunorubicin, asparaginase)

PVP; PVP-16 (Platinol, VP-16)

RIDD (recombinant interleukin-2, dacarbazine, DDP)

SMF (streptozocin, mitomycin, fluorouracil)

standard VAC

Stanford V (mechlorethamine, doxorubicin, vinblastine, vincristine, bleomycin, etoposide, prednisone)

STEAM (streptonigrin, thioguanine, cyclophosphamide, actinomycin, mitomycin)

T-10 protocol (methotrexate, doxorubicin, cisplatin, bleomycin, cyclophosphamide, dactinomycin)

T-2 protocol (dactinomycin, doxorubicin, vincristine, cyclophosphamide, radiation)

TAD (thioguanine, ara-C, daunorubicin)

tamoxifen citrate & DTIC

TC (thioguanine, cytarabine)

TCF (Taxol, cisplatin, fluorouracil)

TEC (thiotepa, etoposide, carboplatin)

TEMP (tamoxifen, etoposide, mitoxantrone, Platinol)

TIP (Taxol, isosfamide [with mesna rescue], Platinol)

TIT (methotrexate, cytarabine, hydrocortisone)

TOAP (thioguanine, Oncovin, [cytosine] arabinoside, prednisone)

topo/CTX (topotecan, cyclophosphamide [with mesna rescue])

TPCH (thioguanine, procarbazine, CCNU, hydroxyurea)

TPDCV (thioguanine, procarbazine, DCD, CCNU, vincristine)

trastuzumab & paclitaxel

V-TAD (VePesid, thioguanine, ara-C, daunorubicin)

V-CAP III (VP-16-213, cyclophosphamide, Adriamycin, Platinol)

VA (vincristine, actinomycin D)

Antineoplastics, Chemotherapy Protocols (cont.)

VAAP (vincristine, asparaginase, Adriamycin, prednisone)

VAB; VAB-I (vinblastine, actinomycin D, bleomycin)

VAB-6 (vinblastine, actinomycin D, bleomycin, cyclophosphamide, cisplatin)

VAB-II (vinblastine, actinomycin D, bleomycin, cisplatin)

VAB-III (vinblastine, actinomycin D, bleomycin, cisplatin, chlorambucil, cyclophosphamide)

VAB-V (vinblastine, actinomycin D, bleomycin, cyclophosphamide, cisplatin)

VABCD (vinblastine, Adriamycin, bleomycin, CCNU, DTIC)

VAC (vincristine, Adriamycin, cisplatin)

VAC (vincristine, Adriamycin, cyclophosphamide)

VAC pulse; VAC standard (vincristine, actinomycin D, cyclophosphamide)

VACA (vincristine, actinomycin D, cyclophosphamide, Adriamycin)

VACAD (vincristine, actinomycin D, cyclophosphamide, Adriamycin, dacarbazine)

VACAdr (vincristine, actinomycin D, cyclophosphamide, Adriamycin)

VACAdr-IfoVP (vincristine, actinomycin D, cyclophosphamide, Adriamycin, ifosfamide, VePesid)

VACP (VePesid, Adriamycin, cyclophosphamide, Platinol)

VAD (vincristine, Adriamycin, dactinomycin)

VAD (vincristine, Adriamycin, dexamethasone)

VAD/V (vincristine, Adriamycin, dexamethasone, verapamil)

VAdrC (vincristine, Adriamycin, cyclophosphamide)

VAFAC (vincristine, amethopterin, fluorouracil, Adriamycin, cyclophosphamide)

Indications

Antineoplastics, Chemotherapy Protocols (cont.)

VAI (vincristine, actinomycin D, ifosfamide)

VAM (vinblastine, Adriamycin, mitomycin)

VAM (VP-16-213, Adriamycin, methotrexate)

VAMP (vincristine, actinomycin, methotrexate, prednisone)

VAMP (vincristine, Adriamycin, methylprednisolone)

VAMP (vincristine, amethopterin, mercaptopurine, prednisone)

VAP (vinblastine, actinomycin D, Platinol)

VAP (vincristine, Adriamycin, prednisone)

VAP (vincristine, Adriamycin, procarbazine)

VAP (vincristine, asparaginase, prednisone)

VAT (vinblastine, Adriamycin, thiotepa)

VATD; VAT-D (vincristine, ara-C, thioguanine, daunorubicin)

VATH (vinblastine, Adriamycin, thiotepa, Halotestin)

VAV (VP-16-213, Adriamycin, vincristine)

VB (vinblastine, bleomycin)

VBA (vincristine, BCNU, Adriamycin)

VBAP (vincristine, BCNU, Adriamycin, prednisone)

VBC (VePesid, BCNU, cyclophosphamide)

VBC (vinblastine, bleomycin, cisplatin)

VBCMP (vincristine, BCNU, cyclophosphamide, melphalan, prednisone)

VBD (vinblastine, bleomycin, DDP)

VBM (vincristine, bleomycin, methotrexate)

VBMCP (vincristine, BCNU, melphalan, cyclophosphamide, prednisone)

VBMF (vincristine, bleomycin, methotrexate, fluorouracil)

Antineoplastics, Chemotherapy Protocols (cont.)

VBP (vinblastine, bleomycin, Platinol)

VC (VePesid, carboplatin)

VC (vinorelbine, cisplatin)

VCAP (vincristine, cyclophosphamide, Adriamycin, prednisone)

VCF (vincristine, cyclophosphamide, fluorouracil)

VCMP (vincristine, cyclophosphamide, melphalan, prednisone)

VCP (vincristine, cyclophosphamide, prednisone)

VD (vinorelbine, doxorubicin)

VDA (vincristine, daunorubicin, asparaginase)

VDP (vinblastine, dacarbazine, Platinol)

VDP (vincristine, daunorubicin, prednisone)

VeIP (Velban, ifosfamide [with mesna rescue], Platinol)

VIC (VePesid, ifosfamide [with mesna rescue], carboplatin)

VIC (vinblastine, ifosfamide, CCNU)

VIE (vincristine, ifosfamide, etoposide)

vinblastine sulfate & estramustine

vinorelbine tartrate & cisplatin

vinorelbine tartrate & paclitaxel

VIP (vinblastine, ifosfamide [with mesna rescue], Platinol)

VIP; VIP-1; VIP-2 (VePesid, ifosfamide [with mesna rescue], Platinol)

VIP-B (VP-16, ifosfamide, Platinol, bleomycin)

VLP (vincristine, L-asparaginase, prednisone)

VM (vinblastine, mitomycin)

VM-26PP (teniposide, procarbazine, prednisone)

VMAD (vincristine, methotrexate, Adriamycin, actinomycin D)

VMCP (vincristine, melphalan, cyclophosphamide, prednisone)

VMP (VePesid, mitoxantrone, prednimustine)

Antineoplastics, Chemotherapy Protocols (cont.)
  VOCAP (VP-16-213, Oncovin, cyclophosphamide, Adriamycin, Platinol)
  VP (VePesid, Platinol)
  VP (vincristine, prednisone)
  VP + A (vincristine, prednisone, asparaginase)
  VP-L-asparaginase (vincristine, prednisone, L-asparaginase)
  VPB (vinblastine, Platinol, bleomycin)
  VPBCPr (vincristine, prednisone, vinblastine, chlorambucil, procarbazine)
  VPCA (vincristine, prednisone, cyclophosphamide, ara-C)
  VPCMF (vincristine, prednisone, cyclophosphamide, methotrexate, fluorouracil)
  VPP (VePesid, Platinol)

Antiparkinsonian Agents
Antiparkinsonian Agents, Anticholinergic Agents
  Akineton
  Anaspaz
  Artane
  atropine sulfate
  belladonna extract
  Bellafoline
  benztropine mesylate
  biperiden HCl
  biperiden lactate
  Cogentin
  Cystospaz
  Cystospaz-M
  Disipal Ⓒ
  Donnamar
  Ed-Spaz
  ethopropazine HCl
  Gastrosed
  hyoscyamine sulfate
  Kemadrin
  Levbid
  Levsin
  Levsinex
  NuLev

Antiparkinsonian Agents, Anticholinergic Agents (cont.)
  orphenadrine HCl
  Parsidol
  procyclidine HCl
  Sal-Tropine
  Symax-SR
  Trihexy-2; Trihexy-5
  trihexyphenidyl HCl
Antiparkinsonian Agents, Dopaminergic Agents
  amantadine HCl
  brasofensine maleate
  bromocriptine mesylate
  cabergoline
  Carbex
  Dopar
  Dostinex
  Eldepryl
  Larodopa
  levodopa
  Mirapex
  N-Graft
  neural dopaminergic cells (or precursors), porcine fetal
  NeuroCell-PD
  Parlodel
  pergolide mesylate
  Permax
  PMS-Bromocriptine Ⓒ
  pramipexole dihydrochloride
  Requip
  ropinirole HCl
  selegiline HCl
  Sertoli cells, porcine
  Sinemet 10/100; Sinemet 25/100; Sinemet 25/250
  Sinemet CR
  Symmetrel
Antiparkinsonian Agents, Other
  Altropane
  Apokinon
  apomorphine HCl
  carbidopa
  Comtan
  entacapone
  iodine I 123 murine MAb to alpha-fetoprotein (AFP)
  Lodosyn
  Rilutek

Indications

Antiparkinsonian Agents, Other (cont.)
riluzole
Tasmar
tolcapone
Zydis

Antiprotozoals
[see also: Antibiotics]
Antiprotozoals, Amebicides
dehydroemetine
diloxanide furoate
Flagyl
Flagyl IV
Flagyl IV RTU
Furamide
Humatin
Hydrocortisone Iodoquinol 1%
iodoquinol
Mebadin
Metro I.V.
metronidazole
paromomycin sulfate
Prevacid
Protostat
Vytone
Yodoxin
Antiprotozoals, Antimalarials
Aralen HCl
Aralen Phosphate
atovaquone
chloroguanide HCl
chloroquine HCl
chloroquine phosphate
Daraprim
Fansidar
Halfan
halofantrine HCl
hydroxychloroquine sulfate
Lariam
Malarone; Malarone Pediatric
mefloquine HCl
Mephaquin
Plaquenil Sulfate
primaquine phosphate
pyrimethamine
Quilimmune-M
quinidine gluconate
quinine sulfate

Antiprotozoals, Other
Antrypol
Arsobal
Belganyl
eflornithine HCl
Fourneau 309
Germanin
Lampit
melarsoprol
Moranyl
Naganol
Naphuride
nifurtimox
Ornidyl
Pentostam
sodium stibogluconate
suramin sodium

Antisecretories
Antisecretories, Gastrointestinal
[see also: Antacids; Peptic Ulcer and Gastric Reflux Agents]
A-Spas S/L
Aciphex
Anaspaz
Cystospaz
Cystospaz-M
Donnamar
Ed-Spaz
esomeprazole magnesium
Gastrosed
glycopyrrolate
hyoscyamine sulfate
lansoprazole
Levbid
Levsin
Levsin PB
Levsin with Phenobarbital
Levsin/SL
Levsinex
Nexium
NuLev
omeprazole
pantoprazole
pantoprazole sodium
Pantozol
Prilosec
rabeprazole sodium
Robinul

Antisecretories, Gastrointestinal (cont.)
Robinul Forte
Sal-Tropine
Symax-SR
Antisecretories, Hyperhidrosis
Anaspaz
Cystospaz
Cystospaz-M
Donnamar
Ed-Spaz
Gastrosed
hyoscyamine sulfate
Levbid
Levsin
Levsinex
Symax-SR
Antisecretories, Respiratory
[see also: Antihistamines, Systemic; Respiratory System Agents]
Anaspaz
atropine sulfate
Cystospaz
Cystospaz-M
Donnamar
Ed-Spaz
Gastrosed
hyoscyamine sulfate
Levbid
Levsin
Levsinex
Sal-Tropine
Symax-SR
Antipsychotics [see: Psychotherapeutics, Antipsychotics]

Antiseptics
[see also: Dermatological Preparations, Acne Products, Topical; Mouth and Throat Preparations; Ophthalmologicals, Contact Lens Preparations; Vaginal Preparations, Antiseptic Cleansers]
alcohol
benzalkonium chloride (BAC)
Castellani Paint Modified
chlorhexidine gluconate
chlorobutanol
chloroxylenol

Antiseptics (cont.)
Erygel
gentian violet
hexachlorophene
hexylresorcinol
ichthammol
iodine
isopropyl alcohol
Lugol
Ovide
phenol
pHisoHex
potassium iodide
povidone-iodine
Septi-Soft
Septisol
Strong Iodine
thimerosal
Tinver
triclosan
Versiclear
Xerac AC

Antispasmodics
[see also: Urinary Tract Agents, Antispasmodics]
A-Spas S/L
Anaspaz
Antispas
Antispasmodic
Antrocol
Arco-Lase Plus
atropine sulfate
Barbidonna; Barbidonna No. 2
Bel-Phen-Ergot SR
Bellacane
Bellacane SR
belladonna extract
Bellafoline
Bellergal-S
Bentyl
Butibel
Byclomine
Cafatine-PB
Chardonna-2
clidinium bromide
Clindex
Cystospaz
Cystospaz-M

Antispasmodics (cont.)
dexpanthenol
Di-Spaz
Dibent
dicyclomine HCl
Donna-Sed
Donnamar
Donnatal
Donnatal No. 2
Ed-Spaz
Enlon Plus
Folergot-DF
Gastrosed
glycopyrrolate
hyoscyamine hydrobromide
hyoscyamine sulfate
Hyosophen
Ilopan
Ilopan-Choline
Kutrase
Levbid
Levsin
Levsin PB
Levsin with Phenobarbital
Levsin/SL
Levsinex
Librax
Logen
Lomanate
Lomotil
Lonox
Malatal
methscopolamine bromide
Motofen
NuLev
Pamine
Phenerbel-S
Pro-Banthīne
propantheline bromide
Quarzan
Robinul
Robinul Forte
Sal-Tropine
Scopace
scopolamine hydrobromide
Spasmolin
Susano
Symax-SR
tizanidine HCl
Transderm Scōp

Antispasmodics (cont.)
Zanaflex

Antituberculosis Agents
[*see also: Antibiotics*]
aminosalicylate sodium (*p*-aminosal-
icylate sodium)
aminosalicylic acid (4-aminosalicylic
acid)
aminosidine
BCG vaccine (bacillus Calmette-
Guérin)
Capastat Sulfate
capreomycin sulfate
clofazimine
cycloserine (L-cycloserine)
ethambutol HCl
ethionamide
Gabbromicina
isoniazid
Lamprene
Laniazid
Laniazid C.T.
Myambutol
Nydrazid
Paromomycin
Paser
Priftin
pyrazinamide (PZA)
Rifadin
Rifamate
rifampin
rifapentine
Rifater
Rimactane
Seromycin
streptomycin sulfate
Tice BCG
Trecator-SC

Antitussives
Antitussives, Narcotic
acetaminophen & hydrocodone
bitartrate
Actagen-C Cough
Actifed with Codeine Cough
Allerfrin with Codeine

Antitussives, Narcotic (cont.)
Ambenyl Cough
Amgenal Cough
Anaplex HD
Aprodine with Codeine
Atuss EX
Atuss G
Atuss HD
Bromanate DC Cough
Bromanyl
Bromotuss with Codeine
Bromphen DC with Codeine Cough
Brompheniramine DC Cough
Brontex
Calcidrine
Calmylin with Codeine Ⓒ🄰🄽
Cheracol Cough
Chlorgest-HD
Co-Tuss V
Codamine
Codegest Expectorant
Codehist DH
codeine phosphate
codeine sulfate
Codiclear DH
Codimal DH
Conex with Codeine
Cophene XP
Cotridin Ⓒ🄰🄽
Cotridin Expectorant Ⓒ🄰🄽
Cyclofed Pediatric
Cycofed Pediatric
Decohistine DH
Deconamine CX
Decongestant Expectorant
Deconsal Pediatric
Deproist Expectorant with Codeine
Detussin
Detussin Expectorant
Dihistine Expectorant
Dilaudid Cough
Dimetane-DC Cough
Donatussin DC
ED-TLC; ED Tuss HC
Endagen-HD
Endal Expectorant
Endal-HD; Endal-HD Plus
Entuss-D
Entuss-D Jr.
Entuss Expectorant

Antitussives, Narcotic (cont.)
Guiatuss AC
Guiatuss DAC
Guiatussin DAC
Guiatussin with Codeine Expectorant
H-Tuss-D
Histex HC
Histinex HC
Histinex PV
Histussin D
Histussin HC
HycoClear Tuss
Hycodan
Hycomine
Hycomine Compound
Hycotuss Expectorant
Hydro-PC
hydrocodone bitartrate
hydrocodone bitartrate & acetaminophen
hydrocodone polistirex
Hydrocodone Compound
Hydrocodone CP; Hydrocodone HD
Hydrocodone GF
Hydrocodone PA
Hydromet
Hyphed
Iodal HD
Iophen-C
Iotussin HC
Isoclor Expectorant
Kwelcof
Levall 5.0
Marcof Expectorant
Myphetane DC Cough
Mytussin AC Cough
Mytussin DAC
Naldecon CX Adult
Novagest Expectorant with Codeine
Novahistine DH
Novahistine Expectorant
Nucofed
Nucofed Expectorant; Nucofed
   Pediatric Expectorant
Nucotuss Expectorant; Nucotuss
   Pediatric Expectorant
Oncet
P-V-Tussin
Pancof-HC
Pancof-XL; Pancof XP

Indications

Antitussives, Narcotic (cont.)

Para-Hist HD
Pediacof
Pedituss Cough
Pentazine VC with Codeine
Phenergan VC with Codeine
Phenergan with Codeine
Phenhist DH with Codeine
Phenhist Expectorant
Pherazine VC with Codeine
Pherazine with Codeine
Pneumotussin
Pneumotussin HC
Poly-Histine CS
Prometh VC with Codeine
Prometh with Codeine
Promethazine VC with Codeine
Promethist with Codeine
Protuss
Protuss-D
Robafen AC Cough
Robafen DAC
Robitussin A-C
Robitussin-DAC
Rolatuss Expectorant
Rolatuss with Hydrocodone
Romilar AC
Ru-Tuss with Hydrocodone
Ryna-C
Ryna-CX
S-T Forte 2
SRC Expectorant
Statuss Expectorant
Statuss Green
T-Koff
Triacin-C Cough
Triafed with Codeine
Triaminic Expectorant DH
Triaminic Expectorant with Codeine
Tricodene Cough and Cold
Trifed-C Cough
Tussafed HC
Tussafin Expectorant
Tussanil DH
Tussar SF; Tussar-2
Tussend
Tussi-Organidin NR; Tussi-Organidin-S NR
Tussigon
Tussionex Pennkinetic

Antitussives, Narcotic (cont.)

Tussirex
Tyrodone
Unituss HC
Vanex Expectorant
Vanex-HD
Vetuss HC
Vicodin Tuss

Antitussives, Non-narcotic

Anaplex DM Cough
Anatuss
Aquatab C
Aquatab DM
Atuss DM
benzonatate
Bromadine-DM
Bromadine-DX
Bromarest DX Cough
Bromatane DX Cough
Bromfed-DM Cough
Bromphen DX Cough
brompheniramine maleate & pseudoephedrine HCl & dextromethorphan hydrobromide
caramiphen edisylate
carbetapentane citrate
carbetapentane tannate
Carbinoxamine Compound
Carbodec DM
Cardec-DM
Coldec DM
Cophene-X
dextromethorphan
dextromethorphan hydrobromide
dextromethorphan hydrobromide & brompheniramine maleate & pseudoephedrine HCl
dextromethorphan polistirex
Dimetane-DX Cough
Donatussin
Duratuss DM
Fenesin DM
Guaifenex DM
Histine DM; Histinex DM
Humibid DM
Humibid DM Sprinkle
Iobid DM
Iohist DM
Iophen-DM
Liqui-Histine DM

Antitussives, Non-narcotic (cont.)
MED-Rx DM
Monafed DM
MorphiDex
Muco-Fen-DM
Myphetane DX Cough
Ordrine AT
PanMist-DM
Phenameth DM
Phenergan with Dextromethorphan
Pherazine DM
Poly-Histine DM
Profen Forte DM
Profen II DM
Prometh with Dextromethorphan
Promethazine DM
Protuss DM
Pseudo-Car DM
pseudoephedrine HCl & dextromethorphan hydrobromide & brompheniramine maleate
Rentamine Pediatric
Rescaps-D S.R.
Respa-DM
Rondamine-DM
Rondec-DM
Rynatuss
Sildec-DM
Siltapp with Dextromethorphan HBr Cold & Cough
Tannic-12
Tessalon
Touro CC
Touro DM
Tri-Tannate Plus Pediatric
Tusquelin
Tuss-Ornade
Tuss-Allergine Modified T.D.
Tuss-Tan
Tussafed
Tussafed-LA
Tussi-Organidin DM NR; Tussi-Organidin DM-S NR
Tussi-12
Tusso-DM
Tussogest

Antitoxin [see: Antidotes]

Antivenin
[see also: Immunizing Agents, Immune Extracts]

Antivenin (cont.)
antivenin (*Latrodectus mactans*)
antivenin (*Micrurus fulvius*) (equine)
antivenin (Crotalidae) polyvalent (equine)
antivenin (Crotalidae) polyvalent immune Fab (ovine)
antivenin (Crotalidae) purified (avian)
CroFab

Antivirals
Antivirals, Systemic
[see also: HIV Infections, Viral]
abacavir succinate
abacavir sulfate
acyclovir
acyclovir sodium
adefovir dipivoxil
amantadine HCl
Apo-Acyclovir ⓒⒶⓃ
atevirdine mesylate
Aztec
Combivir
Crixivan
Cytovene
didanosine
Doxovir
emtricitabine
Epivir
Epivir-HBV
famciclovir
Famvir
Flumadine
Fortovase
ganciclovir
ganciclovir sodium
Genvir
HAART (highly active antiretroviral therapy)
Heptovir ⓒⒶⓃ
Hivid
indinavir sulfate
interferon alfa-2b (IFN-α2)
interferon alfa-n1
Intron A
Invirase
Kaletra

Indications

Antivirals, Systemic (cont.)
  lamivudine
  lopinavir
  lysine (L-lysine)
  Norvir
  oseltamivir phosphate
  Ostavir
  Papirine
  PEG-Intron
  peginterferon alfa-2b
  Picovir
  pleconaril
  Preveon
  Rebetol
  Rebetron
  Relenza
  Retrovir
  ribavirin
  rimantadine HCl
  ritonavir
  saquinavir
  saquinavir mesylate
  stavudine
  Symmetrel
  Tamiflu
  tenofovir disoproxil fumarate (teno-
    fovir DF)
  Trizivir
  tuvirumab
  valacyclovir HCl
  valganciclovir HCl
  Valtrex
  vidarabine
  Videx
  Videx EC
  Virazole
  Viread
  Wellferon
  zalcitabine
  zanamivir
  Zeffix
  Zerit
  Ziagen
  zidovudine (ZDV)
  Zovirax
Antivirals, Topical
  [see also: Ophthalmologicals, Antibiotics]
  acyclovir
  acyclovir sodium
  Alferon N

Antivirals, Topical (cont.)
  Denavir
  docosanol (n-docosanol)
  Herplex
  idoxuridine (IDU)
  interferon alfa-n3
  penciclovir
  trifluridine
  Viroptic
  Zovirax

Asthma Agents
[see also: Corticosteroids, Systemic;
    Respiratory System Agents]
Asthma Agents, Inhalants
  AccuNeb
  Adrenalin Chloride
  Advair
  AeroBid; AeroBid-M
  Airet
  Airomir ⒸⒶⓃ
  albuterol
  albuterol sulfate
  Alti-Flunisolide ⒸⒶⓃ
  Alti-Ipratropium ⒸⒶⓃ
  Alupent
  Apo-Beclomethasone ⒸⒶⓃ
  Apo-Cromolyn ⒸⒶⓃ
  Apo-Ipravent ⒸⒶⓃ
  Apo-Salvent ⒸⒶⓃ
  Atrovent
  Azmacort
  Becloforte Inhaler ⒸⒶⓃ
  beclomethasone dipropionate (BDP)
  Beclovent
  Beclovent Inhaler ⒸⒶⓃ
  Beta-2
  bitolterol mesylate
  Brethaire
  Bronalide ⒸⒶⓃ
  Bronkometer
  Bronkosol
  budesonide
  Combivent
  cromolyn sodium
  Dexacort Phosphate
  dexamethasone sodium phosphate
  Duo-Medihaler
  DuoNeb

Asthma Agents, Inhalants (cont.)

edodekin alfa
epinephrine
epinephrine bitartrate
epinephrine HCl
Flovent
flunisolide
fluticasone propionate
Foradil
formoterol fumarate
Gen-Ipratropium ⒸⒶⓃ
Intal
ipratropium bromide
isoetharine
isoetharine HCl
isoetharine mesylate
isoproterenol HCl
isoproterenol sulfate
Isuprel
levalbuterol HCl
Maxair
Medihaler-Iso
metaproterenol sulfate
mometasone furoate
nedocromil sodium
Novo-Salmol ⒸⒶⓃ
Nu-Beclomethasone ⒸⒶⓃ
Oxeze ⒸⒶⓃ
phenylephrine bitartrate
pirbuterol acetate
Proventil
Proventil HFA
Pulmicort
QVAR
racepinephrine HCl
salbutamol
salbutamol sulfate
Salbutamol Nebuamp ⒸⒶⓃ
salmeterol xinafoate
Serevent
terbutaline sulfate
Tilade
Tornalate
Tri-Nasal
triamcinolone acetonide
Vanceril; Vanceril Double Strength
Ventolin
Ventolin ⒸⒶⓃ
Ventolin HFA
Xopenex

Asthma Agents, Systemic

A-Hydrocort
A-Methapred
Accolate
Accurbron
Adlone
Adrenalin Chloride
Aerolate Sr.; Aerolate Jr.; Aerolate III
albuterol sulfate
alpha$_1$-antitrypsin (AAT), recombinant
Alupent
Amcort
aminophylline
Ana-Guard
Ana-Kit
Apo-Orciprenaline ⒸⒶⓃ
Apo-Prednisone ⒸⒶⓃ
Aquaphyllin
Aristocort
Aristocort Forte
Articulose L.A.
Asmalix
Atolone
Berotec
Brethine
Bricanyl
Bronchial
Brondelate
Bronkodyl
Choledyl SA
Contramid
Cordox
Cortef
dehydroepiandrosterone sulfate (DHEAS)
Deltasone
depMedalone 40; depMedalone 80
Depo-Medrol
Depoject
Depopred-40; Depopred-80
Dilor
Dilor 400
Dilor-G
Duralone-40; Duralone-80
Dy-G
Dyflex-G
Dyline-GG
dyphylline
dyphylline & guaifenesin

Indications

Asthma Agents, Systemic (cont.)

Elixomin
Elixophyllin
Elixophyllin GG
Elixophyllin-KI
ephedrine HCl
ephedrine sulfate
ephedrine tannate
epinephrine
epinephrine HCl
Epinephrine Pediatric
ethylnorepinephrine HCl
fenoterol
fructose-1,6-diphosphate (FDP)
Glyceryl-T
guaifenesin & dyphylline
hydrocortisone (HC)
hydrocortisone acetate (HCA)
hydrocortisone sodium phosphate
hydrocortisone sodium succinate
Hydrocortone
Hydrocortone Acetate
Hydrocortone Phosphate
Hydrophed
Iophylline
isoproterenol HCl
isoproterenol sulfate
Isuprel
Kenacort
Kenaject-40
Kenalog-10; Kenalog-40
Lanophyllin
levalbuterol
Liquid Pred
Lufyllin
Lufyllin 400
Lufyllin-EPG
Lufyllin-GG
M-Prednisol-40; M-Prednisol-80
Marax
Marax-DF
Medralone 40; Medralone 80
Medrol
Metaprel
metaproterenol sulfate
methylprednisolone
methylprednisolone acetate
methylprednisolone sodium succinate
Meticorten
montelukast sodium

Asthma Agents, Systemic (cont.)

Mudrane
Mudrane GG
Mudrane GG-2
Norisodrine with Calcium Iodide
omalizumab
Orasone
orciprenaline sulfate
oxtriphylline
Panasol-S
Panfil G
Phyllocontin
Prednicen-M
prednisone
Proventil
Quadrinal
Quibron; Quibron-300
Quibron-T
Quibron-T/SR
Respbid
Singulair
Slo-bid
Slo-phyllin
Slo-phyllin GG
Solu-Cortef
Solu-Medrol
Sterapred; Sterapred DS
Sus-Phrine
Sustaire
Synophylate-GG
T-Phyl
Tac-3
Tac-40
terbutaline sulfate
Theo-24
Theo-Dur
Theo-Sav
Theo-X
Theobid
Theochron
Theoclear-80
Theoclear L.A.
Theolair; Theolair-SR
Theolate
Theomax DF
Theophyllin KI
theophylline (TH)
Theospan-SR
Theostat 80
Theovent

Asthma Agents, Systemic (cont.)
  Tri-Kort
  Triam Forte
  Triam-A
  triamcinolone
  triamcinolone acetonide
  Triamolone 40
  Triamonide 40
  Trilog
  Trilone
  Tristoject
  Truphylline
  Uni-Dur
  Uniphyl
  Volmax
  Xolair
  zafirlukast
  zileuton
  Zyflo
Anxiolytics [see: Psychotherapeutics, Anxiolytics]
Arrhythmias [see: Cardiac Agents, Antiarrhythmics]
Attention Deficit Hyperactivity Disorder (ADHD) [see: Central Nervous System Stimulants]
Benign Prostatic Hypertrophy (BPH) [see: Prostatic Hyperplasia Agents]

Biliary Tract Agents
  Actigall
  Chenix
  chenodiol
  cholestyramine resin
  dehydrocholic acid
  desoxycholic acid
  Digestozyme
  flumecinol
  LoCholest; LoCholest Light
  Moctanin
  monoctanoin
  Prevalite
  Questran; Questran Light
  Stanate
  stannsoporfin
  Urso
  ursodiol
  Zixoryn

Bipolar Disorder [see: Psychotherapeutics, Antidepressants; Psychotherapeutics, Antimanic]

Blood Expanders and Substitutes
  albumin, human
  Albuminar-5; Albuminar-25
  Albutein 5%; Albutein 25%
  Buminate 5%; Buminate 25%
  dextran 40
  dextran 70
  dextran 75
  Gendex 75
  Gentran 40
  Gentran 70
  hemoglobin, recombinant human (rHb1.1)
  Hemolink
  Hemopure
  Hespan
  hetastarch
  Hextend
  intravascular perfluorochemical emulsion
  LiquiVent
  10% LMD
  Macrodex
  Oxygent
  Pentaspan
  pentastarch
  perflubron
  Plasbumin-5; Plasbumin-25
  plasma protein fraction
  Plasma-Plex
  Plasmanate
  Plasmatein
  PolyHeme
  Protenate
  Rheomacrodex
Bronchodilators [see: Asthma agents; Respiratory System Agents]
Burns [see: Wound Treatment]
Cancer [see: Antineoplastics]

Cardiac Agents
  [see also: Antihypertensives; Diuretics]

Indications

Cardiac Agents, Antianginals

acebutolol HCl
Adalat
Adalat CC; Adalat Oros
Adalat XL ⒸⒶⓃ
amlodipine
amlodipine besylate
Apo-Diltiaz ⒸⒶⓃ
Apo-Diltiaz CD ⒸⒶⓃ
Apo-Diltiaz SR ⒸⒶⓃ
Apo-Metoprolol ⒸⒶⓃ
Apo-Metoprolol L ⒸⒶⓃ
Apo-Atenolol ⒸⒶⓃ
atenolol
bepridil HCl
Betachron E-R
Calan
Calan SR
Cardene
Cardizem
Cardizem CD
Cardizem SR
Cardizem XL
Cartia XT
celiprolol HCl
Corgard
Covera-HS
dalteparin sodium
Deponit
Dilacor XR
Dilatrate-SR
diltiazem HCl
diltiazem malate
enoxaparin sodium
erythrityl tetranitrate
Fragmin
Gen-Metoprolol ⒸⒶⓃ
Gen-Verapamil ⒸⒶⓃ
Gen-Acebutolol ⒸⒶⓃ
Imdur
Inderal
Inderal LA
Ismo
Isoptin
Isoptin SR
Isordil
isosorbide dinitrate
isosorbide mononitrate
Isotrate ER
Lopressor

Cardiac Agents, Antianginals (cont.)

Lovenox
metoprolol succinate
metoprolol tartrate
mibefradil dihydrochloride
Minitran
Monoket
nadolol
nicardipine HCl
Nifedical XL
nifedipine
NitroTab
Nitrek
Nitro-Bid
Nitro-Bid IV
Nitro-Derm
Nitro-Dur
Nitro-Time
Nitrodisc
Nitrogard
nitroglycerin
Nitroglyn
Nitrol
Nitrolingual Pumpspray
Nitrong
NitroQuick
Nitrostat
Norvasc
Novo-Diltiazem CD ⒸⒶⓃ
Novo-Metoprol ⒸⒶⓃ
Nu-Diltiaz-CD ⒸⒶⓃ
pentaerythritol tetranitrate (PETN)
PMS-Pindolol ⒸⒶⓃ
Posicor
Procardia
Procardia XL
propranolol HCl
ranolazine HCl
Rhoxal-diltiazem CD ⒸⒶⓃ
Sectral
Selecor
Sorbitrate
Tenormin
Tiamate
Tiazac
Toprol-XL
Transderm-Nitro
Tridil

Cardiac Agents, Antianginals (cont.)
Trinipatch ⒸⒶⓃ
Vascor
verapamil HCl
Verelan

Cardiac Agents, Antiarrhythmics
Adenocard
adenosine
Alti-Amiodarone ⒸⒶⓃ
Amio-Aqueous
amiodarone HCl
Apo-Diltiaz ⒸⒶⓃ
Apo-Diltiaz CD ⒸⒶⓃ
Apo-Diltiaz SR ⒸⒶⓃ
Apo-Propafenone ⒸⒶⓃ
Betachron E-R
Betapace
Betapace AF
bretylium tosylate
Bretylol
Brevibloc
Calan
Calan SR
Cardioquin
Cardizem
Cardizem CD
Cardizem SR
Cardizem XL
Cartia XT
cifenline succinate
Cipralan
Cordarone
Corvert
Covera-HS
Crystodigin
Digitek
digitoxin
digoxin
Digoxin Injection C.S.D. ⒸⒶⓃ
Digoxin Pediatric Injection C.S.D. ⒸⒶⓃ
Dilacor XR
diltiazem HCl
diltiazem malate
disopyramide phosphate
dofetilide
esmolol HCl
Ethmozine
flecainide acetate

Cardiac Agents, Antiarrhythmics (cont.)
Gen-Verapamil ⒸⒶⓃ
Gen-Amiodarone ⒸⒶⓃ
ibutilide fumarate
Inderal
Inderal LA
Isoptin
Isoptin SR
Lanoxicaps
Lanoxin
lidocaine HCl
LidoPen
mexiletine HCl
Mexitil
moricizine HCl
Norpace
Norpace CR
Novo-Diltiazem CD ⒸⒶⓃ
Novo-Amiodarone ⒸⒶⓃ
Pacerone
PMS-Sotalol ⒸⒶⓃ
procainamide HCl
Procanbid
Pronestyl
Pronestyl-SR
propafenone HCl
propranolol HCl
Quinaglute
Quinalan
Quinidex
quinidine gluconate
quinidine polygalacturonate
quinidine sulfate
Quinora
Rhoxal-amiodarone ⒸⒶⓃ
Rhoxal-diltiazem CD ⒸⒶⓃ
RSD-921
Rythmol
sotalol HCl
Tambocor
Tiamate
Tiazac
Tikosyn
tocainide HCl
Tonocard
verapamil HCl
Verelan
Xylocaine HCl IV for Cardiac Arrhythmias

Indications

Cardiac Agents, Congestive Heart Failure Agents

Accupril
Accuretic
Aldactazide
Aldactone
amiloride HCl
Apo-Furosemide (CAN)
Apo-Hydro (CAN)
Aquatensen
bumetanide
Bumex
Capoten
Capozide 25/15; Capozide 25/25; Capozide 50/15; Capozide 50/25
captopril
captopril & hydrochlorothiazide
carvedilol
chlorthalidone
cilazapril
Clorpres
Combipres 0.1; Combipres 0.2; Combipres 0.3
Coreg
Corgenic
Crystodigin
Demadex
Demi-Regroton
Digitek
digitoxin
digoxin
Digoxin Injection C.S.D. (CAN)
Digoxin Pediatric Injection C.S.D. (CAN)
dobutamine HCl
Dobutrex
dopamine HCl
Dyazide
Dyrenium
Edecrin
Edecrin Sodium
enalapril maleate
enalapril maleate & hydrochlorothiazide
enalaprilat
Enbrel
Enduron
Esidrix
etanercept
ethacrynate sodium
ethacrynic acid

Cardiac Agents, Congestive Heart Failure Agents (cont.)

Ezide
furosemide
gemopatrilat
Hydro-Par
hydrochlorothiazide (HCT; HCTZ)
hydrochlorothiazide & captopril
hydrochlorothiazide & enalapril maleate
hydrochlorothiazide & triamterene
HydroDIURIL
Hygroton
inamrinone lactate
Inocor
Intropin
Lanoxicaps
Lanoxin
Lasix
levosimendan
lisinopril
Maxzide
methyclothiazide
metolazone
Microzide
Midamor
milrinone lactate
Moduretic
moxonidine
Mykrox
Natrecor
nesiritide citrate
Novo-Hydrazide (CAN)
Novo-Semide (CAN)
omapatrilat
Oretic
Physiotens
Primacor
Primacor in 5% Dextrose
Prinivil
Prinzide
Prinzide 12.5; Prinzide 25
quinapril HCl
Simdax
spironolactone
Thalitone
torsemide
triamterene
triamterene & hydrochlorothiazide
Vanlev

Cardiac Agents, Congestive Heart Failure Agents (cont.)
Vaseretic 5-12.5; Vaseretic 10-25
Vasotec
Vasotec I.V.
vesnarinone
Zaroxolyn
Zestoretic
Zestril

Cardiac Agents, Vasopressors
Adrenalin Chloride
Ana-Guard
Aramine
dobutamine HCl
Dobutrex
dopamine HCl
dopamine HCl in 5% dextrose
ephedrine sulfate
epinephrine
epinephrine HCl
Epinephrine Pediatric
EpiPen; EpiPen Jr.
Intropin
isoproterenol HCl
Isuprel
Levophed
mephentermine sulfate
metaraminol bitartrate
methoxamine HCl
midodrine HCl
Neo-Synephrine
norepinephrine bitartrate
phenylephrine HCl
ProAmatine
Sus-Phrine
Vasoxyl
Wyamine Sulfate

Cardiac Agents, Other
alprostadil
Antrin
Apo-Pravastatin Ⓒᴬᴺ
Berinert-P
C1-esterase-inhibitor, human
coenzyme Q_{10}
Foltx
Indocin I.V.
indomethacin sodium trihydrate
Lin-Pravastatin Ⓒᴬᴺ
monoclonal antibody 5G1.1-SC
motexafin lutetium

Cardiac Agents, Other (cont.)
Pravachol
pravastatin sodium
Prostin VR Pediatric
simvastatin
tenecteplase
TNKase
Vasoprost
Zocor

Central Nervous System Stimulants
Adderall
Alertec Ⓒᴬᴺ
amphetamine aspartate
amphetamine sulfate
Cafcit
caffeine
caffeine & sodium benzoate
caffeine citrate
citrated caffeine
Concerta
Cylert
d-methylphenidate HCl (d-MPH)
Desoxyn
Dexedrine
dexmethylphenidate HCl
dextroamphetamine saccharate
dextroamphetamine sulfate
Dextrostat
Dopram
doxapram HCl
Metadate CD
Metadate ER
methamphetamine HCl
Methylin
Methylin ER
methylphenidate
methylphenidate HCl (MPH)
modafinil
Neocaf
Oxydess II
PemADD
PemADD CT
pemoline
Provigil
Ritadex
Ritalin

Indications

**Central Nervous System Stimu-
lants (cont.)**
Ritalin-SR
sodium benzoate & caffeine
Spancap No. 1
Chelating Agents [see: Antidotes,
Chelating Agents]
Chemonucleolytic Agents [see:
Enzymes, Proteolytic]
Chemotherapy Protocols [see: Anti-
neoplastics, Chemotherapy Protocols]
Cholelithics [see: Biliary Tract Agents]
Cholesterol-lowering Agents [see:
Lipid-lowering Agents]
**Chronic Obstructive Pulmonary
Disease (COPD)** [see: Respiratory
System Agents]
Cold Sores and Fever Blisters [see:
Mouth and Throat Preparations]
Congestive Heart Failure [see: Car-
diac Agents, Congestive Heart Failure
Agents]
Contraceptives [see: Gynecological
Agents, Contraceptives; Vaginal
Preparations, Contraceptives]

Contrast Media
Contrast Media, Paramagnetic
AngioMark
Combidex
Feridex
ferristene
ferucarbotran
ferumoxides
ferumoxsil
ferumoxtran-10
gadodiamide
gadofosveset trisodium
gadopentetate dimeglumine
gadoteridol
gadoversetamide
GastroMARK
Magnevist
mangafodipir trisodium
mangofodipir trisodium
MS-325
Omniscan
Optimark
perflubron

**Contrast Media, Paramagnetic
(cont.)**
ProHance
Resovist
Teslascan
Contrast Media, Radiopaque
Amipaque
Anatrast
Angio-Conray
Angiovist 282
Angiovist 292; Angiovist 370
arcitumomab
Baricon
barium sulfate
Baro-cat
Barobag
Baroflave
Barosperse
Barosperse, Liquid
Bear-E-Bag Pediatric
Bear-E-Yum CT
Bear-E-Yum GI
Bilivist
Bilopaque
CEA-Scan
Cholebrine
Cholografin Meglumine
Conray 325
Conray 400
Conray; Conray 30; Conray 43
Cysto-Conray; Cysto-Conray II
Cystografin; Cystografin Dilute
diatrizoate meglumine
diatrizoate sodium
Dionosil Oily
Enecat
Enhancer
Entrobar
Epi-C
ethiodized oil
Ethiodol
Flo-Coat
Gastrografin
HD 200 Plus
HD 85
Hexabrix
Hypaque-76
Hypaque-Cysto
Hypaque-M 75; Hypaque-M 90

Contrast Media, Radiopaque (cont.)
Hypaque Meglumine 30%; Hypaque
  Meglumine 60%
Hypaque Sodium
Hypaque Sodium 20%
Hypaque Sodium 25%; Hypaque
  Sodium 50%
Imager ac
Intropaste
iocetamic acid
iodamide meglumine
iodipamide meglumine
iodixanol
iohexol
iopamidol
iopanoic acid
iopromide
iosulfan blue
iothalamate meglumine
iothalamate sodium
iotrolan
ioversol
ioxaglate meglumine
ioxaglate sodium
ipodate calcium
ipodate sodium
Isovue-M 200; Isovue-M 300
Isovue-128; Isovue-200; Isovue-250;
  Isovue-300; Isovue-370
Liqui-Coat HD
Liquipake
Lymphazurin 1%
MD-60; MD-76
MD-76 R
MD-Gastroview
Medebar Plus
Medescan
metrizamide
Novopaque
OctreoScan
Omnipaque
Optiray 160; Optiray 240; Optiray
  300; Optiray 320; Optiray 350
Oragrafin Calcium
Oragrafin Sodium
oxidronate sodium
polyvinyl chloride, radiopaque
Prepcat
propyliodone
Quick AC Enema Kit

Contrast Media, Radiopaque (cont.)
Reno-30
Reno-Dip; Reno-60
RenoCal-76
Renografin-60
Renografin-76
Renovist; Renovist II
Renovue-Dip; Renovue-65
Sinografin
Sitzmarks
Telepaque
Tomocat
Tonopaque
tyropanoate sodium
Ultravist
Urovist Cysto
Urovist Meglumine DIU/CT
Urovist Sodium 300
Vascoray
Visipaque

Contrast Media, Ultrasound
albumin, human (sonicated with
  chlorofluorocarbons)
Albunex
Definity
EchoGen
Echovist ⒸⒶⓃ
Filmix
galactose
Imagent US
Levovist ⒸⒶⓃ
microbubble contrast agent
Optison
palmitic acid
perflenapent
perflexane
perflisopent
perflutren
Sonazoid

Corticosteroids, Systemic
[see also: Asthma Agents; Gout
  Agents; Immunosuppressants;
  Rheumatic Disease Agents]
A-Hydrocort
A-Methapred
ACTH
ACTH-80
Acthar

Indications

Corticosteroids, Systemic (cont.)

Adlone
Alti-Dexamethasone (CAN)
Amcort
Apo-Prednisone (CAN)
Aristocort
Aristocort Forte
Aristospan Intra-articular
Articulose-50
Articulose L.A.
Atolone
Betaject (CAN)
betamethasone
betamethasone acetate
betamethasone sodium phosphate
Cel-U-Jec
Celestone
Celestone Phosphate
Celestone Soluspan
Cortef
corticotropin
cortisone acetate
Cortone Acetate
Dalalone
Dalalone D.P.
Dalalone L.A.
Decadron
Decadron-LA
Decadron Phosphate
Decadron with Xylocaine
Decaject
Decaject-L.A.
Delta-Cortef
Deltasone
depMedalone 40; depMedalone 80
Depo-Medrol
Depoject
Depopred-40; Depopred-80
Dexameth
dexamethasone
dexamethasone acetate
dexamethasone sodium phosphate
Dexasone
Dexasone L.A.
Dexone
Dexone LA
Duralone-40; Duralone-80
Florinef Acetate
fludrocortisone acetate
H.P. Acthar Gel

Corticosteroids, Systemic (cont.)

Hexadrol
Hexadrol Phosphate
Hydeltra-T.B.A.
Hydeltrasol
hydrocortisone (HC)
hydrocortisone acetate (HCA)
hydrocortisone sodium phosphate
hydrocortisone sodium succinate
Hydrocortone
Hydrocortone Acetate
Hydrocortone Phosphate
Key-Pred 25; Key-Pred 50
Kenacort
Kenaject-40
Kenalog-10; Kenalog-40
Key-Pred-SP
Liquid Pred
M-Prednisol-40; M-Prednisol-80
Medralone 40; Medralone 80
Medrol
methylprednisolone
methylprednisolone acetate
methylprednisolone sodium phosphate
methylprednisolone sodium succinate
Meticorten
Orapred
Orasone
Panasol-S
Pediapred
PMS-Dexamethasone (CAN)
Predalone 50
Predcor-50
Prednicen-M
Prednisol TBA
prednisolone
prednisolone acetate
prednisolone sodium phosphate
prednisolone tebutate
prednisone
Prelone
Solu-Cortef
Solu-Medrol
Solurex
Solurex LA
Sterapred; Sterapred DS
Tac-3
Tac-40
Tri-Kort
Triam Forte

Corticosteroids, Systemic (cont.)
Triam-A
triamcinolone
triamcinolone acetonide
triamcinolone diacetate
triamcinolone hexacetonide
Triamolone 40
Triamonide 40
Trilog
Trilone
Tristoject
Cough [*see: Antitussives*]
Crohn Disease: [*see: Inflammatory Bowel Disease Agents*]
Debriding Agents [*see: Wound Treatment, Cleansing and Debriding Agents*]

Decongestants, Systemic
Aclophen
Actagen-C Cough
Actifed with Codeine Cough
AH-chew
AH-chew D
Allegra-D
Allent
Allerfrin with Codeine
AlleRx
Alumadrine
Ami-Tex LA
Anamine
Anamine T.D.
Anaplex
Anaplex DM Cough
Anaplex HD
Anatuss
Anatuss LA
Andehist
Andehist DM
Aprodine with Codeine
Aquatab C
Aquatab D
Atrohist Pediatric
Atrohist Plus
Atuss DM
Atuss G
Atuss HD
Biohist-LA
Brexin-L.A.
Brofed

Decongestants, Systemic (cont.)
Bromadine-DM
Bromadine-DX
Bromanate DC Cough
Bromarest DX Cough
Bromatane DX Cough
Bromfed
Bromfed-DM Cough
Bromfed-PD
Bromfenex
Bromfenex PD
Bromophen T.D.
Bromphen DC with Codeine Cough
Bromphen DX Cough
brompheniramine maleate & pseudoephedrine HCl & dextromethorphan hydrobromide
Brompheniramine DC Cough
Broncholate
Bronkotuss Expectorant
Calmylin with Codeine ⒸⒶ
Carbinoxamine Compound
Carbiset
Carbiset-TR
Carbodec
Carbodec DM
Carbodec TR
Cardec-DM
Cardec-S
Chlorafed; Chlorafed HS
Chlordrine S.R.
Chlorgest-HD
Chlorphedrine SR
chlorpheniramine maleate & phenylpropanolamine HCl
Claritin-D; Claritin-D 12 Hour; Claritin-D 24 Hour
Codamine
Codegest Expectorant
Codehist DH
Codimal DH
Codimal-L.A.; Codimal-L.A. Half
Coldec DM
Coldloc
Coldloc-LA
Colfed-A
Comhist
Comhist LA
Conex with Codeine
Congess JR

Indications

Decongestants, Systemic (cont.)
    Congess SR
    Contuss
    Cophene No. 2
    Cophene-X
    Cophene XP
    Cotridin ⒸⒶⓃ
    Cotridin Expectorant ⒸⒶⓃ
    Cyclofed Pediatric
    Cycofed Pediatric
    D.A.
    D.A. II
    Dallergy
    Dallergy-JR
    Decohistine DH
    Deconamine
    Deconamine CX
    Deconamine SR
    Decongestabs
    Decongestant
    Decongestant Expectorant
    Deconhist L.A.
    Deconomed SR
    Deconsal II
    Deconsal Pediatric
    Deconsal Sprinkle
    Defen-LA
    Dehistine
    Deproist Expectorant with Codeine
    Despec
    Detussin
    Detussin Expectorant
    Dexaphen S.A.
    dextromethorphan hydrobromide & brompheniramine maleate & pseudoephedrine HCl
    Dihistine Expectorant
    Dimetane-DC Cough
    Dimetane-DX Cough
    Disobrom
    Donatussin
    Donatussin DC
    Drixomed
    Drize
    Dura-Gest
    Dura-Tap/PD
    Dura-Vent
    Dura-Vent/A
    Dura-Vent/DA
    Duralex

Decongestants, Systemic (cont.)
    Duratuss; Duratuss-GP
    E.N.T.
    Ed A-Hist
    ED-TLC; ED Tuss HC
    Endafed
    Endagen-HD
    Endal
    Endal Expectorant
    Endal-HD; Endal-HD Plus
    Enomine
    Entex
    Entex LA
    Entex PSE
    Entuss-D
    Entuss-D Jr.
    ephedrine HCl
    ephedrine sulfate
    ephedrine tannate
    Eudal-SR
    Ex-Histine
    Exgest LA
    Extendryl
    Extendryl JR
    Extendryl SR
    Fedahist
    Gelhist
    GFN/PSE
    GP-500
    Guai-Vent/PSE
    Guaifed
    Guaifed-PD
    guaifenesin & phenylephrine HCl & phenylpropanolamine HCl
    Guaifenex
    Guaifenex PPA 75
    Guaifenex PSE 60; Guaifenex PSE 120; Guaifenex Rx DM
    Guaifenex Rx
    GuaiMAX-D
    Guaipax
    Guaitex
    Guaitex LA
    Guaitex PSE
    Guaivent
    Guaivent PD
    Guiatex LA
    Guiatex PSE
    Guiatuss DAC
    Guiatussin DAC

Decongestants, Systemic (cont.)
H-Tuss-D
Hista-Vadrin
Histade
Histalet
Histalet Forte
Histalet X
Histex HC
Histex SR
Histine DM; Histinex DM
Histinex HC
Histinex PV
Histor-D
Histussin D
Histussin HC
Hycomine
Hycomine Compound
Hydro-PC
Hydrocodone CP; Hydrocodone HD
Hydrocodone PA
Hydrophed
Hyphed
Iodal HD
Iofed
Iofed PD
Iohist D
Iohist DM
Iosal II
Iotussin HC
Isoclor Expectorant
KIE
Klerist-D
Kronofed-A Jr.
Kronofed-A
Levall 5.0
Liqui-Histine-D
Liqui-Histine DM
Liquibid-D
Lodrane LD
Lufyllin-EPG
Marax
Marax-DF
MED-Rx
MED-Rx DM
Mescolor
methscopolamine nitrate
Mudrane
Mudrane GG
Myphetane DC Cough
Myphetane DX Cough

Decongestants, Systemic (cont.)
Mytussin DAC
Naldecon
Naldecon CX Adult
Naldelate
Nalgest
Nasabid
Nasabid SR
Nasatab LA
ND Clear
No-Hist
Nolamine
Norel
Norel Plus
Novafed A
Novagest Expectorant with Codeine
Novahistine DH
Novahistine Expectorant
Nucofed
Nucofed Expectorant; Nucofed
   Pediatric Expectorant
Nucotuss Expectorant; Nucotuss
   Pediatric Expectorant
OMNIhist L.A.
Ordrine AT
Ornade
P-V-Tussin
Palgic-D
Palgic-DS
Pancof-HC
Pancof-XL; Pancof XP
Panmist JR
PanMist-DM
Pannaz
Para-Hist HD
Partuss LA
Pediacof
Pedituss Cough
Phenahist-TR
Phenate
Phenchlor S.H.A.
Phenergan VC
Phenergan VC with Codeine
Phenhist DH with Codeine
Phenhist Expectorant
phenylephrine HCl
phenylephrine HCl & phenylpropa-
   nolamine HCl & guaifenesin
phenylephrine tannate
Phenylfenesin L.A.

Decongestants, Systemic (cont.)

phenylpropanolamine HCl
phenylpropanolamine HCl & chlor-
    pheniramine maleate
phenylpropanolamine HCl & phen-
    ylephrine HCl & guaifenesin
Pherazine VC with Codeine
Polaramine Expectorant
Poly-Histine CS
Poly-Histine-D
Poly-Histine-D Ped Caps
Poly-Histine DM
Prehist
Prehist D
Profen Forte DM
Profen II DM
Profen II; Profen LA
Prometh VC Plain
Prometh VC with Codeine
Promethazine VC
Promethazine VC Plain
Promethazine VC with Codeine
Promethist with Codeine
Protuss-D
Protuss DM
Pseudo-Car DM
Pseudo-Chlor
pseudoephedrine HCl
pseudoephedrine HCl & dextro-
    methorphan hydrobromide &
    brompheniramine maleate
pseudoephedrine sulfate
pseudoephedrine tannate
Quadrinal
R-Tanna 12
R-Tannamine
R-Tannate
R-Tannic-S A/D
Rentamine Pediatric
Resaid
Rescaps-D S.R.
Rescon
Rescon-ED
Rescon JR
Respa-1st
Respahist
Respaire-60; Respaire-120
Rhinatate
Rhinolar-EX; Rhinolar-EX 12
Rinade B.I.D.

Decongestants, Systemic (cont.)

Robafen DAC
Robitussin-DAC
Rolatuss Expectorant
Rolatuss with Hydrocodone
Rondamine-DM
Rondec
Rondec-DM
Rondec-TR
Ru-Tuss DE
Ru-Tuss with Hydrocodone
Rymed
Rymed-TR
Ryna-C
Ryna-CX
Rynatan
Rynatan-12 S
Rynatan-S
Rynatuss
Seldane-D
Semprex-D
Sil-Tex
Sildec-DM
Siltapp with Dextromethorphan
    HBr Cold & Cough
Sinufed
Sinupan
SinuVent
SRC Expectorant
Stahist
Stamoist E
Stamoist LA
Statuss Expectorant
Statuss Green
Sudal 120/600
Sudal 60/500
Syn-Rx
T-Koff
Tamine S.R.
Tanafed
Tannic-12
Tanoral
Theomax DF
Time-Hist
Touro A & H; Touro Allergy
Touro CC
Touro LA
Tri-P
Tri-Phen-Chlor
Tri-Phen-Chlor T.R.

Decongestants, Systemic (cont.)
  Tri-Phen-Mine
  Tri-Phen-Mine S.R.
  Tri-Tannate
  Tri-Tannate Plus Pediatric
  Triacin-C Cough
  Triafed with Codeine
  Triaminic
  Triaminic Expectorant DH
  Triaminic Expectorant with Codeine
  Trifed-C Cough
  Trinalin
  Triotann
  Tritan
  Tusquelin
  Tuss-LA
  Tuss-Ornade
  Tuss-Allergine Modified T.D.
  Tuss-Tan
  Tussafed
  Tussafed HC
  Tussafed-LA
  Tussafin Expectorant
  Tussanil DH
  Tussar SF; Tussar-2
  Tussend
  Tussi-12
  Tussirex
  Tussogest
  Tyrodone
  ULR-LA
  UltraBrom
  UltraBrom PD
  Uni-Decon
  Unituss HC
  V-Dec-M
  Vanex Expectorant
  Vanex Forte
  Vanex Forte-R
  Vanex-HD
  Versacaps
  Vetuss HC
  Xiral
  Zephrex
  Zephrex LA
  Zyrtec-D
Dementia [see: Alzheimer Disease Agents]
Depigmenting Agents [see: Dermatological Preparations, Depigmenting Agents]

Dermatological Preparations
Dermatological Preparations, Acne Products, Systemic
  [see also: Antibiotics; Corticosteroids, Systemic]
  Accutane
  Achromycin V
  cyproterone acetate
  Diane-35 ⓒᴬᴺ
  Dynacin
  E-Base
  E-Mycin
  Ery-Tab
  ERYC
  erythromycin
  erythromycin estolate
  Estrostep 21
  Gen-Cyproterone ⓒᴬᴺ
  Ilosone
  isotretinoin
  Minocin
  minocycline HCl
  Nor-Tet
  Ortho Tri-Cyclen
  Panmycin
  PCE
  PMS-Minocycline ⓒᴬᴺ
  Rhoxal-minocycline ⓒᴬᴺ
  Robimycin
  Robitet
  Sumycin
  Sumycin '250'; Sumycin '500'
  Teline; Teline-500
  Tetracap
  tetracycline HCl
  Tetralan
  Tetralan "250"; Tetralan-500
  Vectrin
Dermatological Preparations, Acne Products, Topical
  [see also: Antibiotics, Topical; Antiseptics; Dermatological Preparations, Keratolytics]
  A/T/S
  adapalene
  Akne-mycin
  Altinac
  Atrisone
  Avita
  azelaic acid

Indications

Dermatological Preparations, Acne Products, Topical (cont.)

Azelex

Benzac AC 2½; Benzac W 2½; Benzac 5; Benzac AC 5; Benzac W 5; Benzac 10; Benzac AC 10; Benzac W 10

Benzac AC Wash 2½; Benzac AC Wash 5; Benzac W Wash 5; Benzac AC Wash 10; Benzac W Wash 10

Benzaclin

5 Benzagel; 10 Benzagel

Benzagel Wash

Benzamycin

Benzashave

Benzox-10

benzoyl peroxide

Brevoxyl

Brevoxyl Cleansing

Brevoxyl Creamy Wash

C/T/S

Cleocin T

Clinda-Derm

clindamycin

clindamycin phosphate

Clindets

Dalacin T ⓒⒶⓃ

Del Aqua-5; Del Aqua-10

Del-Mycin

Desquam-E; Desquam-E 5; Desquam-E 10

Desquam-X 5 Wash; Desquam-X 10 Wash

Desquam-X 5; Desquam-X 10

Differin

Emgel

Erycette

EryDerm 2%

Erygel

Erymax

Erythra-Derm

erythromycin

Finevin

Hyacne

Klaron

Meclan

meclocycline sulfosalicylate

Novacet

Panoxyl

Dermatological Preparations, Acne Products, Topical (cont.)

Panoxyl AQ 2½; Panoxyl 5; Panoxyl AQ 5; Panoxyl 10; Panoxyl AQ 10

Peroxin A 5; Peroxin A 10

Persa-Gel; Persa-Gel W 5%; Persa-Gel W 10%

PROPApH Foaming Face Wash

pyrithione zinc

Rejuva-A ⓒⒶⓃ

Renova

Retin-A

Retin-A Micro

salicylic acid (SA)

Septi-Soft

Septisol

Staticin

Sulfacet-R

sulfacetamide sodium

Sulfoxyl Regular; Sulfoxyl Strong

sulfur, precipitated

sulfur, sublimed

T-Stat

tazarotene

Tazorac

tetracycline HCl

Theramycin Z

Topicycline

tretinoin

Triaz

triclosan

Vanocin

Vanoxide-HC

Vitinoin ⓒⒶⓃ

Dermatological Preparations, Antihyperhidrotics

aluminum chloride

aluminum chlorohydrate

aluminum sulfate

Drysol

formaldehyde solution

Formalyde-10

Lazer Formalyde

Dermatological Preparations, Antiinflammatory Agents

Aclovate

Acticort 100

Aeroseb-Dex

Aeroseb-HC

Ala-Cort

Dermatological Preparations, Anti-inflammatory Agents (cont.)

Ala-Quin
alclometasone dipropionate
Alphatrex
amcinonide
Aristocort
Aristocort A
Aristocort Intralesional
Aristospan Intralesional
Beta-Val
betamethasone benzoate
betamethasone dipropionate
betamethasone dipropionate & clotrimazole
betamethasone dipropionate, augmented
betamethasone sodium phosphate
betamethasone valerate
Betatrex
Capex
Carmol HC
Celestoderm-V; Celestoderm-V/2 (CAN)
Celestone Soluspan
Cetacort
clobetasol propionate
clocortolone pivalate
Cloderm
clotrimazole & betamethasone dipropionate
Cordran
Cordran SP
Cormax
Corque
Cort-Dome
Cortate (CAN)
cortisone acetate
Cortisporin
Cortone Acetate
Cutivate
Cyclocort
Dalalone
Dalalone L.A.
Decadron-LA
Decadron Phosphate
Decaject
Decaject-L.A.
Delta-Tritex
depMedalone 40; depMedalone 80
Depo-Medrol

Dermatological Preparations, Anti-inflammatory Agents (cont.)

Depoject
Depopred-40; Depopred-80
Derma-Smoothe/FS
Dermacort
Dermatop
desonide
DesOwen
Desoxi (CAN)
desoximetasone
dexamethasone
dexamethasone acetate
dexamethasone sodium phosphate
Dexasone
Dexasone L.A.
Dexone
Dexone LA
diclofenac potassium
diflorasone diacetate
dimethyl sulfoxide (DMSO)
Diprolene
Diprolene AF
Diprosone
Duralone-40; Duralone-80
Elocom (CAN)
Elocon
Enzone
Epifoam
1+1-F Creme
Finevin
Florone
Florone E
fluocinolone acetonide
fluocinonide
Fluonex
Fluonid
flurandrenolide
Flurosyn
Flutex
fluticasone propionate
FS Shampoo
Fungoid-HC
1% HC
halcinonide
halobetasol propionate
Halog
Halog-E
Hexadrol Phosphate
Hi-Cor 1.0; Hi-Cor 2.5

Indications

Dermatological Preparations, Anti-inflammatory Agents (cont.)

Hycort
Hydeltra-T.B.A.
HydroTex
Hydrocort
hydrocortisone (HC)
hydrocortisone acetate (HCA)
hydrocortisone buteprate
hydrocortisone butyrate
hydrocortisone probutate
hydrocortisone valerate
Hydrocortisone Iodoquinol 1%
Hydrocortone Acetate
Hytone
Hytone 1%
Kemsol ⓒᴬᴺ
Kenaject-40
Kenalog
Kenalog-H
Kenalog-10; Kenalog-40
Kenonel
Kutapressin
LactiCare-HC
Lida-Mantle-HC
Lidex
Lidex-E
liver derivative complex
Locoid
Lotrisone
Luxiq
Lyderm ⓒᴬᴺ
M-Prednisol-40; M-Prednisol-80
Mantadil
Maxiflor
Maxivate
Medralone 40; Medralone 80
methylprednisolone acetate
mometasone furoate
Myco-Biotic II
Myco-Triacet II
Mycogen II
Mycolog-II
Myconel
Mytrex
N.G.T.
Nasonex
Neo-Cortef
NeoDecadron
Nutracort

Dermatological Preparations, Anti-inflammatory Agents (cont.)

Olux
orgotein
OxSODrol
Pandel
Pedi-Cort V Creme
Penecort
Pramosone
prednicarbate
Prednisol TBA
prednisolone tebutate
Protopic
Psorcon E
S-T Cort
Solurex
Solurex LA
Synacort
Synalar
Synalar-HP
Synemol
Tac-3
tacrolimus
Teladar
Temovate
Temovate Emollient
Texacort
Topicort
Topicort LP
Tri-Kort
Tri-Statin II
Triacet
Triam-A
triamcinolone acetonide
triamcinolone diacetate
triamcinolone hexacetonide
Triamonide 40
Triderm
Tridesilon
Trilog
U-Cort
Ultravate
Valisone
Valisone Reduced Strength
Vanoxide-HC
ViaFoam
Vytone
Westcort
Zemaphyte
Zone-A Forte

Dermatological Preparations, Depigmenting Agents

Alustra
Glyquin
hydroquinone
Lustra; Lustra-AF
Melanex
Melpaque HP
Melquin HP
Nuquin HP
Solaquin Forte
Viquin Forte

Dermatological Preparations, Dermatitis Herpetiformis Agents

dapsone

Dermatological Preparations, Emollients and Protectants

[see also: Wound Treatment, Vulneraries]

Accuzyme
allantoin
aloe
aluminum acetate
Alustra
ammonium lactate (lactic acid neutralized with ammonium hydroxide)
ascorbic acid (L-ascorbic acid; vitamin C)
bismuth subnitrate
Carmol HC
cocoa butter
cod liver oil
colloidal oatmeal
Cosmederm-7 (CAN)
Derma-Smoothe/FS
dimethicone
glycerin
glycolic acid
Glyquin
Gordon's Urea 40%
Lac-Hydrin
lactic acid
Lactinol
Lactinol-E
lanolin
Lustra; Lustra-AF
mineral oil
Panafil
Panafil White

Dermatological Preparations, Emollients and Protectants (cont.)

Papain Urea Chlorophyllin
Papain Urea Debriding
Peruvian balsam
petrolatum
propylene glycol
shark liver oil
silicone
urea
vitamin A
vitamin A palmitate
vitamin E
zinc oxide

Dermatological Preparations, Hair and Scalp Agents

Ala-Scalp
betamethasone valerate
Capitrol
chloroxine
coal tar
Drithocreme; Drithocreme HP 1%; Dritho-Scalp
eflornithine HCl
finasteride
ketoconazole
Luxiq
minoxidil
Nizoral
Olux
phenol
povidone-iodine
Propecia
pyrithione zinc
Sal-Oil-T
salicylic acid (SA)
sulfur, precipitated
Vaniqa

Dermatological Preparations, Keratolytic Agents

[see also: Dermatological Preparations, Acne Products, Topical; Dermatological Products, Wart and Corn Removers]

Alustra
Bensal HP
Castellani Paint Modified
Emersal
Finevin
glycolic acid

Indications

Dermatological Preparations, Keratolytic Agents (cont.)

Glyquin
Lustra; Lustra-AF
Mono-Chlor
monochloroacetic acid
resorcinol
salicylic acid (SA)
silver nitrate
Tinver
Tri-Chlor
trichloroacetic acid
Versiclear

Dermatological Preparations, Photodamaged Skin Agents

Actinex
Altinac
5-aminolevulinic acid HCl (5-ALA HCl)
Avita
diclofenac potassium
Levulan Kerastick
masoprocol
Rejuva-A ⒸⒶ
Renova
Retin-A
Retin-A Micro
Solage
Solaraze
tretinoin
Vitinoin ⒸⒶ

Dermatological Preparations, Psoriasis Agents, Systemic

acitretin
Amevive
calcitriol (1,25-hydroxycholecalciferol; 1,25-hydroxyvitamin D_3)
etretinate
Folex PFS
methotrexate (MTX)
methotrexate sodium
methoxsalen (8-methoxsalen)
Oxsoralen-Ultra
P-53
Rheumatrex
Rocaltrol
Soriatane
Tegison
Trexall

Dermatological Preparations, Psoriasis Agents, Topical

[see also: Dermatological Preparations, Hair and Scalp Agents]
Anthra-Derm
anthralin
calcipotriene
coal tar
Dovonex
Drithocreme; Drithocreme HP 1%; Dritho-Scalp
Lasan
Lasan HP-1
maxacalcitol
mercury, ammoniated
methenamine sulfosalicylate
methoxsalen (8-methoxsalen)
MG217 Dual Treatment
Miconal
Prezios
Sal-Oil-T
salicylic acid (SA)
Unguentum Bossi
Zetar Emulsion

Dermatological Preparations, Rosacea Agents

MetroCream
MetroGel; MetroLotion
metronidazole
Noritate

Dermatological Preparations, Vitiligo Agents

Benoquin
methoxsalen (8-methoxsalen)
monobenzone
8-MOP
Oxsoralen
trioxsalen
Trisoralen

Dermatological Preparations, Wart and Corn Removers

[see also: Dermatological Preparations, Keratolytics]
Bichloracetic Acid
cantharidin
Condylox
dichloroacetic acid
DuoPlant
Gordofilm
Paplex Ultra

Dermatological Preparations, Wart and Corn Removers (cont.)
Podocon-25
podofilox
Podofin
podophyllum
podophyllum resin
salicylic acid (SA)
Verr-Canth
Verrex
Wartec ⒸⒶⒷ

Dermatological Preparations, Other
aminobenzoate potassium
Dermprotective Factor (DPF)
Glylorin
monolaurin
Potaba
SERPACWA (Skin Exposure Reduction Paste Against Chemical Warfare Agents)
TopiCare

Diabetes Agents
Diabetes Agents, Insulin
AERx
Humalog
Humalog Mix 50/50
Humalog Mix 75/25
Humalog Mix25 ⒸⒶⒷ
Humulin R Regular U-500 (concentrated)
insulin
insulin aspart
insulin glargine
insulin lispro
insulin lispro protamine
Lantus
NovoLog
NovoPen 1.5
Oralgen; Oralin
Regular Iletin II U-500 (concentrated)

Diabetes Agents, Oral Agents
acetohexamide
Actos
Alti-Metformin HCl ⒸⒶⒷ
Amaryl
Apo-Glyburide ⒸⒶⒷ
Avandia

Diabetes Agents, Oral Agents (cont.)
Basen
bromocriptine mesylate
chlorpropamide
Diaβeta (or DiaBeta)
Diab II
Diabinese
Diapid
Dymelor
Ergoset
Euglucon ⒸⒶⒷ
Gen-Gliclazide ⒸⒶⒷ
Gen-Glybe ⒸⒶⒷ
Gen-Metformin ⒸⒶⒷ
gliclazide
glimepiride
glipizide
GlucoNorm ⒸⒶⒷ
Glucophage; Glucophage XR
Glucotrol; Glucotrol XL
Glucovance
Glustat
glyburide
Glynase
Glyset
IGF-1/BP3 complex
INS-1
lypressin
metformin HCl
Micronase
Micronized Glyburide
miglitol
moxonidine
nateglinide
Novo-Glyburide ⒸⒶⒷ
Novo-Metformin ⒸⒶⒷ
Oralgen; Oralin
Orinase
Physiotens
pioglitazone HCl
pramlintide acetate
Prandase ⒸⒶⒷ
Prandin
Precose
repaglinide
Rezulin
rosiglitazone maleate
Starlix
Symlin
tolazamide

Indications

Diabetes Agents, Oral Agents (cont.)
tolbutamide
Tolinase
troglitazone
voglibose
Diabetes Agents, Related Disorders
alprostadil, liposomal
Alredase
Apligraf
Apo-Domperidone (CAN)
Axokine
becaplermin
Cytolex
Dermagraft; Dermagraft-TC
domperidone
epalrestat
graftskin
Locilex
memantine
Motilium (CAN)
Novo-Domperidone (CAN)
pexiganan acetate
pimagedine HCl
Regranex
tolrestat

Diagnostic Agents
Diagnostic Agents for Home Use
Accu-Chek Advantage
Advance
Advanced Care Cholesterol Test
Answer One-Step; Answer Plus;
    Answer Quick & Simple
Answer Ovulation
Azo Test Strips
Bili-Labstix
Biosafe HbA1c
Biosafe PSA
Biosafe Total Cholesterol
Biosafe Total Cholesterol Panel
Biosafe TSH
Biotel kidney
BTA Stat Test
Chemstrip 2 GP; Chemstrip 2 LN;
    Chemstrip 4 the OB; Chemstrip
    6; Chemstrip 7; Chemstrip 8;
    Chemstrip 9; Chemstrip 10 with
    SG; Chemstrip uGK
Chemstrip bG

Diagnostic Agents for Home Use (cont.)
Chemstrip uG
Clearblue Easy
Clearplan Easy
Clinistix
Clinitest
ColoCare
Color Ovulation Test
Combistix
Conceive Pregnancy
Confide
Dextrostix
Diascan
Diastix
Dr. Brown's Home Drug Testing System
e.p.t. Quick Stick
Easy A1C
EZ Detect
Fact Plus
First Choice
First Response Ovulation Predictor
First Response; First Response Early Result
Fortel Plus
Glucofilm
Glucometer Encore; Glucometer Elite
Glucostix
Hema-Check
Hema-Combistix
HemeSelect Collection
Hemoccult II Dispenserpak; Hemoccult II Dispenserpak Plus
Home Access Hepatitis C Check
Home Access; Home Access Express
Keto-Diastix
Ketostix
Labstix
Midstream Pregnancy Test
Multistix; Multistix 2; Multistix 7;
    Multistix 8 SG; Multistix 9; Multistix 9 SG; Multistix 10 SG;
    Multistix SG
N-Multistix; N-Multistix SG
Nimbus; Nimbus Quick Strip
One Step Midstream Pregnancy Test
One Touch
OraSure
OvuGen

Diagnostic Agents for Home Use (cont.)
OvuKIT Self-Test
OvuQuick Self-Test
ProTime
Pregnosis
QTest
Quickscreen
RapidVue
Uristix; Uristix 4

Diagnostic Agents for Professional Use
[see also: Contrast Media; Ophthalmologicals, Diagnostic Agents; Radiopharmaceuticals]
Abbott TestPack Plus hCG-Urine Plus
Acetest
Acthrel
AcuTect
AD7C
Adenoscan
adenosine
AlaSTAT
Albay
Albunex
Albustix
allergenic extracts (aqueous, glycerinated, or alum-precipitated)
Allpyral
Altropane
aminohippurate sodium
Amplicor Chlamydia
Amplicor HIV-1 Monitor
Amplicor MTB
Aplisol
Aplitest
arbutamine
arginine (L-arginine)
ASPIRINcheck
Azostix
Bactigen B Streptococcus-CS
Bactigen Meningitis Panel
Bactigen N meningitis
Bactigen Salmonella-Shigella
Baros
bentiromide
benzylpenicillin
benzylpenicilloyl polylysine
BiliCheck

Diagnostic Agents for Professional Use (cont.)
BioCox
Biocult-GC
BTA Rapid Urine Test
Calypte
Candida albicans skin test antigen
CandidaSure
Candin
capromab pendetide
carbon C 13 urea
carbon C 14 urea
Cardiac T
Cardio-Green (CG)
Cardiolite
CAST (Color Allergy Screening Test)
Center-Al
Chemstrip K
Chemstrip Micral
Chlamydiazyme
Chymex
Clearview Chlamydia
coccidioidin
Color Allergy Screening Test (CAST)
ColoScreen
Combidex
Conceive Ovulation Predictor
corticorelin ovine triflutate
Cortrosyn
cosyntropin
Crypto-LA
Culturette 10 Minute Group A Strep ID
Definity
depreotide
Detect-A-Strep
DiaScreen
dipyridamole
Dopascan
Entero-Test; Entero-Test Pediatric
Evans blue
Fetal Fibronectin Test
Fibrimage
FlexPack HP
Flu OIA
Fortel Midstream
Gadolite
Gastro-Test
Gastroccult
GenESA

Indications

Diagnostic Agents for Professional Use (cont.)

Geref
GlucaGen Diagnostic Kit
glucagon
Glucagon Diagnostic Kit
glucose, liquid
gonadorelin acetate
Gonozyme Diagnostic
Helicosol
Hemastix
Hematest
HemeSelect Reagent
Hemoccult
Hemoccult II
Hemoccult SENSA; Hemoccult II
    SENSA
HercepTest
histamine phosphate
Histolyn-CYL
histoplasmin
HIVAB HIV-1 EIA; HIVAB HIV-1/
    HIV-2 EIA; HIVAB HIV-2 EIA
HIVAG-1
Human T-Lymphotropic Virus Type
    I EIA
Hybrid Capture II Chlamydia Test
Hyskon
Ictotest
imciromab pentetate
Immunex CRP
ImmunoCAP Specific IgE
ImmuRAID-AFP
ImmuRAID-hCG
Impact Rubella
indium In 111 IGIV pentetate
indium In 111 pentetreotide
indium In 111 satumomab pendetide
indocyanine green
inulin
iodine I 123 murine MAb to human
    chorionic gonadotropin (hCG)
iodine I 131 6B-iodomethyl-19-nor-
    cholesterol
Isocult for Bacteriuria
Isocult for Candida
Isocult for N gonorrhoeae and Can-
    dida
Isocult for Neisseria gonorrhoeae
Isocult for Staphylococcus aureus

Diagnostic Agents for Professional Use (cont.)

Isocult for Streptococcal pharyngitis
Isocult for T vaginalis and Candida
k82 ImmunoCap
Kinevac
latex agglutination test
LCx *Neisseria gonorrhoeae* Assay
LeuTech
LeukoScan
LymphoScan
Macroscint
mespiperone C 11
methacholine chloride
methylene blue (MB)
Metopirone
metyrapone
MicroTrak Chlamydia trachomatis
MicroTrak HSV 1/HSV 2 Culture
    Identification/Typing Test
MicroTrak HSV 1/HSV 2 Direct
    Specimen Identification/Typing
    Test
MicroTrak Neisseria gonorrhoeae
    Culture Confirmation Test
Microstix-3
Miraluma
Mono-Diff
Mono-Latex
Mono-Plus
Mono-Sure
Mono-Test
Mono-Vacc Test (O.T.)
Monospot
Monosticon Dri-Dot
MSTA (Mumps Skin Test Antigen)
Multitest CMI
mumps skin test antigen (MSTA)
Myoscint
Myoview
NeoTect
Neurolite
NG-29
NicCheck I
NicCheck II
Nimbus Plus
Nitrazine
NMP-22
nofetumomab merpentan
OctreoScan 111

Diagnostic Agents for Professional Use (cont.)

OncoTrac
OncoScint CR/OV
Optison
OraSure HIV-1
Orinase Diagnostic
Osteomark
P-748
Parathar
pentagastrin
Peptavlon
Perchloracap
perflutren
Persantine IV
Pharmalgen
potassium perchlorate
PreVue B. burgdorferi Antibody Detection Assay
Pre-Pen
Pre-Pen/MDM
ProstaScint
protirelin
Provocholine
Pylori-Check
Pyloriset
PYtest
QTest Ovulation
Quantaffirm
QuickVue H. pylori gII
QuickVue Influenza Test
QuickVue Pregnancy Test
R-gene 10
Recombigen HIV-1 LA Test
Resovist
Respiracult-Strep
Rheumatex
Rheumaton
Riba 3.0 SIA
RIGScan
rose bengal
Rubazyme
SalEst
secretin
Secretin Ferring
Sentinel
sermorelin acetate
Sickledex
simethicone
sincalide

Diagnostic Agents for Professional Use (cont.)

sodium iodide I 123
Somatrel
SonoRx
Spherulin
Stat-Crit
Strep Detect
Streptonase-B
Streptozyme
Sure Cell Chlamydia Test
Sure Cell Herpes (HSV) Test
Sure Cell Pregnancy
Sure Cell Streptococci
T.R.U.E. Test
technetium (^{99m}Tc) dimercaptosuccinic acid
technetium (^{99m}Tc) methylenediphosphonate
technetium Tc 99m albumin aggregated
technetium Tc 99m antimelanoma murine MAb
technetium Tc 99m apcitide
technetium Tc 99m arcitumomab
technetium Tc 99m bectumomab
technetium Tc 99m biciromab
technetium Tc 99m bicisate
technetium Tc 99m disofenin
technetium Tc 99m furifosmin
technetium Tc 99m medronate
technetium Tc 99m mertiatide
technetium Tc 99m murine MAb to human alpha-fetoprotein (AFP)
technetium Tc 99m murine MAb to human chorionic gonadotropin (hCG)
technetium Tc 99m oxidronate
technetium Tc 99m sestamibi
technetium Tc 99m siboroxime
technetium Tc 99m succimer
technetium Tc 99m sulesomab
technetium Tc 99m teboroxime
technetium Tc 99m tetrofosmin
teriparatide
Test Pack
Thypinone
Thyrel-TRH
Thyrogen
thyrotropin

Indications

Diagnostic Agents for Professional Use (cont.)

thyrotropin alfa
Thytropar
Tine Test PPD
tolbutamide sodium
tolonium chloride
TPM Test
Trichophyton extract
tuberculin
Tuberculin Tine Test, Old
Tubersol
UBT Breath Test for H. pylori
UCG Beta Slide Monoclonal II
UCG Slide
Unistep hCG
Uricult
Venomil
Verluma
Virogen Herpes
Virogen Rotatest
xylose (D-xylose)

Diet Aids [see: Weight Reduction Agents]

Digestive Enzymes [see: Enzymes, Digestive]

Diuretics

[see also: Antihypertensives, Diuretics; Cardiac Agents, Congestive Heart Failure Agents]

acetazolamide
acetazolamide sodium
ammonium chloride
caffeine
chlorothiazide
citrated caffeine
Daranide
Dazamide
Diamox
dichlorphenamide
Diurese
Diurigen
Diuril
Ismotic
isosorbide
Metahydrin
Naqua
Sodium Diuril
urea

Diuretics (cont.)

Ureaphil

Dressings [see: Hemostatics; Wound Treatment, Medicated Dressings]

Electrolytes

Aminosyn 3.5% M; Aminosyn II 3.5% M
Aminosyn 7% (8.5%) with Electrolytes; Aminosyn II 7% (8.5%, 10%) with Electrolytes
Aminosyn-HBC 7%
Aminosyn II 3.5% M in 5% Dextrose; Aminosyn II 4.25% M in 10% Dextrose
betaine HCl
calcium carbonate
calcium chloride
calcium citrate
calcium gluconate (calcium D-gluconate)
calcium glycerophosphate
calcium lactate
calcium lactobionate
Cena-K
Cystadane
5% Dextrose and Electrolyte #48; 5% Dextrose and Electrolyte #75; 10% Dextrose and Electrolyte #48
50% Dextrose with Electrolyte Pattern A (or N)
Dialyte Pattern LM
Effer-K
Effervescent Potassium
FreAmine HBC 6.9%
FreAmine III 3% (8.5%) with Electrolytes
Gen-K
HepatAmine
Hyperlyte; Hyperlyte CR; Hyperlyte R
Isolyte E (G; H; M; P; R; S) with 5% Dextrose
Isolyte E; Isolyte S; Isolyte S pH 7.4
Isolyte S pH 7.4
K-vescent
K+ 8; K+ 10
K+ Care
K+ Care ET
K-Dur 10; K-Dur 20

Electrolytes (cont.)
  K-G Elixir
  K-Lease
  K-Lor
  K-Lyte; K-Lyte DS
  K-Lyte/Cl
  K-Lyte/Cl; K-Lyte/Cl 50
  K-Norm
  K-Tab
  Kaochlor 10%; Kaochlor S-F
  Kaon
  Kaon-Cl 20%
  Kaon-Cl; Kaon-Cl 10
  Kay Ciel
  Kaylixir
  Klor-Con 8; Klor-Con 10; Klor-Con
    M10; Klor-Con M20
  Klor-Con; Klor-Con/25
  Klor-Con/EF
  Klorvess
  Klotrix
  Kolyum
  Lypholyte; Lypholyte II
  magnesium chloride
  magnesium gluconate
  magnesium sulfate
  Micro-K LS
  Micro-K; Micro-K 10
  Multilyte-20; Multilyte-40
  NephrAmine 5.4%
  Normosol-M and 5% Dextrose; Nor-
    mosol-R and 5% Dextrose
  Normosol-R; Normosol-R pH 7.4
  Nutrilyte; Nutrilyte II
  Plasma-Lyte A pH 7.4; Plasma-Lyte
    R; Plasma-Lyte 56; Plasma-Lyte 148
  Plasma-Lyte M (R; 56; 148) and 5%
    Dextrose
  Plegisol
  Potasalan
  potassium acetate
  potassium bicarbonate
  potassium chloride (KCl)
  potassium citrate
  potassium gluconate
  potassium phosphate, dibasic
  potassium phosphate, monobasic
  ProcalAmine
  RenAmin
  Rum-K

Electrolytes (cont.)
  Slow-K
  sodium acetate
  sodium bicarbonate
  sodium chloride (NaCl)
  sodium lactate (SL)
  sodium phosphate, dibasic
  sodium phosphate, monobasic
  Ten-K
  TPN Electrolytes; TPN Electrolytes
    II; TPN Electrolytes III
  Tracelyte; Tracelyte II; Tracelyte
    with Double Electrolytes; Trace-
    lyte II with Double Electrolytes
  Travasol 3.5% (5.5%, 8.5%) with
    Electrolytes
  5% Travert and Electrolyte No. 2;
    10% Travert and Electrolyte No. 2
  Tri-K
  Twin-K
  Uro-KP-Neutral
Emphysema [see: *Respiratory System*
  Agents]
Endometriosis [see: *Gynecological*
  Agents, Endometriosis Agents]
Enuresis [see: *Urinary Tract Agents,*
  Enuresis Agents]

Indications

Enzymes
Enzymes, Digestive
  amylase
  Arco-Lase Plus
  bile salts
  cellulase
  Cotazym
  Cotazym-S
  Creon
  Creon 10
  Creon 20
  Digepepsin
  Digestozyme
  Donnazyme
  Gustase Plus
  Ilozyme
  Ku-Zyme
  Ku-Zyme HP
  Kutrase
  lactase enzyme
  lipase

Enzymes, Digestive (cont.)
Lipram-CR20
Lipram-PN10
Lipram-PN16
Lipram-UL12
Lipram-UL18
Lipram-UL20
Pancrease; Pancrease MT 4; Pancrease MT 10; Pancrease MT 16; Pancrease MT 20
pancreatin
Pancrecarb MS-8
pancrelipase
pepsin
protease
Protilase
Ultrase; Ultrase MT 12; Ultrase MT 18; Ultrase MT 20
Viokase
Zymase

Enzymes, Proteolytic
[see also: Wound Treatment, Cleansing and Debriding Agents]
Accuzyme
ananain
bromelains
Chymodiactin
chymopapain
collagenase
comosain
Dermuspray
Elase
Elase-Chloromycetin
fibrinolysin, human
Granulderm
Granulex
GranuMed
Panafil
Panafil White
papain
Papain Urea Chlorophyllin
Papain Urea Debriding
Santyl
sutilains
trypsin, crystallized
Vianain

Enzymes, Thrombolytic
[see also: Thrombolytic Agents]
Abbokinase
Abbokinase Open-Cath

Enzymes, Thrombolytic (cont.)
anistreplase
Eminase
Kabikinase
r-ProUK
Retavase
reteplase
saruplase
Streptase
streptokinase (SK)
urokinase

Enzymes, Other
Adagen
agalsidase alfa
agalsidase beta
Aldurazyme
alglucerase
alpha-galactosidase A
CC-Galactosidase
Ceredase
Cerezyme
FABRase
Fabrazyme
imiglucerase
laronidase
Lysodase
PEG-glucocerebrosidase
pegademase bovine
Replagal
sacrosidase
Sucraid

Epilepsy [see: Anticonvulsants]

Erectile Dysfunction [see: Sexual Dysfunction Agents, Male]

Estrogens [see: Hormones, Estrogens]

Expectorants
Ami-Tex LA
ammonium chloride
Anatuss
Anatuss LA
Andehist DM
Aquatab C
Aquatab D
Aquatab DM
Atuss EX
Atuss G
Bronchial
Broncholate

Expectorants (cont.)
   Brondelate
   Bronkotuss Expectorant
   Brontex
   Calcidrine
   calcium iodide
   Calmylin with Codeine ⓒᴬᴺ
   Cheracol Cough
   Co-Tuss V
   Codegest Expectorant
   Codiclear DH
   Coldloc
   Coldloc-LA
   Conex with Codeine
   Congess JR
   Congess SR
   Contuss
   Cophene-X
   Cophene XP
   Cotridin Expectorant ⓒᴬᴺ
   Cyclofed Pediatric
   Cycofed Pediatric
   Deconamine CX
   Decongestant Expectorant
   Deconsal II
   Deconsal Pediatric
   Deconsal Sprinkle
   Defen-LA
   Deproist Expectorant with Codeine
   Despec
   Detussin Expectorant
   Dihistine Expectorant
   Dilaudid Cough
   Dilor-G
   Donatussin
   Donatussin DC
   Dura-Gest
   Dura-Vent
   Duratuss DM
   Duratuss-G
   Duratuss; Duratuss-GP
   Dy-G
   Dyflex-G
   Dyline-GG
   dyphylline & guaifenesin
   Elixophyllin GG
   Elixophyllin-KI
   Endal
   Endal Expectorant
   Enomine

Expectorants (cont.)
   Entex
   Entex LA
   Entex PSE
   Entuss-D
   Entuss-D Jr.
   Entuss Expectorant
   Eudal-SR
   Exgest LA
   Fenesin
   Fenesin DM
   GFN/PSE
   glycerol, iodinated
   Glyceryl-T
   GP-500
   Guai-Vent/PSE
   Guaifed
   Guaifed-PD
   guaifenesin
   guaifenesin & dyphylline
   guaifenesin & phenylephrine HCl &
      phenylpropanolamine HCl
   Guaifenex
   Guaifenex DM
   Guaifenex LA
   Guaifenex PPA 75
   Guaifenex PSE 60; Guaifenex PSE
      120; Guaifenex Rx DM
   Guaifenex Rx
   GuaiMAX-D
   Guaipax
   Guaitex
   Guaitex LA
   Guaitex PSE
   Guaivent
   Guaivent PD
   Guiatex LA
   Guiatex PSE
   Guiatuss AC
   Guiatuss DAC
   Guiatussin DAC
   Guiatussin with Codeine Expectorant
   Histalet X
   Humibid DM
   Humibid DM Sprinkle
   Humibid L.A.
   Humibid Sprinkle
   HycoClear Tuss
   Hycotuss Expectorant
   Hydrocodone GF

Indications

Expectorants (cont.)
Iobid DM
Iophen
Iophen-C
Iophen-DM
Iophylline
Iosal II
Isoclor Expectorant
KIE
Kwelcof
Levall 5.0
Liquibid-D
Liquibid; Liquibid-1200
Lufyllin-EPG
Lufyllin-GG
Marcof Expectorant
MED-Rx
MED-Rx DM
Monafed
Monafed DM
Muco-Fen-DM
Muco-Fen-LA
Mudrane
Mudrane GG
Mudrane GG-2
Mytussin AC Cough
Mytussin DAC
Naldecon CX Adult
Nasabid
Nasabid SR
Nasatab LA
Norel
Norisodrine with Calcium Iodide
Novagest Expectorant with Codeine
Novahistine Expectorant
Nucofed Expectorant; Nucofed
    Pediatric Expectorant
Nucotuss Expectorant; Nucotuss
    Pediatric Expectorant
Organidin NR
P-V-Tussin
Pancof-XL; Pancof XP
Panfil G
Panmist JR
PanMist-DM
Par Glycerol
Partuss LA
Pediacof
Pedituss Cough
Phenhist Expectorant

Expectorants (cont.)
phenylephrine HCl & phenylpropa-
    nolamine HCl & guaifenesin
Phenylfenesin L.A.
phenylpropanolamine HCl & phen-
    ylephrine HCl & guaifenesin
Pima
Pneumomist
Pneumotussin
Pneumotussin HC
Polaramine Expectorant
potassium guaiacolsulfonate
potassium iodide
Profen Forte DM
Profen II DM
Profen II; Profen LA
Protuss
Protuss-D
Protuss DM
Quadrinal
Quibron; Quibron-300
R-Gen
Respa-DM
Respa-GF
Respa-1st
Respaire-60; Respaire-120
Robafen AC Cough
Robafen DAC
Robitussin A-C
Robitussin-DAC
Rolatuss Expectorant
Romilar AC
Ru-Tuss DE
Rymed
Rymed-TR
Ryna-CX
Sil-Tex
Sinufed
Sinumist-SR
Sinupan
SinuVent
Slo-phyllin GG
SRC Expectorant
SSKI
Stamoist E
Stamoist LA
Statuss Expectorant
Sudal 120/600
Sudal 60/500
Syn-Rx

Expectorants (cont.)
Synophylate-GG
terpin hydrate
Theolate
Theophyllin KI
Touro CC
Touro DM
Touro Ex
Touro LA
Triaminic Expectorant DH
Triaminic Expectorant with Codeine
Tuss-LA
Tussafed HC
Tussafed-LA
Tussafin Expectorant
Tussanil DH
Tussar SF; Tussar-2
Tussi-Organidin DM NR; Tussi-
    Organidin DM-S NR
Tussi-Organidin NR; Tussi-Organi-
    din-S NR
Tusso-DM
ULR-LA
V-Dec-M
Vanex Expectorant
Versacaps
Vicodin Tuss
Zephrex
Zephrex LA

Fertility Agents [see: Gynecological
    Agents, Fertility Stimulants]

Gallbladder Disease and Gallstones
    [see: Biliary Tract Agents]

**Gastroesophageal Reflux Disease
    (GERD)** [see: Antisecretories, Gas-
    trointestinal; Peptic Ulcer and Gastric
    Reflux Agents]

Glucocorticoids [see: Corticosteroids,
    Systemic; Dermatological Preparations,
    Anti-inflammatory Agents; Ophthal-
    mologicals, Anti-inflammatory]

Gout Agents
[see also: Analgesics, Nonsteroidal;
    Corticosteroids, Systemic]
allopurinol
Anturane
Benemid ⒸⒶⓃ

Gout Agents (cont.)
Benuryl ⒸⒶⓃ
Col-Probenecid
ColBenemid
colchicine
colchicine & probenecid
Probalan
Proben-C
probenecid
probenecid & colchicine
Purinol ⒸⒶⓃ
sulfinpyrazone
Zyloprim

Gynecological Agents
[see also: Hormones; Vaginal Prepara-
    tions]

**Gynecological Agents, Abortifa-
    cients**
carboprost tromethamine
dinoprostone
Hemabate
Mifegyne
Mifeprex
mifepristone
Prostin E2

**Gynecological Agents, Contracep-
    tives, Emergency Postcoital**
Alesse
Aviane-28
Enpresse
Levlen
Levlite
levonorgestrel
Levora 0.15/30
Lo/Ovral
Low-Ogestrel
Mifeprex
mifepristone
Nordette
Ogestrel
Ovral
Ovrette
Plan B
Preven
Tri-Levlen
Triphasil
Trivora-28

Indications

Gynecological Agents, Contraceptives, Oral

Alesse
Apri
Aviane-28
Brevicon
Cyclessa
Demulen 1/35; Demulen 1/50
Desogen
Enpresse
Estrostep 21
Estrostep Fe
Genora 0.5/35; Genora 1/35
Genora 1/50
Jenest-28
Levlen
Levlite
levonorgestrel
Levora 0.15/30
Lo/Ovral
Loestrin 21 1/20; Loestrin 21 1.5/30
Loestrin Fe 1/20; Loestrin Fe 1.5/30
Low-Ogestrel
Marvelon ⒸⒶⓃ
Microgestin Fe 1/20; Microgestin Fe 1.5/30
Micronor
Minesse
Mircette
Modicon
N.E.E. 1/35
Necon 0.5/35; Necon 1/35
Necon 1/50
Necon 10/11
Nelova 0.5/35E; Nelova 1/35E
Nelova 1/50M
Nelova 10/11
Nor-Q.D.
Nordette
norelgestromin
Norethin 1/35E
Norethin 1/50M
norethindrone
Norinyl 1 + 35
Norinyl 1 + 50
Nortrel
Ogestrel
Ortho 0.5/35; Ortho 1/35 ⒸⒶⓃ
Ortho 7/7/7 ⒸⒶⓃ
Ortho-Cept

Gynecological Agents, Contraceptives, Oral (cont.)

Ortho-Cyclen
Ortho Evra
Ortho-Novum 1/35
Ortho-Novum 1/50
Ortho-Novum 10/11
Ortho-Novum 7/7/7
Ortho Tri-Cyclen
Ovcon-35
Ovcon-50
Ovral
Ovrette
Tri-Levlen
Tri-Norinyl
Triphasil
Trivora-28
Yasmin
Zovia 1/35E; Zovia 1/50E

Gynecological Agents, Contraceptives, Parenteral

Depo-Provera
levonorgestrel
Lunelle
Norplant

Gynecological Agents, Endometriosis Agents

Alti-MPA ⒸⒶⓃ
Amen
Aygestin
Curretab
Cycrin
danazol
Danocrine
goserelin acetate
leuprolide acetate
Lupron Depot
medroxyprogesterone acetate (MPA)
Mifeprex
mifepristone
nafarelin acetate
norethindrone
norethindrone acetate
Novo-Medrone ⒸⒶⓃ
Provera
Synarel
Zoladex
Zoladex LA ⒸⒶⓃ

Gynecological Agents, Fertility Stimulants
A.P.L.
Antagon
cetrorelix acetate
Cetrotide
Chorex-5; Chorex-10
choriogonadotropin alfa
Choron-10
Clomid
clomiphene citrate
Factrel
Fertinex
Follistim
follitropin alfa
follitropin beta
ganirelix acetate
gonadorelin acetate
gonadorelin HCl
gonadotropin, chorionic
Gonal-F
Gonic
Humegon
Lutrepulse
menotropins
Metrodin
Milophene
Novarel
Ovidrel
Pergonal
Pregnyl
Profasi
Puregon (CAN)
Repronex
Serophene
urofollitropin

Gynecological Agents, Labor Stimulants
carbetocin
carboprost tromethamine
Cervidil
dinoprostone
Duratocin (CAN)
ergonovine maleate
Ergotrate Maleate
Hemabate
Methergine
methylergonovine maleate
oxytocin
Pitocin

Gynecological Agents, Labor Stimulants (cont.)
Prepidil
Syntocinon

Gynecological Agents, Labor Suppressants
ritodrine HCl
Yutopar

Gynecological Agents, Lactation Suppressants
bromocriptine mesylate
cabergoline
Dostinex
Parlodel
PMS-Bromocriptine (CAN)

Gynecological Agents, Menopause Agents
[see also: Mineral Replacement, Calcium]
Activella
alendronate sodium
Allelix
Alora
Aquest
Bondronat
Bonviva
C.E.S. (CAN)
Calcimar
calcitonin (salmon)
Cenestin
Climara
CombiPatch
Delestrogen
depAndrogyn
depGynogen
Depo-Estradiol Cypionate
Depo-Testadiol
DepoGen
Depotestogen
Didrocal (CAN)
Dioval XX; Dioval 40
Duo-Cyp
Duratestrin
E2II
Esclim
Estalis 140/50; Estalis 250/50 (CAN)
Estinyl
Estra-L 20
Estra-L 40
Estrace

Gynecological Agents, Menopause Agents (cont.)

Estraderm
Estradiol Transdermal System
Estrasorb
Estratab
Estratest; Estratest H.S.
Estring
Estro-Cyp
Estrogel ⓒ
Estrogenic Substance Aqueous
Estrone 5
Estrone Aqueous
Evista
femhrt 1/5
FemPatch
Fortical
Fosamax
Gynodiol
Gynogen L.A. 20
Kestrone 5
Livial
Macritonin
Menest
Menogen; Menogen H.S.
Menorest
Menrium 5-2; Menrium 5-4; Menrium 10-4
Miacalcin
Oesclim ⓒ
Ogen
Ortho Dienestrol
Ortho-Est
Ortho-Prefest
Osteocalcin
parathyroid hormone (1-84), recombinant human
PMB 200; PMB 400
PMS-Conjugated Estrogens ⓒ
Premarin
Premarin with Methyltestosterone
Premphase
Prempro
raloxifene HCl
Salmonine
Slow Fluoride
sodium fluoride
Test-Estro Cypionates
tibolone
Vagifem

Gynecological Agents, Menopause Agents (cont.)

Valergen 20; Valergen 40
Valertest No. 1
Vivelle; Vivelle-Dot
Xyvion

Hemorrhoidal Agents

[see also: Analgesics, Topical; Antihistamines, Topical; Dermatological Preparations, Anti-inflammatory]
Analpram-HC
Anogesic
Anucort HC
Anumed HC
Anusol-HC
Anusol-HC 1
Anuzinc ⓒ
Cort-Dome High Potency
Dermol HC
Hemorrhoidal HC
Hemril-HC
hydrocortisone (HC)
hydrocortisone acetate (HCA)
phenol
Pramoxine HC
Proctocort
ProctoCream-HC
ProctoCream-HC 2.5%
Proctodan-HC ⓒ
Proctofoam-HC
Rectacort

Hemostatics

[see also: Wound Treatment, Medicated Dressings]
acetylhydrolase
Alphanate
AlphaNine
AlphaNine SD
Amicar
aminocaproic acid
anti-inhibitor coagulant complex
antihemophilic factor (AHF)
Antihemophilic Factor (Porcine) Hyate:C
aprotinin

Hemostatics (cont.)
AquaMEPHYTON
Autoplex T
Avitene Hemostat
Bebulin VH
Benefix
Bioclate
calcium alginate fiber
cellulose, oxidized
collagen sponge, absorbable
Cyklokapron
DDAVP
desmopressin acetate
eptacog alfa (activated)
Ethamolin
ethanolamine oleate
factor IX complex
factor VIIa, recombinant
factor VIII SQ, recombinant
factor XIII, plasma-derived
Feiba VH Immuno
Fibrogammin P
gelatin film, absorbable
gelatin powder, absorbable
gelatin sponge, absorbable
Gelfilm; Gelfilm Ophthalmic
Gelfoam
Helistat
Helixate
Hemaseel HMN
Hemofil M
Hemonyne
Hemopad
Hemotene
Humate-P
Koāte-DVI
Koāte-HP
Kogenate
Kogenate FS
Konakion
Konyne 80
Mephyton
microfibrillar collagen hemostat (MCH)
Monoclate P
Mononine
NiaStase Ⓒᴬᴺ
nonacog alfa
NovoSeven
Oxycel

Hemostatics (cont.)
Pafase
phytonadione (vitamin K$_1$)
Profilate HP
Profilnine SD
Proplex T
Recombinate
ReFacto
Stimate
Surgicel
thrombin
Thrombin-JMI
Thrombinar
Thrombogen
Thrombostat
tranexamic acid
Trasylol
Herpes Simplex [see: Mouth and Throat Preparations]

HIV Infections
[see also: Antibiotics; Antifungals; Antidiarrheal Agents, Intestinal Antibacterials; Antiemetics and Antinauseants; Antiprotozoals; Antituberculosis Agents; Antivirals; Immunizing Agents; Immunostimulants]
HIV Infections, Bacterial
aminosidine
azithromycin
Biaxin
Biaxin XL
clarithromycin
diethylhomospermine (DEHOP; DEHSPM)
ethambutol HCl
Gabbromicina
gentamicin sulfate
isoniazid
Laniazid
Laniazid C.T.
letrazuril
Maitec
Myambutol
Mycobutin
Nydrazid
Paromomycin
Pneumo 23 Ⓒᴬᴺ
pneumococcal vaccine, polyvalent

Indications

HIV Infections, Bacterial (cont.)
Pneumovax 23
Pnu-Imune 23
Priftin
pyrazinamide (PZA)
rifabutin
Rifadin
Rifamate
rifampin
rifapentine
Rifater
Rimactane
Synsorb Cd
Trecator-SC
Zithromax

HIV Infections, Fungal
Abelcet
AmBisome
Amphocin
Amphotec
amphotericin B cholesteryl
amphotericin B deoxycholate
amphotericin B lipid complex
  (ABLC)
Apo-Fluconazole ⒸⒶⓃ
Apo-Ketoconazole ⒸⒶⓃ
Diflucan
fluconazole
Fungizone
itraconazole
ketoconazole
Nizoral
Sporanox

HIV Infections, Parasitic
albendazole
atovaquone
azithromycin
Bactrim IV
Bactrim Pediatric
Bactrim; Bactrim DS
Biaxin
Biaxin XL
clarithromycin
Cotrim Pediatric
Cotrim; Cotrim D.S.
Daraprim
Mepron
NeuTrexin
NebuPent
Pentacarinat

HIV Infections, Parasitic (cont.)
Pentam 300
pentamidine isethionate
Pneumopent
pyrimethamine
Septra
Septra DS
Septra IV
sulfadiazine
sulfamethoxazole (SMX; SMZ)
Sulfatrim
trimethoprim (TMP)
trimetrexate glucuronate
Zithromax

HIV Infections, Viral
[see also: Antivirals, Systemic]
abacavir succinate
abacavir sulfate
acemannan
activated cellular therapy (ACT)
adefovir dipivoxil
Agenerase
AIDS vaccine
AIDSVax
Alferon LDO
Ampligen
amprenavir
amprenavir & indinavir sulfate
amprenavir & lamivudine & zidovudine
amprenavir & nelfinavir mesylate
amprenavir & saquinavir
Anticort
AR-177
atevirdine mesylate
Aztec
benzimidavir
Bravavir
calanolide A
Carrisyn
CD4, recombinant soluble human
  (rCD4)
celgosivir HCl
cidofovir
Combivir
Coviracil
Crixivan
crofelemer
cytolin
Cytovene

HIV Infections, Viral (cont.)
- delavirdine mesylate
- dextran sulfate
- didanosine
- didanosine & nevirapine & zidovudine
- didanosine & zidovudine
- docosanol (n-docosanol)
- efavirenz
- efavirenz & lamivudine & zidovudine
- emtricitabine
- Epivir
- filgrastim
- fomivirsen sodium
- Fortovase
- Forvade
- foscarnet sodium
- Foscavir
- ganciclovir
- ganciclovir sodium
- Genevax-HIV
- gp120 (glycoprotein 120) antigens
- gp160 (glycoprotein 160) antigens
- HAART (highly active antiretroviral therapy)
- HIV immunotherapeutic (HIV-IT); HIV therapeutic
- HIV-1 peptide vaccine
- Hivid
- hypericin
- Inactivin
- indinavir sulfate
- indinavir sulfate & amprenavir
- inosine pranobex
- interferon alfa-n3
- interleukin-10 (IL-10)
- Invirase
- Isoprinosine
- Kaletra
- lamivudine
- lamivudine & saquinavir mesylate & ritonavir
- lamivudine & zidovudine & amprenavir
- lamivudine & zidovudine & efavirenz
- Lidakol
- lodenosine
- lopinavir
- MultiKine
- nelfinavir mesylate

HIV Infections, Viral (cont.)
- nelfinavir mesylate & amprenavir
- nevirapine
- nevirapine & zidovudine & didanosine
- Norvir
- Novapren
- Panavir
- pentafuside
- poly I: poly C12U
- Preveon
- probucol
- procaine HCl
- Protovir
- Receptin
- Remune
- Rescriptor
- Retrovir
- ritonavir
- ritonavir & lamivudine & saquinavir mesylate
- ritonavir & zidovudine & saquinavir mesylate
- saquinavir
- saquinavir & amprenavir
- saquinavir mesylate
- saquinavir mesylate & ritonavir & lamivudine
- saquinavir mesylate & ritonavir & zidovudine
- Savvy
- Scriptene
- sevirumab
- sorivudine
- stavudine
- Sustiva
- T-cell gene therapy
- TAT antagonist
- tenofovir disoproxil fumarate (tenofovir DF)
- Tenovil
- tetrachlorodecaoxide
- thymopentin
- Timunox
- tipranavir disodium
- tirilazad mesylate
- trichosanthin
- Trizivir
- tucaresol
- tumor necrosis factor (TNF)

Indications

HIV Infections, Viral (cont.)

Uendex
Valcyte
valganciclovir HCl
VaxSyn HIV-1
vidarabine
Videx
Videx EC
VIMRxyn
Vira-A
Viracept
Viramune
Viread
Virend
Vistide
Vitrasert
Vitravene
zalcitabine
Zerit
Ziagen
zidovudine (ZDV)
zidovudine & amprenavir & lamivudine
zidovudine & didanosine
zidovudine & didanosine & nevirapine
zidovudine & efavirenz & lamivudine
zidovudine & saquinavir mesylate & ritonavir
Zintevir

HIV Infections, Other Related Disorders

Alferon N
alitretinoin
alitretinoin & interferon
amikacin
9-aminocamptothecin (9-AC)
Androderm
AndroGel
Androgel-DHT
Atragen
Avonex
Betaseron
bexarotene
Cachexon
Caelyx ⒸⒶⓃ
Coactinon
crofelemer
Cryptaz

HIV Infections, Other Related Disorders (cont.)

Cryptosporidium parvum bovine colostrum IgG concentrate
DaunoXome
daunorubicin citrate, liposomal
diethylhomospermine (DEHOP; DEHSPM)
dihydrotestosterone (DHT)
docosanol (*n*-docosanol)
doxorubicin HCl, liposome-encapsulated (LED)
dronabinol
edodekin alfa
emivirine
epoetin alfa (EPO)
Epogen
gallium nitrate
Geref
L-glutathione, reduced
Hepandrin
Immuno-C
interferon & alitretinoin
interferon alfa
interferon alfa-2a (IFN-αA; rIFN-A)
interferon alfa-2b (IFN-α2)
interferon beta (IFN-B)
interferon beta-1a
interferon beta-1b
Intron A
Lidakol
LymphoCide
Marinol
Megace
megestrol acetate
memantine
MiKasome
monoclonal antibody LL2, humanized
monoclonal antibody to CD22 antigen on B-cells, radiolabeled
Nipent
nitazoxanide (NTZ)
Omniferon
Onxol
Oxandrin
oxandrolone
paclitaxel
Panretin
pentostatin
phenylhydrazone

HIV Infections, Other Related Disorders (cont.)
poloxamer 331
Procrit
Proleukin
Protox
Provir
R-Frone
rifalazil
rIFN-beta
Roferon-A
sermorelin acetate
Sporidin-G
SU-5416
Targretin
Taxol
testosterone
thalidomide
Thalomid
TheraDerm
topotecan HCl
Valcyte
valganciclovir HCl
Veldona
Virulizin

Hormones
[see also: Gynecological Agents]
Hormones, Anabolic/Androgenic
Anadrol-50
Andro L.A. 200
Androderm
AndroGel
Androgel-DHT
Android
Android-10; Android-25
Androlone-D 200
Andropository-200
Androtest-SL
Deca-Durabolin
Delatestryl
depAndro 100; depAndro 200
depAndrogyn
Depo-Testadiol
Depo-Testosterone
Depotest 100; Depotest 200
Depotestogen
Diane-35 ⒸⒶⓃ
dihydrotestosterone (DHT)

Hormones, Anabolic/Androgenic (cont.)
Duo-Cyp
Durabolin
Duratest 100; Duratest 200
Duratestrin
Durathate-200
Estratest; Estratest H.S.
Everone 200
fluoxymesterone
Halotestin
Hepandrin
Histerone 100
Hybolin Decanoate-50; Hybolin Decanoate-100
Hybolin Improved
Menogen; Menogen H.S.
Methitest
methyltestosterone
nandrolone decanoate
nandrolone phenpropionate
Neo-Durabolic
Oreton Methyl
Oxandrin
oxandrolone
oxymetholone
Premarin with Methyltestosterone
stanozolol
Tesamone
Teslac
Test-Estro Cypionates
Testandro
Testoderm TTS
Testoderm; Testoderm with Adhesive
testolactone
Testopel
testosterone
testosterone cypionate
testosterone enanthate
testosterone propionate
Testosterone Aqueous
Testred
TheraDerm
TheraDerm-MTX
Tostrex
Valertest No. 1
Virilon
Winstrol
Hormones, Estrogens
Activella

Hormones, Estrogens (cont.)
- Alora
- Aquest
- C.E.S. ⓒᴬᴺ
- Cenestin
- chlorotrianisene
- Climara
- CombiPatch
- Delestrogen
- depAndrogyn
- depGynogen
- Depo-Estradiol Cypionate
- Depo-Testadiol
- DepoGen
- Depotestogen
- Diane-35 ⓒᴬᴺ
- dienestrol
- Dioval XX; Dioval 40
- Duo-Cyp
- Duratestrin
- E2II
- E2III
- Enovid
- Esclim
- Estalis 140/50; Estalis 250/50 ⓒᴬᴺ
- Estinyl
- Estra-L 20
- Estra-L 40
- Estrace
- Estraderm
- estradiol
- estradiol cypionate (E_2C)
- estradiol hemihydrate
- estradiol valerate
- Estradiol Transdermal System
- estradiol-17β
- Estrasorb
- Estratab
- Estratest; Estratest H.S.
- Estring
- Estro-Cyp
- Estrogel ⓒᴬᴺ
- Estrogenic Substance Aqueous
- estrogens, conjugated
- estrogens, esterified
- estrone
- Estrone 5
- Estrone Aqueous
- estropipate
- ethinyl estradiol

Hormones, Estrogens (cont.)
- femhrt 1/5
- FemPatch
- Gynodiol
- Gynogen L.A. 20
- Kestrone 5
- Lunelle
- Menest
- Menogen; Menogen H.S.
- Menorest
- Menrium 5-2; Menrium 5-4; Menrium 10-4
- mestranol
- Oesclim ⓒᴬᴺ
- Ogen
- Ortho Dienestrol
- Ortho-Est
- Ortho-Prefest
- PMB 200; PMB 400
- PMS-Conjugated Estrogens ⓒᴬᴺ
- Premarin
- Premarin Intravenous
- Premarin with Methyltestosterone
- Premphase
- Prempro
- quinestrol
- sodium estrone sulfate
- Tace
- Test-Estro Cypionates
- TheraDerm-MTX
- Vagifem
- Valergen 20; Valergen 40
- Valertest No. 1
- Vivelle; Vivelle-Dot

Hormones, Hypothalamic
- buserelin acetate
- deslorelin
- Factrel
- Gn-RH (gonadotropin-releasing hormone)
- gonadorelin acetate
- gonadorelin HCl
- gonadotropin-releasing hormone (Gn-RH)
- goserelin acetate
- histrelin
- histrelin acetate
- LH-RH (luteinizing hormone–releasing hormone)
- Lupron Depot

Hormones, Hypothalamic (cont.)
  Lupron Depot-Ped
  Lupron Depot–3 month; Lupron
    Depot–4 month
  Lupron; Lupron Pediatric
  luteinizing hormone–releasing hor-
    mone (LH-RH)
  Lutrepulse
  nafarelin acetate
  octreotide acetate
  ProMaxx-100
  Reducin
  Sandostatin
  Sandostatin LAR Depot
  Somagard
  somatostatin (SS)
  Supprelin
  Suprefact ⓒⒶⓃ
  Suprefact; Suprefact Depot ⓒⒶⓃ
  Synarel
  Zecnil
  Zoladex
  Zoladex LA ⓒⒶⓃ
Hormones, Pancreatic
  GlucaGen Emergency Kit
  glucagon
  Glucagon Emergency Kit
Hormones, Pituitary
  Apo-Desmopressin ⓒⒶⓃ
  Cortrosyn
  cosyntropin
  DDAVP
  desmopressin acetate
  Diapid
  Genotropin
  Genotropin MiniQuick
  Geref
  Humatrope
  lypressin
  Norditropin
  Norditropin SimpleXx
  Nutropin
  Nutropin AQ
  Nutropin Depot
  oxytocin
  pegvisomant
  Pitocin
  Pitressin
  Protropin
  Protropin II

Hormones, Pituitary (cont.)
  Saizen
  sermorelin acetate
  Serostim
  somatrem
  somatropin
  Somavert
  Stimate
  Syntocinon
  Umatrope
  vasopressin (VP)
Hormones, Progestins
  Activella
  Alti-MPA ⓒⒶⓃ
  Amen
  Aygestin
  CombiPatch
  Crinone
  Curretab
  Cycrin
  Depo-Provera
  desogestrel
  drospirenone
  Enovid
  Estalis 140/50; Estalis 250/50 ⓒⒶⓃ
  ethynodiol diacetate
  femhrt 1/5
  gestodene
  hydroxyprogesterone caproate
  Hylutin
  Hyprogest 250
  levonorgestrel
  Lin-Megestrol ⓒⒶⓃ
  Lunelle
  medroxyprogesterone acetate (MPA)
  Megace
  megestrol acetate
  Mirena
  norethindrone
  norethindrone acetate
  norethynodrel
  norgestimate
  norgestrel
  Novo-Medrone ⓒⒶⓃ
  Ortho-Prefest
  Premphase
  Prempro
  Proclim ⓒⒶⓃ
  Progestasert
  progesterone

Hormones, Progestins (cont.)
  Prometrium
  Provera

Hypercalcemia Agents
  Actonel
  alendronate sodium
  Aredia
  Bondronat
  Bonefos ⓒ
  Bonviva
  Calcimar
  calcitonin (human)
  calcitonin (salmon)
  Cibacalcin
  clodronate disodium
  Didronel
  disodium clodronate tetrahydrate
  etidronate disodium
  Fortical
  Fosamax
  gallium nitrate
  Ganite
  ibandronate sodium
  Miacalcin
  Ostac ⓒ
  Osteo-D
  Osteocalcin
  pamidronate disodium
  risedronate sodium
  Salmonine
  secalciferol
  Skelid
  tiludronate disodium
  zoledronic acid
  Zometa
Hyperhidrosis [see: Dermatological Preparations, Antihyperhidrotics]

Hyperkalemia Agents
  Kayexalate
  sodium polystyrene sulfonate
  SPS
Hyperlipidemia [see: Lipid-lowering Agents]

Hyperphosphatemia Agents
  calcium acetate
  calcium carbonate
  Lambda
  lanthanum carbonate
  MagneBind 400 Rx
  PhosLo
  R & D Calcium Carbonate/600
  Renagel
  sevelamer HCl
Hyperuricemia [see: Gout Agents]
Hypoglycemics [see: Diabetes Agents]

Immunizing Agents
  [see also: Immunostimulants]
Immunizing Agents, Bacterial Vaccines
  Acel-Imune
  Acel-P ⓒ
  ActHIB
  ActHIB/Tripedia
  Adacel ⓒ
  BCG vaccine (bacillus Calmette-Guérin)
  Certiva
  cholera vaccine
  Comvax
  diphtheria & tetanus toxoids & acellular pertussis (DTaP) vaccine, adsorbed
  diphtheria & tetanus toxoids & whole-cell pertussis vaccine (DTwP)
  diphtheria & tetanus toxoids, adsorbed (DT; Td)
  diphtheria toxoid, adsorbed
  Hemophilus b conjugate vaccine
  HibTITER
  ImmuCyst ⓒ
  Infanrix
  lipoprotein OspA, recombinant
  LYMErix
  meningococcal polysaccharide vaccine, group A
  meningococcal polysaccharide vaccine, group C
  meningococcal polysaccharide vaccine, group W-135

Immunizing Agents, Bacterial Vaccines (cont.)

meningococcal polysaccharide vaccine, group Y
Menomune-A/C/Y/W-135
mixed respiratory vaccine (MRV)
MRV
OmniHIB
OncoTICE ⒸⒶⓃ
PedvaxHIB
pertussis vaccine, adsorbed
plague vaccine
Pneumo 23 ⒸⒶⓃ
pneumococcal vaccine, 7-valent
pneumococcal vaccine, polyvalent
Pneumovax 23
Pnu-Imune 23
Prevnar
ProHIBiT
Quilimmune-P
SPL-Serologic types I and III
StaphVAX
staphage lysate (SPL)
tetanus toxoid
tetanus toxoid, adsorbed
Tetramune
Tice BCG
Tri-Immunol
TriHIBit
Tripedia
Typherex
Typherix ⒸⒶⓃ
Typhim Vi
typhoid vaccine
typhoid Vi capsular polysaccharide vaccine
Typhoid Vaccine (AKD)
Typhoid Vaccine (H-P)
Vivotif Berna

Immunizing Agents, Immune Extracts

antivenin (*Latrodectus mactans*)
antivenin (*Micrurus fulvius*) (equine)
antivenin (Crotalidae) polyvalent (equine)
diphtheria antitoxin

Immunizing Agents, Immunoglobulins

antithymocyte globulin (ATG)

Immunizing Agents, Immunoglobulins (cont.)

Atgam
BayTet
BayGam
BayHep B
BayRab
BayRho-D Full Dose; BayRho-D Mini-Dose
CytoGam
cytomegalovirus immune globulin (CMV-IG), human
Gamimune N
Gammagard S/D
Gammar-P I.V.
Gamulin Rh
globulin, immune
H-BIG
hepatitis B immune globulin (HBIG)
HIV immune globulin (HIVIG)
HIV-IG
Hypermune RSV
Imogam
Imogam Rabies-HT
Iveegam
lymphocyte immune globulin (LIG)
MICRhoGAM
Mini-Gamulin Rh
Nabi-HB
Nashville Rabbit Antithymocyte Serum
Panglobulin
Polygam
Polygam S/D
rabies immune globulin (RIG)
RespiGam
respiratory syncytial virus immune globulin (RSV-IG)
$Rh_0(D)$ immune globulin
RhoGAM
Sandoglobulin
tetanus immune globulin (TIG)
varicella-zoster immune globulin (VZIG)
Venoglobulin-I
Venoglobulin-S
WinRho SD
WinRho SDF

Immunizing Agents, Viral Vaccines

[see also: *HIV Infections, Viral*]

Indications

Immunizing Agents, Viral Vaccines (cont.)
AIDS vaccine
AIDSVax
Arilvax
Attenuvax
Avaxim; Avaxim Pediatric ⓒⒶⓃ
Biavax II
ChimeriVax
Comvax
Engerix-B
FluMist
Fluogen
FluShield
Fluvirin
Fluzone
Genevax-HIV
gp120 (glycoprotein 120) antigens
Havrix
Hepagene
hepatitis A vaccine, inactivated
hepatitis B virus vaccine, inactivated
HIV-1 peptide vaccine
Imovax
influenza virus vaccine
IPOL
Japanese encephalitis (JE) virus vaccine
JE-VAX
M-M-R II
M-R-Vax II
measles & rubella virus vaccine, live
measles, mumps & rubella virus vaccine, live
measles virus vaccine, live
Meruvax II
mumps virus vaccine, live
Mumpsvax
Orimune
poliovirus vaccine, inactivated (IPV)
poliovirus vaccine, live oral (OPV)
Priorix ⓒⒶⓃ
RabAvert
rabies vaccine
Recombivax HB
Remune
Rotamune
RotaShield
rotavirus vaccine
rubella & mumps virus vaccine, live

Immunizing Agents, Viral Vaccines (cont.)
rubella virus vaccine, live
thymalfasin
Twinrix
Vaqta
varicella virus vaccine
Varivax
Vaxigrip ⓒⒶⓃ
yellow fever vaccine
YF-Vax
Zadaxin

Immunizing Agents, Immunostimulating Adjuncts
aldesleukin
ancestim
Avonex
Betaseron
diethyldithiocarbamate
diphtheria CRM_{197} conjugate
filgrastim
Infergen
interferon alfa
interferon beta-1a
interferon beta-1b
Intron A
levamisole HCl
Maxamine
Neupogen
Omniferon
Proleukin
R-Frone
Rebetron
Rebif ⓒⒶⓃ
rIFN-beta
Roferon-A
Stemgen ⓒⒶⓃ
tetrachlorodecaoxide
Veldona
Wellferon
Wellferon ⓒⒶⓃ

Immunostimulants
[see also: HIV Infections; Immunizing Agents]
acetylcysteine (N-acetylcysteine)
Actimmune
Aldara
Alferon LDO

Immunostimulants (cont.)

Alferon N
Aliminase
Ampligen
beta alethine
Beta LT
Betafectin
BLyS protein
cilmostim
coenzyme Q_{10}
Copaxone
disaccharide tripeptide glycerol
    dipalmitoyl
Ergamisol
Fluimucil
glatiramer acetate
Iamin
ImmTher
imiquimod
Imreg-1
Imuthiol
interferon alfa
interferon alfa-2a (IFN-αA; rIFN-A)
interferon alfa-2b (IFN-α2)
interferon alfa-n1
interferon alfa-n3
interferon alfacon-1
interferon beta (IFN-B)
interferon gamma-1b
interleukin-4 receptor (IL-4R)
Leucomax
Leucotropin
Leukine
Linomide
lisofylline (LSF)
Macstim
Megagen
megakaryocyte growth and develop-
    ment factor, pegylated, recombi-
    nant human
milodistim
molgramostim
Neumega
Nuvance
oprelvekin
oxothiazolidine carboxylate (L-2-
    oxothiazolidine-4-carboxylic acid)
PGG glucan
Pixykine
poly I: poly C12U

Immunostimulants (cont.)

prezatide copper acetate
Procysteine
regramostim
Remune
roquinimex
sargramostim
Stimulon
T-cell gene therapy
thalidomide
Thalomid
thymopentin
Timunox
tucaresol
Vendona

Immunosuppressants

[see also: Antineoplastics; Corticoster-
    oids, Systemic; Rheumatic Disease
    Agents]
abetimus sodium
alemtuzumab
anti-human thymocyte immuno-
    globulin, rabbit
antithymocyte globulin (ATG)
Atgam
azathioprine
azathioprine sodium
basiliximab
Campath
CellCept
Centara
cyclosporine
daclizumab
Gengraf
Imuran
lymphocyte immune globulin (LIG)
muromonab-CD3
mycophenolate mofetil
mycophenolate mofetil HCl
Nashville Rabbit Antithymocyte
    Serum
Neoral
Orthoclone OKT3
priliximab
Prograf
Protopic
Rapamune
Sandimmune

Immunosuppressants (cont.)
Sandimmune Neoral (CAN)
SangCya
Simulect
sirolimus
tacrolimus
Thymoglobulin
triptolide
Zenapax
Impotence [see: Sexual Dysfunction Agents, Male]
Incontinence [see: Urinary Tract Agents, Urinary Retention Agents]

Inflammatory Bowel Disease Agents

[see also: Dermatological Preparations, Anti-inflammatory; Hemorrhoidal Agents]
Aliminase
alosetron HCl
aminosalicylic acid (4-aminosalicylic acid)
anakinra
Antegren
Antril
Asacol
Azulfidine
Azulfidine EN-tabs
balsalazide disodium
budesonide
Canasa
Colazal
Colomed
Cortenema
Cortifoam
Dipentum
Entocort (CAN)
FIV-ASA
infliximab
Lotronex
mesalamine
natalizumab
olsalazine sodium
Pamisyl
Pentasa
Remicade
Rezipas

Inflammatory Bowel Disease Agents (cont.)
Rowasa
Salofalk (CAN)
short chain fatty acids
sulfasalazine
tegaserod
Zelmac
Intestinal Parasites [see: Anthelmintics; Antiprotozoals]
Keratolytics [see: Dermatological Preparations, Keratolytic Agents]
Kidney Stones [see: Urinary Tract Agents, Antiurolithic]
Labor Stimulants and Suppressants [see: Gynecological Agents, Labor Stimulants; Gynecological Agents, Labor Suppressants]
Lactation Suppressants [see: Gynecological Agents, Lactation Suppressants]

Laxatives

Apo-Lactulose (CAN)
barley malt soup extract
bisacodyl
calcium polycarbophil
carboxymethylcellulose sodium
casanthranol
cascara fluidextract, aromatic
cascara sagrada
castor oil
cellulose
Chronulac
Constilac
Constulose
Duphalac
Evalose
glycerin
Heptalac
Kristalose
lactulose
magnesia, milk of
magnesium citrate
magnesium sulfate
methylcellulose
mineral oil
MiraLax
Osmoglyn
phenolphthalein

Laxatives (cont.)
   phenolphthalein, yellow
   polycarbophil
   polyethylene glycol (PEG)
   prucalopride HCl
   prucalopride succinate
   psyllium husk
   psyllium hydrophilic mucilloid
   senna
   sennosides
   sodium phosphate, dibasic
   sodium phosphate, monobasic
Laxatives, Pre-procedure Bowel
   Evacuants
   bisacodyl
   Clysodrast
   Co-Lav
   Colovage
   CoLyte
   Go-Evac
   GoLYTELY
   MiraLax
   NuLytely
   OCL
   polyethylene glycol (PEG)
   polyethylene glycol–electrolyte solu-
      tion (PEG-ES)
   senna
   Visicol
Laxatives, Stool Softeners
   docusate calcium
   docusate sodium
Leukemia [see: Antineoplastics]
Lice [see: Pediculicides and Scabicides]

Lipid-lowering Agents
   Advicor
   Apo-Gemfibrozil ⒸⒶⓃ
   Apo-Pravastatin ⒸⒶⓃ
   atorvastatin calcium
   Atromid-S
   Baycol
   bezafibrate
   cerivastatin sodium
   CholestaGel
   cholestyramine resin
   Cholestyramine Light
   Choloxin
   clofibrate

Lipid-lowering Agents (cont.)
   colesevelam HCl
   Colestid
   colestipol HCl
   Crestor
   dextrothyroxine sodium
   fenofibrate
   fluvastatin sodium
   Gemcor
   gemfibrozil
   Gen-Fenofibrate Micro ⒸⒶⓃ
   lecithin
   Lescol
   Lescol XL
   Lin-Pravastatin ⒸⒶⓃ
   Lipidil Supra ⒸⒶⓃ
   Lipitor
   LoCholest; LoCholest Light
   Lopid
   lovastatin
   Mevacor
   niacin (vitamin B_3)
   Niacor
   Niaspan
   Nicolar
   nicotinic acid (vitamin B_3)
   Novo-Gemfibrozil ⒸⒶⓃ
   PMS-Bezafibrate ⒸⒶⓃ
   PMS-Fenofibrate Micro ⒸⒶⓃ
   Pravachol
   pravastatin sodium
   Prevalite
   probucol
   Questran; Questran Light
   rosuvastatin calcium
   simvastatin
   Tricor
   Welchol
   Zocor
Manic-Depressive Disorder [see:
   Psychotherapeutics, Antidepressants;
   Psychotherapeutics, Antimanic]
Mast Cell Stabilizers [see: Allergy and
   Anaphylaxis Agents; Asthma Agents,
   Inhalants; Nasal Preparations, Antial-
   lergic; Ophthalmologicals, Antiallergic]
Menopause Agents [see: Gynecologi-
   cal Agents, Menopause Agents]

Indications

Mineral Replacement
Mineral Replacement, Calcium
[*see also: Gynecological Agents,
Menopause Agents*]
Adeflor M
calcium
calcium carbonate
calcium gluceptate
calcium glycerophosphate
calcium lactate
Calphosan
Citracal Prenatal
Enfamil Natalins Rx
Ester-C Plus, Extra Potency
Forcaltonin
Lactocal-F
MagneBind 400 Rx
Marnatal-F
Materna
Mission Prenatal Rx
Mynatal
Mynatal FC
Mynatal P.N.
Mynatal P.N. Forte
Mynatal Rx
Mynate 90 Plus
NataFort
NatalCare Plus
Natalins
Natalins Rx
Natarex Prenatal
Nestabs CFB; Nestabs FA
Niferex-PN Forte
O-Cal f.a.
Par-F
Par-Natal Plus 1 Improved
Pramilet FA
PreCare Conceive
PreCare Prenatal
PremesisRx
Prenatal H.P.
Prenatal Maternal
Prenatal MR 90
Prenatal Plus Iron
Prenatal Plus with Betacarotene
Prenatal Plus; Prenatal Plus
Improved
Prenatal Rx
Prenatal Rx with Betacarotene
Prenatal Z

Mineral Replacement, Calcium
(cont.)
Prenatal-1 + Iron
Prenate Advance; Prenate 90
Prenate Ultra
Strong Start
Stuartnatal Plus
Mineral Replacement, Fluoride
ADC with Fluoride
Adeflor M
Apatate with Fluoride
Chewable Multivitamins with Fluo-
ride
Chewable Triple Vitamins with Flu-
oride
Florvite
Florvite + Iron
Florvite + Iron; Half Strength
Florvite + Iron
Florvite; Florvite Half Strength
Fluoritab
Flura
Flura-Drops
Karidium
Luride
Multivitamin with Fluoride
Mulvidren-F
Neosten
O-Cal f.a.
Pediaflor
Pharmaflur; Pharmaflur df; Phar-
maflur 1.1
Poly-Vi-Flor
Poly-Vi-Flor with Iron
Polytabs-F
Polyvitamin Fluoride
Polyvitamin Fluoride with Iron
Polyvitamin with Iron and Fluoride
Polyvitamins with Fluoride and Iron
sodium fluoride
Soluvite C.T.
Soluvite-f
Tri-Flor-Vite with Fluoride
Tri-Vi-Flor
Tri-Vi-Flor with Iron
Tri Vit with Fluoride
Tri-Vitamin with Fluoride
Tri-A-Vite F
Triple Vitamin ADC with Fluoride
Trivitamin Fluoride

Mineral Replacement, Fluoride (cont.)
Vi-Daylin/F ADC
Vi-Daylin/F ADC + Iron
Vi-Daylin/F Multivitamin
Vi-Daylin/F Multivitamin + Iron
Mineral Replacement, Iron
[see also: Anemia Agents, Iron]
Adeflor M
B-C with Folic Acid Plus
Bacmin
Berocca Plus
Berplex Plus
carbonyl iron
Cevi-Fer
Citracal Prenatal
Enfamil Natalins Rx
Estrostep Fe
Ferrex PC; Ferrex PC Forte
ferrous fumarate
ferrous gluconate
ferrous sulfate
ferrous sulfate, dried
Florvite + Iron
Florvite + Iron; Half Strength
   Florvite + Iron
Formula B Plus
iron
Lactocal-F
Loestrin Fe 1/20; Loestrin Fe 1.5/30
Marnatal-F
Materna
Microgestin Fe 1/20; Microgestin Fe
   1.5/30
Mission Prenatal Rx
Mynatal
Mynatal FC
Mynatal P.N.
Mynatal P.N. Forte
Mynatal Rx
Mynate 90 Plus
NataChew
NataFort
NatalCare Plus
Natalins
Natalins Rx
Natarex Prenatal
Nestabs CFB; Nestabs FA
Niferex-PN
Niferex-PN Forte

Mineral Replacement, Iron (cont.)
Nu-Iron V
O-Cal f.a.
Par-F
Par-Natal Plus 1 Improved
Poly-Vi-Flor with Iron
polysaccharide-iron complex
Polyvitamin Fluoride with Iron
Polyvitamin with Iron and Fluoride
Polyvitamins with Fluoride and Iron
Pramilet FA
PreCare Conceive
PreCare Prenatal
Prenatal H.P.
Prenatal Maternal
Prenatal MR 90
Prenatal Plus Iron
Prenatal Plus with Betacarotene
Prenatal Plus; Prenatal Plus
   Improved
Prenatal Rx
Prenatal Rx with Betacarotene
Prenatal Z
Prenatal-1 + Iron
Prenate Advance; Prenate 90
Prenate Ultra
Senilezol
Strong Start
Stuartnatal Plus
Theragran Hematinic
Tri-Vi-Flor with Iron
Ultra-Natal
Vi-Daylin/F ADC + Iron
Vi-Daylin/F Multivitamin + Iron
Vitafōl; Vitafōl-PN
Zenate, Advanced Formula
Zodeac-100
Mineral Replacement, Magnesium
MagneBind 400 Rx
magnesium
magnesium amino acid chelate
magnesium carbonate
magnesium gluconate
magnesium oxide
Mineral Replacement, Zinc
zinc gluconate
zinc sulfate
Zinca-Pak
Zincate

Indications

Mineral Replacement, Trace Elements

ammonium molybdate
Chroma-Pak
chromic chloride
Chromium Chloride
ConTE-Pak-4
cupric sulfate
M.T.E.-4; M.T.E.-5; M.T.E.-6;
M.T.E.-7; M.T.E.-4 Concentrated;
M.T.E.-5 Concentrated; M.T.E.-6
Concentrated
manganese chloride
manganese sulfate
Molypen
MulTE-Pak-4; MulTE-Pak-5
Multiple Trace Element with Selenium; Multiple Trace Element
with Selenium Concentrated
Multiple Trace Element; Multiple
Trace Element Concentrated;
Multiple Trace Element Neonatal;
Multiple Trace Element Pediatric
Multitrace-5 Concentrate
Neotrace-4
P.T.E.-4; P.T.E.-5
PedTE-Pak-4
Pedtrace-4
Sele-Pak
selenious acid
Selepen
Trace Metals Additive in 0.9% NaCl
Tracelyte; Tracelyte II; Tracelyte
with Double Electrolytes; Tracelyte II with Double Electrolytes

Mineral Replacement, Multiple (not listed)

B-C with Folic Acid Plus
Bacmin
Berocca Plus
Berplex Plus
Cezin-S
Eldercaps
Ferrex PC; Ferrex PC Forte
Florvite + Iron
Florvite + Iron; Half Strength
Florvite + Iron
Formula B Plus
Hemocyte Plus
Lactocal-F

Mineral Replacement, Multiple (not listed) (cont.)

Marnatal-F
Materna
Megaton
Mynatal
Mynatal FC
Mynatal P.N. Forte
Mynatal Rx
NataTab CFe; NataTab FA
NatalCare Plus
Niferex-PN; Niferex-PN Forte
O-Cal f.a.
Par-F
Poly-Vi-Flor with Iron
Polyvitamin Fluoride with Iron
Pramilet FA
PreCare Conceive
PreCare Prenatal
Prenatal Maternal
Strovite Advance
Strovite Plus; Strovite Forte
Theragran Hematinic
Ultra-Natal
Vicon Forte
Zincvit
Zodeac-100

Mouth and Throat Preparations

[see also: Antiseptics]

acidulated phosphate fluoride (sodium
fluoride & hydrofluoric acid)
Actisite
Americaine Anesthetic Lubricant
amlexanox
Anestacon
Aphthasol
Apo-Benzydamine Ⓒᴬᴺ
Apo-Chlorhexidine Ⓒᴬᴺ
Arestin
articaine HCl
Astracaine; Astracaine Forte Ⓒᴬᴺ
Atrisorb FreeFlow GTR Barrier
benzocaine
benzydamine HCl
carbamide peroxide
Carisolv Ⓒᴬᴺ
cevimeline HCl
chlorhexidine gluconate

Mouth and Throat Preparations (cont.)
chlorobutanol
chlorophyllin
choline salicylate
Citanest Forte
Dey-Pak Sodium Chloride 3% & 10%
docosanol (n-docosanol)
doxycycline hyclate
Duo-Trach Kit
Evoxac
Fluoride Loz
Fluorinse
Flura-Loz
Gel-Kam
itraconazole
Karigel; Karigel-N
Kenalog in Orabase
lidocaine HCl
Luride SF
minocycline HCl
Minute-Gel
Mycostatin
Nilstat
nystatin
Nystex
Orabase HCA
OraDisc
Oralease
Oralone Dental
Orarinse
Peridex
PerioChip
PerioGard
Periostat
phenol
Phos-Flur
pilocarpine HCl
Point-Two
Pontocaine HCl
povidone-iodine
PreviDent
PreviDent 5000 Plus
PreviDent Rinse
Ravocaine & Novocaine with Levophed
Salagen
Septocaine
sodium chloride (NaCl)
sodium fluoride

Mouth and Throat Preparations (cont.)
sodium hypochlorite
Sporanox
stannous fluoride
Stop
Tantrum
tetracaine HCl
tetracycline HCl
Thera-Flur; Thera-Flur-N
triamcinolone acetonide
Trilisate
Xylocaine
Xylocaine 10% Oral
Xylocaine Viscous
MRI Contrast Media [see: Contrast Media, Paramagnetic]

Indications

Multiple Sclerosis Agents
Antegren
bovine myelin
mitoxantrone HCl
Myloral
natalizumab
Novantrone
paclitaxel

Muscle Relaxants
[see also: Psychotherapeutics, Anxiolytics; Sedatives and Hypnotics]
Muscle Relaxants, Skeletal
Anectine
Apo-Diazepam ⒸⒶ⒩
Arduan
atracurium besylate
baclofen (L-baclofen)
Banflex
botulinum toxin, type B
carisoprodol
chlorphenesin carbamate
chlorzoxazone
cisatracurium besylate
cyclobenzaprine HCl
Dantrium
dantrolene sodium
Diazemuls ⒸⒶ⒩
diazepam

Muscle Relaxants, Skeletal (cont.)

Dizac
doxacurium chloride
Flexaphen
Flexeril
Flexoject
Flexon
gallamine triethiodide
Lioresal
Maolate
metaxalone
methocarbamol
metocurine iodide
Metubine Iodide
Mivacron
mivacurium chloride
Myobloc
Myolin
Nimbex
Norcuron
Norflex
Norgesic; Norgesic Forte
Nuromax
orphenadrine citrate
Orphengesic; Orphengesic Forte
pancuronium bromide
Paraflex
Parafon Forte DSC
Pavulon
pipecuronium bromide
Quelicin
rapacuronium bromide
Raplon
Remular-S
Rhoxal-orphenadrine ⒸⒶⓃ
Robaxin
Robaxisal
rocuronium bromide
Skelaxin
Sodol Compound
Soma
Soma Compound
Soma Compound with Codeine
succinylcholine chloride
Tracrium
tubocurarine chloride
Valium
Valium Roche Oral ⒸⒶⓃ
vecuronium bromide
Zemuron

Muscle Relaxants, Smooth

Cyclan
cyclandelate
Cyclospasmol
Cyclospasmol ⒸⒶⓃ
flavoxate HCl
Genabid
papaverine HCl
Pavabid
Pavagen TD
Pavarine
Pavatine
Paverolan
Urispas

Muscle Stimulants

ambenonium chloride
carbachol
edrophonium chloride
Enlon
Enlon Plus
guanidine HCl
IGF-1/BP3 complex
Mestinon
Mytelase
neostigmine bromide
neostigmine methylsulfate
Prostigmin
pyridostigmine bromide
Regonol
Reversol
SomatoKine
Tensilon

Narcolepsy [see: Central Nervous System Stimulants]

Nasal Preparations
Nasal Preparations, Antiallergic

[see also: Allergy and Anaphylaxis Agents; Antihistamines, Topical]
Alti-Ipratropium ⒸⒶⓃ
Apo-Cromolyn ⒸⒶⓃ
Astelin
Atrovent
azelastine HCl
cromolyn sodium
ipratropium bromide

Nasal Preparations, Antiallergic (cont.)

levocabastine HCl

Livostin (CAN)

pheniramine maleate

Nasal Preparations, Anti-inflammatory

Alti-Flunisolide (CAN)

Apo-Beclomethasone (CAN)

Apo-Flunisolide (CAN)

beclomethasone dipropionate (BDP)

Beconase

Beconase AQ

budesonide

Dexacort Phosphate

dexamethasone sodium phosphate

Flonase

flunisolide

fluticasone propionate

Nasacort

Nasacort AQ

Nasalide

Nasarel

Nu-Beclomethasone (CAN)

Rhinocort

Rhinocort (CAN)

Rhinocort Aqua

triamcinolone acetonide

Vancenase

Vancenase AQ

Nasal Preparations, Decongestants

Adrenalin Chloride

Benzedrex

ephedrine sulfate

epinephrine HCl

naphazoline HCl

oxymetazoline HCl

phenylephrine HCl

propylhexedrine

tetrahydrozoline HCl

Tyzine

Nasal Preparations, Moisturizers

sodium chloride (NaCl)

Nausea [see: Antiemetics and Antinauseants]

Nutritional Agents

5% Alcohol and 5% Dextrose in Water; 10% Alcohol and 5% Dextrose in Water

Aminess 5.2%

Aminosyn 3.5% (5%, 7%, 8.5%, 10%); Aminosyn (pH6) 10%; Aminosyn II 3.5% (5%, 7%, 8.5%, 10%, 15%); Aminosyn-PF 7% (10%)

Aminosyn 3.5% M; Aminosyn II 3.5% M

Aminosyn 7% (8.5%) with Electrolytes; Aminosyn II 7% (8.5%, 10%) with Electrolytes

Aminosyn-HBC 7%

Aminosyn II 3.5% in 5% (25%) Dextrose; Aminosyn II 4.25% in 10% (20%, 25%) Dextrose; Aminosyn II 5% in 25% Dextrose

Aminosyn II 3.5% M in 5% Dextrose; Aminosyn II 4.25% M in 10% Dextrose

Aminosyn-RF 5.2%

BranchAmin 4%

Carnitor

choline

choline chloride

cysteine HCl (L-cysteine HCl)

D-2.5-W; D-5-W; D-10-W; D-20-W; D-25-W; D-30-W; D-40-W; D-50-W; D-60-W; D-70-W

dextrose

5% Dextrose and Electrolyte #48; 5% Dextrose and Electrolyte #75; 10% Dextrose and Electrolyte #48

50% Dextrose with Electrolyte Pattern A (or N)

Dialyte Pattern LM

Dianeal Peritoneal Dialysis Solution with 1.1% Amino Acids

Extraneal Peritoneal Dialysis Solution

fat emulsion, intravenous

Foltx

FreAmine HBC 6.9%

FreAmine III 3% (8.5%) with Electrolytes

FreAmine III 8.5%; FreAmine III 10%

glutamic acid (L-glutamic acid)

Indications

Nutritional Agents (cont.)
glycine
HepatAmine
icodextrin
Infuvite Pediatric
inositol
Intrachol
Intralipid 10%; Intralipid 20%
Iodopen
Isolyte E (G; H; M; P; R; S) with
　5% Dextrose
levocarnitine
Liposyn II 20%; Liposyn III 20%
lysine (L-lysine)
M.V.I. Neonatal
NephrAmine 5.4%
Normosol-M and 5% Dextrose; Nor-
　mosol-R and 5% Dextrose
Novamine; Novamine 15%
Nutrineal Peritoneal Dialysis Solu-
　tion with 1.1% Amino Acid
Plasma-Lyte M (R; 56; 148) and 5%
　Dextrose
ProcalAmine
ProSol 20%
RenAmin
sodium iodide
Strovite Advance
sugar, invert (50% dextrose & 50%
　fructose)
threonine (L-threonine)
Travasol 2.75% in 5% (10%, 25%)
　Dextrose; Travasol 4.25% in 5%
　(10%, 25%) Dextrose
Travasol 3.5% (5.5%, 8.5%) with
　Electrolytes
Travasol 5.5% (8.5%, 10%)
5% Travert and Electrolyte No. 2;
　10% Travert and Electrolyte No. 2
TrophAmine 6%; TrophAmine 10%
VitaCarn
**Obsessive-Compulsive Disorder
(OCD)** [see: Psychotherapeutics,
Antiobsessional]

Ophthalmologicals
Ophthalmologicals, Antiallergic
[see also: Antihistamines, Topical]
Alamast

**Ophthalmologicals, Antiallergic
(cont.)**
Alocril
Alomide
antazoline phosphate
azelastine HCl
Crolom
cromolyn sodium
Emadine
emedastine difumarate
ketotifen fumarate
levocabastine HCl
Livostin
lodoxamide tromethamine
Naphoptic-A
nedocromil sodium
olopatadine HCl
Opticrom 4%
Optivar
Patanol
pemirolast potassium
pheniramine maleate
Vasocon-A
Zaditor
Ophthalmologicals, Antibiotics
[see also: Antibiotics, Topical]
AK-Chlor
AK-Spore
AK-Spore H.C.
AK-Sulf
AK-Trol
AK-Poly-Bac
AKTob
bacitracin zinc
bacitracin zinc & neomycin sulfate
　& polymyxin B sulfate
bacitracin zinc & polymyxin B sulfate
Bleph-10
Blephamide
Cetamide
Cetapred
Chibroxin
chloramphenicol
chlorobutanol
Chloromycetin
Chloromycetin Hydrocortisone
Chloroptic
Chloroptic S.O.P.
chlortetracycline HCl
Ciloxan

Ophthalmologicals, Antibiotics (cont.)

ciprofloxacin HCl
Cortisporin
Defy
Dexacidin
dexamethasone & neomycin sulfate & polymyxin B sulfate
Dexasporin
erythromycin
FML-S
Garamycin
Genoptic
Genoptic S.O.P.
Gentacidin
Gentak
gentamicin sulfate
gramicidin
gramicidin & neomycin sulfate & polymyxin B sulfate
Herplex
idoxuridine (IDU)
Ilotycin
Isopto Cetamide
Isopto Cetapred
levofloxacin
Maxitrol
Metimyd
Natacyn
natamycin
neomycin sulfate
neomycin sulfate & polymyxin B sulfate & bacitracin zinc
neomycin sulfate & polymyxin B sulfate & dexamethasone
neomycin sulfate & polymyxin B sulfate & gramicidin
Neosporin
Neotricin HC
norfloxacin
Ocuflox
Ocusulf-10
Ocutricin
ofloxacin
oxytetracycline HCl
PMS-Tobramycin ⒸⒶⓃ
PMS-Polytrimethoprim ⒸⒶⓃ
Poly-Pred
polymyxin B sulfate
polymyxin B sulfate & bacitracin zinc

Ophthalmologicals, Antibiotics (cont.)

polymyxin B sulfate & bacitracin zinc & neomycin sulfate
polymyxin B sulfate & gramicidin & neomycin sulfate
polymyxin B sulfate & neomycin sulfate & dexamethasone
polymyxin B sulfate & trimethoprim sulfate
Polytrim
Pred-G
Pred-G S.O.P.
Quixin
Sab-Cortimyxin ⒸⒶⓃ
silver nitrate
silver protein, mild
Sodium Sulamyd
Storz-N-P-D
Storz-Sulf
Sulf-10
sulfacetamide sodium
sulfisoxazole diolamine
Sulster
Terak with Polymyxin B Sulfate
Terra-Cortril
Terramycin with Polymyxin B
tetracycline HCl
TobraDex
tobramycin
Tobrex
Tomycine ⒸⒶⓃ
trifluridine
trimethoprim sulfate & polymyxin B sulfate
Triple Antibiotic
Vasocidin
Vasocine
Vasosulf
vidarabine
Vira-A
Viroptic

Ophthalmologicals, Antiglaucoma

acetazolamide
acetazolamide sodium
Adsorbocarpine
Akarpine
AKBeta
AKPro
Alphagan; Alphagan P

Indications

Ophthalmologicals, Antiglaucoma (cont.)

Alti-Timolol Ⓒᴬᴺ
Apo-Dipivefrin Ⓒᴬᴺ
Apo-Levobunolol Ⓒᴬᴺ
apraclonidine HCl
Azopt
Beta-Tim Ⓒᴬᴺ
Betagan Liquifilm
BetaSite
betaxolol HCl
Betaxon
Betimol
Betoptic; Betoptic S
bimatoprost
brimonidine tartrate
brinzolamide
carbachol
Carboptic
carteolol HCl
Cosopt
demecarium bromide
Diamox
dipivefrin HCl
dorzolamide HCl
E-Pilo-1; E-Pilo-2; E-Pilo-4; E-Pilo-6
echothiophate iodide
Epifrin
Epinal
epinephrine bitartrate
epinephrine borate
epinephrine HCl
epinephryl borate
Eserine Sulfate
GlaucTabs
Glaucon
Humorsol
Iopidine
isoflurophate
isopropyl unoprostone
Isopto Carbachol
Isopto Carpine
latanoprost
levobetaxolol HCl
levobunolol HCl
Lumigan
Med Timolol Ⓒᴬᴺ
methazolamide
metipranolol HCl
MZM

Ophthalmologicals, Antiglaucoma (cont.)

Neptazane
Novo-Timol Ⓒᴬᴺ
Ocupress
Ocusert Pilo-20; Ocusert Pilo-40
OptiPranolol
P_1E_1; P_2E_1; P_4E_1; P_6E_1
P_3E_1
Phospholine Iodide
physostigmine
physostigmine salicylate
physostigmine sulfate
Pilagan
Pilocar
pilocarpine
pilocarpine HCl
pilocarpine nitrate
Pilopine HS
Piloptic-½; Piloptic-1; Piloptic-2; Piloptic-3; Piloptic-4; Piloptic-6
Pilopto-Carpine
Pilostat
PMS-Dipivefrin Ⓒᴬᴺ
PMS-Levobunolol Ⓒᴬᴺ
Propine
Rescula
Rhoxal-timolol Ⓒᴬᴺ
Sab-Betaxolol Ⓒᴬᴺ
Storzine 2
Timodal Ⓒᴬᴺ
timolol
timolol hemihydrate
timolol maleate
Timoptic
Timoptic-XE
Travatan
travoprost
Trusopt
unoprostone isopropyl
Xalatan
Xalcom

Ophthalmologicals, Anti-inflammatory

AK-Dex
AK-Pred
AK-Spore H.C.
AK-Trol
Acular; Acular PF
AK-Neo-Dex

Ophthalmologicals, Anti-inflammatory (cont.)
Alrex
Blephamide
Cetapred
Chloromycetin Hydrocortisone
Cortisporin
Decadron Phosphate
Dexacidin
dexamethasone
dexamethasone & neomycin sulfate & polymyxin B sulfate
dexamethasone sodium phosphate
Dexasporin
diclofenac sodium
Diodex ⓒ
Econopred; Econopred Plus
Eflone
Flarex
Fluor-Op
fluorometholone
fluorometholone acetate
flurbiprofen sodium
FML S.O.P.
FML; FML Forte
FML-S
HMS
hydrocortisone (HC)
hydrocortisone acetate (HCA)
Inflamase Mild; Inflamase Forte
Isopto Cetapred
Lotemax
loteprednol etabonate
Maxidex
Maxitrol
medrysone
Metimyd
Neo-Dexair
Neo-Dexameth
NeoDecadron
neomycin sulfate & polymyxin B sulfate & dexamethasone
Neotricin HC
Ocufen
PMS-Dexamethasone ⓒ
PMS-Fluorometholone ⓒ
Poly-Pred
polymyxin B sulfate & neomycin sulfate & dexamethasone
Pred-G

Ophthalmologicals, Anti-inflammatory (cont.)
Pred-G S.O.P.
Pred Mild; Pred Forte
prednisolone acetate
prednisolone sodium phosphate
Profenal
R.O.-Dexsone ⓒ
Sab-Cortimyxin ⓒ
Spersadex ⓒ
Storz-N-D
Storz-N-P-D
Sulster
suprofen
Surodex
Terra-Cortril
TobraDex
Vasocidin
Vasocine
Vexol
Vofenal ⓒ
Voltaren Ophtha ⓒ
Voltaren Ophthalmic
Zenapax
Ophthalmologicals, Contact Lens Preparations
[see also: Antiseptics]
hydrogen peroxide
sodium chloride (NaCl)
Ophthalmologicals, Decongestants
AK-Con
AK-Dilate
Albalon
Mydfrin 2.5%
Nafazair
naphazoline HCl
Naphcon Forte
Naphoptic-A
Neo-Synephrine
oxymetazoline HCl
Phenoptic
phenylephrine HCl
Storzfen
tetrahydrozoline HCl
Vasocon Regular
Vasocon-A
Vasosulf
Ophthalmologicals, Diagnostic Agents
AK-Fluor

Indications

Ophthalmologicals, Diagnostic Agents (cont.)
Cardio-Green (CG)
Flu-Oxinate
Fluor-I-Strip; Fluor-I-Strip A.T.
Fluoracaine
fluorescein
fluorescein sodium
Fluorescite
Fluoresoft
fluorexon
Flurate
Fluress
Ful-Glo
Funduscein-10; Funduscein-25
Healon Yellow
Ophthifluor
Schirmer Tear Test
Sno-Strips

Ophthalmologicals, Local Anesthetics
[see also: Anesthetics, Local]
Alcaine
benoxinate HCl
Flu-Oxinate
Fluoracaine
Flurate
Fluress
Ophthaine
Ophthetic
Pontocaine HCl
proparacaine HCl
tetracaine HCl

Ophthalmologicals, Miotics
acetylcholine chloride
Adsorbocarpine
Akarpine
carbachol
Carbastat
Carboptic
dapiprazole HCl
demecarium bromide
echothiophate iodide
Eserine Sulfate
Humorsol
isoflurophate
Isopto Carbachol
Isopto Carpine
Miochol-E
Miostat

Ophthalmologicals, Miotics (cont.)
Ocusert Pilo-20; Ocusert Pilo-40
Phospholine Iodide
physostigmine
physostigmine salicylate
physostigmine sulfate
Pilagan
Pilocar
pilocarpine
pilocarpine HCl
pilocarpine nitrate
Pilopine HS
Piloptic-½; Piloptic-1; Piloptic-2;
    Piloptic-3; Piloptic-4; Piloptic-6
Pilopto-Carpine
Pilostat
Rēv-Eyes
Storzine 2

Ophthalmologicals, Moisturizers, Lubricants, and Emollients
Albalon
boric acid
carboxymethylcellulose sodium
collagen
glycerin
Herrick Lacrimal Plug
hydroxypropyl cellulose
hydroxypropyl methylcellulose
methylcellulose
polyethylene glycol (PEG)
polyvinyl alcohol (PVA)
Punctum Plug
Restasis
silicone
TearSaver Punctum Plugs
vitamin A

Ophthalmologicals, Mydriatics and Cycloplegics
AK-Dilate
AK-Homatropine
AK-Pentolate
atropine sulfate
Atropine Care
Atropine-1
Atropisol
Cyclogyl
Cyclomydril
cyclopentolate HCl
homatropine hydrobromide
hydroxyamphetamine hydrobromide

Ophthalmologicals, Mydriatics and Cycloplegics (cont.)
Isopto Atropine
Isopto Homatropine
Isopto Hyoscine
Murocoll-2
Mydfrin 2.5%
Mydriacyl
Neo-Synephrine
Opticyl
Paredrine
Paremyd
Pentolair
Phenoptic
phenylephrine HCl
scopolamine hydrobromide
Storzfen
Tropi-Storz
Tropicacyl
tropicamide

Ophthalmologicals, Surgical Preparations
AdatoSil 5000
AMO Vitrax
Amvisc; Amvisc Plus
Betadine 5% Sterile Ophthalmic Prep
Catarase 1:5000
chymotrypsin
gelatin film, absorbable
gelatin powder, absorbable
gelatin sponge, absorbable
Gelfilm; Gelfilm Ophthalmic
Gelfoam
glycerin
Healon Yellow
Healon; Healon GV
Healon5 (CAN)
hyaluronate sodium
hydroxypropyl methylcellulose
Occucoat
Ophthalgan
polydimethylsiloxane
povidone-iodine
Profenal
silver protein, mild
Staarvisc
suprofen
Viscoat

Ophthalmologicals, Other
aminocaproic acid

Ophthalmologicals, Other (cont.)
AMO Endosol; AMO Endosol Extra
B-Salt Forte
Botox
botulinum toxin, type A
BSS; BSS Plus
Caprogel
cyclosporine
Dysport
fomivirsen sodium
Galardin
glucose, liquid
Glucose-40
ilomastat
Lu-Tex
matrix metalloproteinase (MMP) inhibitors
motexafin lutetium
Optimmune
Optrin
PhotoPoint
prinomastat
Purlytin
rostaporfin
Salagen
Sandimmune
sodium chloride (NaCl)
Succus Cineraria Maritima
tin etiopurpurin dichloride
tyloxapol
verteporfin
Visudyne
Vitrase
Vitravene

Organ Transplant Rejection [see: Immunosuppressive Agents]

Osteoarthritis [see: Antiarthritics; Analgesics, Nonsteroidal]

Osteoporosis [see: Gynecological Agents, Menopause Agents; Mineral Replacement, Calcium]

Otologicals
[see also: Anesthetics, Local; Antibiotics, Topical; Antiseptics; Dermatological Preparations, Anti-inflammatory]
AK-Spore H.C.
AA-HC Otic
Acetasol

Indications

Otologicals (cont.)
Acetasol HC
acetic acid
Allergen Ear Drops
Americaine Otic
AntibiŌtic
Antibiotic Ear Solution
Antibiotic Ear Suspension
antipyrine
Auralgan Otic
Auroto Otic
benzocaine
boric acid
Borofair Otic
carbamide peroxide
Cerumenex
chloramphenicol
chlorobutanol
Chloromycetin Otic
chloroxylenol
Cipro HC Otic
ciprofloxacin
colistin sulfate
Coly-Mycin S Otic
Cortatrigen Modified
Cortic
Cortisporin Otic
Cortisporin-TC
Cresylate
Drotic
Ear-Eze
Floxin Otic
hydrocortisone (HC)
hydrocortisone acetate (HCA)
LazerSporin-C
neomycin sulfate
Octicare
ofloxacin
Oti-Med
Otic-Care
Otic Domeboro
OtiTricin
Otobiotic Otic
Otocain
Otocalm
Otocort
Otomar-HC
Otomycet-HC
Otomycin-HPN Otic
Otosporin

Otologicals (cont.)
Pediotic
Pedotic
PMS-Dexamethasone ⓒⒶⓃ
polymyxin B sulfate
Tri-Otic
trolamine polypeptide oleate-condensate
Tympagesic
UAD Otic
VōSol HC Otic
VōSol Otic
Vasotate HC
Zoto-HC
Paget Disease [see: *Hypercalcemia Agents*]
Panic Disorder [see: *Psychotherapeutics, Antipanic*]
Parasites, Intestinal [see: *Anthelmintics; Antiprotozoals*]
Parkinson Disease [see: *Antiparkinsonian Agents*]

Pediculicides and Scabicides
Acticin
bioallethrin
crotamiton
Elimite
Eurax
G-Well
lindane
malathion
Ovide
permethrin
piperonyl butoxide
pyrethrins
Scabene

Peptic Ulcer and Gastric Reflux Agents
[see also: *Antacids; Antisecretories, Gastrointestinal*]
Aciphex
Alti-Famotidine ⓒⒶⓃ
anisotropine methylbromide
Apo-Cimetidine ⓒⒶⓃ
Apo-Ranitidine ⓒⒶⓃ

Peptic Ulcer and Gastric Reflux Agents (cont.)

Arthrotec
Axid
Banthīne
Cantil
Carafate
cimetidine
cimetidine HCl
cisapride
Cytotec
Daricon
enprostil
esomeprazole magnesium
famotidine
Gardrin
Gastrozepine
Gen-Ranitidine (CAN)
Hp-PAC (CAN)
Iamin
lansoprazole
Losec (CAN)
Losec 1-2-3 A (CAN)
Losec 1-2-3 M (CAN)
mepenzolate bromide
methantheline bromide
misoprostol
Nexium
nizatidine
Novo-Nizatidine (CAN)
Novo-Ranidine (CAN)
omeprazole
oxyphencyclimine HCl
Panto IV (CAN)
Pantoloc (CAN)
pantoprazole
pantoprazole sodium
Pantozol
Pathilon
Pepcid
Pepcid RPD
pirenzepine HCl
PMS-Nizatidine (CAN)
PMS-Ranitidine (CAN)
PMS-Sucralfate (CAN)
Prepulsid (CAN)
Prevacid
Prevpac
Prilosec
Propulsid

Peptic Ulcer and Gastric Reflux Agents (cont.)

Protonix
Protonix I.V.
Pylorid (CAN)
rabeprazole sodium
ranitidine
ranitidine bismuth citrate
ranitidine HCl
Rhoxal-ranitidine (CAN)
Rhoxal-famotidine (CAN)
roxatidine acetate HCl
Roxin
sucralfate
Tagamet
tridihexethyl chloride
Tritec
Zantac
Zantac EFFERdose
Zantac GELdose

Indications

Peripheral Vasodilators

beraprost
beraprost sodium
cilostazol
Cyclan
cyclandelate
Cyclo-Prostin
Cyclospasmol
Cyclospasmol (CAN)
epoprostenol
ethaverine HCl
Flolan
flunarizine HCl
Genabid
isoxsuprine HCl
niacin (vitamin B_3)
Niacor
Niaspan
Nicolar
nicotinic acid (vitamin B_3)
papaverine HCl
Pavabid
Pavagen TD
Pavarine
Pavatine
Paverolan
pentoxifylline
Pletal

Peripheral Vasodilators (cont.)
   Priscoline HCl
   Remodulin
   Sibelium
   tolazoline HCl
   Trental
   treprostinil sodium
   Vasodilan
   Voxsuprine
Plasma Expanders [see: Blood
   Expanders and Substitutes]

Platelet Aggregation Inhibitors
[see also: Cardiac Agents]
abciximab
Aggrastat
Aggrenox
Alti-Ticlopidine ⒸⒶⓃ
Apo-Ticlopidine ⒸⒶⓃ
aspirin
beraprost
beraprost sodium
cilostazol
clopidogrel bisulfate
dipyridamole
Easprin
eptifibatide
Gen-Ticlodipine ⒸⒶⓃ
Integrilin
LeukArrest
Persantine
Plavix
Pletal
PMS-Ticlopidine ⒸⒶⓃ
Remodulin
ReoPro
Rhoxal-ticlopidine ⒸⒶⓃ
rovelizumab
Ticlid
ticlopidine HCl
tirofiban HCl
treprostinil sodium
vitamin E
ZORprin
Progestins [see: Hormones, Progestins]

Prostatic Hyperplasia Agents
Alti-Doxazosin ⒸⒶⓃ
Apo-Doxazosin ⒸⒶⓃ
Apo-Terazosin ⒸⒶⓃ
Cardura
doxazosin mesylate
finasteride
Flomax
Gen-Doxazosin ⒸⒶⓃ
HP-4
Hytrin
Hytrin ⒸⒶⓃ
Novo-Terazosin ⒸⒶⓃ
PMS-Terazosin ⒸⒶⓃ
PPRT-321
Proscar
tamsulosin HCl
terazosin HCl
Psoriasis [see: Dermatological Prepara-
   tions, Psoriasis Agents]

Psychotherapeutics
Psychotherapeutics, Antidepressants
   Alti-Fluoxetine ⒸⒶⓃ
   Alti-Nortriptylene Hydrochloride ⒸⒶⓃ
   amitriptyline HCl
   amoxapine
   Anafranil
   Apo-Moclobemide ⒸⒶⓃ
   Apo-Nefazodone ⒸⒶⓃ
   Apo-Sertraline ⒸⒶⓃ
   Apo-Amitriptylene ⒸⒶⓃ
   Asendin
   Aventyl HCl
   benactyzine HCl
   bupropion HCl
   Catatrol
   Celexa
   Cipralex
   citalopram hydrobromide
   clomipramine HCl
   CO Fluoxetine ⒸⒶⓃ
   deramciclane
   desipramine HCl
   Desyrel
   dothiepin HCl
   doxepin HCl
   duloxetine
   duloxetine HCl

Psychotherapeutics, Antidepressants (cont.)
Edronax
Effexor
Effexor XR
Elavil
Etrafon; Etrafon 2–10; Etrafon-A; Etrafon-Forte
fluoxetine HCl
fluvoxamine maleate
Gamma-OH
Gen-Fluoxetine (CAN)
Gen-Fluvoxamine (CAN)
imipramine HCl
imipramine pamoate
isocarboxazid
Limbitrol DS 10-25
Ludiomil
Luvox
Manerix (CAN)
maprotiline HCl
Marplan
mirtazapine
moclobemide
Nardil
nefazodone HCl
Norpramin
nortriptyline HCl
Novo-Fluvoxamine (CAN)
Novo-Moclobemide (CAN)
Novo-Sertraline (CAN)
Novo-Triptyn (CAN)
Nu-Fluvoxamine (CAN)
Nu-Moclobemide (CAN)
Pamelor
Parnate
paroxetine HCl
Paxil
Paxil CR
phenelzine sulfate
PMS-Fluvoxamine (CAN)
PMS-Moclobemide (CAN)
Prothiaden
protriptyline HCl
Prozac
Prozac Weekly
reboxetine
reboxetine mesylate
Remeron

Psychotherapeutics, Antidepressants (cont.)
Rhoxal-fluoxetine (CAN)
sertraline HCl
Serzone
Serzone-5HT$_2$ (CAN)
Sinequan
Surmontil
Tofranil
Tofranil-PM
tranylcypromine sulfate
trazodone HCl
Triavil
Triavil 4-50
trimipramine maleate
venlafaxine HCl
Vestra
viloxazine
Vivactil
Wellbutrin
Wellbutrin SR
Zoloft
Zoloft (CAN)

Psychotherapeutics, Antimanic
Apo-Lithium (CAN)
Atretol
carbamazepine
Carbatrol
Carbolith (CAN)
Depakote
Depakote ER
Depitol
Duralith (CAN)
Epitol
Eskalith
Eskalith CR
Gen-Carbamazepine CR (CAN)
Lithane (CAN)
lithium carbonate
lithium citrate
Lithobid
Lithonate
Lithotabs
olanzapine
PMS-Carbamazepine CR (CAN)
PMS-Lithium Carbonate (CAN)
PMS-Lithium Citrate (CAN)
Tegretol
Tegretol-XR
Zyprexa

Indications

Psychotherapeutics, Antiobsessional
Alti-Fluoxetine ⒸⒶⓃ
Anafranil
Apo-Sertraline ⒸⒶⓃ
clomipramine HCl
CO Fluoxetine ⒸⒶⓃ
fluoxetine HCl
fluvoxamine maleate
Gen-Fluoxetine ⒸⒶⓃ
Gen-Fluvoxamine ⒸⒶⓃ
Luvox
Novo-Fluvoxamine ⒸⒶⓃ
Novo-Sertraline ⒸⒶⓃ
Nu-Fluvoxamine ⒸⒶⓃ
paroxetine HCl
Paxil
PMS-Fluvoxamine ⒸⒶⓃ
Prozac
Rhoxal-fluoxetine ⒸⒶⓃ
sertraline HCl
Zoloft
Zoloft ⒸⒶⓃ

Psychotherapeutics, Antipanic
alprazolam
Apo-Sertraline ⒸⒶⓃ
Novo-Sertraline ⒸⒶⓃ
Pagoclone
paroxetine HCl
sertraline HCl
Xanax
Zoloft
Zoloft ⒸⒶⓃ

Psychotherapeutics, Antipsychotics
acetophenazine maleate
Apo-Fluphenazine ⒸⒶⓃ
Apo-Haloperidol LA ⒸⒶⓃ
Apo-Loxapine ⒸⒶⓃ
Apo-Perphenazine ⒸⒶⓃ
Apo-Prochlorazine ⒸⒶⓃ
Apo-Thioridazine ⒸⒶⓃ
Apo-Trifluoperazine ⒸⒶⓃ
chlorpromazine
chlorpromazine HCl
clozapine
Clozaril
Compazine
Etrafon; Etrafon 2–10; Etrafon-A;
    Etrafon-Forte
fluphenazine decanoate
fluphenazine enanthate

Psychotherapeutics, Antipsychotics (cont.)
fluphenazine HCl
Geodon
Haldol
Haldol Decanoate 50; Haldol Deca-
    noate 100
haloperidol
haloperidol decanoate
haloperidol lactate
Haloperidol LA ⒸⒶⓃ
iloperidone
Loxapac ⒸⒶⓃ
loxapine
loxapine HCl
loxapine succinate
Loxitane
Loxitane C
Loxitane IM
Mellaril
Mellaril-S
mesoridazine besylate
Moban
Modecate; Modecate Concentrate ⒸⒶⓃ
Moditen Enanthate ⒸⒶⓃ
Moditen HCl ⒸⒶⓃ
molindone HCl
Navane
Nu-Prochlor ⒸⒶⓃ
olanzapine
Orap
Ormazine
Permitil
perphenazine
pimozide
PMS-Fluphenazine ⒸⒶⓃ
PMS-Fluphenazine Decanoate ⒸⒶⓃ
PMS-Haloperidol ⒸⒶⓃ
PMS-Haloperidol LA ⒸⒶⓃ
prochlorperazine
prochlorperazine bimaleate
prochlorperazine edisylate
prochlorperazine maleate
prochlorperazine mesylate
Prolixin
Prolixin Decanoate
Prolixin Enanthate
promazine HCl
Prozine-50
quetiapine fumarate

Psychotherapeutics, Antipsychotics (cont.)
rauwolfia serpentina
reserpine
Rho-Fluphenazine Decanoate ⓒ
Risperdal
risperidone
Serentil
Seroquel
Sparine
Stelazine
Stemetil ⓒ
thioridazine HCl
thiothixene
thiothixene HCl
Thorazine
Triavil
Triavil 4-50
trifluoperazine HCl
triflupromazine HCl
Trilafon
Vesprin
ziprasidone HCl
ziprasidone mesylate
Zomaril
Zyprexa

Psychotherapeutics, Anxiolytics
[see also: Sedatives and Hypnotics]
acecarbromal
alprazolam
Alti-Clobazam ⓒ
Anxanil
Apo-Diazepam ⓒ
Apo-Lorazepam ⓒ
Apo-Oxazepam ⓒ
Apo-Trifluoperazine ⓒ
Atarax
Atarax 100
Ativan
BuSpar
buspirone HCl
chlordiazepoxide
chlordiazepoxide HCl
chlormezanone
Clindex
clobazam
clorazepate dipotassium
deramciclane
Diazemuls ⓒ
diazepam

Psychotherapeutics, Anxiolytics (cont.)
Dizac
E-Vista
Equagesic
Equanil
Frisium
Gen-Xene
halazepam
hydroxyzine HCl
hydroxyzine pamoate
Hyzine-50
Librax
Libritabs
Librium
Limbitrol DS 10-25
Lin-Buspirone ⓒ
lorazepam
Menrium 5-2; Menrium 5-4; Menrium 10-4
meprobamate
Meprospan
Micrainin
Miltown
Miltown-600
Mitran
Neuramate
Novo-Lorazem ⓒ
Novoxapam ⓒ
oxazepam
Paxarel
PMB 200; PMB 400
prazepam
Quiess
Reposans-10
Riva-Lorazepam ⓒ
Serax
Stelazine
Trancopal
Tranxene
Tranxene-SD
trifluoperazine HCl
Valium
Valium Roche Oral ⓒ
Vistacon
Vistaquel 50
Vistaril
Vistazine 50
Xanax

Psychotherapeutics, Other
  Cephulac
  Cholac
  Enulose
  fluoxetine HCl
  lactulose
  ritanserin
  Sarafem
Radiopaque Contrast Media [*see:*
  Contrast Media, Radiopaque]

Radiopharmaceuticals
  [*see also: Diagnostic Agents*]
  AcuTect
  Bexxar
  Cardiolite
  CEA-Cide
  chromic phosphate P 32
  Cotara
  depreotide
  Fibrimage
  Gd-Tex
  ibritumomab tiuxetan
  ImmuRAID-AFP
  ImmuRAID-hCG
  ImmuRAIT-LL2
  indium In 111 IGIV pentetate
  indium In 111 pentetreotide
  indium In 111 satumomab pendetide
  iodine I 123 murine MAb to alpha-
    fetoprotein (AFP)
  iodine I 123 murine MAb to human
    chorionic gonadotropin (hCG)
  iodine I 131 6B-iodomethyl-19-nor-
    cholesterol
  iodine I 131 Lym-1 MAb
  iodine I 131 murine MAb IgG$_2$a to
    B cell
  iodine I 131 murine MAb to alpha-
    fetoprotein (AFP)
  iodine I 131 murine MAb to human
    chorionic gonadotropin (hCG)
  iodine I 131 radiolabeled B1 MAb
  iodine I 131 tositumomab
  Iodotope
  LeuTech
  LeukoScan
  LymphoScan
  Macroscint

Radiopharmaceuticals (cont.)
  mespiperone C 11
  Metastron
  Miraluma
  motexafin gadolinium
  Myoview
  NeoTect
  Neurolite
  nofetumomab merpentan
  OctreoScan 111
  OncoTrac
  Oncolym
  OncoScint CR/OV
  palladium Pd 103
  Phosphocol P 32
  Quadramet
  samarium Sm 153 lexidronam
  sodium iodide (^{131}I)
  sodium iodide I 123
  sodium iodide I 131
  sodium phosphate P 32
  strontium chloride Sr 89
  technetium (^{99m}Tc) dimercaptosuc-
    cinic acid
  technetium (^{99m}Tc) methylenedi-
    phosphonate
  technetium Tc 99m albumin aggre-
    gated
  technetium Tc 99m antimelanoma
    murine MAb
  technetium Tc 99m apcitide
  technetium Tc 99m arcitumomab
  technetium Tc 99m bectumomab
  technetium Tc 99m biciromab
  technetium Tc 99m bicisate
  technetium Tc 99m disofenin
  technetium Tc 99m furifosmin
  technetium Tc 99m medronate
  technetium Tc 99m mertiatide
  technetium Tc 99m murine MAb to
    human alpha-fetoprotein (AFP)
  technetium Tc 99m murine MAb to
    human chorionic gonadotropin
    (hCG)
  technetium Tc 99m oxidronate
  technetium Tc 99m sestamibi
  technetium Tc 99m siboroxime
  technetium Tc 99m succimer
  technetium Tc 99m sulesomab
  technetium Tc 99m teboroxime

Radiopharmaceuticals (cont.)
technetium Tc 99m tetrofosmin
Theraseed
Verluma
Xcytrin
Zevalin

Respiratory System Agents

[see also: *Allergy and Anaphylaxis
Agents; Antisecretories, Respiratory;
Antituberculosis Agents; Asthma
Agents; Expectorants*]
AccuNeb
acetylcysteine (*N*-acetylcysteine)
acetylcysteine sodium
Advair
AeroBid; AeroBid-M
Aeropin
Airet
Airomir (CAN)
alatrofloxacin mesylate
albuterol
albuterol sulfate
Alec
alpha$_1$-proteinase inhibitor (alpha$_1$ PI)
Alti-Ipratropium (CAN)
Apo-Ipravent (CAN)
Apo-Oflox (CAN)
Apo-Salvent (CAN)
Atrovent
Avelox
Azmacort
beclomethasone dipropionate (BDP)
Beclovent
beractant
budesonide
calfactant
Cipro
ciprofloxacin
colfosceril palmitate
Combivent
Contramid
Curosurf
Delaprem
dextran sulfate
dornase alfa
DuoNeb
Exosurf
Exosurf Neonatal

Respiratory System Agents (cont.)
Flovent
Floxin
flunisolide
fluticasone propionate
Foradil
formoterol fumarate
gatifloxacin
Gen-Ipratropium (CAN)
heparin, 2-0-desulfated
hexoprenaline sulfate
HP-3
Infasurf
INOmax
ipratropium bromide
KL4 surfactant
levalbuterol
levalbuterol HCl
Levaquin
levofloxacin
LiquiVent
lomefloxacin HCl
Maxaquin
Mezlin
mezlocillin sodium
moxifloxacin HCl
Mucomyst
Mucomyst 10
Mucosil-10; Mucosil-20
Neuprex
nitric oxide
Novo-Salmol (CAN)
ofloxacin
orgotein
OxSODrol
palivizumab
perflubron
phosphatidylglycerol
poractant alfa
Prolastin
protirelin
Proventil
Proventil HFA
Pseudostat
Pulmicort
Pulmozyme
salbutamol
salbutamol sulfate
Salbutamol Nebuamp (CAN)
Sclerosol

Indications

Respiratory System Agents (cont.)
 sparfloxacin
 Spiriva
 Surfaxin
 Survanta
 Synagis
 talc, sterile aerosol
 Tequin
 Thymone
 tiotropium
 trovafloxacin mesylate
 Trovan
 Uendex
 Vanceril; Vanceril Double Strength
 Ventolin
 Ventolin ⒸⒶⓃ
 Ventolin HFA
 Volmax
 Xopenex
 Zagam

Rheumatic Disease Agents
 [see also: Analgesics; Antiarthritics;
   Corticosteroids, Systemic]
 AE-941
 amiprilose HCl
 anakinra
 Antril
 Arava
 auranofin
 Aurolate
 aurothioglucose
 azathioprine
 azathioprine sodium
 Azulfidine EN-tabs
 Bispan
 Cuprimine
 Depen
 Enbrel
 etanercept
 Folex PFS
 gold sodium thiomalate
 hydroxychloroquine sulfate
 Imuran
 infliximab
 IPL-423
 Kineret
 leflunomide
 methotrexate (MTX)

Rheumatic Disease Agents (cont.)
 methotrexate sodium
 monoclonal antibody 5G1.1-SC
 orgotein
 OxSODrol
 penicillamine
 Plaquenil Sulfate
 Prosorba Column
 protein A
 Remicade
 Rheumatrex
 Ridaura
 Solganal
 sulfasalazine
 T-cell receptor (TCR) peptide
 Therafectin
 Trexall
Rosacea [see: Dermatological Prepara-
   tions, Rosacea Agents]
Sarcoma [see: Antineoplastics]
Schizophrenia [see: Psychotherapeu-
   tics, Antipsychotics]

Sedatives and Hypnotics
 [see also: Psychotherapeutics, Anxiolyt-
   ics]
**Sedatives and Hypnotics, Barbitur-
ates**
 acetaminophen & butalbital & caf-
   feine
 Alurate
 Amaphen
 amobarbital sodium
 Amytal Sodium
 Anoquan
 Antispasmodic
 Antrocol
 aprobarbital
 Arco-Lase Plus
 aspirin & butalbital & caffeine
 Axocet
 Barbidonna; Barbidonna No. 2
 Bel-Phen-Ergot SR
 Bellacane
 Bellacane SR
 Bellatal
 Bellergal-S
 Bucet
 Bupap

Sedatives and Hypnotics, Barbiturates (cont.)
- butabarbital
- butabarbital sodium
- butalbital
- butalbital & acetaminophen & caffeine
- butalbital & aspirin & caffeine
- Butalbital Compound
- Butex Forte
- Butibel
- Butisol Sodium
- Cafatine-PB
- Chardonna-2
- Dolgic
- Donna-Sed
- Donnatal
- Donnatal No. 2
- Endolor
- Esgic
- Esgic-Plus
- Femcet
- Fioricet
- Fiorinal
- Fiorpap
- Fiortal
- Folergot-DF
- Gustase Plus
- Hyosophen
- Isocet
- Lanorinal
- Levsin PB
- Levsin with Phenobarbital
- Lufyllin-EPG
- Luminal Sodium
- Malatal
- Margesic
- Marten-Tab
- Mebaral
- Medigesic
- mephobarbital
- Mudrane
- Mudrane GG
- Nembutal
- Nembutal Sodium
- pentobarbital
- pentobarbital sodium
- Phenerbel-S
- phenobarbital
- phenobarbital sodium

Sedatives and Hypnotics, Barbiturates (cont.)
- Phrenilin
- Phrenilin Forte
- Pyridium Plus
- Quadrinal
- Repan
- Repan CF
- secobarbital sodium
- Seconal Sodium
- Sedapap
- Solfoton
- Spasmolin
- Susano
- Tencon
- Triad
- Tuinal

Sedatives and Hypnotics, Benzodiazepines
- alprazolam
- Alti-Clobazam (CAN)
- Apo-Diazepam (CAN)
- Apo-Lorazepam (CAN)
- Apo-Oxazepam (CAN)
- Apo-Temazepam (CAN)
- Ativan
- clobazam
- clorazepate dipotassium
- Dalmane
- Diazemuls (CAN)
- diazepam
- Dizac
- Doral
- flurazepam HCl
- Frisium
- Gen-Xene
- halazepam
- Halcion
- lorazepam
- midazolam HCl
- Mogadon
- nitrazepam
- Novo-Lorazem (CAN)
- Novoxapam (CAN)
- oxazepam
- prazepam
- quazepam
- Restoril
- Riva-Lorazepam (CAN)
- Serax

Indications

Sedatives and Hypnotics, Benzodiazepines (cont.)
temazepam
Tranxene
Tranxene-SD
triazolam
Valium
Valium Roche Oral Ⓒ
Versed
Xanax

Sedatives and Hypnotics, Nonprescription Sleep Aids
diphenhydramine HCl
Flextra-DS
Magsal
pyrilamine maleate

Sedatives and Hypnotics, Other
acecarbromal
Alti-Zopiclone Ⓒ
Ambien
Apo-Methoprazine Ⓒ
Aquachloral
chloral hydrate
dexmedetomidine HCl
dichloralphenazone (chloral hydrate & phenazone)
Diprivan
droperidol
Duradrin
Equagesic
esopiclone
estazolam
Estorra
ethchlorvynol
Gamma-OH
Gen-Zopiclone Ⓒ
glutethimide
Imovane Ⓒ
Inapsine
Isocom
Isopap
Largon
Levoprome
meprobamate
methotrimeprazine
methotrimeprazine maleate
Micrainin
Midchlor
Midrin
Migratine

Sedatives and Hypnotics, Other (cont.)
Paral
paraldehyde
Paxarel
Placidyl
Precedex
propiomazine HCl
propofol
ProSom
sodium oxybate
Sonata
Starnoc Ⓒ
valerian (*Valeriana officinalis*)
Xyrem
zaleplon
zolpidem tartrate
zopiclone

Senile Dementia [*see: Alzheimer Disease Agents*]

Sex Hormones [*see: Hormones; Gynecological Agents; Vaginal Preparations*]

Sexual Dysfunction Agents, Male

alprostadil
Alprox-TD
aminobenzoate potassium
Aphrodyne
apomorphine HCl
Caverject
Cialis
Dayto Himbin
Edex
Invicorp
Muse
Plaquase
Potaba
sildenafil citrate
tadalafil
Topiglan
Uprima
vasoactive intestinal polypeptide (VIP)
Vasomax
Viagra
Yocon

Sexual Dysfunction Agents, Male (cont.)
   yohimbe (*Corynanthe johimbe; Pausinystalia johimbe*)
   yohimbine HCl
   Yohimex
Shampoos [see: *Dermatological Preparations, Hair and Scalp Agents*]

Smoking Cessation Aids
   benzocaine
   bupropion HCl
   Habitrol
   lobeline sulfate
   NicErase-SL
   Nicorette DS
   nicotine
   nicotine polacrilex
   Nicotrol
   Nicotrol NS
   ProStep
   Zyban
Steroids [see: *Corticosteroids, Systemic; Dermatological Preparations, Anti-inflammatory Agents; Ophthalmologicals, Anti-inflammatory; Hormones, Anabolic/Androgenic*]
Surfactants, Lung [see: *Respiratory System Agents*]

Thrombolytic Agents
   [see also: *Enzymes, Thrombolytic*]
   Abbokinase
   Abbokinase Open-Cath
   Activase
   Agrylin
   alteplase
   Arixtra
   Eminase
   fondaparinux sodium
   Kabikinase
   lanoteplase
   r-ProUK
   saruplase
   Streptase
   streptokinase (SK)
   tenecteplase

Thrombolytic Agents (cont.)
   Tenecteplase
   TNKase
   urokinase
   xemilofiban HCl
Thrush [see: *Mouth and Throat Preparations*]

Thyroid Agents
   Armour Thyroid
   Cytomel
   Eltroxin
   Levo-T
   Levothroid
   Levothroid ⒸⒶⓃ
   levothyroxine sodium (T_4)
   Levoxyl
   liothyronine sodium (T_3)
   liotrix
   Lugol
   methimazole
   potassium iodide
   S-P-T
   Strong Iodine
   Synthroid
   Tapazole
   Thyrar
   Thyro-Block
   thyroid
   Thyroid Strong
   Thyrolar-0.25; -0.5; -1; -2; -3
   thyrotropin
   Thytropar
   Triacana
   triiodothyroacetic acid (TRIAC)
   Triostat
   Unithroid
Total Parenteral Nutrition (TPN) [see: *Nutritional Agents*]
Tuberculosis [see: *Antituberculosis Agents*]
Ulcerative Colitis [see: *Inflammatory Bowel Disease Agents*]
Ulcers, Decubitus [see: *Diabetes Agents, Related Disorders; Wound Treatment*]
Ulcers, Gastric [see: *Antacids; Antisecretories, Gastrointestinal; Peptic Ulcer and Gastric Reflux Agents*]

Indications

Ultrasound Contrast Media [see:
Contrast Media, Ultrasound]

Urinary Tract Agents
Urinary Tract Agents, Analgesics
Atrosept
Azo-Sulfisoxazole
Baridium
Cystex
Dolsed
Geridium
Phenazo ⒸⒶⓃ
phenazopyridine HCl
phenyl salicylate
Prosed/DS
Pyridiate; Pyridate No. 2
Pyridium
Pyridium Plus
salicylamide
sodium salicylate (SS)
Trac Tabs 2X
UAA
Uridon Modified
Urimar-T
Urimax
Urinary Antiseptic No. 2
Urised
Uristat
Uritin
Urobiotic-250
Urodine
Urogesic
Urogesic Blue

Urinary Tract Agents, Antineoplastics
[see also: Antineoplastics]
BCG vaccine (bacillus Calmette-
   Guérin)
doxorubicin HCl
eflornithine HCl
ImmuCyst ⒸⒶⓃ
OncoTICE ⒸⒶⓃ
Pacis
Photofrin
Platinol-AQ
Regressin
TheraCys
Tice BCG
Valstar

Urinary Tract Agents, Antineoplastics (cont.)
Valtaxin ⒸⒶⓃ

Urinary Tract Agents, Antibacterials
[see also: Antibiotics]
Apo-Norflox ⒸⒶⓃ
Apo-Oflox ⒸⒶⓃ
Atrosept
Azo-Sulfisoxazole
Cinobac
cinoxacin
Cipro
ciprofloxacin
cycloserine (L-cycloserine)
Cystex
Dolsed
enoxacin
Floxin
fosfomycin tromethamine
Furadantin
Furalan
gatifloxacin
Hiprex
Levaquin
levofloxacin
lomefloxacin HCl
Macrobid
Macrodantin
Mandameth
Mandelamine
Maxaquin
Methblue 65
methenamine
methenamine hippurate
methenamine mandelate
methylene blue (MB)
Mezlin
mezlocillin sodium
Monurol
nalidixic acid
NegGram
nitrofurantoin
norfloxacin
Noroxin
Novo-Norfloxacin ⒸⒶⓃ
ofloxacin
Penetrex
piperacillin sodium
Pipracil
Primsol

Urinary Tract Agents, Antibacterials (cont.)
Prosed/DS
Riva-Norfloxacin Ⓒ
Seromycin
sulfamethizole
sulfamethoxazole (SMX; SMZ)
sulfisoxazole
Tequin
Trac Tabs 2X
trimethoprim (TMP)
UAA
Urex
Uridon Modified
Urimar-T
Urimax
Urinary Antiseptic No. 2
Urised
Urisedamine
Uritin
Uro-Phosphate
Urobak
Urobiotic-250
Urogesic Blue
Urolene Blue
Uroqid-Acid No. 2

Urinary Tract Agents, Antispasmodics
[see also: Antispasmodics]
A-Spas S/L
Anaspaz
atropine sulfate
Atrosept
belladonna extract
Cystospaz
Cystospaz-M
Ditropan
Ditropan XL
Dolsed
Donnamar
Ed-Spaz
flavoxate HCl
Gastrosed
hyoscyamine (L-hyoscyamine)
hyoscyamine sulfate
Levbid
Levsin
Levsin PB
Levsin with Phenobarbital
Levsin/SL

Urinary Tract Agents, Antispasmodics (cont.)
Levsinex
NuLev
oxybutynin chloride
PMS-Oxybutynin Ⓒ
Prosed/DS
Pyridium Plus
Sal-Tropine
Symax-SR
Trac Tabs 2X
UAA
Uridon Modified
Urimar-T
Urimax
Urinary Antiseptic No. 2
Urised
Urisedamine
Urispas
Uritin
Urogesic Blue

Urinary Tract Agents, Antiurolithic
Calcibind
cellulose sodium phosphate (CSP)
Cystagon
cysteamine bitartrate
magnesium hydroxycarbonate
Renacidin
Renacidin Irrigation
Thiola
tiopronin

Urinary Tract Agents, Cystitis Agents
Apo-Norflox Ⓒ
Apo-Oflox Ⓒ
Cipro
ciprofloxacin
dimethyl sulfoxide (DMSO)
Elmiron
enoxacin
Floxin
gatifloxacin
Levaquin
levofloxacin
lomefloxacin HCl
Maxaquin
norfloxacin
Noroxin

Indications

Urinary Tract Agents, Cystitis Agents (cont.)
Novo-Norfloxacin (CAN)
ofloxacin
Penetrex
pentosan polysulfate sodium
Rimso-50
Riva-Norfloxacin (CAN)
Tequin

Urinary Tract Agents, Enuresis Agents
Apo-Desmopressin (CAN)
collagen
DDAVP
desmopressin acetate
Detrol
Detrol LA
Hylagel Uro
imipramine HCl
Tofranil
tolterodine tartrate

Urinary Tract Agents, pH Modifiers
ammonium chloride
ascorbic acid (L-ascorbic acid; vitamin C)
Bicitra
citric acid
Citrolith
Cytra-2
Cytra-3
Cytra-K
Cytra-LC
K-Lyte (CAN)
K-Phos M.F.
K-Phos Neutral
K-Phos No. 2
K-Phos Original
M-Caps
methionine (DL-methionine)
Neut
Oracit
Pedameth
PMS-Dicitrate (CAN)
Polycitra
Polycitra-K
Polycitra-LC
potassium acid phosphate
potassium citrate
racemethionine
sodium acid phosphate

Urinary Tract Agents, pH Modifiers (cont.)
sodium bicarbonate
sodium biphosphate
sodium citrate
Uracid
Uracyst-S; Uracyst-S Concentrate (CAN)
Urimar-T
Uro-Phosphate
Urocit-K
Urogesic Blue

Urinary Tract Agents, Urinary Retention Agents
bethanechol chloride
Duvoid
Myotonachol
neostigmine methylsulfate
PMS-Bethanechol Chloride (CAN)
Prostigmin
Urecholine

Urinary Tract Agents, Other
acetohydroxamic acid (AHA)
Durasphere
FemSoft
Lambda
lanthanum carbonate
Lithostat
Miniguard
Resectisol
sorbitol

Vaccines [see: Immunizing Agents]

Vaginal Preparations
Vaginal Preparations, Antibacterial
[see also: Antibiotics, Topical]
Alasulf
aminacrine HCl
AVC
Cleocin
clindamycin phosphate
D.I.T.I.-2
Dalacin (CAN)
Dayto Sulf
Deltavac
Gyne-Sulf
MetroGel Vaginal
metronidazole
Nidagel (CAN)
Savvy

Vaginal Preparations, Antibacterial (cont.)
sulfabenzamide
sulfacetamide
sulfanilamide
sulfathiazole
sulfisoxazole
Sultrin Triple Sulfa
Triple Sulfa
Trysul
V.V.S.
Vagisec Plus

Vaginal Preparations, Antifungal
[see also: Antifungals, Topical]
Amino-Cerv pH 5.5
butoconazole nitrate
clotrimazole (CLT)
Gynazole-1
miconazole nitrate
Monistat Dual-Pak
Mycelex-G
Mycelex Twin Pack
Mycostatin
nystatin
sodium propionate
Terazol 3
Terazol 7
terconazole
tioconazole

Vaginal Preparations, Antiseptic Cleansers
[see also: Antiseptics]
povidone-iodine
Vagisec Douche

Vaginal Preparations, Contraceptives
levonorgestrel
Mirena
nonoxynol 9
octoxynol 9
Progestasert
progesterone
Prostin E2
Savvy

Vaginal Preparations, Other
Cervidil
Crinone
Estrace
Estring
Ogen
Ortho Dienestrol

Vaginal Preparations, Other (cont.)
Premarin
PRO-2000
Vagifem

Varicose Vein Agents
adenosine phosphate
morrhuate sodium
Scleromate
sodium tetradecyl (STD) sulfate
Sotradecol
Verruca [see: Dermatological Preparations, Wart and Corn Removers]

Vitamin Replacement
Vitamin Replacement, Vitamin A
ADC with Fluoride
Aquasol A
beta carotene
Chewable Triple Vitamins with Fluoride
Del-Vi-A
NataChew
Soluvite-f
Tri-Flor-Vite with Fluoride
Tri-Vi-Flor
Tri-Vi-Flor with Iron
Tri Vit with Fluoride
Tri-Vitamin with Fluoride
Tri-A-Vite F
Triple Vitamin ADC with Fluoride
Trivitamin Fluoride
Vi-Daylin/F ADC
Vi-Daylin/F ADC + Iron
vitamin A
vitamin A palmitate

Vitamin Replacement, B Vitamins
[see also: Anemia Agents, B Vitamins]
aminobenzoic acid (4-aminobenzoic acid)
Apatate with Fluoride
B-C with Folic Acid
B-Plex
Berocca
calcium pantothenate (calcium D-pantothenate; vitamin B_5)
Citracal Prenatal

Vitamin Replacement, B Vitamins (cont.)

cyanocobalamin (vitamin B_{12})
folic acid
Foltx
Formula B
hydroxocobalamin
liver, desiccated; liver extracts
MagneBind 400 Rx
Nascobal
NataChew
niacin (vitamin B_3)
niacinamide (vitamin B_3)
Nicolar
nicotinic acid (vitamin B_3)
PremesisRx
pyridoxine HCl (vitamin B_6)
riboflavin (vitamin B_2)
thiamine HCl (vitamin B_1)

Vitamin Replacement, Vitamin C

acerola (*Malpighia glabra; M. punicifolia*)
ADC with Fluoride
Anemagen
ascorbic acid (L-ascorbic acid; vitamin C)
B Complex with C and B-12
B-C with Folic Acid
B-Plex
Berocca
calcium ascorbate (vitamin C)
Cenolate
Cevalin
Cevi-Fer
Chewable Triple Vitamins with Fluoride
Chromagen
Contrin
Ester-C Plus, Extra Potency
Fero-Folic-500
Ferotrinsic
Foltrin
Formula B
Fumatinic
Hemocyte Plus
Iberet-Folic-500
Key-Plex
Livitrinsic-f

Vitamin Replacement, Vitamin C (cont.)

Lypholized Vitamin B Complex & Vitamin C with B_{12}
Nephplex Rx
Nephro-Vite Rx
Nephro-Vite Rx + Fe
Nephrocaps
Nephron FA
Neurodep
Pronemia Hematinic
rose (*Rosa acicularis; R. canina; R. rugosa* and other species)
sodium ascorbate (vitamin C)
Soluvite-f
Strovite
Tri-Flor-Vite with Fluoride
Tri-Vi-Flor
Tri-Vi-Flor with Iron
Tri Vit with Fluoride
Tri-Vitamin with Fluoride
Tri-A-Vite F
TriHemic 600
Trinsicon
Triple Vitamin ADC with Fluoride
Trivitamin Fluoride
Vi-Daylin/F ADC
Vi-Daylin/F ADC + Iron
Vicam

Vitamin Replacement, Vitamin D

ADC with Fluoride
alfacalcidol (1α-hydroxycholecalciferol; 1α-hydroxyvitamin D_3)
calcifediol (25-hydroxycholecalciferol; 25-hydroxyvitamin D_3)
Calciferol
Calcijex
calcitriol (1,25-hydroxycholecalciferol; 1,25-hydroxyvitamin D_3)
Calderol
Chewable Triple Vitamins with Fluoride
cholecalciferol (vitamin D_3)
DHT
dihydrotachysterol (DHT)
doxercalciferol
Drisdol
ergocalciferol (vitamin D_2)
Hectorol
Hytakerol

Vitamin Replacement, Vitamin D (cont.)
NataChew
One-Alpha ⓒᴬᴺ
paricalcitol
Rocaltrol
Soluvite-f
Tri-Flor-Vite with Fluoride
Tri-Vi-Flor
Tri-Vi-Flor with Iron
Tri Vit with Fluoride
Tri-Vitamin with Fluoride
Tri-A-Vite F
Triple Vitamin ADC with Fluoride
Trivitamin Fluoride
Vi-Daylin/F ADC
Vi-Daylin/F ADC + Iron
Zemplar

Vitamin Replacement, Vitamin E
Aquavit-E
TriHemic 600
vitamin E

Vitamin Replacement, Other
aminobenzoate potassium
AquaMEPHYTON
bioflavonoids (vitamin P)
Ester-C Plus, Extra Potency
eucalyptus (*Eucalyptus globulus*)
hesperidin
Konakion
Mephyton
phytonadione (vitamin K_1)
Potaba
rutin

Vitamin Replacement, Multiple (not listed)
Adeflor M
B-C with Folic Acid Plus
Bacmin
Berocca Parenteral Nutrition
Berocca Plus
Berplex Plus
Cefol
Cernevit-12
Cezin-S
Chewable Multivitamins with Fluoride
Eldercaps
Enfamil Natalins Rx
Ferrex PC; Ferrex PC Forte

Vitamin Replacement, Multiple (not listed) (cont.)
Florvite
Florvite + Iron
Florvite + Iron; Half Strength Florvite + Iron
Florvite; Florvite Half Strength
Formula B Plus
Infuvite Pediatric
Lactocal-F
M.V.I. Neonatal
M.V.I. Pediatric
M.V.I.-12
Marnatal-F
Materna
Mission Prenatal Rx
Multi-12; Multi-12 Pediatric ⓒᴬᴺ
Multi Vitamin Concentrate
Multivitamin with Fluoride
Mulvidren-F
Mynatal
Mynatal FC
Mynatal P.N.
Mynatal P.N. Forte
Mynatal Rx
Mynate 90 Plus
NataTab CFe; NataTab FA
NataFort
NatalCare Plus
Natalins
Natalins Rx
Natarex Prenatal
Nestabs CFB; Nestabs FA
Niferex-PN
Niferex-PN Forte
Nu-Iron V
O-Cal f.a.
Par-F
Par-Natal Plus 1 Improved
Poly-Vi-Flor
Poly-Vi-Flor with Iron
Polytabs-F
Polyvitamin Fluoride
Polyvitamin Fluoride with Iron
Polyvitamin with Iron and Fluoride
Polyvitamins with Fluoride and Iron
Pramilet FA
PreCare Conceive
PreCare Prenatal
Prenatal H.P.

Indications

Vitamin Replacement, Multiple (not listed) (cont.)
Prenatal Maternal
Prenatal MR 90
Prenatal Plus Iron
Prenatal Plus with Betacarotene
Prenatal Plus; Prenatal Plus Improved
Prenatal Rx
Prenatal Rx with Betacarotene
Prenatal Z
Prenatal-1 + Iron
Prenate Advance; Prenate 90
Prenate Ultra
Soluvite C.T.
Strong Start
Strovite Advance
Strovite Plus; Strovite Forte
Stuartnatal Plus
Theragran Hematinic
Ultra-Natal
Vi-Daylin/F Multivitamin
Vi-Daylin/F Multivitamin + Iron
Vicon Forte
Vitafōl; Vitafōl-PN
Zenate, Advanced Formula
Zincvit
Zodeac-100
Vitiligo [see: *Dermatological Preparations, Vitiligo Agents*]

Weight Reduction Agents
Weight Reduction Agents, CNS Modifiers
[see also: *Central Nervous System Stimulants*]
Adipex-P
Adipost
benzphetamine HCl
Bontril
Bontril PDM
dexfenfluramine HCl
Didrex
diethylpropion
diethylpropion HCl
Dital
Dyrexan-OD
Fastin
fenfluramine HCl

Weight Reduction Agents, CNS Modifiers (cont.)
Ionamin
Mazanor
mazindol
Melfiat-105
Meridia
Obenix
Obephen
Oby-Cap
phendimetrazine tartrate
phentermine HCl
Phentrol 2; Phentrol 4; Phentrol 5
Pondimin
Prelu-2
Redux
Rexigen Forte
Sanorex
sibutramine HCl
Tenuate
Zantryl
Weight Reduction Agents, Digestion Modifiers
bromocriptine mesylate
Ergoset
orlistat
Xenical
Weight Reduction Agents, Nonprescription Diet Aids
benzocaine
phenylpropanolamine HCl

Wound Treatment
Wound Treatment, Cleansing and Debriding Agents
Accuzyme
ananain
collagenase
comosain
Debrisan
Dermuspray
desoxyribonuclease
dextranomer
Elase
Elase-Chloromycetin
fibrinolysin, human
Granulderm
Granulex
GranuMed

Wound Treatment, Cleansing and Debriding Agents (cont.)
Panafil
Panafil White
papain
Papain Urea Chlorophyllin
Papain Urea Debriding
Santyl
sutilains
trypsin, crystallized
Vianain

Wound Treatment, Medicated Dressings
[see also: Antibiotics, Topical; Hemostatics]
AcryDerm Strands
Adcon-L
Adcon-P
Apligraf
Biobrane
Biobrane-L
cadexomer iodine
carbohydrate polymer gel
DuraGen
Emdogain
Flexderm
Flexzan; Flexzan Extra

Wound Treatment, Medicated Dressings (cont.)
Furacin Soluble Dressing
Hydrocol
Iamin
mafenide
mafenide acetate
nitrofurazone
povidone-iodine
prezatide copper acetate
scarlet red
Scarlet Red Ointment Dressings
Sorbsan
Sulfamylon

Wound Treatment, Vulneraries
[see also: Dermatological Preparations, Emollients and Protectants]
allantoin
chlorophyllin
ersofermin
Ossigel
Panafil
Panafil White
Papain Urea Chlorophyllin
scarlet red
Scarlet Red Ointment Dressings

Indications

XRef Investigational Code Names to Generic Names

A code name is a temporary identification assigned to a product by the manufacturer. The number or letter-number combination is used while the substance is undergoing testing, before a generic name is given. Code names appearing in this list cross-reference to the assigned generic name (3916 entries) or are designated "generic not yet assigned" (201 entries), which indicates that testing is ongoing or has been discontinued within the past five years. Both generic names and code names appearing here without generic names are listed alphabetically in *Saunders Pharmaceutical Word Book*. Additional information may be obtained there.

10275-S epitiostanol
106223 cefamandole nafate
10 80 07 omoconazole nitrate
10-EDAM edatrexate
110264 cefaparole
125 I NM-113 iomethin I 125
1263W94 benzimidavir
1263W94 maribavir
129Y83 colfosceril palmitate
12C velaresol
1314 TH ethionamide
131 I NM-113 iomethin I 131
1380U baquiloprim
141W94 amprenavir
1589 RB pefloxacin
1592U89 abacavir succinate
1592U89 abacavir sulfate
15AU81 generic not yet assigned—
  see main list
16726 symetine HCl
16842 bitoscanate
1709 CERM niaprazine
177 J.D. aminocaproic acid
1875 CERM fepromide
18894 nifungin
194-B zolamine HCl
20025 clorprenaline HCl
205 E calcium dobesilate
21401-Ba tribenoside
21679-CH malethamer
22-708 endralazine mesylate

24281 mitocarcin
249-16 deditonium bromide
2-5410-3A iodixanol
256U87 HCl valacyclovir HCl
26383 thiphencillin potassium
26P aliflurane
27165 temefos
27-400 cyclosporine
28002 epipropidine
29060-LE vinblastine sulfate
2936 proscillaridin
29866 levopropoxyphene napsylate
30038CB minaprine HCl
3-01003 guanoxan sulfate
3-01029 guanoclor sulfate
30109 noracymethadol HCl
30639 polyethadene
311C90 zolmitriptan
3123L puromycin
31518 pyrroliphene HCl
31595C mitosper
31814 heteronium bromide
32-046 edetate dipotassium
32379 dromostanolone propionate
32645 vinleurosine sulfate
33006 acetohexamide
33355 mestranol
33379 flurandrenolide
33876 anthelmycin
34977 capreomycin sulfate
349 C59 moxipraquine

35483 cyclothiazide
36781 vinrosidine sulfate
36-801 etifoxine
37 162 R.P. suproclone
37231 vincristine sulfate
38000 clometherone
38253 cephalothin sodium
38389 levopropylcillin potassium
38489 nortriptyline HCl
38851 bolmantalate
39435 cephaloglycin
3 MS hydroxytoluic acid
3TC lamivudine
40 045 articaine
40045 trimetazidine
40602 cephaloridine
4091 C.B. benfurodil hemisuccinate
41071 cefalonium
41-123 clazolam
41 982 RP pefloxacin mesylate
42-348 lifibrate
42406 metoquizine
42-548 mazindol
4306 CB clorazepate dipotassium
4311 CB clorazepate monopotassium
43-663 guanoxabenz
43-715 proquazone
43853 clobenoside
44089 valproic acid
44106 toquizine
44328 dexproxibutene
46083 cefazolin sodium
46236 dobutamine HCl
46-790 fluproquazone
46 R.P. benzylsulfamide
47-210 (as sodium) tetriprofen
47599 pyrazofurin
47657 apramycin
47663 tobramycin
48-674 furacrinic acid
49040 vinglycinate sulfate
4909 RP chlorproethazine HCl
49825 nylestriol
4A65 imidocarb HCl
4-C-32 ticlopidine HCl
5048 dimethisterone
5052 acetylcysteine
5054 prodilidine HCl
5058 oxybutynin chloride
506U nelarabine

5071 megestrol acetate
5107 chloral betaine
516 MD cinnarizine
5190 amidephrine mesylate
51W89 cisatracurium besylate
520C9x22 generic not yet assigned—
see main list
52230 pyrrolnitrin
524W91 emtricitabine
53183 aranotin
53-32C ticlopidine HCl
5373 melengestrol acetate
53858 fenoprofen
566C atovaquone
566C80 atovaquone
57C65 cloguanamil
589C tucaresol
59156 enpromate
5A8 generic not yet assigned—see
main list
5G1.1-SC generic not yet assigned—
see main list
5IUDR idoxuridine
60284 cyclophenazine HCl
611 C 65 thenium closylate
640/1 cefuracetime
640/359 cefuroxime
64716 cinoxacin
65-318 bidimazium iodide
66-269 pretamazium iodide
66873 cephalexin
673-082 nexeridine HCl
67314 monensin
68618 mycophenolic acid
69323 fenoprofen calcium
711 SE pipratecol
7162 RP trimipramine
7432-S ceftibuten
776C85 eniluracil
786-723 anilopam HCl
79907 lergotrile
79 T61 lucanthone HCl
7-OMEN menogaril
80066 bufilcon A
8088 C.B. benfotiamine
8102 CB bamifylline HCl
83636 lergotrile mesylate
8599 R.P. mesylate fonazine mesylate
882C generic not yet assigned—see
main list

88BV59 votumumab
935U83 raluridine
[99mTc]-P246 technetium Tc 99m apcitide
A-118 sultroponium
A-12253A nebramycin
A-147627.1 atrasentan HCl
A-157378.0 lopinivir
A-16612 teroxalene HCl
A-16686 ramoplanin
A-174606.0 valomaciclovir stearate
A-17624 ditolamide
A-182091.0 omaciclovir
A-185980.1 fiduxosin HCl
A-19120 paragyline HCl
A-19757 encyprate
A-1981-12 prodilidine HCl
A-20968 piposulfan
A-2205 profadol HCl
A-2371 plicamycin
A-2655 dioxamate
A-27053 chromonar HCl
A-272 rutamycin
A-3217 ocfentanil HCl
A-32686 proscillaridin
A-3331 brifentanil HCl
A-33547 remoxipride
A-33547.HCl·H₂O remoxipride HCl
A-3508.HCl mirfentanil HCl
A-35957 altrenogest
A-3665.HCl trefentanil HCl
A-4020 Linz midodrine HCl
A 40664 (as tartrate) raclopride
A-41-304 desoximetasone
A-4166 nateglinide
A-4180 isometamidium chloride
A-4492 pentamorphone
A 46 745 gestrinone
A-4696 actaplanin
A-4828 trofosfamide
A-53986 fostedil
A-5610 azelastine HCl
A 5MP adenosine phosphate
A-60386X beractant
A-61589 docebenone
A-65006 lansoprazole
A-71100 voglibose
A-7283 guanoctine HCl
A-73001 seratrodast
A-75200 mesylate napitane mesylate

A-77000 pazinaclone
A-8103 pipobroman
A-81229 alemcinal
A-82 nitroxoline
A-85761.0 atreleuton
A-8999 aspartocin
A-93431.1 adrogolide HCl
AA-2414 seratrodast
AA-673 amlexanox
AA-861 docebenone
AAFC flurocitabine
AB08 doxycycline fosfatex
AB-100 uredepa
AB-103 benzodepa
AB-132 meturedepa
AB-A 663 cimaterol
Abbott-147627 atrasentan HCl
Abbott-16900 teflurane
Abbott-19957 lorbamate
Abbott-22370 trimetozine
Abbott-24091 berythromycin
Abbott-34842 butamben picrate
Abbott-35616 clorazepate dipotassium
Abbott-36581 butamirate citrate
Abbott-38579 protirelin
Abbott-38642 fosfonet sodium
Abbott-39083 clorazepate monopotassium
Abbott-40728 cetocycline HCl
Abbott-41070 gonadorelin acetate
Abbott-43326 carteolol HCl
Abbott-43818 leuprolide acetate
Abbott 44090 valproate sodium
Abbott-44747 astromicin sulfate
Abbott-45975 terazosin HCl
Abbott-46811 cefsulodin sodium
Abbott-47631 estazolam
Abbott-48999 cefotiam HCl
Abbott-50192 (HCl) cefmenoxime HCl
Abbott-50711 divalproex sodium
Abbott-56268 clarithromycin
Abbott-56619 difloxacin HCl
Abbott-56620 sarafloxacin HCl
Abbott-57135 sarafloxacin HCl
Abbott-61827 tosufloxacin
Abbott-62254 temafloxacin HCl
Abbott-64077 zileuton
Abbott-64662 enalkiren
Abbott 70569.1 tiagabine HCl

Abbott 70569 HCl tiagabine HCl
Abbott-72517 zankiren HCl
Abbott-73001 seratrodast
Abbott-76120 urokinase alfa
Abbott-76745 fenleuton
Abbott-81229.0 alemcinal
Abbott-84538 ritonavir
Abbott-85761 atreleuton
ABC 12/3 doxofylline
ABOB moroxydine
ABS-205 generic not yet assigned—
  see main list
ABT-001 seratrodast
ABT-091 omaciclovir
ABT-120 urokinase alfa
ABT-229 alemcinal
ABT-378 lopinavir
ABT-431 adrogolide HCl
ABT-538 ritonavir
ABT-569 tiagabine HCl
ABT-606 valomaciclovir stearate
ABT-627 atrasentan HCl
ABT-719 generic not yet assigned—
  see main list
ABT-761 atreleuton
ABT-980 fiduxosin HCl
ABX-CBL generic not yet assigned—
  see main list
ABX-IL8 generic not yet assigned—
  see main list
AC001 amlintide
AC0137 pramlintide acetate
AC 1198 dimethadione
AC 1370 cefpimizole
AC 263,780 cimaterol
AC-2993 generic not yet assigned—
  see main list
AC 3810 bamifylline HCl
AC4464 torsemide
AC-528 dioxation
AC-601 buramate
ACC-9089 flestolol sulfate
ACC-9653-010 fosphenytoin sodium
ACEA 1021 licostinel
AD 106 cicrotoic acid
AD-32 valrubicin
AD-439 generic not yet assigned—see
  main list
AD-519 generic not yet assigned—see
  main list

AD-810 zonisamide
ADD-3878 ciglitazone
ADR-033 tripamide
ADR-529 dexrazoxane
AE-705W neutramycin
AE-9 feclobuzone
AE-941 generic not yet assigned—see
  main list
AF-0150 perflexane
AF102B cevimeline HCl
AF-1161 trazodone HCl
AF 1934 (lysine) bendazac
AF-2139 dapiprazole HCl
AF 2838 bindarit
AF-438 (as citrate) oxolamine
AF-634 proxazole citrate
AF-864 benzydamine HCl
AG-1343 nelfinavir mesylate
AG-1549 generic not yet assigned—
  see main list
AG-1749 lansoprazole
AG-3 chromonar HCl
AG331 metesind glucuronate
AG-3340 prinomastat
AG 58107 ioxitalamic acid
AG-EE 623 ZW repaglinide
Agent M-01 sucrosofate potassium
AGN 190168 tazarotene
AGN 190342-LF brimonidine tartrate
AGN 191024 generic not yet
  assigned—see main list
AGN 192013 alitretinoin
AGN 20 metamfazone
AGN 511 (as HCl) prazitone
AGN 616 fantridone HCl
AGR-1240 minaprine
AH 19065 ranitidine HCl
AH 22216 lamtidine
AH 23844 lavoltidine succinate
AH 23844A lavoltidine succinate
AH 25352X sufotidine
AH 3923 salmefamol
AH 5158A labetalol HCl
AH 8165D fazadinium bromide
AHR-10282B bromfenac sodium
AHR-10718 suricainide maleate
AHR-1118 pridefine HCl
AHR-11190-B zacopride HCl
AHR-11325-D rocastine HCl
AHR-11748 dezinamide

AHR-1680 fenpipalone
AHR-224 pyroxamine maleate
AHR-2277 (as HCl) lenperone
AHR-2438B polignate sodium
AHR-3000 butaperazine
AHR-3002 fenfluramine HCl
AHR-3015 cintazone
AHR-3018 apazone
AHR-3053 carbocysteine
AHR-3070-C metoclopramide HCl
AHR-438 metaxalone
AHR-4698 isosorbide mononitrat
AHR-504 glycopyrrolate
AHR-5531C dazopride fumarate
AHR-5850D amfenac sodium
AHR-6134 cloroperone HCl
AHR-619 doxapram HCl
AHR 6646 duoperone fumarate
AHR-8559 fluzinamide
AHR-857 sulfameter
AHR-9377 tampramine fumarate
AHR-9434 nepafenac
AI-27,303 cetamolol HCl
AICA orazamide
AIT-082 leteprinim potassium
A IX demecycline
AJ-2615 monatepil maleate
AL02145 apraclonidine HCl
AL02725 pyrithione sodium
Al-0361 hydroxyphenamate
AL 0559 fenamole
AL-1021 carperone
AL1577A levobetaxolol HCl
AL 20 (as HCl) clemizole
AL-3432A emedastine difumarate
AL-3789 anecortave acetate
AL-4862 brinzolamide
AL-6221 travoprost
AL-6515 nepafenac
AL-721 generic not yet assigned—see main list
AL 842 deterenol HCl
ALCA alcloxa
ALDA aldioxa
Allergan 211 idoxuridine
ALO 1401-02 betaxolol HCl
ALO 2184 resocortol butyrate
ALO4943A olopatadine HCl
ALRT 1057 alitretinoin
AL-T150 oxyfilcon A

AL-T30 vinafocon A
ALT-711 generic not yet assigned—see main list
ALVAC-120TMG generic not yet assigned—see main list
ALVAC-HIV 1 generic not yet assigned—see main list
ALX-0600 generic not yet assigned—see main list
ALX1-11 parathyroid hormone (1-84), recombinamt human
AM-1155 gatifloxacin
AM-684-Beta relomycin
AMA 1080(2Na) carumonam sodium
AMD-3100 generic not yet assigned—see main list
AMI-121 ferumoxsil
AMI-25 ferumoxides
AMI-7228 generic not yet assigned—see main list
AMR-69 pirfenidone
AN021 tizanidine HCl
AN-051 dezinamide
AN 1317 perimetazine
AN 1324 glybuzole
anesthetic compound no. 347 enflurane
ANP 246 clofexamide
ANP 3260 clofezone
antibiotic 241a biniramycin
antibiotic 273a$_1$ paldimycin
antibiotic A-5283 natamycin
antifoam A simethicone
antifoam AF simethicone
AO-128 voglibose
AO-407 hydrofilcon A
AOD-9604 generic not yet assigned—see main list
AOMA surfomer
AO-PLUTO mesifilcon A
AP-1903 generic not yet assigned—see main list
AP 67 chlorthenoxazine
APC-2059 generic not yet assigned—see main list
APC-366 generic not yet assigned—see main list
API-GP3 motexafin gadolinum
APL 400-020 generic not yet assigned—see main list

APM aspartame
APSAC anistreplase
AQ-110 tretoquinol
AR 12008 trapidil
AR-121 nystatin liposomal
AR-177 generic not yet assigned—see main list
ARC I-K-1 methopholine
ARDF 26 gliquidone
AS-013 generic not yet assigned—see main list
AS 101 arsanilic acid
AS-17665 nifurthiazole
ASA 158/5 (as phosphate) benproperine
ASL-279 dopamine HCl
ASL-601 acecainide HCl
ASL-603 bretylium tosylate
ASL-607 pentastarch
ASL-8052 esmolol HCl
Asta 3746 ciclonium bromide
Astra 1512 prilocaine HCl
Astra 1572 iron sorbitex
AT-101 isosorbide
AT-125 acivicin
AT-2266 enoxacin
AT 327 tipepidine
AT-4140 sparfloxacin
ATI 01 sinapultide
ATM-027 generic not yet assigned—see main list
AW 10 sitogluside
AW 105-843 naftifine HCl
AW 14′2333 perlapine
AW-14′2446 clodazon HCl
AY-11,440 clogestone acetate
AY-11,483 estrofurate
AY-15,613 citenamide
AY-20,385 nequinate
AY-20,694 dexpropranolol HCl
AY-21,011 practolol
AY-21,367 furobufen
AY-21,554 talopram HCl
AY-22,124 intriptyline HCl
AY-22,214 taclamine HCl
AY-22,241 actodigin
AY-22,284A alrestatin sodium
AY-22,469 deprostil
AY-22989 sirolimus
AY-23,028 butaclamol HCl

AY-23,289 prodolic acid
AY-23,713 pirandamine HCl
AY-23,946 tandamine HCl
AY-24,031 gonadorelin HCl
AY-24,169 dexclamol HCl
AY-24,236 etodolac
AY-24,269 proroxan HCl
AY-24,559 doxaprost
AY-24,856 pareptide sulfate
AY-25,329 azaclorzine HCl
AY-25,712 acifran
AY-27,110 ciladopa HCl
AY-27,255 vinpocetine
AY-27,773 tolrestat
AY-28,228 atiprosin maleate
AY-28,768 pelrinone HCl
AY-30,715 pemedolac
AY4166 nateglinide
AY-5312 chlorhexidine HCl
AY-5710 magaldrate
AY-6108 ampicillin
AY-61122 methallibure
AY-61123 clofibrate
AY-62014 butriptyline HCl
AY-62021 clopenthixol
AY-62022 medrogestone
AY 6204 (as HCl) pronetalol
AY-64043 propranolol HCl
AY-6608 pentagastrin
AY-8682 cyheptamide
AZQ diaziquone
AZT-P-ddI zidovudine + didanosine
B 10610 iodoxamic acid
B 11420 iopronic acid
B 1312 (as HCl) bupranolol
B 1464 guanacline sulfate
B1 61.012 sargramostim
B19036/7 gagobenate dimeglumine
B1Q 16 hedaquinium chloride
B2036-PEG pegvisomant
B-2311 morinamide
B28-Asp-Insulin insulin aspart
B-35251 mitocromin
B-360 paroxypropione
B-4130 iodamide
B-436 prenylamine
B992 stannsoporfin
Ba 13155 (as tartrate) meladrazine
Ba-20684 etonitazene
Ba-29038 boldenone undecylenate

Ba-29837 deferoxamine HCl
Ba-30803 benzoctamine HCl
BA 32644 niridazole
Ba-32968 delfantrine
Ba-33112 deferoxamine mesylate
Ba-34,276 (as HCl) maprotiline
Ba-34,647 baclofen
BA 36278A cephacetrile sodium
Ba-39,089 oxprenolol HCl
Ba-40088 proxibutene
Ba 41166/E rifampin
BA 4164-8 diflumidone sodium
Ba-41795 codactide
BA 4197 flucrylate
BA 4223 triflumidate
BA 7602-06 talniflumate
BA 7604-02 talosalate
BA 7605-06 talmetacin
BAQD 10 dequalinium chloride
BASF 43915 pelretin
BASF 47011 doretinel
BASF 52404 linarotene
BAX 1400Z dimethadione
BAX 1515 sutilains
BAX 1526 chymopapain
BAX 2739Z bamifylline HCl
BAX 422Z albutoin
BAY 12-8039 moxifloxacin HCl
BAY 1500 mefruside
BAY 1521 noxiptiline
BAY 2353 niclosamide
BAY 4059 Va brotianide
BAY 4503 propiram fumarate
BAY 5097 clotrimazole
BAY 9002 naftalofos
Bay a 1040 nifedipine
BAY B 4231 glisoxepide
Bay d 1107 etofenamate
BAY d 8815 (HCl) amidantel
Bay e 5009 nitrendipine
BAY e 9736 nimodipine
Bayer 1362 butaperazine
Bayer 1420 propanidid
Bayer 205 suramin sodium
Bayer 21199 coumaphos
Bayer 2502 nifurtimox
Bayer 3231 triaziquone
Bayer 5360 metronidazole
Bayer 9015 niclofolan
Bayer 9037 quintiofos

Bayer 9053 phoxim
Bayer A 128 aprotinin
Bayer L 1359 metrifonate
BAY g 2821 muzolimine
Bay g 5421 acarbose
Bay g 6575 nafazatrom
BAY h 2049 daniquidone
Bay h 4502 bifonazole
Bay h 5757 febantel
BAY i 3930 isomalt
BAY i 7433 copovithane
Bay k 5552 nisoldipine
BAY m 1099 miglitol
BAYNAC fenfluthrin
BAY o 1248 emiglitate
Bay o 9867 monohydrate ciprofloxacin HCl
Bay q 3939 ciprofloxacin
Bay q 4218 butaprost
BAY q 7821 ipsapirone HCl
BAY V1 4718 etisomicin
BAY V1 6045 flumethrin
BAY Va 1470 xylazine HCl
Bay VA 9387 etisazole
BAY Va 9391 olaquindox
Bay Vi 9142 toltrazuril
BAY Vk 4999 fuzlocillin
Bay Vl 1704 cyfluthrin
Bay Vn 6528 fenfluthrin
Bay Vp 2674 enrofloxacin
BAY w 6228 cerivastatin sodium
BAY w 6240 factor VIII (rDNA)
BAY X 1352 nerelimomab
BAY y 7432 ecadotril
BB-10010 nagrestipen
BB-2516 marimastat
BB-2893 generic not yet assigned—see main list
BB-882 lexipafant
BB-94 batimastat
BB-K8 amikacin sulfate
BBM-2478A elsamitrucin
BC-105 pizotyline
BCH 10652 generic not yet assigned—see main list
BCH-4556 troxacitabine
BCM mannomustine
BCX-1470 generic not yet assigned—see main list

BCX 2600 stiripentol
BCX-34 peldesine
BD 40A formoterol fumarate
BDF5896 moxonidine
BDH 1298 megestrol acetate
BDH 1921 melengestrol acetate
Be-100 ibuprofen piconol
Be-1293 xipamide
BE 419 ioglycamic acid
BE5895 moxonidine
BEC-2 mitumomab
BG 8301 teceleukin
BG8967 bivalirudin
BG9273 alefacept
BG9712 alefacept
BGM-24 generic not yet assigned—
   see main list
BIBR 277 SE telmisartan
BIBV 308 SE terbogrel
BIIP 20 XX apaxifylline
BI-L-239 enofelast
BILA 2011 BS palinavir
BIM-23014C lanreotide acetate
BIMT 17 flibanserin
BIMT 17 BS flibanserin
BIRG 0587 nevirapine
BIRM-270 ontazolast
BI-RR-0001 enlimomab
BIRR004 tremacamra
BL 191 pentoxifylline
BL-3912A dimoxamine HCl
BL-4162a anagrelide HCl
BL-5111 tiodazosin
BL-5572M proxorphan tartrate
BL-5641A etintidine HCl
BL-P 1322 cephapirin sodium
BL-P 1462 suncillin sodium
BL-P 1761 sarpicillin
BL-P 1780 sarmoxicillin
BLP-25 generic not yet assigned—see
   main list
BL-P 804 hetacillin
BL-R 743 intrazole
BL-S578 cefadroxil
BL-S640 cefatrizine
BL-S786 ceforanide
BM01.004 metipranolol
BM02.015 torsemide
BM 06.019 epoetin beta
BM 06.022 reteplase

BM 13.177 sulotroban
BM 13.505 daltroban
BM 14.190 carvedilol
BM 15.075 bezafibrate
BM 21.0955·Na·H$_2$O ibandronate
   sodium
BM 22.145 isosorbide mononitrate
BM 41.332 ciamexon
BM 41.440 ilmofosine
BM 51052 carazolol
BMS 180048 avitriptan fumarate
BMS 180048-02 avitriptan fumarate
BMS-180194 lobucavir
BMS-180291 ifetroban
BMS-180291-02 ifetroban sodium
BMS 180549 ferumoxtran-10
BMS-181158 mequinol
BMS-181173 gusperimus trihy-
   drochloride
BMS-181339-01 paclitaxel
BMS-182751 satraplatin
BMS-186091 ammonium lactate
BMS-186295 irbesartan
BMS-186716 omapatrilat
BMS-186716-01 omapatrilat
BMS-189921 gemopatrilat
BMS-200475-01 entecavir
BMS 200980 lanoteplase
BMS-204756-07 brasofensine maleate
BMS-205603-01 uracil
BMS-206584-01 gatifloxacin
BMS-217380-01 tesmilifene HCl
BMS 232632 generic not yet
   assigned—see main list
BMS-234475 generic not yet
   assigned—see main list
BMY-05763-1-D dexsotalol HCl
BMY 13754 nefazodone HCl
BMY 13805-1 gepirone HCl
BMY 13859-1 tiospirone HCl
BMY-21891 belfosdil
BMY-25182 cefbuperazone
BMY-25801-01 batanopride HCl
BMY-26517 pemirolast potassium
BMY-27857 stavudine
BMY-28090 elsamitrucin
BMY-28100-03-800 cefprozil
BMY-28142 cefepime
BMY-28142 2HCl·H$_2$O cefepime HCl
BMY-30056 halobetasol propionate

BMY-30120 chlorhexidine phosphanilate
BMY-33419 tesmilifene HCl
BMY-40327 modecainide
BMY 40481 etoposide phosphate
BMY-40900 didanosine
BMY-41606 vapreotide
BMY-42215-1 gusperimus trihydrochloride
BMY-45594 satraplatin
BN-1270 cicletanine
BOF-A2 emitefur
BP 1.02; S.049 ecadotril
BP-1184 guanoctine HCl
BP 400 pimethixene
BRL-1241 methicillin sodium
BRL 12594 ticarcillin cresyl sodium
BRL-1288 benapryzine HCl
BRL-1341 ampicillin
BRL 13856 clopirac
BRL 14151 clavulanic acid
BRL 14151K clavulanate potassium
BRL 14777 nabumetone
BRL-1621 cloxacillin sodium
BRL-1702 dicloxacillin
BRL 17421 (as sodium) temocillin
BRL-2039 floxacillin
BRL-2064 carbenicillin disodium
BRL 2288 ticarcillin disodium
BRL 2333 amoxicillin
BRL 2333AB-B amoxicillin sodium
BRL 2534 azidocillin
BRL 26921 anistreplase
BRL-284 levopropylcillin potassium
BRL 29060 paroxetine
BRL 30892 denbufylline
BRL-3475 carbenicillin phenyl sodium
BRL 34915 cromakalim
BRL-38227 levcromakalim
BRL 38705 epsiprantel
BRL-39123 penciclovir
BRL-39123-D penciclovir sodium
BRL 40015 diproteverine
BRL-42810 famciclovir
BRL 43694 granisetron
BRL 43694A granisetron HCl
BRL 4664 nonabine
BRL 4910A mupirocin
BRL 4910F mupirocin calcium
BRL-49653-C rosiglitazone maleate

BRL 61063 cipamfylline
BRL-804 hetacillin
BRL 8988 HCl talampicillin HCl
BS 100-141 guanfacine HCl
B.S. 6534 bufenadrine
BS 6748 xyloxemine
BS 6987 deptropine citrate
BS 7161D (as HCl) pytamine
B.S. 7173-D xylocoumarol
BS 749 metacetamol
B.S. 7561 (as HCl) tixadil
B.S. 7573-a acridorex
BS 7723 (as maleate) tropirine
BS 7977 D (as dihydrochloride) xipranolol
BSH borocaptate sodium B 10
BSSG sitogluside
BT 621 (as HCl) todralazine
BTI-322 generic not yet assigned—see main list
BTPABΛ, PFT bentiromide
BTS 13622 hexaprofen
BTS 17345 fluprofen
BTS 18,322 flurbiprofen
BTS 24332 esflurbiprofen
BTS 49 465 flosequinan
BTS 54524 sibutramine HCl
BTS 7706 debropol
BU-2231A talisomycin
BW 12C generic not yet assigned—see main list
BW 207U xenalipin
BW 234U dihydrochloride rimcazole HCl
BW 248U sodium acyclovir sodium
BW256U valacyclovir
BW 301U isethionate piritrexim isethionate
BW 325U trifenagrel
BW 33A atracurium besylate
BW 33-T-57 methisazone
BW 356-C-61 gloxazone
BW 430C lamotrigine
BW-467-C-60 bethanidine sulfate
BW 49-210 diaveridine
BW-524W91 emtricitabine
BW 532U cinflumide
BW 56-158 allopurinol
BW 56-72 trimethoprim
BW-57-322 azathioprine

BW 57-323 thiamiprine
BW 58-271 rolodine
BW-61-32 stilbazium iodide
BW 63-90 butacetin
BW 647U HCl bipenamol HCl
BW 64-9 butoxamine HCl
BW 72U trimethoprim sulfate
BW 759U ganciclovir
BW 825C acrivastine
BW A256C palatrigine
BW A509U zidovudine
BW A515U desciclovir
BW A770U mesylate crisnatol mesylate
BW A938U dichloride doxacurium chloride
BW B109OU mivacurium chloride
Bx 311 cinoxolone
BX 341 bifluranol
BX 363A (as disodium salt) cicloxolone
BX 591 acefluranol
BX 650A ipsalazide
BX 661A balsalazide; balsalazide disodium
BY 1023 pantoprazole
BZ 55 carbutamide
C-1 edrecolomab
C-11925 phanquone
C-12669 demecolcine
C-1428 cyclarbamate
C 1656 clometacin
C-225 cetuximab
C-238 pridinol
C242-DM1 generic not yet assigned—see main list
C-3 capobenate sodium
C-3 capobenic acid
C-4 imciromab pentetate
C-434 trimedoxime bromide
C-49802B-Ba oxaprotiline HCl
c7E3 abciximab
Ca 1022 carbutamide
CA-7 brinolase
CAB-2001 trafermin
CAM-807 bialamicol HCl
CARN 750 acemannan
CAS 276 molsidomine
CAS 936 pirsidomine
CB 1048 chlornaphazine

CB 10615 nifurmazole
CB 11380 nifurizone
CB 11 (as HCl) phenadoxone
CB 12592 subendazole
CB-154 bromocriptine
CB-154 mesylate bromocriptine mesylate
CB 1664 aceprometazine
CB 1678 propiomazine
CB 2201 amfepentorex
CB-30038 minaprine
CB 302 ferric fructose
CB 3025 melphalan
CB 304 azaribine
CB 309 fenabutene
CB-311 somatropin
CB 313 mitotane
CB-337 meglutol
CB 3697 racefemine
CB 4260 nortetrazepam
CB 4261 tetrazepam
CB 4857 menitrazepam
CB 4985 acequinoline
CB 7432 idoxifene
CB 804 bucloxic acid
CBP-1011 generic not yet assigned—see main list
CCA lobenzarit sodium
CCD 1042 ganaxolone
C.C.I. 12923 minaxolone
CCI 15641 cefuroxime axetil
CCI 18773 cloticasone propionate
CCI 18781 fluticasone propionate
CCI 23628 cefuroxime pivoxetil
CCI 4725 clobetasol propionate
CCI 5537 clobetasone butyrate
CCRG-81045 temozolomide
CD 271 adapalene
CDDD 1815 alprenoxime HCl
CDDD 2803 adaprolol maleate
CDDD 3602 tematropium methylsulfate
CDDD 5604 loteprednol etabonate
CDP-571 generic not yet assigned—see main list
CEN 000029 priliximab
CEP-151 mecasermin
CEP 1538 modafinil
CEPH (as HCl) todralazine
CERM 1978 bepridil HCl

CERM 730 amoproxan
CG 201 bevonium metilsulfate
CG-315E tramadol HCl
GCA 18809 azamethiphos
CGA-23654 nitroscanate
CGA 72662 cyromazine
CGP-14221/E cefotiam HCl
CGP 14,458 halobetasol propionate
CGP 21690E oxiracetam
CGP 2175C metoprolol fumarate
CGP-2175E metoprolol tartrate
CGP 23339AE pamidronate disodium
CGP 25827A formoterol fumarate
CGP 30694 edatrexate
CGP 32349 formestane
CGP 39393 desirudin
CGP 42446 zoledronic acid
CGP 42446A zoledronate disodium
CGP 42446B zoledronate trisodium
CGP 45840B diclofenac potassium
CGP 48933 valsartan
CGP-61755 generic not yet assigned—see main list
CGP-64128A generic not yet assigned—see main list
CGP-69846A generic not yet assigned—see main list
CGP-7174/E cefsulodin sodium
CGP 7760B prenalterol HCl
CGP 9000 cefroxadine
CGS 10078B bendacalol mesylate
CGS 10746B pentiapine maleate
CGS 10787D prinomide tromethamine
CGS 13080 pirmagrel
CGS 13429A batelapine maleate
CGS 13945 pentopril
CGS 14824A HCl benazepril HCl
CGS 14831 benazeprilat
CGS 15040A serazapine HCl
CGS 16617 libenzapril
CGS 16949A fadrozole HCl
CGS 18416A zoniclezole HCl
CGS 19755 selfotel
CGS 20267 letrozole
CGS 25019C moxilubant maleate
CGS 26214 axitirome
CGS 5391B (anhydrous) enolicam sodium
CGS 7135A azaloxan fumarate
CGS 7525A aptazapine maleate

CH 3565 triclosan
CHX-100 masoprocol
CHX-3673 amlexanox
CI-100 acetosulfone sodium
CI-1003 suramin hexasodium
CI-1004 darbufelone mesylate
CI-1006 diethylnorspermine
CI-1008 pregabalin
CI-1011 avasimibe
CI-1012 generic not yet assigned—see main list
CI-1014 zenarestat
CI-1019 igmesine HCl
CI-1020 generic not yet assigned—see main list
CI-107 argipressin tannate
CI-301 bialamicol HCl
CI-336 carbocloral
CI-366 ethosuximide
CI-379 benzilonium bromide
CI-395 phencyclidine HCl
CI 403A pararosaniline pamoate
CI-406 oxymetholone
CI-416 triclofenol piperazine
CI-419 fenimide
CI 427 prodilidine HCl
CI-433 clamoxyquin HCl
CI 440 flufenamic acid
CI-456 diapamide
CI-473 mefenamic acid
CI-501 cycloguanil pamoate
CI-515 guanoxyfen sulfate
CI-546 alipamide
CI 556 acedapsone
CI-572 profadol HCl
CI-581 ketamine HCl
CI-583 meclofenamic acid
CI-633 clioxanide
CI-634 tiletamine HCl
CI-636 sulfacytine
CI-642 butirosin sulfate
CI 673 vidarabine
CI-686 HCl trebenzomine HCl
CI-705 methaqualone
CI-716 zolazepam HCl
CI-718 bentazepam
CI-719 gemfibrozil
CI-720 gemcadiol
CI-781 zometapine
CI 787 tioperidone HCl

CI-825 pentostatin
CI-874 indeloxazine HCl
CI-879 pramiracetam HCl
CI-879 **(sulfate)** pramiracetam sulfate
CI-880 amsacrine
CI-881 ametantrone acetate
CI-882 sparfosate sodium
CI-888 procaterol HCl
CI-897 tebuquine
CI-898 trimetrexate
CI-904 diaziquone
CI-906 quinapril HCl
CI-907 indolapril HCl
CI-908 dezaguanine
CI-908 **mesylate** dezaguanine mesylate
CI-909 tiazofurin
CI-911 rolziracetam
CI-912 zonisamide
CI-914 imazodan HCl
CI-9148 cysteamine HCl
CI-919 enoxacin
CI-920 fostriecin sodium
CI 925 moexipril HCl
CI-928 quinaprilat
CI-942 piroxantrone HCl
CI-945 gabapentin
CI-946 ralitoline
CI-958 ledoxantrone trihydrochloride
CI-960 **HCl** clinafloxacin HCl
CI-970 tacrine HCl
CI-977 enadoline HCl
CI-978 sparfloxacin
CI-979 milameline HCl
CI-980 mivobulin isethionate
CI-981 atorvastatin calcium
CI-982 fosphenytion sodium
CI-983 cefdinir
CI-991 troglitazone
CIBA 1906 thiambutosine
CJ-11,974 ezlopitant
CJ 91B olsalazine sodium
CK-0383 verofylline
CK-0569 **(as the base)** ipexidine
  mesylate
CK-1752A sematilide HCl
CL09 icomethasone enbutate
CL 10304 aminocaproic acid
CL 106359 triamcinolone acetonide
  sodium phosphate
CL 108,756 brocresine

CL 112,302 buprenorphine HCl
CL 115,347 viprostol
CL 118,532 triptorelin
CL 12,625 natamycin
CL-1388R guanadrel sulfate
CL 13,900 puromycin
CL 14377 methotrexate
CL 16,536 puromycin HCl
CL 184,116 porfimer sodium
CL 184,824 alovudine
CL-1848C etoxadrol HCl
CL 186,815 biapenem
CL 203,821 cetaben sodium
CL 205925 iprocinodine HCl
CL 206,214 butamisole HCl
CL 206,576 sulbenox
CL 206,797 cypothrin
CL 216,942 bisantrene HCl
CL 217,658 imcarbofos
CL 220,075 bicifadine HCl
CL 22415 demecycline
CL 227,193 piperacillin sodium
CL 232,315 mitoxantrone HCl
CL 2422 guancydine
CL 25477 azetepa
CL 26193 simtrazene
CL 27,071 descinolone acetonide
CL 273,547 ocinaplon
CL 273,703 maduramicin
CL 274,471 colestolone
CL 284,635 cefixime
CL 284,846 zaleplon
CL 286,558 zeniplatin
CL 287,088 nemadectin
CL 287,110 enloplatin
CL 287,389 nilvadipine
CL 291,894 somagrebove
CL 297,939 bisoprolol
CL 297,939 bisoprolol fumarate
CL 298,741 tazobactam
CL 301,423 moxidectin
CL 307,579 tazobactam sodium
CL 307,782 levoleucovorin calcium
CL 318,952 verteporfin
Cl 337 azaserine
CL 34433 triamcinolone hexacetonide
CL 34699 amcinonide
CL 36467 methotrimeprazine
CL 369 ketamine HCl
CL 39743 methotrimeprazine

CL 39808 thozalinone
CL 399 tiletamine HCl
CL 40881 ethambutol HCl
CL 48156 imidoline HCl
CL 5,279 nithiamide
CL 53415 cyproximide
CL 54131 piperamide maleate
CL 54998 brocresine
Cl-583.Na salt meclofenamate sodium
CL 59112 roletamide
CL 61965 triamcinolone acetonide
    sodium phosphate
CL 62,362 loxapine
CL-639C dioxadrol HCl
Cl-64,976 zilantel
CL 65205 boxidine
CL 65336 tranexamic acid
CL 65,562 triflocin
Cl-661 oxiramide
CL 67,772 amoxapine
Cl-683 ripazepam
CL 71563 loxapine succinate
Cl-775 bevantolol HCl
Cl-808 vidarabine phosphate
Cl-808 sodium vidarabine sodium
    phosphate
CL 81,587 avoparcin
CL 82,204 fenbufen
CL 83,544 felbinac
Cl-845 pirmenol HCl
CL 84,633 nimidane
CL-867 piridicillin sodium
Cl-871 piracetam
CL 88,893 clazolimine
CL 90,748 azolimine
CL-911C dexoxadrol HCl
CL-912C levoxadrol HCl
CL 98984 cinodine HCl
CLY-503 simfibrate
CM 31-916 ceftiofur sodium
CMA-676 gemtuzumab ozogamicin
CN-10,395 ethosuximide
CN-14,329-23A cycloguanil pamoate
CN-15,573-23A pararosaniline pamoate
CN-15,757 azaserine
CN-16146 carbocloral
CN-17,900-2B clamoxyquin HCl
CN-1883 acedapsone
CN-20,172-3 benzilonium bromide

CN-25,253-2 phencyclidine HCl
CN-27,554 flufenamic acid
CN-34,799-5A guanoxyfen sulfate
CN-35355 mefenamic acid
CN-36,337 diapamide
CN-38,474 alipamide
CN 38703 methaqualone
CN-52,372-2 ketamine HCl
CN-54521-2 tiletamine HCl
CN-5834-5931B triclofenol piperazine
CN 59,567 clioxanide
CNS 1102 aptiganel HCl
CNS-5161 generic not yet assigned—
    see main list
CO 405 butidrine
Code 7277 ferumoxtran-10
compound 109168 nifluridide
compound 112531 vindesine
compound 113878 ciprefadol succi-
    nate
compound 113935 pentomone
compound 122587 drobuline
compound 133314 trioxifene mesylate
compound 24266 pentetate calcium
    trisodium Yb 169
compound 42339 acronine
compound 469 isoflurane
compound 49510 paricalcitol
compound 497 dieldrin
compound 53616 frentizole
compound 56063 melizame
compound 57926 sinefungin
compound 68-198 diamfenetide
compound 79891 narasin
compound 81929 dobutamine
compound 83405 cefamandole
compound 83846 aprindine HCl
compound 85287 nibroxane
compound 89218 nisoxetine
compound 904 alexidine
compound 90459 benoxaprofen
compound 90606 isamoxole
compound 93819 fluretofen
compound 99170 aprindine
compound 99638 cefaclor
compound LY 131126 butopamine
compound S zidovudine
COP-1 glatiramer acetate
CP-0127 deltibant
CP-101,606-27 traxoprodil mesylate

CP-10,188 fenclonine
CP-10,303-8 quinterenol sulfate
CP-10,423-16 pyrantel pamoate
CP-10,423-18 pyrantel tartrate
CP 1044 J3 bufexamac
CP-11,332-1 quinazosin HCl
CP-116,517-27 alatrofloxacin mesylate
CP-118,954-11 icopezil maleate
CP-12,009-18 morantel tartrate
CP-12,252-1 thiothixene HCl
CP-12,299-1 prazosin HCl
CP-12,521-1 piquizil HCl
CP-12,574 tinidazole
CP-13,608 tesicam
CP-14,185-1 hoquizil HCl
CP-14,368-1 lometraline HCl
CP-14,445-16 oxantel pamoate
CP-148,623 pamaqueside
CP-15,464-2 carbenicillin indanyl sodium
CP-15,467-61 lithium carbonate
CP 1552 S milacemide HCl
CP-15,639-2 carbenicillin disodium
CP-15,973 sudoxicam
CP-16,171 piroxicam
CP-16,171-85 piroxicam olamine
CP-16,533-1 verapamil
CP 172 AP clopirac
CP-18,524 tibric acid
CP-19,106-1 trimazosin HCl
CP-20,961 avridine
CP-22,341 temodox
CP-22,665 flumizole
CP-24,314-1 pirbuterol HCl
CP-24,314-14 pirbuterol acetate
CP-24,441-1 tametraline HCl
CP-24,877 drinidene
CP-25,673 tiazuril
CP-26,154 tolimidone
CP-27,634 gliamilide
CP-28,720 glipizide
CP-31,081 polydextrose
CP-32,387 pirolate
CP-336,156-CB lasofoxifene tartrate
CP-33,994-2 pirbenicillin sodium
CP-34,089 sulprostone
CP-36,584 flutroline
CP-38,754 plauracin
CP-424,391-18 capromorelin tartrate
CP-44,001-1 nantradol HCl

CP-45,634 sorbinil
CP-45,899-2 sulbactam sodium
CP-45,899-99 sulbactam benzathine
CP-47,904 sulbactam pivoxil
CP-48,810-27 fanetizole mesylate
CP-48,867-9 ristianol phosphate
CP-49,952 sultamicillin
CP-50,556-1 levonantradol HCl
Cp-51,974-1 sertraline HCl
CP-52,640-2 cefoperazone sodium
CP-54,802 alitame
CP-556S suloctidil
CP-57,361-01 zaltidine HCl
CP-62,993 azithromycin
CP-65703 ampiroxicam
CP-66,248 tenidap
CP-66,248-2 tenidap sodium
CP-70,429 sulopenem
CP-70,490-09 enazadrem phosphate
CP-72,133 ilonidap
CP-72,467-2 englitazone sodium
CP-73,049 binfloxacin
CP-73,850 zopolrestat
CP-76,136-27 danofloxacin mesylate
CP-80,794 terlakiren
CP-86,325-2 darglitazone sodium
CP-88,059 ziprasidone
CP-88,059-1 ziprasidone HCl
CP-88,059-27 ziprasidone mesylate
CP-88,818 tiqueside
CP-93,393-1 sunepitron HCl
CP-99,219-27 trovafloxacin mesylate
CPC-111 generic not yet assigned—
    see main list
CPC-211 sodium dichloroacetate
Cpd 109514 nabilone
Cpd. 5411 iopentol
CPI-1189 generic not yet assigned—
    see main list
CPT-11 irinotecan
CR/662 tipepidine
CRL 40476 modafinil
CS-045 troglitazone
CS-151 crofilcon A
CS-514 pravastatin sodium
CS-622 temocapril HCl
CS-807 cefpodoxime proxetil
CS-92 generic not yet assigned—see
    main list
CSAG-144 mebeverine HCl

CT 1501R lisofylline
CT-2584 generic not yet assigned—see main list
CTC-96 generic not yet assigned—see main list
CTLA4-Ig generic not yet assigned—see main list
CTP-37 generic not yet assigned—see main list
CTR 6110 nitrodan
CTX lornoxicam
CV-11974 candesartan
CV 57533 xenyhexenic acid
CV 58903 xenazoic acid
CVT-124 generic not yet assigned—see main list
CVT-313 generic not yet assigned—see main list
CVT-510 generic not yet assigned—see main list
CY-116 aminocaproic acid
CY-1503 generic not yet assigned—see main list
CY 153 acexamic acid
CY-1899 generic not yet assigned—see main list
CY 216 nadroparin calcium
CY2301 generic not yet assigned—see main list
CY 39 psilocybine
CYT-103 ^{111}In indium In 111 satumomab pendetide
CYT-103-Y-90 generic not yet assigned—see main list
CYT-356 capromab pendetide
CYT-424 samarium Sm 153 lexidronam pentasodium
D 00079 anoxomer
D-1262 cloxypendyl
D-1593 diapamide
D-1721 alipamide
D-1959 HCl reproterol HCl
D-20761 cetrorelix acetate
D2083 desonide
D-2163 generic not yet assigned—see main list
D 237 cloforex
D-254 pipazethate
D-365 verapamil
D 4028 enprofylline

D 47 sulbentine
d4T stavudine
D 7093 mesna
D-775 homofenazine
D-9998 flupirtine maleate
DA 1773 sodium picosulfate
DA 2370 feprazone
DA-398 epirizole
DA 688 gefarnate
DA-708 teflurane
DA-808 nafcaproic acid
DA-893 roflurane
DA-914 nafiverine
DA-992 naftypramide
DAB-389 generic not yet assigned—see main list
DAC decitabine
D.A.T. acetiamine
DATC tiocarlide
DAU6215CL itasetron
DBV buformin
DCH 21 (as sodium salt) exiproben
DCL Hb hemoglobin crosfumaril
DETF trichlorfon
DF 118 dihydrocodeine bitartrate
DH-524 fenmetozole HCl
DH-581 probucol
DIM-SA succimer
DIN 608 nateglinide
DK-7419 argatroban
DL 152 bietaserpine
DL-164 tiodonium chloride
DL-588 napactadine HCl
DL-8280 ofloxacin
dl HM-PAO exametazime
dl HM-PAO hexametazime
DMI desipramine HCl
DMP-115 perflutren
DMP 266 efavirenz
DMP 450 generic not yet assigned—see main list
DMP 504 generic not yet assigned—see main list
DMP 754 roxifiban acetate
DMP 777 generic not yet assigned—see main list
DMP 840 bisnafide dimesylate
DMSC doxycycline fosfatex
DN-2327 pazinaclone
DO6 lexipafant

DPDP fodipir
DR-3355 levofloxacin
DS 103-282 tizanidine HCl
DS-4152 tecogalan sodium
DT-3 detrothyronine
DT-327 clopamide
DTI-015 generic not yet assigned—see main list
DTPA-SMS pentetreotide
D-Trp LHRH-PEA deslorelin
DU-21220 ritodrine
DU-21445 tiprenolol HCl
DU 22550 (as sulfate) caproxamine
DU23000 fluvoxamine maleate
DU-23187 quincarbate
DU-6958a sitafloxacin
DuP 128 lecimibide
DuP 753 losartan potassium
Dup 785 brequinar sodium
DuP 921 sibopirdine
DUP 937 teloxantrone HCl
DUP 941 losoxantrone
DuP 996 linopirdine
DV-1006 cetraxate HCl
DW-61 flavoxate HCl
DW-62 dimefline HCl
DW 75 norleusactide
DX-8951f exatecan mesylate
DyDTPA-BMA sprodiamide
E-0659 azelastine HCl
E-1000 amiloxate
E-106-E (as cyclamate) furfenorex
E 141 ethamsylate
E-2020 donepezil HCl
E25 generic not yet assigned—see main list
E-2663 bentiromide
E-3810 rabeprazole sodium
E 39 inproquone
E-52 pentafilcon A
E-614 tripamide
E 9002 naftalofos
EA-166 guanoxyfen sulfate
EDU edoxudine
EE₃ME mestranol
EF-27 generic not yet assigned—see main list
EF9 temoporfin
EGTA egtazic acid
EGYT 201 bencyclane fumarate

EHB 776 foscarnet sodium
EL10 dehydroepiandrosterone
EL349 somidobove
EL737 ractopamine HCl
EL-857 apramycin
EL870 tilmicosin
EL-970 fampridine
EL-974 ticarbodine
ELD 950 eledoisin
EMBAY 8440 praziquantel
EMD 15 700 nitrefazole
EMD 19698 (as hydrogen maleate) peratizole
EMD 33 512 bisoprolol
EMD 9806 pramiverine
EN-1010 pyrrocaine
EN-141 josamycin
EN-15304 naloxone HCl
EN-1620A nalmexone HCl
EN-1639A (as HCl) naltrexone
EN-1661L bisobrin lactate
EN-1733A molindone HCl
EN-2234A nalbuphine HCl
EN-313 moricizine
EN-970 fluquazone
ENA-713 rivastigmine
ENT-20852 butonate
ENT-23969 carbaril
ENT-25567 naftalofos
ENT 29,106 nimidane
EPI-2010 generic not yet assigned—see main list
EPOCH epoetin beta
ES 304 nicofuranose
ET-394 tribromsalan
ET-495 piribedil
ETTN propatyl nitrate
EU-1063 proquinolate
EU-1085 leniquinsin
EU-1093 buquinolate
EU-1806 nafronyl oxalate
EU-2826 benurestat
EU-2972 nolinium bromide
EU-3120 acodazole HCl
EU-3325 triafungin
EU-3421 oxifungin HCl
EU-4093 azumolene sodium
EU-4200 piribedil
EU-4534 flurofamide
EU-4584 tolfamide

EU-4891 diacetolol HCl
EU-4906 sitogluside
EU-5306 pefloxacin
EUDR edoxudine
EV2-7 sevirumab
EX 10-029-C elantrine
EX 10-781 metizoline HCl
EX 12-095 eterobarb
EX 4355 desipramine HCl
EX 4810 ambuside
Ex 4883 rolicyprine
EXP-105-1 amantadine HCl
EXP 126 rimantadine HCl
EXP 338 midaflur
EXP 999 metopimazine
F 1500 succisulfone
F 1983 pyrovalerone HCl
F28249α nemadectin
F-368 dantrolene
F-413 clodanolene
F-440 dantrolene sodium
F-605 (as the sodium) clodanolene
F 6066 cyclofenil
F-691 furodazole
F-776 orpanoxin
F-853 nitrafudam HCl
Fa 402 fentonium bromide
FBA 1420 propanidid
FBA 4059 brotianide
FBB 4231 glisoxepide
FBB 6896 clenpirin
FC-1157a toremifene citrate
FC 41-12 perflenapent + perflisopent
FCE 20124 reboxetine mesylate
FCE 21336 cabergoline
FCF 89 roquinimex
FER-1443 ticlatone
FG-10571 panadiplon
FG 5111 melperone
FGN-1 exisulind
FI 5852 oxabolone cipionate
F.I. 6146 buzepide metiodide
FI 6337 metergoline
FI 6339 (as the base) daunorubicin HCl
F.I. 6426 stallimycin HCl
F.I. 6654 caroxazone
F.I. 6820 brofoxine
FK 027 cefixime
FK-201 quinotolast

FK 235 nilvadipine
FK-366 zenarestat
FK 482 cefdinir
FK-506 tacrolimus
FK-565 generic not yet assigned—see main list
FK 749 ceftizoxime sodium
FKS-508 cevimeline HCl
FLA 731 remoxipride
FLA 731(−) remoxipride HCl
FP-GP1 motexafin gadolinum
FPL 12924AA remacemide HCl
FPL 58668KC probicromil calcium
FPL 59002 nedocromil
FPL 59002KC nedocromil calcium
FPL 59002KP nedocromil sodium
FPL 59360 minocromil
FPL 60278 dopexamine
FPL 60278AR dopexamine HCl
FPL.670 cromolyn sodium
FP-LP1 motexafin lutetium
FR 13749 ceftizoxime sodium
FR 17027 cefixime
FR-74366 zenarestat
FS069 perflutren
(−)-FTC emtricitabine
FTC-(−)
FTY-720 generic not yet assigned—see main list
FU-02 fumoxicillin
FUT-175 nafamostat mesylate
FWH 399 troxonium tosilate
G-101 erythromycin salnacedin
G-201 salnacedin
G-203 fluocinonide
G-24480 dimpylate
G-25178 prodeconium bromide
G-25766 clorindione
G 26,872 phenbutazone sodium glycerate
G 30320 clofazimine
G-3139 generic not yet assigned—see main list
G-32883 carbamazepine
G-33040 opipramol HCl
G-33182 chlorthalidone
G 34586 clomipramine HCl
G-35020 desipramine HCl
G 35259 ketipramine fumarate
G-4 dichlorophen

G-704,650 alendronate sodium

GBC-590 generic not yet assigned—
see main list

GD-0039 tridolgosir HCl

GEA 654 alaproclate

GEM 132 generic not yet assigned—
see main list

GEM 231 generic not yet assigned—
see main list

GEM 91 trecovirsen sodium

GER-11 pimagedine HCl

GF 120918A elacridar

GG-167 zanamivir

GG-745 dutasteride

GI147211C lurtotecan dihydrochloride

GI 198745 dutasteride

GI262570X farglitazar

GI 87084B remifentanil HCl

GL-701 dehydroepiandrosterone

GLQ 223 trichosanthin

GMC 89-107 regramostim

GN1600 argatroban

Go 1213 atolide

Go 1733 suloxifen oxalate

Go 2782 iproxamine HCl

Go 3026A ciclafrine HCl

Go-560 febarbamate

Go 919 piprozolin

GOE 3450 gabapentin

Goedecke 3282 ozolinone

GP-1-110 acadesine

gp120 generic not yet assigned—see
main list

GP-121 phencyclidine HCl

gp 160 generic not yet assigned—see
main list

GP-2-121-3 arbutamine HCl

GP 31406 depramine

GP 45840 diclofenac sodium

GP 51084 glibutimine

GPA-878 metazamide

GPI-1046 generic not yet assigned—
see main list

GPI-200 iometopane I 123

GPI-5000 generic not yet assigned—
see main list

GR109714X lamivudine

GR 114297A picumeterol fumarate

GR 114297X (picumeterol) picumeterol fumarate

GR 116526X isotretinoin anisatil

GR 121167X zanamivir

GR 122311X ranitidine bismuth citrate

GR 138950C saprisartan potassium

GR 20263 ceftazidime

GR 205171A vofopitant dihydrochloride

GR 2/1214 clobetasone butyrate

GR 2/1574 alfadolone

GR 2/234 alfaxalone

GR 2/443 (as propionate) doxibetasol

GR 2/925 clobetasol propionate

Gr 30921 mitoquidone

GR 32191 vapiprost HCl

GR 32191B vapiprost HCl

GR 33207 ovandrotone albumin

GR 33343 G salmeterol xinafoate

GR 33343 X salmeterol

GR 38032F ondansetron HCl

GR 412 dodeclonium bromide

GR 43175C sumatriptan succinate

GR 43659X lacidipine

GR50360A fluparoxan HCl

GR 50692 cefempidone

GR 53992B (GX 1296B) teludipine
HCl

GR 63178K fosquidone

GR 68755C alosetron HCl

GR 81225C galdansetron HCl

GR 85548A naratriptan HCl

GR 87442 N luroseron mesylate

GR92132 troglitazone

GR 69153X cefetecol

GRF1-44 generic not yet assigned—
see main list

GS-0504 cidofovir

GS-0840 adefovir dipivoxil

GS-1278 tenofovir

GS-1339 dymanthine HCl

GS 2147 sancycline

GS-2876 methacycline

GS-2989 meclocycline

GS-3065 doxycycline

GS-3159 carbenicillin potassium

GS 393 generic not yet assigned—see
main list

GS-4104 oseltamivir phosphate

GS-4331-05 tenofovir disoproxil
fumarate

GS-6244 carbadox

Code Names

GS-6742 sulfomyxin
GS-7443 mequidox
GS 840 adefovir dipivoxil
GS-95 thiethylperazine maleate
GT16-026A sevelamer HCl
GT31-104HB colesevelam HCl
GV 104326B sanfetrinem sodium
GV 118819X sanfetrinem cilexetil
GV 150526X gavestinel
GW-1536 generic not yet assigned—
see main list
GW-2570 generic not yet assigned—
see main list
GW275175 generic not yet
assigned—see main list
GW 433908A fosamprenavir sodium
GW 433908G fosamprenavir calcium
GW-80126 seprilose
H 102/09 HCl zimeldine HCl
H 104/08 pamatolol sulfate
H 133/22 prenalterol I ICl
H 154/82 felodipine
H 168/68 omeprazole
H 168/68 sodium omeprazole sodium
H199/18 magnesium trihydrate
esomeprazole magnesium
H 365 paroxypropione
H 3774 alibendol
H 4132 dotefonium bromide
H 4170 tolpiprazole
H 4723 clobazam
H 56/28 alprenolol HCl
H65-RTA zolimomab aritox
H 93/26 succinate metoprolol succi-
nate
HA-1A nebacumab
HB 115 nifurprazine
HB 419 glyburide
H.B.F. 386 cactinomycin
HBY097 generic not yet assigned—
see main list
HC 1528 decoquinate
HC 20,511 fumarate ketotifen fuma-
rate
HE-200 generic not yet assigned—see
main list
HF 1854 clozapine
HF 1927 dibenzepin HCl
HF-2159 clothiapine
HF 241 bufeniode

HGP-1 loteprednol etabonate
HGP-2 adaprolol maleate
HGP-30W generic not yet assigned—
see main list
HGP-5 alprenoxime HCl
HGP-6 tematropium methylsulfate
HH105 butetamate
HH 197 butamirate citrate
HI-236 generic not yet assigned—see
main list
HL 267 dipenine bromide
HL 362 colforsin
HL 523 (as HCl) tiformin
HMD oxymetholone
HMR 3480 generic not yet
assigned—see main list
HMR-3647 generic not yet
assigned—see main list
HMR 4004 generic not yet
assigned—see main list
HNK-20 generic not yet assigned—
see main list
Hoe 045 articaine
HOE 062 roxatidine acetate HCl
HOE 077 lufironil
Hoe 105 citenazone
HOE 118 piretanide
HOE 140 icatibant acetate
HOE 18 680 embutramide
HOE 216V luxabendazole
HOE 280 ofloxacin
HOE 296 ciclopirox olamine
HOE 296b ciclopirox
Hoe 296 V resorantel
HOE 304 desoximetasone
HOE 36801 etifoxine
HOE 39-893d penbutolol sulfate
HOE 42-440 tiamenidine HCl
HOE440 tiamenidine
Hoe 473 aclantate
HOE 490 glimepiride
HOE 498 ramipril
HOE 760 roxatidine acetate HCl
HOE 766 buserelin acetate
HOE 777 prednicarbate
Hoe 881V fenbendazole
HOE 893d penbutolol sulfate
HOE 984 nomifensine maleate
Hoechst 10495 norpipanone
Hoechst 10582 normethadone

HP 029 velnacrine maleate
HP 128 suronacrine maleate
HP 1598 guanoxyfen sulfate
HP 290 quilostigmine
HP-3 generic not yet assigned—see main list
HP 3522 brocrinat
HP-4 generic not yet assigned—see main list
HP 494 fluradoline HCl
HP 522 brocrinat
HP 549 isoxepac
HP 749 besipirdine HCl
HP 873 iloperidone
HPEK-1 tetroquinone
hPTH 1-34 (acetate salt) teriparatide acetate
HR111V-sulfate cefquinome sulfate
HR 221 (as sodium) cefodizime
HR 376 clobazam
HR 756 cefotaxime sodium
HR 810 sulfate cefpirome sulfate
HR 930 fosazepam
HRP 543 dazepinil HCl
HRP 913 neflumozide HCl
HS-592 clemastine
HSP 2986 pramiverine
HT-11 cloperastine
HTF 919 tegaserod
HTO tritiated water
HU-1124 generic not yet assigned—see main list
HU-211 dexanabinol
Hu23F2G rovelizumab
HUF-2446 clodazon HCl
HWA 285 propentofylline
HWA-486 leflunomide
HY-185 carbocloral
123I labeled IMP iofetamine HCl I 123
123I-M123 iofetamine HCl I 123
I-2105 afovirsen sodium
I-653 desflurane
IA-307 acetosulfone sodium
IB-367 generic not yet assigned—see main list
IBT-9302 heparinase III
IC-351 tadalafil
ICI 118,587 xamoterol
ICI 118,630 goserelin
ICI 125,211 tiotidine

ICI 128,436 ponalrestat
ICI 136,753 tracazolate
ICI 139603 tetronasin
ICI 141,292 epanolol
ICI 156,834 cefotetan
ICI 176,334 bicalutamide
ICI 182,780 fulvestrant
ICI 194,660 meropenem
ICI 204,219 zafirlukast
ICI 204,636 quetiapine fumarate
ICI 28257 clofibrate
ICI 29661 pyrimitate
ICI 32865 etoglucid
ICI-33,828 methallibure
ICI 35,868 propofol
ICI 38174 (as HCl) pronetalol
ICI 45520 propranolol HCl
ICI 45763 (as HCl) toliprolol
ICI 46,474 tamoxifen citrate
ICI 46683 oxyclozanide
I.C.I. 47,319 dexpropranolol HCl
ICI 48213 cyclofenil
ICI 50,123 pentagastrin
I.C.I. 50,172 practolol
I.C.I. 54,450 fenclozic acid
ICI 54,594 (as sodium salt) brofezil
ICI 55,052 nequinate
ICI 55,897 clobuzarit
ICI 58,834 viloxazine HCl
ICI 59118 razoxane
ICI 66,082 atenolol
ICI 80,008 (as sodium salt) fluprostenol sodium
ICI 80,996 cloprostenol sodium
ICI 81,008 fluprostenol sodium
ICI 8173 quindoxin
ICI D1033 anastrozole
ICI-U.S. 457 octazamide
ICN-1256 tocladesine
ICN-542 ribaminol
ICRF 159 razoxane
ICRF-187 dexrazoxane
IDEC-102 rituximab
IDEC-129 ibritumomab tiuxetan
IDEC-151 clenoliximab
IDEC-C2B8 rituximab
IDEC-CE9.1 generic not yet assigned—see main list
IDEC-Y2B8 ibritumomab tiuxetan
IL-17803A (as HCl) acebutolol

Code Names

IL-19552 pipotiazine palmitate
IL 22811 HCl meptazinol HCl
IL 5902 spiramycin
IL 6001 trimipramine
IL-6302 mesylate fonazine mesylate
IM-862 generic not yet assigned—see main list
IMI-28 epirubicin HCl
IMI 30 idarubicin HCl
IMI 58 esorubicin HCl
IMMU-4 arcitumomab
IMMU-LL2 bectumomab
IMMU-MN3 sulesomab
IN 1060 cyprolidol HCl
IN 29-5931B triclofenol piperazine
IN 379 pimetine HCl
IN 461 benzindopyrine HCl
IN 511 phenyramidol HCl
IN 836 fenyripol HCl
INA-X14 insulin aspart
INF-1837 flufenamic acid
INF-3355 mefenamic acid
INF 4668 meclofenamic acid
INGN-201 generic not yet assigned—see main list
INS-1 generic not yet assigned—see main list
insulin X14 insulin aspart
IP-2105 afovirsen sodium
IP 302 sodium citicoline sodium
IP 456 pagoclone
IPA riboprine
IPL-576 generic not yet assigned—see main list
IR-501 generic not yet assigned—see main list
IR-502 generic not yet assigned—see main list
IS 2596 domoxin
I.S. 499 poldine methylsulfate
ISIS-13312 generic not yet assigned—see main list
ISIS 2105 afovirsen sodium
ISIS-2302 generic not yet assigned—see main list
ISIS 2503 generic not yet assigned—see main list
ISIS 3521 generic not yet assigned—see main list

ISIS-5132 generic not yet assigned—see main list
isomer A zuclomiphene
isomer B enclomiphene
ISV-205 generic not yet assigned—see main list
ISV-208 generic not yet assigned—see main list
Janssen R 4929 benzetimide HCl
JAV 852 benfosformin
JB-8181 desipramine HCl
JD-96 vinylbital
JF-1 nalmefene
JL-1078 dihexyverine HCl
JL 512 fenadiazole
JM-216 satraplatin
JM-8 carboplatin
JM-83 oxaliplatin
JM-9 iproplatin
JO-1784 igmesine HCl
JTT-501 generic not yet assigned—see main list
K 11941 alfaprostol
K 12148 lifibrol
K-17 thalidomide
K-1900 nimorazole
K-38 glycyclamide
K-386 glycyclamide
K 4024 glipizide
K 4277 indoprofen
K 9147 tolciclate
Kabi 2234 tolterodine
KABI 925 emylcamate
KAT 256 (as HCl) clobutinol
KB-944 fostedil
KB 95 benzpiperylon
K-F 224 naftoxate
KL-255 (as HCl) bupranolol
Ko 1173 Cl mexiletine HCl
KO 1366 bunitrolol
Ko 592 (as HCl) toliprolol
KP-363 butenafine HCl
KRM-1648 rifalazil
KS 33 oxyridazine
KVX-478 amprenavir
KW-110 aceglutamide aluminum
KW-2189 pibrozelesin hydrobromide
KW4679 olopatadine HCl
KWD 2019 terbutaline sulfate
L1 deferiprone

L-1573 cysteamine
L-1633 sodium dibunate
L-1718 osalmid
L-1777 medazomide
L 2197 benzarone
L-2214 benzbromarone
L 2329 benziodarone
L 2642 etabenzarone
L-3428 amiodarone
L-364,718 devazepide
L-4269 pyridarone
L-5103 **Lepetit** rifampin
L-5418 diftalone
L 542 mercurobutol
L-554 tritoqualine
L 566 dibemethine
L 5818 **(as HCl)** coumazoline
L-6257 oxetorone fumarate
L-627 biapenem
L-637,510 nelezaprine maleate
L-6400 fluazacort
L-647,339 naxagolide HCl
L-668,019 verlukast
L-669,455 dexibuprofen lysine
L-67 prilocaine HCl
L-735,524 indinavir sulfate
L-749 salacetamide
L 75 1362B colforsin
L-8 lypressin
L 8027 nictindole
L-9394 butoprozine HCl
LA-012 **(as HCl)** quatacaine
LA 1221 **(as HCl)** butalamine
LA III diazepam
LA 391 sodium picosulfate
La 6023 metformin
LAC-43 bupivacaine HCl
LAS 30451 pancopride
LAS 31025 arofylline
LAS 31416 almotriptan
LAS 3876 almagate
LAS 9273 clebopride
LAS W-090 ebastine
LB 125 cyprodenate
LB 20304a gemifloxacin mesylate
LB-46 pindolol
LB-502 furosemide
LC 44 flupentixol
LD 2351 **(as hydrobromide)**
  butopiprine

LD 2480 piprocurarium iodide
LD 2630 difencloxazine HCl
LD 2988 folescutol
LD 3055 oxypyrronium bromide
LD 335 propyromazine bromide
LD 3394 fenozolone
LD 3612 paraflutizide
LD 4644 pipebuzone
LD 935 dipiproverine HCl
LDI-200 generic not yet assigned—
  see main list
LDP-02 generic not yet assigned—see
  main list
Leo 1031 prednimustine
Leo 114 polyestradiol phosphate
levo-BC-2605 oxilorphan
levo-BC-2627 butorphanol
levo-BC-2627 **tartrate** butorphanol
  tartrate
levo-BL-4566 moxazocine
LEX-032 generic not yet assigned—
  see main list
LFA3TIP alefacept
LG100057 alitretinoin
LG100069 bexarotene
LGD1057 alitretinoin
LGD 1069 bexarotene
LJ 206 carbocysteine
LJC 10,141 felbinac
LJ C10,627 biapenem
LJP-394 abetimus sodium
LL 1530 nadoxolol
LL-705W neutramycin
LM-1404 lortalamine
LM 176 cobamamide
LM 192 viquidil
LM 2717 clobazam
LM-427 rifabutin
LM-94 hymecromone
L.N. 107 broparestrol
l-OHP oxaliplatin
LP-2307 generic not yet assigned—
  see main list
LS-121 nafronyl oxalate
LS 2616 roquinimex
LS 519 C12 pirenzepine HCl
Lu 10-171-B citalopram hydrobromide
Lu 23-174 sertindole
Lu 26-054-0 escitalopram oxalate
LU3-010 talopram HCl

LVD dextran 40
LY031537 ractopamine HCl
LY 048 740 avilamycin
LY061188 cephalexin HCl
LY097964 cefetamet
LY099094 vindesine sulfate
LY104208 vinzolidine sulfate
LY 108380 doxpicomine HCl
LY110140 fluoxetine HCl
LY 119863 vinepidine sulfate
LY120363 flumezapine
LY121019 cilofungin
LY 122512 anitrazafen
LY 12271-72 viroxime
LY 122772 enviroxime
LY 123508 lorzafone
LY 127123 enviradene
LY 127623 metkephamid acetate
LY 127809 pergolide mesylate
LY 127935 moxalactam disodium
LY 135837 indecainide HCl
LY137998 somatropin
LY 139037 nizatidine
LY 139381 ceftazidime
LY 139603 tomoxetine HCl
LY 141894 amflutizole
LY 146032 daptomycin
LY 150378 clofilium phosphate
LY 150720 picenadol HCl
LY156758 raloxifene HCl
LY163502 quinelorane HCl
LY163892 monohydrate loracarbef
LY167005 proinsulin human
LY170053 olanzapine
LY170680 sulukast
LY171555 quinpirole HCl
LY171883 tomelukast
LY 174008 dobutamine tartrate
LY 175326 isomazole HCl
LY177370 tilmicosin
LY177370 phosphate tilmicosin
  phosphate
LY177837 somidobove
LY186641 sulofenur
LY 186655 tibenelast sodium
LY188011 gemcitabine
LY188011 HCl gemcitabine HCl
LY 195115 indolidan
LY 201116 ameltolide

LY206243 lactobionate levdobuta-
  mine lactobionate
LY207506 dobutamine lactobionate
LY210448 HCl dapoxetine HCl
LY 213829 tazofelone
LY215229 HCl seproxetine HCl
LY231514 pemetrexed disodium
LY 237216 dirithromycin
LY237733 amesergide
LY246708 xanomeline
LY246708 tartrate xanomeline tartrate
LY248686 HCl duloxetine HCl
LY253351 tamsulosin HCl
LY264618 lometrexol sodium
LY275585 insulin lyspro
LY277359 zatosetron maleate
LY281067 sergolexole maleate
LY287041 tazomeline citrate
LY293404 rismorelin porcine
LY294468 sulfate efegatran sulfate
LY295337 basifungin
LY300502 bexlosteride
LY303366 anidulafungin
LY307640 sodium rabeprazole sodium
LY-315535 generic not yet assigned—
  see main list
LY320236 izonsteride
LY326869 moxonidine
LY333328 diphosphate oritavancin
  diphosphate
LY 333334 teriparatide
LY335348 denileukin diftitox
LY353381·HCl arzoxifene HCl
LYO31537 ractopamine HCl
M-1028 (Meiji) haloprogin
M-14 rifamycin
M-141 spectinomycin HCl
M 285 cyprenorphine HCl
M. 5050 diprenorphine
M-811 salverine
M. 99 (as HCl) etorphine
MA 1277 zolertine HCl
MA 1291 quipazine maleate
MA 1337 cloperidone HCl
MA-1443 letimide HCl
MA-540 quinuclium bromide
MA-593 salethamide maleate
MAB35 indium In 111 altumomab
  pentetate

MAK 195 F generic not yet assigned—see main list
MAS-1 polyglyconate
Material A pentetate calcium trisodium Yb 169
MAY nelzarabine
M&B 15497 decoquinate
M&B 16942A diacetolol HCl
M&B 17803A (as HCl) acebutolol
M&B 22948 zaprinast
M&B 33153 oxoprostol
M&B 39831 temozolomide
M&B 5062 A amicarbalide
M&B 782 (as isethionate) propamidine
MB 800 (as isethionate) pentamidine
M&B 9302 clorgiline
MBR-4164-8 diflumidone sodium
MBR-4197 flucrylate
MBR 4223 triflumidate
MC 903 calcipotriene
MCE metergoline
MCI-9038 argatroban
McN-1075 fenmetramide
McN-1107 clominorex
McN-1210 pyrinoline
McN-1231 fluminorex
McN-1546 flumetramide
McN-1589 mixidine
McN-2378 mefenidil
McN-2378-46 mefenidil fumarate
McN-2453 azepindole
McN-2559 tolmetin
McN-2559-21-98 tolmetin sodium
McN-2783-21-98 zomepirac sodium
McN-3113 xilobam
McN-3377-98 fenobam
McN-3495 pirogliride tartrate
McN-3716 methyl palmoxirate
McN-3802-21-98 palmoxirate sodium
McN-3802 (anhydrous free acid) palmoxirate sodium
McN 3935 linogliride
McN-3935 linogliride fumarate
McN-4097-12-98 fenoctimine sulfate
McN-4853 topiramate
McN-742 aminorex
McN-A-2673-11 etoperidone HCl
McN-A-2833 perindopril

McN-A-2833-109 perindopril erbumine
McN-JR-13,558-11 fetoxylate HCl
McN-JR-15,403-11 difenoxin
McN-JR-1625 haloperidol
McN-JR-16,341 penfluridol
McN-JR-2498 trifluperidol
McN-JR-4263-49 fentanyl citrate
McN-JR-4584 benperidol
McN-JR-4749 droperidol
McN-JR-4929-11 benzetimide HCl
McN-JR-6218 fluspirilene
McN-JR-6238 pimozide
McN-JR-7242-11 difluanine HCl
McN-JR-7904 lidoflazine
McN-JR-8299-11 tetramisole HCl
McN-R-1162-22 potassium glucaldrate
McN-R-1967 fenretinide
McN-R-726-47 poldine methylsulfate
McN-R-73-Z rotoxamine
McN-X-181 valnoctamide
McN-X-94 capuride
MD 141 ethamsylate
MD 2028 fluanisone
MD 67350 (as maleate) cinepazide
MD-805 argatroban
mda-7 generic not yet assigned—see main list
MDL 101,731 tezacitabine
MDL 11,939 glemanserin
MDL 14,042 lofexidine HCl
MDL 16,455A fexofenadine HCl
MDL 17,043 enoximone
MDL 18,962 plomestane
MDL 19,205 piroximone
MDL 19,744 tipentosin HCl
MDL-201129 beraprost sodium
MDL-201229 beraprost
MDL 257 zindotrine
MDL 26,024G0 tetrazolast meglumine
MDL 26,479 suritozole
MDL 28,574A celgosivir HCl
MDL 458 deflazacort
MDL 473 rifapentine
MDL 507 teicoplanin
MDL 62,198 ramoplanin
MDL 62,769 rifamexil
MDL 71,754 vigabatrin
MDL 71,782 A eflornithine HCl
MDL 72,222 bemesetron

MDL 72,422 tropanserin HCl
MDL 72,974A mofegiline HCl
MDL 73,005EF binospirone mesylate
MDL 73,147EF dolasetron mesylate
MDL 73,745 zifrosilone
MDL 73,945 camiglibose
MDX-210 generic not yet assigned—
see main list
MDX-240 generic not yet assigned—
see main list
MDX-447 generic not yet assigned—
see main list
MDX-RA generic not yet assigned—
see main list
MEDI 493 palivizumab
MER-29 triparanol
MER-41 clomiphene citrate
MF 934 rufloxacin
M.G. 13054 fenquizone
M.G. 13608 domiodol
M.G. 143 sulmarin
M.G. 1559 xenbucin
Mg 4833 fencibutirol
M.G. 5454 guaiapate
MG 559 metamfepramone
M.G. 5771 butixirate
M.G. 624 stilonium iodide
M.G. 652 oxamarin HCl
M.G. 8823 exaprolol HCl
M.G. 8926 (as HCl) droprenilamine
MGI-114 generic not yet assigned—
see main list
MH-532 phenprobamate
MI-216 iothalamic acid
Mi-85 apazone
MIM D2A21 generic not yet
assigned—see main list
MIV-606 valomaciclovir stearate
MJ 10061 benzbromarone
MJ 12,175-170 tiprinast meglumine
MJ 12,880-1 tipropidil HCl
MJ 13,105-1 bucindolol HCl
MJ 13401-1-3 fenprinast HCl
MJ 13,754-1 nefazodone HCl
MJ 1986 indriline HCl
MJ 1987 mesuprine HCl
MJ 1988 quazodine
MJ 1992 soterenol HCl
MJ 1998 metalol HCl
MJ 1999 sotalol HCl

MJ 4309-1 oxybutynin chloride
MJ 505 phenyramidol HCl
MJ 9022-1 buspirone HCl
MJ 9067-1 encainide HCl
MJ 9184-1 zinterol HCl
MJF 10,938 xipamide
MJF 11567-3 cefadroxil
MJF-12264 tegafur
MJF 12637 suloctidil
MJF 9325 ifosfamide
MK-0462 rizatriptan benzoate
MK-0663 etoricoxib
MK-0677 ibutamoren mesylate
MK-0681 trientine HCl
MK-0699 rofecoxib
MK-0787 imipenem
MK-0826 ertapenem sodium
MK-0869 aprepitant
MK-0936 abamectin
MK-0991 caspofungin acetate
MK-130 (as the base) cyclobenza-
prine HCl
MK-188 zeranol
MK-196 indacrinone
MK-208 famotidine
MK-217 alendronate sodium
MK-233 dexibuprofen lysine
MK-240 protriptyline HCl
MK-250 emylcamate
MK-329 devazepide
MK-341 tranilast
MK-351 methyldopa
MK-360 thiabendazole
MK-366 norfloxacin
MK-383 tirofiban HCl
MK-397 eprinomectin
MK-401 clorsulon
MK-417 sezolamide HCl
MK-422 enalaprilat
MK-458 naxagolide HCl
MK-462 rizatriptan benzoate
MK-476 montelukast sodium
MK-507 dorzolamide HCl
MK-521 lisinopril
MK 57 methyldesorphine
MK-591 quiflapon sodium
MK-595 ethacrynic acid
MK-621 efrotomycin
MK-639 indinavir sulfate

MK-663 generic not yet assigned—see main list
MK-678 seglitide acetate
MK-733 simvastatin
MK790 levomethadyl acetate HCl
MK-791 cilastatin sodium
MK-793 diltiazem maleate
MK-801 dizocilpine maleate
MK-803 lovastatin
MK-826 generic not yet assigned—see main list
MK-869 generic not yet assigned—see main list
MK-906 finasteride
MK-966 rofecoxib
MK-A462 rizatriptan sulfate
MKC-442 generic not yet assigned—see main list
ML-1024 theofibrate
ML 1034 celucloral
ML-1129 beraprost sodium
ML-1229 beraprost
ML-3000 generic not yet assigned—see main list
MO-1255 encyprate
MO-911 pargyline HCl
MP-10013 iogulamide
MP-1051 silodrate
MP-1177 gadoversetamide
MP-1196 versetamide
MP-1554 technetium Tc 99m furifosmin
MP-1727 indium In 111 pentetreotide
MP 2032 iocarmic acid
MP 2032-meglumine iocarmate meglumine
MP-271 iosefamic acid
MP 302 (with ioxaglate sodium) ioxaglate meglumine
MP 328 ioversol
MP-351 generic not yet assigned—see main list
MP 4006 albumin, aggregated
MP 4018 stannous pyrophosphate
MP-537 iomethin I 125
MP-537 iomethin I 131
MP-600 betiatide
MP-6026 ioglucol
MP-620 iocetamic acid
MP 7010 stannous sulfur colloid

MP-8000 ioglucomide
MPV-1248 atipamezole
MPV-1440 dexmedetomidine
MPV-253 AII detomidine HCl
MPV-785 medetomidine HCl
MR6S4 sevoflurane
MRL 38 hexadiline
MRL-41 clomiphene citrate
MRP-10 pentetate calcium trisodium Yb 169
MRX-115 perflutren
MS-325 generic not yet assigned—see main list
MS 325168A fosveset
MSI-78 pexiganan acetate
MSL-109 sevirumab
MTS 263 tropenziline bromide
MUC-1 generic not yet assigned—see main list
MX-6 generic not yet assigned—see main list
MY-25 (as bitartrate) metergotamine
MY-33-7 (as HCl) lotucaine
MY-5116 repirinast
MYC 8003 mocimycin
MZ-144 rimazolium metilsulfate
N-0252 laurocapram
N-0923 generic not yet assigned—see main list
N-137 carbetimer
N-3 methetoin
N-399 xenytropium bromide
N-553 (as HCl) tolperisone
N-7009 flupentixol
N-7020 meprotixol
N-714 chlorprothixene
N-746 clopenthixol
NA-119 bromamid
NA 274 bromhexine HCl
NA-66 pimeclone
NAB 365 clenbuterol
NASH borocaptate sodium B 10
NAT-327 trimoxamine HCl
NAT-333 fenspiride HCl
NB 68 dacuronium bromide
NBI-3001 generic not yet assigned—see main list
NC-123 mesoridazine
NC 1264 thonzonium bromide
NC 150 phenazopyridine HCl

NC-1968 fungimycin
NC-7197 esproquin HCl
NCNU pentamustine
ND 50 octopamine
NDC 0082-4155 daunorubicin HCl
NDR 263 propenzolate HCl
NDR 304 ethyl dibunate
NDR-5061A aletamine HCl
NDR-5523A trimoxamine HCl
NDR-5998A fenspiride HCl
NE-10064 azimilide dihydrochloride
NE 11740 tebufelone
NE-1530 generic not yet assigned—
see main list
NE-19550 olvanil
NE-58095 risedronate sodium
NE 97221 piridronate sodium
NESP darbepoetin alfa
NF-1010 nifurdazil
NF-1088 nifurquinazol
NF-1120 nifurimide
NF-1425 furazolium tartrate
NF-161 nifursemizone
NF-246 nifuradene
NF-602 levofuraltadone
NF-71 nifurmerone
NF-84 nifuraldezone
NF-902 (as HCl) levofuraltadone
NF-963 furazolium chloride
NG-29 generic not yet assigned—see
main list
NIB nabitan HCl
NIH 2933 dimepheptanol
NIH 7574 benzethidine
NIH 7607 etonitazene
NIH 7667 noracymethadol HCl
NIH 7672 methopholine
NIH 8805 buprenorphine HCl
NK 1006 bekanamycin
NK 204 basifungin
NK-631 peplomycin sulfate
NKK-105 malotilate
NKT-01 gusperimus trihydrochloride
NMP-22 generic not yet assigned—
see main list
NN-304 insulin detemir
NNC-05-0328 tiagabine HCl
NO-05-0328 tiagabine HCl
NPAP prajmalium bitartrate
NPT 15392 nosantine

NS 2214 brasofensine maleate
NS-2710 generic not yet assigned—
see main list
NS-75A cetrorelix acetate
NSC-246131 valrubicin
NSC-266046 oxaliplatin
NSC 362856 temozlolomide
NSC 613792 lodenosine
NSC-614491 tocladesine
NSC 659772 alitretinoin
NSD 1055 brocresine
Nu-1779 betaprodine
Nu-1932 betameprodine
NU-2121 nicotinyl alcohol
NU-445 sulfisoxazole diolamine
NXX-066 quilostigmine
NY-198 lomefloxacin HCl
NZ-1001 generic not yet assigned—
see main list
ODA 914 demoxytocin
(–)-OddC troxacitabine
OGT-918 generic not yet assigned—
see main list
OHM-11771 nitric oxide
l-OHP oxaliplatin
OK-B7 generic not yet assigned—see
main list
OM 401 generic not yet assigned—
see main list
OM-977 etaminile
OMDS dipyrithione
OMS No 1825 azamethiphos
ONYX-015 generic not yet
assigned—see main list
OP 21-23 parnaparin sodium
OPB-2045 olanexidine HCl
OPC-1085 carteolol HCl
OPC-13013 cilostazol
OPC-14117 generic not yet
assigned—see main list
OPC-14597 aripiprazole
OPC-17116 grepafloxacin HCl
OPC-18790 toborinone
OPC-21 cilostazol
OPC-31 aripiprazole
OPC-8212 vesnarinone
(–)-OR-1259 levosimendan
OR-611 entacapone
ORF 10131 norgestimate
ORF 11676 nalmefene

ORF 15244 thymopentin
ORF 15817 edoxudine
ORF 15927 rioprostil
ORF 16600 bemarinone HCl
ORF 17070 histrelin
ORF 18704 pelretin
ORF 20257 doretinel
ORF 20485 tepoxalin
ORF 22164 atosiban
ORF 22867 bemoradan
Orf-32541 iturelix
ORF-8063 triflubazam
ORF 9326 nisterime acetate
ORG 10172 danaparoid sodium
ORG 2969 desogestrel
ORG 3236 etonogestrel
ORG-33062 generic not yet assigned—see main list
ORG 3770 mirtazapine
Org 4428 beloxepin
Org 6216 rimexolone
ORG7417 resocortol butyrate
Org 817 epimestrol
ORG 9426 rocuronium bromide
Org 9487 rapacuronium bromide
Org GB 94 mianserin HCl
Org NA 97 pancuronium bromide
ORG NC 45 vecuronium bromide
Org OD 14 tibolone
OST-577 generic not yet assigned—see main list
P 071 cetirizine HCl
P-081 generic not yet assigned—see main list
P-1011 dicloxacillin sodium
P-113 saralasin acetate
P-12 oxacillin sodium
P-1306 glyparamide
P-1496 zeranol
P-1560 taleranol
P-165 azaserine
P-1742 fluperolone acetate
P-1779 althiazide
P-1888 isosulfan blue
P-2105 epithiazide
P-248 levopropylcillin potassium
P-25 cloxacillin sodium
P-2525 polythiazide
P-2530 methalthiazide
P-2647 benzquinamide

P-280 bibapcitide
P-286 ioxaglic acid
P-301 hydroxyphenamate
P-3232 somfasepor
P-3693A doxepin HCl
P-3895 somfasepor
P-3896 guanisoquin sulfate
P-4125 isosulfan blue
P-414 generic not yet assigned—see main list
P-4385B clothixamide maleate
P-4599 cidoxepin HCl
P-463 fenamole
P-4657 B thiothixene
P-50 ampicillin
P-5227 pinoxepin HCl
P53 tetrofosmin
P-54 generic not yet assigned—see main list
P-5604 loteprednol etabonate
P-638 puromycin
P 7 lauroguadine
P-71 lycetamine
P 71-0129 fendosal
P-7138 nifurpirinol
P 720549 isoxepac
P-748 generic not yet assigned—see main list
P 76 2494A fluradoline HCl
P 76 2543 dazepinil HCl
P 78 3522 brocrinat
P79 3913 neflumozide HCl
P829 depreotide
P83 6029A velnacrine maleate
PA-144 plicamycin
PA-1648 rifalazil
PAA-3854 clamoxyquin HCl
PAA-701 bialamicol HCl
PAM-MR-1165 acedapsone
PAM-MR-807-23a cycloguanil pamoate
PAMN (as methonitrate) prampine
PASIT glyprothiazol
PAT fenamole
PB-005 dehydroepiandrosterone sulfate
PB 89 (as HCl) fominoben
p-BIDA butilfenin
PC1020 acetate prezatide copper acetate
PC-1421 piperacetazine

Code Names

PC-603 iproclozide
PCI-0120 motexafin gadolinium
PCI-0123 motexafin lutetium
PD 107779 enoxacin
PD-110843 zonisamide
PD 81565 pentostatin
PD 90,695-73 dezaguanine mesylate
PD-93 piromidic acid
PDB prifinium bromide
PE1-1 tuvirumab
pentapeptide DSDPR pentigetide
PF-26 mepramidil
PFA-186 salicylate meglumine
PG 430 febuverine
PG-501 mazaticol
PH 218 edogestrone
PHXA41 latanoprost
pierrel-TQ 86 azipramine HCl
PIXY321 milodistim
PK 10169 enoxaparin
PM 1807 fenimide
PM-185184 secnidazole
PM-1952 fenacetinol
PM-3944 flucetorex
PM-671 ethosuximide
PMD-387 crilvastatin
PN 200-110 isradipine
PNCRM7 generic not yet assigned—
  see main list
PNU-101387G sonepiprazole mesylate
PNU-140690E tipranavir disodium
PNU-155950E reboxetine mesylate
PNU-180638E almotriptan malate
PNU-200583E tolterodine tartrate
POLI 67 tetrydamine
POR 8 ornipressin
PP 563 cyhalothrin
PPI-002 generic not yet assigned—
  see main list
PPI-149 abarelix
PPRT-321 generic not yet assigned—
  see main list
PR-0818-156A verilopam HCl
PR-122 redox phenytoin
PR-225 redox acyclovir
PR-239 redox penicillin G
PR-320 molecusol & carbamazepine
PR-3847 teroxalene HCl
PR-741-976A somantadine HCl
PR-870-714A veradoline HCl

PR-877-530L flavodilol maleate
PR 879-317A oxamisole HCl
PR 934-423A remacemide HCl
PR-G 138-CL (as HCl)
  ciclosidomine
PRO 2000 generic not yet assigned—
  see main list
PRO 367 generic not yet assigned—
  see main list
PRO 542 generic not yet assigned—
  see main list
protease 1 brinolase
PS-1286 pararosaniline pamoate
PS 2383 trimetozine
PSC-833 valspodar
PT-14 generic not yet assigned—see
  main list
PT-9 betahistine HCl
PU-239 benzilonium bromide
PY 108-068 darodipine
PZ 1511 carpipramine dihydrochloride
PZ68 pentosan polysulfate sodium
Q-12 technetium Tc 99m furifosmin
QB-1 cloquinozine
QS-21 generic not yet assigned—see
  main list
QZ-2 methaqualone
R093877 prucalopride HCl
R 10.100 ethonam nitrate
R-106056 rivoglitazone
R106-1 basifungin
R108512 prucalopride succinate
R 10,948 diamocaine cyclamate
R 11,333 bromperidol
R-121919 generic not yet assigned—
  see main list
R 12,563 (as HCl) dexamisole
R 12,564 levamisole HCl
R 1303 carbofenotion
R-13423 dicloxacillin
R 13,558 fetoxylate HCl
R-13,672 haloperidol decanoate
R 1406 phenoperidine
R-148 methaqualone
R 14,827 econazole nitrate
R 14,889 miconazole nitrate
R 14,950 flunarizine HCl
R 15,403 (as HCl) difenoxin
R-15,454 (as nitrate salt) isoconazole
R 15,556 orconazole nitrate

R **1575** cinnarizine
R **15,889** lorcainide HCl
R-**1625** haloperidol
R **16,341** penfluridol
R **16,470 (as HCl)** dexetimide
R **1658** moperone
R **1707** glafenine
R **17,147** cyclobendazole
R **17,635** mebendazole
R **17,889** flubendazole
R **17,934** nocodazole
R **18,553** loperamide HCl
R **1881** metribolone
R **18,910** fluperamide
R **1929** azaperone
R **19,317** rodocaine
R **2028** fluanisone
R **2113** desoximetasone
R **2159** anisopirol
R **2167** fluanisone
R **22,700 (as HCl)** rodocaine
R **23,050** salantel
R **2323** gestrinone
R **23,633** fludazonium chloride
R **23,979** enilconazole
R **2453** demegestone
R-**2498** trifluperidol
R-**25,061** suprofen
R-**25,160** cliprofen
R **25,540** imafen HCl
R **25,831 (as the free base)** carnidazole
R **26,412** sulnidazole
R **27,500** sepazonium chloride
R **28,096 (as HCl)** carnidazole
R **2858** moxestrol
R-**28,644** azaconazole
R **28,930** fluspiperone
R **2962** amiperone
R **29,764** clopimozide
R **29,860** nitramisole HCl
R **30,730** sufentanil
R **31,520** closantel
R **3248** aceperone
R **33,204** declenperone
R **3345** pipamperone
R **3365** piritramide
R **33,799** carfentanil citrate
R **33800** sufentanil citrate
R **33,812** domperidone

R **34,000** doconazole
R **34,009** milenperone
R **34,301** halopemide
R-**34,803** etibendazole
R **34,995** lofentanil oxalate
R **35,443** oxatomide
R **38,198** buterizine
R**3827** abarelix
R **39,209** alfentanil HCl
R **39,500** parconazole HCl
R **3959** clometacin
R **4082** propyperone
R **41,400** ketoconazole
R-**41,468** ketanserin
R-**42,470** terconazole
R-**4263** fentanyl citrate
R **4318** floctafenine
R **43,512** astemizole
R **4444** duometacin
R-**45,486** flumeridone
R-**4584** benperidol
R-**46,541** bromperidol decanoate
R **46,846** tubulozole HCl
R **4714** oxiperomide
R-**47,465** pirenperone
R-**4749** droperidol
R **48** chlornaphazine
R **4845** bezitramide
R **5046** cinperene
R **50,547** levocabastine HCl
R **50 970** metrenperone
R **51 163** tameridone
R **51,211** itraconazole
R-**51,469** mioflazine HCl
R **5147** spiperone
R **516** cinnarizine
R-**51,619** cisapride
R **5188** spiroxatrine
R-**52** mannosulfan
R **52,245** setoperone
R-**53,200** altanserin tartrate
R **5385** acoxatrine
R **54,718** transcainide
R-**548** tricetamide
R **55104** erbulozole
R **55,667** ritanserin
R **5808** spiramide
R**58425** loperamide oxide
R **58735** sabeluzole
R **60844** irtemazole

R 610 racemoramide
R 6109 spirilene
R 6218 fluspirilene
R 6238 pimozide
R62,690 clazuril
R 62 818 lorcinadol
R 6438 antazonite
R64,433 diclazuril
R 64 766 risperidone
R 64947 noberastine
R65,824 nebivolol
R 661 buzepide metiodide
R 66905 saperconazole
R 67408 fenclofenac
R 68070 ridogrel
R 72063 loreclezole
R 7242 difluanine HCl
R 7464 propoxate
R 75231 draflazine
R 75251 liarozole HCl
R 77975 pirodavir
R 7904 lidoflazine
R 79598 ocaperidone
R 798 rimiterol hydrobromide
R 8025 antienite
R-803 furaprofen
R 805 nimesulide
R 8141 antienite
R-8193 antafenite
R 8284 proclonol
R 8299 tetramisole HCl
R-830 prifelone
R-830T prifelone
R-835 ibafloxacin
R-837 imiquimod
R 83842 vorozole
R 85246 liarozole fumarate
R-87926 lubeluzole
R-89439 loviride
R 91,274 alniditan dihydrochloride
R 9298 seperidol HCl
R-93877 prucalopride HCl
RA-8 dipyridamole
RA-C-384 iodocetylic acid I 123
RBC-CD4 generic not yet assigned—
  see main list
RC-160 vapreotide
RC-167 niceverine
RC-172 aldioxa
RC-173 alcloxa

RC-27109 nifuroxazide
RC 61-91 ifenprodil
RCH 314 benhepazone
RCM 258 fepentolic acid
RD 11654 ibufenac
RD 17345 fluprofen
RD 2801 pyritidium bromide
Rd 292 fenpentadiol
RD 328 pasiniazid
RD 406 cyprodenate
RD 9338 (as HCl) norbudrine
Rec 15 0122 nifurpipone
Rec 15/1476 fenticonazole nitrate
Rec 7/0267 dimefline HCl
REV 3659-(S) pivopril
REV 6000A delapril HCl
RFS-2000 rubitecan
RG 12561 dalvastatin
RG 270 iomeglamic acid
RG 83606 diltiazem HCl
RGG0853,E1A generic not yet
  assigned—see main list
RGH 1106 pipecuronium bromide
rgp160 generic not yet assigned—see
  main list
rgp160 MN generic not yet
  assigned—see main list
RGW-2938 prinoxodan
RH-32,565 uredofos
RH-565 uredofos
RHC 2871 eclazolast
RHC 2906 flordipine
RHC 3659-(S) pivopril
RHC 3988 quazolast
rhuMAb CD18 erlizumab
rhuTNFR:Fc etanercept
RI-64 pifexole
Riker 52G aprotinin
Riker 594 sulthiame
Riker 595 butaperazine
Riker 601 triaziquone
RIT 1140 apicycline
RJW 49004 cedelizumab
RJW 60235 becaplermin
r-metHuG-CSF filgrastim
RMI 10,482A metizoline HCl
RMI 16,238 eterobarb
RMI 16,289 enclomiphene
RMI 16,312 zuclomiphene
RMI 80,029 elantrine

RMI 8090DJ quindecamine acetate
RMI 81,182EF cilobamine mesylate
RMI 81,968 medroxalol
RMI 81,968 A medroxalol HCl
RMI 83,027 rolicyprine
RMI 83,047 ambuside
RMI 9,384A desipramine HCl
RMI 9918 terfenadine
RMP-7 lobradimil
Ro 01-6794/706 dextrorphan HCl
Ro 03-7355/000 avizafone
Ro 03-8799 pimonidazole
Ro 09-1978/000 capecitabine
Ro 10-1670/000 acitretin
Ro 10-6338 bumetanide
Ro 106-6271/297 semparatide acetate
Ro107-9070/194 valganciclovir HCl
Ro 10-9070 amdinocillin
Ro 10-9071 amdinocillin pivoxil
Ro 10-9359 etretinate
Ro 11-1163/000 moclobemide
Ro 11-1430 motretinide
Ro 11-1781/023 tiapamil HCl
Ro 12-0068/000 tenoxicam
Ro 13-5057 aniracetam
Ro 13-6438/006 quazinone
RO 13-8996 oxiconazole nitrate
Ro-13-9297 lornoxicam
Ro 13-9904 ceftriaxone sodium
Ro 14-4767/000 amorolfine
Ro 14-9706/000 sumarotene
RO 1-5155 nicotinyl alcohol
Ro 15-1570/000 etarotene
Ro 15-1788/000 flumazenil
Ro 16-6028/000 bretazenil
Ro 1-6794 dextrorphan
Ro 17-2301/006 carumonam sodium
Ro 18-0647/002 orlistat
Ro 1-9334/19 dehydroemetine
Ro 1-9569 tetrabenazine
Ro 19-6327/000 lazabemide
Ro 19-6327/001 lazabemide HCl
Ro 20-5720/000 carprofen
Ro 21-0702 flurocitabine
Ro 21-3981/001 midazolam maleate
Ro 21-3981/003 midazolam HCl
Ro 21-5535 calcitriol
Ro 21-5998 mefloquine
Ro 21-5998/001 mefloquine HCl
Ro 21-6937/000 trimoprostil

Ro 21-8837/001 estramustine phosphate sodium
Ro 22-1319/003 piquindone HCl
Ro 22-2296/000 estramustine
Ro 22-3747/000 tiacrilast
Ro 22-3747/001 tiacrilast sodium
Ro 22-7796 cifenline
Ro 22-7796/001 cifenline succinate
Ro 22-8181 interferon alfa-2a
Ro 22-9000 alfaprostol
Ro 2-2985 lasalocid
Ro 23-0731/000 sedecamycin
Ro 23-3544/000 ablukast
Ro 23-3544/001 ablukast sodium
Ro 23-6019 teceleukin
Ro 23-6240/000 fleroxacin
Ro 2-3773 clidinium bromide
Ro 24-2027/000 zalcitabine
Ro 24-5913 cinalukast
Ro 24-7375 dacliximab
Ro 24-7472/000 edodekin alfa
Ro-25-8315/000 pegnartograstim
Ro 2-9757 fluorouracil
Ro 2-9915 flucytosine
Ro-31-2848/006 cilazapril
Ro 31-3113 cilazaprilat
Ro-31-3948/000 romazarit
Ro 31-8959/000 saquinavir
Ro 31-8959/003 saquinavir mesylate
Ro 32-3555/000 cipemastat
Ro 4-0403 chlorprothixene
Ro 40-5967/001 mibefradil dihydrochloride
Ro 40-7592 tolcapone
Ro 4-1544-6 sodium stibocaptate
Ro 4-1778/1 methopholine
Ro 4-2130 sulfamethoxazole
Ro 42-1611 arteflene
Ro 4-3780 isotretinoin
RO 4-3816 alcuronium chloride
Ro 4-4393 sulfadoxine
Ro 4-4602 benserazide
Ro 44-9883/000 lamifiban
Ro 44-9883/023 lamifiban HCl
Ro 45-2081 lenercept
Ro 4-5282 mefenorex HCl
Ro 4-5360 nitrazepam
Ro 4-6467/1 procarbazine HCl
Ro 46-6240/000 napsagatran
Ro 47-0203/029 bosentan

Code Names

Ro 48347 trengestone
Ro 48-3657/001 sibrafiban
Ro 5-0690 chlordiazepoxide HCl
Ro 5-2092 demoxepam
Ro 5-2807 diazepam
Ro 5-3059 nitrazepam
RO 5-3307/1 debrisoquin sulfate
Ro 5-3350 bromazepam
Ro 5-4023 clonazepam
Ro 5-4200 flunitrazepam
Ro 5-4556 medazepam HCl
Ro 5-4645/010 coumermycin sodium
Ro 5-6901 flurazepam HCl
Ro 5-9110/1 dorastine HCl
Ro 5-9754 ormetoprim
Ro 64-0796/002 oseltamivir phosphate
Ro 6-4563 glibornuride
Ro 70-0001/001 semparatide acetate
Ro 7-0207 ornidazole
Ro 7-0582 misonidazole
Ro 7-1554 ipronidazole
Ro 7-4488/1 cuprimyxin
RP 12222 penmesterol
RP 13057 (as the base) daunorubicin HCl
RP 13607 clotioxone
RP 14539 secnidazole
RP 16091 metiazinic acid
RP 19552 pipotiazine palmitate
R.P. 19,583 ketoprofen
R.P. 20 578 bamnidazole
RP 22,050 HCl zorubicin HCl
RP 22410 glisoxepide
RP 2254 glyprothiazol
RP 2259 glybuthiazol
rp24 generic not yet assigned—see main list
RP 2512 (as isethionate) pentamidine
RP 27267 zopiclone
RP 2921 aminothiazole
RP 2987 diethazine HCl
RP 31264 suriclone
RP 3854 melarsoprol
RP 4763 (as sodium salt) difetarsone
RP 5171 proadifen HCl
RP 5337 spiramycin
RP 54274 rulizole
RP 54476 dalfopristin
RP 54563 enoxaparin sodium
RP-54780 oxaliplatin

RP 56976 docetaxel
RP 57669 quinupristin
RP 60475 intoplicine
RP 62203 fanserin
RP 62955 pagoclone
RP 64305 ebastine
RP 6484 etymemazine HCl
RP 6847 oxomemazine
RP 6870 inproquone
RP 7044 methotrimeprazine
RP 7204 cyamemazine
RP 7293 pristinamycin
RP 73401 piclamilast
RP 7891 glybuzole
RP 8595 dimetridazole
RP 8823 metronidazole
RP 8909 periciazine
RP 9159 perimetazine
RP 9671 nosiheptide
RP 9778 protionamide
RP 9921 aprotinin
RP 9955 melarsonyl potassium
RPI-4610 generic not yet assigned—see main list
RR No. 32705 rutamycin
RS-079070/194 valganciclovir HCl
RS-100302-190 sulamserod HCl
RS-10085-197 moexipril HCl
RS-11988 laidlomycin propionate potassium
RS-1301 delmadinone acetate
RS-1320 flunisolide acetate
RS 15385 delequamine
RS-15385-197 delequamine HCl
RS-21361 imiloxan HCl
RS-21592 ganciclovir
RS-21592 sodium ganciclovir sodium
RS-21607-197 azalanstat dihydrochloride
R&S 218-M alletorphine
RS-2208 amadinone acetate
RS-2252 flucloronide
RS-2362 procinonide
RS-2386 ciprocinonide
RS 25259 palonosetron HCl
RS-25560-197 nepicastat HCl
RS-26306 ganirelix acetate
RS-3268R nandrolone cyclotate
RS-3540 naproxen
RS-35887 butoconazole nitrate

RS-35887-00-10-3 butoconazole nitrate
RS-35909-00-00-0 ticabesone propionate
RS-3650 naproxen sodium
RS-3694R cormethasone acetate
RS-37326 anirolac
RS-37449 temurtide
RS-3999 flunisolide
RS-4034 naproxol
RS-40584 flumoxonide
RS-40974-00-00-0 tiopinac
RS-43179 lonapalene
RS-43285 ranolazine HCl
RS-4464 triclonide
RS-44872 sulconazole nitrate
RS-44872-00-10-3 sulconazole nitrate
RS-4691 cloprednol
RS-49014 tazifylline HCl
R&S 5205-M homprenorphine
RS-61443 mycophenolate mofetil
RS-61443-190 mycophenolate mofetil HCl
RS-6245 tazolol HCl
RS-66271-297 semparatide acetate
RS-6818 xanoxate sodium
RS-68439 detirelix acetate
RS-69216 nicardipine HCl
RS-69216-XX-07-0 nicardipine HCl
RS-7337 tixanox
RS-82856 lixazinone sulfate
RS-82917-030 tifurac sodium
RS-84043 fenprostalene
RS-84135 enprostil
RS-85446-007 timobesone acetate
RS-87476-000 lifarizine
RS-8858 oxfendazole
RS-9390 prostalene
RS-94991-298 nafarelin acetate
RSR-13 generic not yet assigned—see main list
RU 15060 tiaprofenic acid
Ru 15750 floctafenine
RU-1697 trenbolon acetate
RU-19110 halofuginone hydrobromide
RU-2267 altrenogest
RU 2323 gestrinone
RU 23908 nilutamide
RU 24756 cefotaxime sodium
RU 27987 trimegestone

RU 28965 roxithromycin
RU35926 milameline HCl
RU 38486 mifepristone
RU 38882 inocoterone acetate
RU 44570 trandolapril
RU 486 mifepristone
RU 882 inocoterone acetate
RU 965 roxithromycin
RUF 331 rufinamide
RWJ 10131 norgestimate
RWJ-10553 norelgestromin
RWJ 15817 edoxudine
RWJ 15927 rioprostil
RWJ 16600 bemarinone HCl
RWJ-17021 topiramate
RWJ 17070 histrelin
RWJ 18704 pelretin
RWJ 20257 doretinel
RWJ 20485 tepoxalin
RWJ 21757 loroxibine
RWJ 22164 atosiban
RWJ 24517 carsatrin succinate
RWJ 24834 linarotene
RWJ-25213 levofloxacin
RWJ 26251 cladribine
RWJ 28299 immune globulin intravenous pentetate
RWJ 37796 mazapertine succinate
RX 6029-M HCl buprenorphine HCl
Rx 67408 fenclofenac
RX77989 pentamorphone
R-(−)-YM-12617 tamsulosin HCl
S-041 gadodiamide
S-043 sprodiamide
S 10036 fotemustine
S-1210 bietaserpine
S-1320 budesonide
S 1530 nimetazepam
S-16820 prifelone
S-210 morsuximide
S-222 ditazole
S-2395 tertatolol
S-2539F phenothrin
S-25930 ibafloxacin
S26308 imiquimod
S 314 fusafungine
S 4105 medibazine
S-4522 rosuvastatin calcium
S 5614 HCl dexfenfluramine HCl
S-62 chlorphentermine HCl

S 7 fenticlor
S 73 4118 piretanide
S 77 0777 prednicarbate
S-940 naftalofos
S-9490 perindopril
S-9490-3 perindopril erbumine
S-9780 perindoprilat
SA-267 dipenine bromide
SB-075 acetate cetrorelix acetate
SB-202026-A sabcomeline HCl
SB-207266-A piboserod HCl
SB-209247 ticolubant
SB 209509-AX frovatriptan succinate
SB 209763 felvizumab
SB-210396 generic not yet assigned—
see main list
SB-214857-A lotrafiban HCl
SB-217969 generic not yet assigned—
see main list
SB-218842 tidembersat
SB-223030 idoxifene
SB-223412-A talnetant HCl
SB-265805-S gemifloxacin mesylate
SB 7505 ibopamine
SBW-22 ketorfanol
SC 10363 megestrol acetate
SC 11585 oxandrolone
SC 11800 ethynodiol diacetate
SC-12350 nitralamine HCl
SC-12937 azacosterol HCl
SC-13504 ropizine
SC-13957 disopyramide phosphate
SC-14207 metogest
SC-14266 canrenoate potassium
SC-16148 silandrone
SC 1749 (as sodium salt) menbutone
SC-18862 aspartame
SC-19198 methynodiol diacetate
SC-21009 norgestomet
SC-23992 prorenoate potassium
SC-25469 pinadoline
SC-26100 difenoximide HCl
SC-26304 dicirenone
SC-26438 pirolazamide
SC-26714 mexrenoate potassium
SC-27123 octriptyline phosphate
SC-27166 nufenoxole
SC-27761 pranolium chloride
SC-29333 misoprostol
SC-31828 disobutamide

SC-32642 metronidazole HCl
SC-32840 oxagrelate
SC-33643 bemitradine
SC-33963 reclazepam
SC-34301 enisoprost
SC-35135 edifolone acetate
SC-36602 actisomide
SC-37681 gemeprost
SC-38390 zinoconazole HCl
SC-39026 lodelaben
SC-40230 bidisomide
SC-4642 norethynodrel
SC-47111 lomefloxacin HCl
SC-47111A lomefloxacin
SC-47111B lomefloxacin mesylate
SC-48834 remiprostol
SC-49483 generic not yet assigned—
see main list
SC-52151 telinavir
SC-52458 forasartan
SC-54684A xemilofiban HCl
SC-55389A droxinavir HCl
SC-55494 daniplestim
SC-57099B orbofiban acetate
SC-58635 celecoxib
SC-59046 deracoxib
SC-59735 tifacogin
SC-65872 valdecoxib
SC-66110 eplerenone
SC-69124 parecoxib
SC-69124A parecoxib sodium
SC-7031 disopyramide
SC-70935 leridistim
SC-7294 propetandrol
SC-7525 bolandiol dipropionate
SC-9376 canrenone
SC-9880 flurogestone acetate
SCE-1365 (Takeda) (base) cef-
menoxime HCl
Sch 1000-Br-monohydrate ipratro-
pium bromide
Sch 10144 tolnaftate
Sch 10159 triclofos sodium
Sch 10304 clonixin
Sch 10595 bupicomide
Sch 10649 azatadine maleate
Sch 11460 betamethasone dipropionate
Sch 11572 meclorisone dibutyrate
Sch 11973 tosifen
Sch 12041 halazepam

Sch 12149 pazoxide
Sch 12169 closiramine aceturate
Sch 12650 dazadrol maleate
Sch 12679 trepipam maleate
Sch 12707 clonixeril
Sch 13166 D fumarate domazoline fumarate
Sch 13430.2KH$_2$PO$_4$ megalomicin potassium phosphate
Sch 13475 sulfate sisomicin sulfate
Sch 13521 flutamide
Sch 13949W Sulfate albuterol sulfate
Sch 14342 betamicin sulfate
Sch 14714 flunixin
Sch 14714 meglumine flunixin meglumine
Sch 14947 rosaramicin
Sch 14947.NaH$_2$PO$_4$ rosaramicin sodium phosphate
Sch 14947 stearate rosaramicin stearate
Sch 15280 azanator maleate
Sch 15427 carmantadine
Sch 15507 dopamantine
Sch 15698 fletazepam
Sch 15719W labetalol HCl
Sch 16134 quazepam
Sch 16524 repromicin
Sch 17894 rosaramicin propionate
Sch 18020W beclomethasone dipropionate
Sch 18667 rosaramicin butyrate
Sch 19741 picotrin diolamine
Sch 19927 dilevalol HCl
Sch 20569 netilmicin sulfate
Sch 209579 maxacalcitol
Sch 21420 isepamicin
Sch 21480 tioxidazole
Sch 22219 alclometasone dipropionate
Sch 22591 pentisomicin
Sch 25298 florfenicol
Sch 2544 cycliramine maleate
SCH 27899 evernimicin
Sch 28316Z indenolol
Sch 29851 loratadine
Sch 30500 interferon alfa-2b
Sch 31353 dexamethasone acefurate
Sch 32088 mometasone furoate
Sch 32481 netobimin
Sch 33844 spirapril HCl

Sch 33861 spiraprilat
SCH 34117 desloratadine
Sch 3444 parapenzolate bromide
Sch 35852 cisconazole
SCH 39166 ecopipam HCl
Sch 39300 molgramostim
Sch 39400 binetrakin
Sch 39720 ceftibuten
SCH 40054 HCl nemazoline HCl
Sch 4358 meprednisone
Sch 4831 betamethasone
Sch 4855 pseudoephedrine sulfate
SCH 52365 temozlolomide
Sch 56592 posaconazole
SCH58235 ezetimibe
SCH-58500 generic not yet assigned—see main list
Sch 6620 prednazate
Sch 6673 acetophenazine maleate
Sch 6783 diazoxide
Sch 7056 acrisorcin
Sch 9384 oxymetazoline HCl
Sch 9724 gentamicin sulfate
Scha-306 cintazone
SCL-70 alofilcon A
SCT 1 salcatonin
SCTZ (as edisylate) clomethiazole
SCY-Er erythromycin salnacedin
SD 1223-01 trazitiline
SD 1248-17 (as HCl) tropatepine
SD 14112 sulclamide
SD 149-01 feneritrol
SD 15803 vincofos
SD 17102 meticrane
SD 1750 dichlorvos
SD 2102-18 acrocinonide
SD 2124-01 procinolol
SD 25 dicarfen
SD 270-07 (as succinate) oxaprazine
SD 270-31 (as disuccinate) oxaflumazine
SD 271-12 clobenzorex
SD 27115 (as cyclamate) furfenorex
SD 286-03 cimemoxin
SD 7859 clofenvinfos
SDZ-212-713 rivastigmine
SDZ 215-811 pentetreotide
SDZ 215-811s pentetreotide
SDZ ASM 981 pimecrolimus
SDZ-CHI-621 basiliximab

SDZ DIN 608 nateglinide
SDZ-ENA-713 rivastigmine
SDZ-HTF-919 tegaserod
SDZ ILE 964 muplestim
SDZ MSL 109 sevirumab
SDZ OST 577 tuvirumab
SDZ PSC 833 valspodar
SE 1702 gliclazide
SeHCAT tauroselcholic acid
SERM 3 arzoxifene HCl
SF 86-327 terbinafine
SF-R11 bovactant
SG-75 nicorandil
SGD 301-76 oxiconazole nitrate
SGP 3 unifocon A
SH 100 oxapium iodide
SH 1040 gestaclone
SH 1051 glicetanile sodium
SH 2.1139/H 248 AB ioxotrizoic acid
SH 213 AB iotroxic acid
SH 240 moxnidazole
SH 263 droxacin sodium
SH 3.1168 gliflumide
SH 567 methenolone acetate
SH 582 gestonorone caproate
SH 601 methenolone enanthate
SH 714 cyproterone acetate
SH 717 glymidine sodium
SH 723 mesterolone
SH 741 clomegestone acetate
SH 742 fluocortolone
SH 770 fluocortolone caproate
SH 818 clocortolone acetate
SH 863 clocortolone pivalate
SH 926 iodamide
SH 968 diflucortolone pivalate
SH B 331 gestodene
SH E 199 etoformin HCl
SH G 318 AB sermetacin
SH H 200 AB ioglicic acid
SH H 239 AB ioseric acid
SH K 203 fluocortin butyl
SH L 451 A gadopentetate dimeglumine
SIB-1508Y altinicline mesylate
SJ 1977 methixene HCl
SK&F 101468-A ropinirole HCl
SK&F 102,362 nilvadipine
SK&F 104353-Q pobilukast edamine
SKF 105657 epristeride

SK&F 106615-A2 atiprimod dihydrochloride
SF&F 106615-I2 atiprimod dimaleate
SK&F 108566 eprosartan
SK&F 108566-J eprosartan mesylate
SK&F 110679 generic not yet assigned—see main list
SK&F 12866 clorethate
SKF 13338 ampyrimine
SK&F 13364-A thyromedan HCl
SK&F 1340 dimefadane
SK&F 14287 idoxuridine
SK&F 14336 clomacran phosphate
SK&F 15601A toliodium chloride
SKF 16046 anisacril
SK&F 18,667 poloxalene
SK&F 1995 dicloralurea
SK&F 20716 periciazine
SK&F 2208 hetaflur
SK&F 24529 lobendazole
SKF 2599 doxenitoin
SK&F 28175 fluotracen HCl
SK&F 29044 parbendazole
SK&F 30310 oxibendazole
SK&F 3050 cortodoxone
SKF 33134-A amiodarone
SK&F 38094 dectaflur
SK&F 38095 olaflur
SK&F 39162 auranofin
SK&F 39186 amicloral
SK&F 40383 carbuterol HCl
SK&F 41558 cefazolin sodium
SK&F 478 diphenidol
SK&F 478-A diphenidol HCl
SK&F 478-J diphenidol pamoate
SK&F 51 octodrine
SK&F 5116 methotrimeprazine
SK&F 525-A proadifen HCl
SK&F 53705-A sulfonterol HCl
SK&F 59962 cefazaflur sodium
SK&F 61636 bromoxanide
SK&F 62698 ticrynafen
SK&F 62979 albendazole
SK&F 63797 dribendazole
SK&F 6539 flurothyl
SK&F 69634 clopipazan mesylate
SK&F 70230-A pipazethate
SK&F 72517 elfazepam
SK&F 7690 benorterone
SK&F 7988 virginiamycin

SK&F 82526-J fenoldopam mesylate
SKF-8318 xenazoic acid
SK&F 8542 triamterene
SK&F 88373-Z ceftizoxime sodium
SKF 8898-A moroxydine
SK&F 92058 metiamide
SK&F 92657-A₂ prizidilol HCl
SK&F 92676-A₃ impromidine HCl
SK&F 92994-A₂ oxmetidine HCl
SK&F 92994-J₂ oxmetidine mesylate
SK&F 93319 icotidine
SK&F 93479 lupitidine HCl
SK&F 93574 donetidine
SK&F 93944 temelastine
SK&F 94836 siguazodan
SK&F 95587 sulotroban
SK&F 96022 pantoprazole
SK&F 96148 daltroban
SKF 9976 (as citrate) oxolamine
SK&F D-39304 cephradine
SK&F D-75073-Z cefonicid monosodium
SK&F D-75073-Z₂ cefonicid sodium
SK&F S-104846-A topotecan HCl
SL 501 chlophedianol HCl
SL 75 177-10 cicloprolol HCl
SL 75.212-10 betaxolol HCl
SL 76 002 progabide
SL 77 499-10 alfuzosin HCl
SL 79.229-00 fengabine
SL 80.0342-00 alpidem
SL 80.0750-23N zolpidem tartrate
SL 81.0142-00 tolgabide
SM-1213 (free base) amiprilose HCl
SM-3997 tandospirone citrate
SM-7338 meropenem
SMP 68-40 pyrabrom
SMP-78 Acid S ambruticin
SMS-201-995 octreotide
SMS-201-995 ac octreotide acetate
SMS-201-995 pa octreotide pamoate
Sms2PA strontium chloride Sr 89
SN-166 (as the sodium salt) glucosulfone
SN-263 sodium amylosulfate
S.N. 44 insulin, dalanated
SN 654 mepartricin
SND-5008 cevimeline HCl
SNI-2011 cevimeline HCl
SNK-508 cevimeline HCl

SNR 1804 clamidoxic acid
SNX-111 ziconotide
SNX-482 generic not yet assigned—see main list
SP-106 nabitan HCl
SP-119 tinabinol
SP-175 nabazenil
SP-204 menabitan HCl
SP-303 crofelemer
SP-304 pirnabine
SP-325 naboctate HCl
SP54 pentosan polysulfate sodium
SP63 otilonium bromide
SPA-S-132 partricin
SPA-S-160 mepartricin
SPA-S-510 piroxicam cinnamate
SPA-S-565 rifametane
SPC-100270 safingol
SPC-100271 safingol HCl
SPC-101210 cedefingol
SPC 297 D azidocillin
SPC3 generic not yet assigned—see main list
SPI-77 mitopodozide
SPM 925 moexipril HCl
SQ 10,269 carbiphene HCl
SQ 10,496 thiazesim HCl
SQ 10,643 cinanserin HCl
SQ 1089 hydroxyurea
SQ 11,302 epicillin
SQ 11436 cephradine
SQ 11725 nadolol
SQ 13050 econazole nitrate
SQ 13,396 iopamidol
SQ 13847 pirquinozol
SQ 14055 tiamulin
SQ 14,225 captopril
SQ 1489 thiram
SQ 15,101 algestone acetophenide
SQ 15,102 amcinafal
SQ 15,112 amcinafide
SQ 15,659 rolitetracycline
SQ 15,860 glyhexamide
SQ 15,874 pipazethate
SQ 16,123 methicillin sodium
SQ 16,150 estradiol enanthate
SQ 16360 fusidate sodium
SQ 16374 methenolone enanthate
SQ 16,401 halquinols
SQ 16,423 oxacillin sodium

SQ 16496 methenolone acetate
SQ 16,603 fusidic acid
SQ 18566 halcinonide
SQ 19844 sincalide
SQ 20009 etazolate HCl
SQ 20824 cicloprofen
SQ 20881 teprotide
SQ 2128 ethoxazene HCl
SQ 21982 iodoxamic acid
SQ 21983 iopronic acid
SQ 22022 (dihydrate) cephradine
SQ 22947 tiamulin fumarate
SQ 26490 naflocort
SQ 26,703 zofenoprilat arginine
SQ 26776 aztreonam
SQ 26962 mebrofenin
SQ 26991 zofenopril calcium
SQ 27,239 tipredane
SQ 27,519 fosinoprilat
SQ 28555 fosinopril sodium
SQ 29,852 ceronapril
SQ 30217 technetium Tc 99m teboroxime
SQ 30836 tigemonam dicholine
SQ-31,000 pravastatin sodium
SQ 32,097 technetium Tc 99m siboroxime
SQ 32,692 gadoteridol
SQ 32,756 sorivudine
SQ 33,248 calteridol calcium
SQ 34,514 lobucavir
SQ34676 entecavir
SQ-6201 uracil
SQ 65396 cartazolate
SQ-7726 uracil
SQ 82291 oximonam
SQ 82531 gloximonam
SQ 82629 oximonam sodium
SQ 83360 pirazmonam sodium
SQ-8493 uracil
SQ 9343 phytate sodium
SQ 9453 dimethyl sulfoxide
SQ 9538 testolactone
SQ 9993 estradiol undecylate
SR-202 mifobate
SR 2508 etanidazole
SR 25990 C clopidogrel
SR 25990 C clopidogrel bisulfate
SR 33557 fantofarone
SR 41319B tiludronate disodium

SR 47436 irbesartan
SR 57746 generic not yet assigned—see main list
SR-7037 belfosdil
SR 720-22 metolazone
SR 96225 adenosine
SR-96669 oxaliplatin
SRG 95213 diazoxide
St 1085 (as the base) midodrine HCl
ST12 dexamethasone dipropionate
St 1411 dimepregnen
ST1512/SO4 hexoprenaline sulfate
ST-155 clonidine HCl
ST-155-BS clonidine
ST 375 tolonidine
St 567-BR (as hydrobromide) alinidine
ST 600 flutonidine
ST-813 oxiconazole nitrate
ST 9067 azintamide
STA-307 tiomesterone
STI571 imatinib mesylate
St. Peter 224 midodrine HCl
SU-101 leflunomide
Su-10568 clortermine HCl
Su-13437 nafenopin
Su-18137 cyproquinate
Su 21524 pirprofen
Su-4885 metyrapone tartrate
SU-5416 generic not yet assigned—see main list
Su-5864 guanethidine sulfate
Su-6518 dimethindene maleate
Su-8341 cyclopenthiazide
Su-9064 metoserpate HCl
SUD919CL2Y pramipexole
SUM 3170 loxapine
SUN 9216 lanoteplase
SUR 2647 sumacetamol
SYD-230 clioxanide
synthetic TRH protirelin
T-1220 piperacillin sodium
T-1249 generic not yet assigned—see main list
T-1551 cefoperazone sodium
T-1982 cefbuperazone
T-20 pentafuside
T-2636 sedecamycin
T-2636A sedecamycin
T2G1s biciromab

TA-3090 clentiazem maleate
TA 5901 cefempidone
TAK-603 generic not yet assigned—see main list
TAP031 (as the base) fertirelin acetate
TAP-144 leuprolide acetate
TAT-3 picoperine
TATBA triamcinolone hexacetonide
TBC-11251 generic not yet assigned—see main list
TBC-1269z bimosiamose disodium
TBC-3B generic not yet assigned—see main list
Tc 924 (DPD) butedronate tetrasodium
Tc99m-MP 4006 technetium Tc 99m albumin aggregated
Tc99m RP-30A technetium Tc 99m sestamibi
Tc-MAG$_3$ technetium Tc 99m mertiatide
TCV-116 candesartan cilexetil
TE-031 clarithromycin
TE 114 tiemonium iodide
tenite butyrate formula 264 H4 cabufocon B
TH 1165a (as hydrobromide salt) fenoterol
TH-1321 protionamide
Th-152 metaproterenol sulfate
TH-2151 hydracarbazine
TH-2180 propanidid
Th 322 metrifudil
TH-9506 generic not yet assigned—see main list
THFES (HM) zeranol
THR 221 (as sodium) cefodizime
TJ-9 generic not yet assigned—see main list
TLC ABLC generic not yet assigned—see main list
TLC C-53 generic not yet assigned—see main list
TLC D-99 generic not yet assigned—see main list
TMB-4 trimedoxime bromide
TNF MAb nerelimomab
TNO-6 spiroplatin
TNP-470 generic not yet assigned—see main list
TP-1 thymostimulin

TP-10 generic not yet assigned—see main list
TP-20 generic not yet assigned—see main list
TP-21 thioridazine
TP-5 thymopentin
TPN-12 sulforidazine
TPS-23 mesoridazine
TR-2378 broperamole
TR-2515 pelanserin HCl
TR-2855 cromitrile sodium
TR-2985 ropitoin HCl
TR-3369 indorenate HCl
TR-4698 rioprostil
TR-495 methaqualone
TR-4979 butaprost
TR-5109 conorphone HCl
TR-5379M xorphanol mesylate
TS 408 hydrocortisone probutate
TSAA-291 oxendolone
TTFD fursultiamine
TVP-1012 rasagiline mesylate
TVX485 etofenamate
TWSB; TWSb sodium stibocaptate
U-100,592 eperezolid
U-100,766 linezolid
U-10,136 alprostadil
U-101.440E irinotecan HCl
U-10,149 lincomycin
U-108342E trecetilide fumarate
U-10,858 minoxidil
U-10,974 flumethasone
U-10,997 mibolerone
U-11100A nafoxidine HCl
U-12,019E methylprednisolone sodium phosphate
U-12,062 dinoprostone
U-12,241 cirolemycin
U-12898 bluensomycin
U-13,933 asperlin
U-14,583 dinoprost
U-14,583E dinoprost tromethamine
U-14,743 porfiromycin
U-15167 nogalamycin
U-15,614 trestolone acetate
U-15,965 lydimycin
U-17312E etryptamine acetate
U-17,323 fluorometholone acetate
U-17835 tolazamide
U-18,409AE spectinomycin HCl

U-18,496 azacitidine
U-18,573 ibuprofen
U-18,573G ibuprofen aluminum
U-19183 sparsomycin
U-19,646 chlorphenesin carbamate
U-19,718 kalafungin
U-19763 bolasterone
U-19,920 cytarabine
U-19920A cytarabine HCl
U-2032 kethoxal
U-20,661 steffimycin
U-21,251 clindamycin
U-22020 indoxole
U-22,550 calusterone
U-22,559A dexoxadrol HCl
U-24,729A mirincamycin HCl
U-24,792 lomofungin
U-24,973A melitracen HCl
U-25,179 E clindamycin palmitate HCl
U-25,873 ranimycin
U-26,225A tramadol HCl
U-26,452 glyburide
U-27,182 flurbiprofen
U-28,009 denofungin
U-28,288D guanadrel sulfate
U-28,508 clindamycin phosphate
U-28,774 ketazolam
U-29,479 scopafungin
U-30,604 zorbamycin
U-31,889 alprazolam
U-31,920 uldazepam
U-32,070E calcifediol
U-32,921 carboprost
U-32,921E carboprost tromethamine
U-33,030 triazolam
U-34,865 diflorasone diacetate
U-36,059 amitraz
U-36,384 carboprost methyl
U-41,123 adinazolam
U-41,123F adinazolam mesylate
U-42,126 acivicin
U-42,585E lodoxamide tromethamine
U-42,718 lodoxamide ethyl
U-42,842 arbaprostil
U-43,120 paulomycin
U-4527 cycloheximide
U-46,785 meteneprost
U-47,931E bromadoline maleate
U-48,753E eclanamine maleate
U-52,047 menogaril

U-53,059 itazigrel
U-53,217 epoprostenol
U-53,217A epoprostenol sodium
U-53,996H tazadolene succinate
U-54,461 bropirimine
U-54,555 metronidazole phosphate
U-54,669F losulazine HCl
U-56,321 timefurone
U-57,930E pirlimycin HCl
U-5956 filipin
U-6013 isoflupredone acetate
U-60,257 piriprost
U-60,257B piriprost potassium
U-61,431F ciprostene calcium
U-62066E spiradoline mesylate
U-63,196 cefpimizole
U-63,196E cefpimizole sodium
U-63287 ciglitazone
U-63,366F trospectomycin sulfate
U-63,557A fıregrelate sodium
U-64279A ceftiofur HCl
U-64279E ceftiofur sodium
U-66858 bunaprolast
U-67,590A methylprednisolone
U-69689E fertirelin acetate
U-6987 carbutamide
U-70138 paldimycin
U-70226E ibutilide fumarate
U-71038 ditekiren
U-72107A pioglitazone HCl
U-72791 cefmetazole
U-72791A cefmetazole sodium
U-73,975 adozelesin
U-74006F tirilazad mesylate
U-75630 ibuprofen piconol
U-76252 cefpodoxime proxetil
U-77,233 ormaplatin
U-7743 mercufenol chloride
U-7750 streptovarycin
U-77779 bizelesin
U-7800 fluprednisolone
U-78875 panadiplon
U-78,938 dexormaplatin
U-80244 carzelesin
U-82127 alexomycin
U-8344 uracil mustard
U-8471 medrysone
U-85,855 alvircept sudotox
U-87201E atevirdine mesylate
U-88943E artilide fumarate

U89 generic not yet assigned—see main list
U-90152S delavirdine mesylate
U-935 amiquinsin HCl
U-95376 premafloxacin
U-98079A itasetron
U-98528E pramipexole
U-9889 streptozocin
UCB 1402 decloxizine
UCB 1474 chlorbenzoxamine HCl
UCB 1549 minepentate
UCB 1967 dropropizine
UCB 2073 etoxeridine
UCB 3928 fedrilate
UCB 4445 buclizine HCl
UDCG-115 pimobendan
UF-021 isopropyl unoprostone
UH-AC 62XX meloxicam
UK-11,443 primidolol
UK-116,044-04 eletriptan hydrobromide
UK-14304-18 brimonidine tartrate
UK-18,892 butikacin
UK-20,349 tioconazole
UK-2054 famotine HCl
UK-2371 memotine HCl
UK-25,842 oxfenicine
UK-31,214 propikacin
UK-31,557 carbazeran
UK-33,274-27 doxazosin mesylate
UK-3540-1 amedalin HCl
UK-3557-15 daledalin tosylate
UK-37,248-01 dazoxiben HCl
UK-38,485 dazmegrel
UK-4271 oxamniquine
UK-48,340-11 amlodipine maleate
UK-48,340-26 amlodipine besylate
UK-49,858 fluconazole
UK-61260-27 nanterinone
UK-61,689 semduramicin
UK-61,689-2 semduramicin sodium
UK-67,994 doramectin
UK-68,798 dofetilide
UK-738 ethybenztropine
UK-73,967 candoxatrilat
UK-76654-2 (as fumarate) zamifenacin
UK-79,300 candoxatril
UK-80067 modipafant
UK-88060 espatropate

UK-92,480-10 sildenafil citrate
UM 952 buprenorphine HCl
UP 106 propizepine
UP 107 bepiastine
UP 164 morniflumate
UP 74 nixylic acid
UP 83 niflumic acid
USV 3659-(S) pivopril
UT-15 treprostinil sodium
VA-10367 generic not yet assigned—see main list
VAS-972 generic not yet assigned—see main list
V-C 13 dichlofenthion
VCP 205 generic not yet assigned—see main list
VK-57 glyprothiazol
VM-26 teniposide
VML 251 frovatriptan succinate
VML-262 generic not yet assigned—see main list
VP-16-213 etoposide
VP 63843 pleconaril
VT-1 generic not yet assigned—see main list
VUAB6453 (SPOFA) metipranolol
VX-105 arginine butyrate
VX-478 amprenavir
VX-497 generic not yet assigned—see main list
VX-710-3 biricodar dicitrate
VX-740 generic not yet assigned—see main list
VX-853-2 timcodar dimesylate
W-1015 nisobamate
W 10168 vifilcon A
W-1372 beloxamide
W 1655 phenazopyridine HCl
W 1760A namoxyrate
W-19053 (as HCl) etidocaine
W 1929 colistimethate sodium
W 2180 suxemerid sulfate
W 2197 pentrinitrol
W 2291A mimbane HCl
W-2354 seclazone
W 2394A pemerid nitrate
W-2395 meseclazone
W 2426 chlorphentermine HCl
W 2900A etozolin
W-2946M reproterol HCl

W-2964M flupirtine maleate
W 2965 A acetryptine
W-2979M azelastine HCl
W 3207B modaline sulfate
W 3366A quindonium bromide
W3395 algestone acetonide
W 3399 quingestrone
W 3566 quinestrol
W 3580B ampyzine sulfate
W-36095 tocainide
W 3623 cyprazepam
W 3676 sulazepam
W 3699 piprozolin
W 37 buformin
W 3746 cetophenicol
W 3976B triampyzine sulfate
W 4020 prazepam
W 42782 iproxamine HCl
W 43026A ciclafrine HCl
W 4425 almadrate sulfate
W 4454A estrazinol hydrobromide
W 4540 quingestanol acetate
W 4565 oxolinic acid
W 4600 algeldrate
W 4701 hexedine
W 4744 mecloqualone
W 4869 prednival
W-5219 proglumide
W 5494A naranol HCl
W-554 felbamate
W 5733 atolide
W 5759A tilidine HCl
W-583 mebutamate
W 5975 betamethasone benzoate
W 6309 difluprednate
W 6412A bunolol HCl
W 6439A suloxifen oxalate
W 6495 oxisuran
W 7000A levobunolol HCl
W 713 tybamate
W 7320 alclofenac
W7783 ambruticin
W 8495 isoxicam
WA 184 sitogluside
W-A 335 danitracen
WAL 2014 FU talsaclidine fumarate
WAY-ACA-147 eldacimibe
WAY-ANA-756 tasosartan
WAY-ARI-509 minalrestat

WAY-GPA-748 pralmorelin dihydro-
chloride
WAY-PDA-641 filaminast
WAY-PEM-420 dexpemedolac
WAY-SEC-579 mirisetron maleate
WE352 triflubazam
We 941 brotizolam
We 973-BS ciclotizolam
WEB 2086 BS apafant
WF-10 tetrachlorodecaoxide
WG-253 rimiterol hydrobromide
WG 537 (as acetate) flumedroxone
WH 5668 propanidid
WHR-1051B biclodil HCl
WHR-1142A lidamidine HCl
WHR-2908A lofepramine HCl
WHR-5020 etofenamate
WHR-539 fenclorac
Win 11,318 bupivacaine HCl
Win 11450 benorilate
Win 11,464 fludorex
Win 11,530 menoctone
Win 11831 lorajmine HCl
Win 13,146 teclozan
Win 1344 gamfexine
Win 13820 becanthone HCl
Win 14833 stanozolol
Win 17625 azastene
Win 17665 topterone
Win 17,757 danazol
Win 1783 isomethadone
Win 18,320 nalidixic acid
Win 18,320-3 nalidixate sodium
Win 18,413-2 solypertine tartrate
Win 18,501-2 oxypertine
Win 18,935 milipertine
Win 19356 clorindanic acid
Win 20,228 pentazocine
Win 20,740 cyclazocine
Win 21,904 alexidine
WIN 22118 pegorgotein
Win 23,200 volazocine
Win 24,540 trilostane
Win 24,933 hycanthone
Win 25,347 nimazone
Win 25,978 amfonelic acid
Win 27147-2 cyclindole
Win 27,914 nivazol
Win 29194-6 carbantel lauryl sulfate
Win 31,665 alpertine

Win 32,729 epostane
Win 32,784 bitolterol mesylate
Win 3406 isoetharine
Win 34,276 ketazocine
Win 34284 oxarbazole
Win 34886 nisbuterol mesylate
Win 35150 flucindole
Win 35,213 rosoxacin
Win 35833 ciprofibrate
Win 38020 arildone
Win 38770 azarole
Win 39103 metrizamide
Win 39424 iohexol
Win 40014 quinfamide
Win 40350 durapatite
Win 40680 amrinone
Win 40808-7 sulfinalol HCl
Win 41464-2 octenidine HCl
Win 41,464-6 octenidine saccharin
Win 41528-2 fezolamine fumarate
Win 42156-2 tonazocine mesylate
Win 42,202 fosarilate
Win 42964-4 zenazocine mesylate
Win 44,441-3 quadazocine mesylate
Win 47,203-2 milrinone
Win 48,049 ofornine
Win 48,098-6 pravadoline maleate
Win 49,016 medorinone
Win 49,375 amifloxacin
Win 49,375-3 amifloxacin mesylate
Win 49,596 zanoterone
Win 5063 racephenicol
Win 5063-2 thiamphenicol
Win 51,181-2 napamezole HCl
Win 51,711 disoxaril
Win 54,177-4 ipazilide fumarate
Win 5563-3 colterol mesylate
WIN 59010 mangafodipir trisodium
Win 59075 tirapazamine
WIN 63843 pleconaril
Win 771 hydroxypethidine
Win 8851-2 tyropanoate sodium
Win 90,000 cicletanine
Win 9154 inositol niacinate
Win 9317 propatyl nitrate
Wl 140 calcium polycarbophil
Wl 287 euprocin HCl
Wl 291 zolamine HCl
WP-973 chlorhexidine phosphanilate
WR 142,490 mefloquine

WR-171669 halofantrine HCl
WR 180,409 enpiroline phosphate
WR-228,258 tebuquine
WR-2721 amifostine
WV 569 (as HCl) norfenefrine
WX 14812 alofilcon A
WX 14822 hydrofilcon A
WX 2412 fungimycin
WX-G250RIT generic not yet
    assigned—see main list
Wy-1359 propiomazine
WY-15,705 ciramadol
WY-15,705 HCl ciramadol HCl
WY-16,225 dezocine
WY-18,251 tilomisole
Wy-2039 etoxeridine
WY-20,788 penamecillin
WY-21,743 oxaprozin
WY-21,894 fentiazac
Wy 21901 indoramin
WY-21,901 HCl indoramin HCl
WY-22811 HCl meptazinol HCl
WY-23,409 ciclazindol
WY-24,081 HCl tiquinamide HCl
WY-24,377 isotiquimide
Wy-2445 carphenazine maleate
WY-25,021 rolgamidine
Wy-2837 potassium aspartate & mag-
    nesium aspartate
Wy-2838 potassium aspartate & mag-
    nesium aspartate
Wy-3263 iprindole
Wy-3277 nafcillin sodium
Wy-3467 diazepam
Wy-3475 norbolethone
Wy-3478 sodium oxybate
Wy-3498 oxazepam
Wy-3707 norgestrel
Wy-3917 temazepam
Wy-4036 lorazepam
WY-4082 lormetazepam
WY-40,972 lutrelin acetate
WY-42,362 HCl recainam HCl
WY-42,362 tosylate recainam tosylate
WY-44,417 sodium apalcillin sodium
WY-44,635 cefpiramide
WY-44,635 sodium cefpiramide
    sodium
WY-45,030 venlafaxine HCl
Wy-4508 cyclacillin

Code Names

WY-460E thiazinamium chloride
WY-47384 gevotroline HCl
WY-47,663 acetate anaritide acetate
WY-47791 HCl carvotroline HCl
WY-47846 HCl zalospirone HCl
WY-48252 ritolukast
WY-48314 lexithromycin
WY-48624 enciprazine HCl
WY-48986 risotilide HCl
WY-50324 HCl adatanserin HCl
WY-5104 levonorgestrel
Wy-806 oxethazaine
Wy-8138 bisoxatin acetate
Wy-8678 guanabenz
WY-8678 acetate guanabenz acetate
WY-90493 RD ardeparin sodium
X-1497 methicillin sodium
XA41 latanoprost
XI-921 iron sucrose
XLG polyglactin 910
XM-72 polybutester
XR-9576 generic not yet assigned—
see main list
XU 62-320 fluvastatin sodium
XZ-450 azithromycin
Y 3642 tinoridine
Y 4153 (as HCl) clocapramine
Y 6124 (as HCl) bufetolol
YC-93 nicardipine HCl
YKP-10A generic not yet assigned—
see main list

YM-08316 formoterol fumarate
YM-09330 cefotetan disodium
YM-12617-1 tamsulosin HCl
YM617 tamsulosin HCl
YN-72 sorivudine
YTR-830H tazobactam
Z 1282 fosfomycin tromethamine
Z 326 fentonium bromide
Z 424 viminol
Z-4828 trofosfamide
Z4942 ifosfamide
Z 6000 troxerutin
ZCE025 indium In 111 altumomab
ZD1033 anastrozole
ZD 1694 raltitrexed
ZD 4522 calcium salt rosuvastatin
calcium
ZD5077 quetiapine fumarate
ZD9238 fulvestrant
ZK 10 720 ioprocemic acid
ZK 132281 ferucarbotran
ZK 30595 drospirenone
ZK 35760 iopromide
ZK 39 482 iotrolan
ZK 57 671 sulprostone
ZK 62498 azelaic acid
ZK 62 711 rolipram
ZK 71 630 iotetric acid
ZK 76 604 pirazolac
ZK 79 112 iotasul
ZM 204,636 quetirapine fumarate

XRef Street Drug Slang to Pharmaceutical Names

Below are 1540 slang terms for illegally abused drugs. These slang terms are cross-referenced to the actual names of drugs, legal or illegal, that appear in the *Saunders Pharmaceutical Word Book*.

A [see: LSD; amphetamines]

A-bomb *marijuana and heroin smoked together in a cigarette* [see: marijuana; heroin]

Acapulco gold; Acapulco red *marijuana from southwest Mexico* [see: marijuana]

ace [see: marijuana; PCP]

acid [see: LSD]

AD [see: PCP]

Adam [see: MDMA]

Adam and Eve *a combination of MDMA and MDEA* [see: MDMA; MDEA]

African black; African bush; African woodbine [see: marijuana]

ah-pen-yen [see: opium]

aimies; amys *amphetamines, amyl nitrite, or Amytal (amobarbital; discontinued 1991)* [see: amphetamine; amyl nitrite; Amytal Sodium; amobarbital; amobarbital sodium]

AIP *heroin from Afghanistan, Iran, and Pakistan* [see: heroin]

airplane [see: marijuana]

Alice B. Toklas *marijuana brownies* [see: marijuana]

all-American drug [see: cocaine]

alpha-ET [see: alpha-ethyltryptamine]

amoeba [see: PCP]

amp [see: amphetamines]

amp joint *a marijuana cigarette laced with a narcotic* [see: marijuana]

amys; aimies *amphetamines, amyl nitrite, or Amytal (amobarbital; discontinued 1991)* [see: amphetamines; amyl nitrite; Amytal Sodium; amobarbital; amobarbital sodium]

angel; angel dust; angel hair; angel mist; angel poke [see: PCP]

Angola [see: marijuana]

animal [see: LSD]

animal trank; animal tranquilizer [see: PCP]

antifreeze [see: heroin]

Apache [see: fentanyl (citrate)]

apple jacks [see: cocaine, crack]

Aries [see: heroin]

aroma of men [see: isobutyl nitrite]

ashes [see: marijuana]

Assassin of Youth *from a 1930s film of the same name* [see: marijuana]

atom bomb *a combination of marijuana and heroin* [see: marijuana; heroin]

atshitshi [see: marijuana]

aunt Hazel [see: heroin]

aunt Mary [see: marijuana]

aunt Nora [see: cocaine]

auntie; auntie Emma [see: opium]

aurora borealis [see: PCP]

baby; baby bhang [see: marijuana]

baby T [see: cocaine, crack]

backbreakers *a combination of LSD and strychnine* [see: LSD; strychnine]

back-to-back *smoking crack after injecting heroin or vice versa* [see: heroin; cocaine, crack]

backwards *various CNS depressants*

bad [see: cocaine, crack]

bad pizza [see: PCP]

bad seed [see: mescaline; heroin; marijuana]

bag *1 to 15 g of heroin; also known as a "deck"* [see: heroin]

bah-say [see: cocaine, crack; coca paste]

bale *1 pound of marijuana* [see: marijuana]

ball [see: cocaine, crack]

ballot [see: heroin]

bam *various CNS depressants or amphetamines* [see: amphetamines]

bambalacha [see: marijuana]

bambs *various CNS depressants*

bammy [see: marijuana]

banano *(Spanish for "banana tree") a marijuana or tobacco cigarette laced with cocaine* [see: marijuana; tobacco; cocaine]

bank bandit pills *various CNS depressants*

bar [see: marijuana]

barb; barbie doll; barbies; barbs *various CNS depressants, primarily barbiturates*

barbs [see: cocaine]

barrels [see: LSD]

base; baseball *from "freebase"* [see: cocaine, crack]

bash [see: marijuana]

basuco *coca paste or coca paste residue sprinkled on a marijuana or tobacco cigarette* [see: coca paste; marijuana; tobacco]

bathtub speed [see: methcathinone]

battery acid [see: LSD]

batu *smokable methamphetamine* [see: methamphetamine HCl]

bazooka *crack or a combination of coca paste and marijuana* [see: cocaine, crack; coca paste; marijuana]

bazulco [see: cocaine]

B-bomb *1940s slang for a Benzedrine inhaler (amphetamine sulfate; discontinued)*

beam me up Scotty *crack dipped in PCP* [see: cocaine, crack; PCP]

beans *amphetamines, various CNS depressants, or mescaline* [see: amphetamines; mescaline]

beast [see: LSD]

beautiful boulders [see: cocaine, crack]

bebe [see: cocaine, crack]

beemers [see: cocaine, crack]

Belushi *a combination of cocaine and heroin (from the actor John Belushi, who died of an overdose)* [see: cocaine; heroin]

belyando spruce [see: marijuana]

bennie; bennies; Benny and the Jets *Benzedrine (amphetamine sulfate; discontinued 1982) or any of the amphetamines* [see: amphetamine sulfate; amphetamines]

benz *Benzedrine (amphetamine sulfate; discontinued 1982) or any of the amphetamines* [see: amphetamine sulfate; amphetamines]

Bernice; Bernie; Bernie's flakes; Bernie's gold dust [see: cocaine]

bhang *an Indian term* [see: marijuana]

big 8 *1/8 kg of crack (about 4½ ounces)* [see: cocaine, crack]

big bag [see: heroin]

big C [see: cocaine]

big chief [see: mescaline]

big D [see: LSD]

big flake [see: cocaine]

big H; big Harry [see: heroin]

big O [see: opium]

big rush [see: cocaine]

Bill Blass [see: cocaine, crack]

Billie hoke [see: cocaine]

bings [see: cocaine, crack]

birdie powder [see: heroin; cocaine]

biscuit *50 rocks of crack* [see: cocaine, crack]

black [see: opium; marijuana]

black acid *LSD or a combination of LSD and PCP* [see: LSD; PCP]

black and white [see: amphetamines]

black Bart [see: marijuana]

black beauties *amphetamines or various CNS depressants* [see: amphetamines]

black beauties *Biphetamine (amphetamine + dextroamphetamine; discontinued 1993)* [see: amphetamines; amphetamine sulfate; dextroamphetamine]

black birds; black bombers [see: amphetamines]

black ganga *marijuana resin* [see: marijuana]

black gold *a high-potency marijuana* [see: marijuana]

black gungi *marijuana from India* [see: marijuana]

black gunion [see: marijuana]

black hash *a combination of opium and hashish* [see: opium; hashish]

black mo; black moat *highly potent marijuana* [see: marijuana]

black mollies [see: amphetamines]

black mote *marijuana mixed with honey* [see: marijuana]

black pearl [see: heroin]

black pill *an opium pill* [see: opium]

black rock [see: cocaine, crack]

black Russian *very potent hashish or a combination of hashish and opium* [see: hashish; opium]

black star [see: LSD]

black stuff [see: heroin]

black stuff; black tar opium *a tar-like opium for smoking* [see: opium]

black sunshine [see: LSD]

black tabs [see: LSD]

black tar [see: heroin; opium]

black tar heroin; black Tootsie Roll *a potent form of heroin from Mexico* [see: heroin]

black whack [see: PCP]

blacks [see: amphetamines]

blanco (Spanish for "white") [see: heroin]

blanket *a marijuana cigarette* [see: marijuana]

block *marijuana or crude opium or a cube of morphine* [see: marijuana; opium; morphine]

blockbusters *Nembutal (pentobarbital; discontinued 1979) or various CNS depressants*

blonde [see: marijuana]

blood madman [see: PCP]

blotter [see: LSD; cocaine]

blotter acid; blotter cube [see: LSD]

blow up *crack cocaine cut (diluted) with lidocaine to increase size and weight* [see: cocaine, crack]

blowcaine *crack cocaine cut (diluted) with powdered cocaine* [see: cocaine, crack; cocaine]

blowing smoke [see: marijuana]

blowout [see: cocaine, crack]

blue *crack or various CNS depressants* [see: cocaine, crack]

blue acid [see: LSD]

blue and clears *Fastin (phentermine HCl), which is a blue and clear capsule filled with blue and white balls* [see: Fastin; phentermine]

blue angels *various CNS depressants*

blue barrels [see: LSD]

blue boy [see: amphetamines]

blue bullets *various CNS depressants*

blue caps [see: mescaline]

blue chairs; blue cheers [see: LSD]

blue de hue *marijuana from Vietnam* [see: marijuana]

blue devil *various CNS depressants*

blue dolls *various CNS depressants*

blue heaven [see: LSD]

blue heavens; bluebirds *Amytal (amobarbital; discontinued 1991), Amytal Sodium (amobarbital sodium), or other depressants* [see: Amytal Sodium; amobarbital; amobarbital sodium]

blue microdot; blue mist; blue moons [see: LSD]

Blue Nitro *gamma butyrolactone (GBL), a precursor to gamma hydroxybutyrate (GHB)* [see: gamma butyrolactone (GBL); gamma hydroxybutyrate (GHB)]

blue sage [see: marijuana]

blue sky bond *high-potency marijuana from Colombia* [see: marijuana]

blue star *a type of blotter LSD* [see: LSD]

blue tabs [see: LSD]

blue tips *various CNS depressants*

blue velvet *a combination of paregoric and tripelennamine, used as a weak heroin substitute*

blue velvet *a combination of terpin hydrate, codeine, and tripelennamine, used as a weak heroin substitute*

Blue Verve *gamma butyrolactone (GBL), a precursor to gamma hydroxybutyrate (GHB)* [see: gamma butyrolactone (GBL); gamma hydroxybutyrate (GHB)]

blue vials [see: LSD]

bluebirds; blue heavens Amytal (amobarbital; discontinued 1991), Amytal Sodium (amobarbital sodium), or other depressants [see: Amytal Sodium; amobarbital; amobarbital sodium]

blues Amytal (amobarbital; discontinued 1991), named for the blue-colored capsules [see: Amytal Sodium; amobarbital; amobarbital sodium]

blues and reds Amytal (amobarbital; discontinued 1991) and Seconal (secobarbital; discontinued 1990) [see: Amytal Sodium; amobarbital; Seconal Sodium; secobarbital]

blunt marijuana or a combination of marijuana and cocaine in a cigar [see: marijuana; cocaine]

boat [see: PCP]

bobo; boubou; bobo bush (Spanish for "fool" or "idiot") [see: marijuana; cocaine, crack]

bohd [see: marijuana; PCP]

Bolivian marching powder [see: cocaine]

bolo (Spanish and Italian for "bolus") [see: cocaine, crack]

bolt [see: butyl nitrite; isobutyl nitrite]

bomb [see: cocaine, crack; heroin; marijuana]

bomber a marijuana cigarette [see: marijuana]

bombido; bombita injectable amphetamines, heroin, or various CNS depressants [see: amphetamines; heroin]

bombita (Spanish for "little bomb") injectable Desoxyn (methamphetamine HCl; discontinued 1980) [see: methamphetamine HCl; amphetamines]

bombs away [see: heroin]

bone marijuana or a $50 piece of crack [see: marijuana; cocaine, crack]

bonecrusher; bones [see: cocaine, crack]

bonita (Spanish for "beautiful") [see: heroin]

boo [see: marijuana]

boom [see: marijuana]

boomers [see: psilocybin; psilocin]

booster inhaled (snorted) cocaine [see: cocaine]

boppers [see: amyl nitrite]

botray [see: cocaine, crack]

bottles [see: amphetamines]

boubou; bobo [see: cocaine, crack]

boulder a $20 piece of crack, or crack in general [see: cocaine, crack]

boulya [see: cocaine, crack]

boy [see: heroin]

bozo [see: heroin]

brain ticklers [see: amphetamines]

breakdowns a $40 piece of crack sold for $20 [see: cocaine, crack]

brick 1 kilo (kg) of marijuana or crack in general [see: marijuana; cocaine, crack]

brick gum [see: heroin]

Britton [see: mescaline]

broccoli [see: marijuana]

brother [see: heroin]

brown [see: heroin; marijuana]

brown and clears Dexedrine (dextroamphetamine sulfate) Spansules (brown and clear capsules) [see: Dexedrine; dextroamphetamine sulfate; amphetamines]

brown bombers [see: LSD]

brown crystal [see: heroin]

brown dots [see: LSD]

brown rhine; brown sugar [see: heroin]

brownies; browns amphetamines, especially Dexedrine Spansules (dextroamphetamine sulfate in brown capsules) [see: Dexedrine; dextroamphetamine sulfate; amphetamines]

bubble gum [see: cocaine; cocaine, crack]

bud [see: marijuana]

buda; budda; buddha potent, high-grade marijuana mixed with opium or crack [see: marijuana; opium; cocaine, crack]

bullet [see: isobutyl nitrite]

bullet bolt various inhalants

bullia capital [see: cocaine, crack]

bullion; bullyon [see: cocaine, crack; marijuana]

bumblebees [see: amphetamines]

bump crack, fake crack, or a $20 dose of ketamine [see: cocaine, crack; ketamine HCl]

bundle [see: heroin]
bunk *fake cocaine* [see: cocaine]
Burese [see: cocaine]
burnie [see: marijuana]
burrito [see: marijuana]
bush [see: cocaine; marijuana]
businessman's LSD; businessman's special; businessman's trip [see: dimethyltryptamine]
busters *various CNS depressants*
busy bee [see: PCP]
butt naked [see: PCP]
butter [see: marijuana; cocaine, crack]
butter flower [see: marijuana]
buttons [see: mescaline]
butu [see: heroin]
buzz bomb *nitrous oxide or a device for inhaling nitrous oxide from small canisters* [see: nitrous oxide]
caballo (Spanish for "horse") [see: heroin]
cabello (Spanish for "hair") [see: cocaine]
cactus; cactus buttons; cactus head [see: mescaline]
Cadillac [see: PCP]
Cadillac express [see: methcathinone]
'caine [see: cocaine; cocaine, crack]
cakes *round disks of crack* [see: cocaine, crack]
California cornflakes [see: cocaine]
California sunshine [see: LSD]
Cam red; Cam trip; Cambodian red *high-potency marijuana from Cambodia* [see: marijuana]
came [see: cocaine]
can *1 oz. of marijuana* [see: marijuana]
Canadian black [see: marijuana]
canamo (Spanish for "hemp") [see: marijuana]
canappa [see: marijuana]
cancelled stick *a marijuana cigarette* [see: marijuana]
candy *illegal drugs in general*
candy C; candy cane; candycaine [see: cocaine]
cannabis tea [see: marijuana]
cap; caps [see: cocaine, crack; LSD; heroin; psilocin; psilocybin]
capital H [see: heroin]

caps; cap [see: cocaine, crack; LSD; heroin; psilocin; psilocybin]
Captain Cody [see: codeine]
carga (Spanish for "weight" or "load") [see: heroin]
carne; carnie (Spanish for "meat") [see: heroin; cocaine]
Carrie; Carrie Nation [see: cocaine]
cartucho (Spanish for "cartridge") *a pack of marijuana cigarettes* [see: marijuana]
cartwheels [see: amphetamines]
Casper the ghost [see: cocaine, crack]
cat [see: methcathinone]
cat valium [see: ketamine HCl]
catnip *a marijuana cigarette* [see: marijuana]
caviar [see: cocaine, crack]
cavite all star [see: marijuana]
C-dust; C-game [see: cocaine]
Cecil [see: cocaine]
chalk [see: methamphetamine HCl; amphetamines]
champagne of drugs [see: cocaine HCl]
chandoo; chandu [see: opium]
charas *marijuana from India* [see: marijuana]
charge [see: marijuana]
Charley; Charlie [see: heroin; cocaine]
chasing the dragon *inhaling vapors of heroin or cocaine (powder or crack) heated on tinfoil* [see: heroin; cocaine; cocaine, crack]
chasing the tiger *smoking heroin* [see: heroin]
cheap basing [see: cocaine, crack]
cheeba; cheeo [see: marijuana]
chemical [see: cocaine, crack]
cheroot *a tobacco and/or marijuana cigar* [see: tobacco; marijuana]
cherry menth [see: gamma hydroxybutyrate (GHB)]
chewies [see: cocaine, crack]
chiba chiba *high-potency marijuana from Colombia* [see: marijuana]
Chicago black; Chicago green [see: marijuana]
chick [see: heroin]
chicken powder [see: amphetamines]

Street Slang

chicle [see: heroin]
chief [see: LSD; mescaline]
chieva [see: heroin]
China cat *high-potency heroin* [see: heroin]
China girl; China town [see: fentanyl (citrate)]
China white *very pure heroin, fentanyl, or a fentanyl analogue used as a heroin substitute* [see: heroin; fentanyl citrate]
Chinese molasses [see: opium]
Chinese red [see: heroin]
Chinese tobacco [see: opium]
chip [see: heroin]
chippy [see: cocaine]
chips *tobacco or marijuana cigarettes laced with PCP* [see: tobacco; marijuana; PCP]
chira [see: marijuana]
chocolate [see: hashish; opium; amphetamines]
chocolate chips [see: LSD]
chocolate ecstasy *crack made brown by adding chocolate milk powder during production* [see: cocaine, crack]
cholly [see: cocaine]
chorals *various CNS depressants*
Chris; cris; Christina; Cristina [see: methamphetamine HCl]
Christmas rolls *various CNS depressants*
Christmas tree *marijuana, various CNS depressants, or amphetamines* [see: marijuana; amphetamines]
Christmas trees *Dexamyl (dextroamphetamine sulfate + amobarbital; discontinued 1980) in green and clear capsules* [see: dextroamphetamine sulfate; amobarbital; amphetamines]
Christy; Cristy *smokable methamphetamine* [see: methamphetamine HCl]
chronic *marijuana or marijuana mixed with crack* [see: marijuana; cocaine, crack]
churus [see: marijuana]
CIBAs *Doriden (glutethimide; discontinued 1990)* [see: glutethimide]
cid [see: LSD]
cigarette paper *a packet of heroin* [see: heroin]
cigarrode cristal [see: PCP]

circles *Rohypnol (flunitrazepam; not marketed in the U.S.)* [see: Rohypnol; flunitrazepam]
citrol *high-potency marijuana from Nepal* [see: marijuana]
clarity [see: MDMA]
clicker *a combination of crack and PCP* [see: cocaine, crack; PCP]
cliffhanger [see: PCP]
climax [see: butyl nitrite; isobutyl nitrite; cocaine, crack; heroin]
climb *a marijuana cigarette* [see: marijuana]
clips *rows of vials heat-sealed together*
cloud; cloud nine [see: cocaine, crack]
coast-to-coast *a reference to truckers' use of amphetamines for long-distance runs* [see: amphetamines]
coca [see: cocaine]
coca paste; cocaine paste *a barely refined cocaine with adulterants* [see: cocaine]
cochornis [see: marijuana]
cocktail *a cigarette laced with cocaine, crack, or marijuana* [see: cocaine; cocaine, crack; marijuana]
coco rocks *dark brown crack made by adding chocolate pudding during production* [see: cocaine, crack]
coco snow *benzocaine used as a cutting agent for crack* [see: cocaine, crack; benzocaine]
coconut [see: cocaine]
Cody [see: codeine]
coffee [see: LSD]
coke [see: cocaine; cocaine, crack]
cola [see: cocaine]
colas *(Spanish for "tails") a reference to the flowering tops of marijuana plants* [see: marijuana]
coli [see: marijuana]
coliflor tostada *(Spanish for "brown or toasted cauliflower")* [see: marijuana]
Colombian [see: marijuana]
Colorado cocktail [see: marijuana]
Columbo [see: PCP]
Columbus black [see: marijuana]
comeback *the benzocaine and mannitol used in the conversion of cocaine to crack* [see: cocaine; cocaine, crack]

conductor [see: LSD]
contact lens [see: LSD]
cookies [see: cocaine, crack]
cooler *a regular cigarette laced with a drug*
coolie *a regular cigarette laced with cocaine* [see: cocaine]
co-pilot [see: amphetamines]
coral *various CNS depressants*
cork the air *inhaling (snorting) powdered cocaine* [see: cocaine]
Corrine [see: cocaine]
cosa (Spanish and Italian for "thing") [see: marijuana]
Cozmo's [see: PCP]
'cotics *from "narcotics"* [see: heroin]
cotton brothers *a combination of cocaine, heroin, and morphine* [see: cocaine; heroin; morphine]
cotton fever *septicemia caused by injecting small amounts of cotton fiber with the drugs*
courage pills *heroin or various CNS depressants* [see: heroin]
crack [see: cocaine, crack]
crack back *a combination of crack and marijuana* [see: cocaine, crack; marijuana]
crack cooler *crack soaked in a wine cooler* [see: cocaine, crack]
crackers [see: cocaine, crack]
crank *various amphetamines, especially methamphetamine, or methcathinone* [see: amphetamines; methamphetamine HCl; methcathinone]
crazy coke; crazy Eddie [see: PCP]
crazy weed [see: marijuana]
cream and crimson *Dalmane (flurazepam HCl), named for the white and red capsules* [see: Dalmane; flurazepam HCl]
crib [see: cocaine, crack]
crimmie *a regular cigarette laced with crack* [see: cocaine, crack]
crink [see: methamphetamine HCl]
cripple *a marijuana cigarette* [see: marijuana]
cris; Chris; Cristina; Christina [see: methamphetamine HCl]
crisscross [see: amphetamines]

Cristina; Christina; cris; Chris [see: methamphetamine HCl]
Cristy; Christy *smokable methamphetamine* [see: methamphetamine HCl]
croak *a combination of crack and methamphetamine* [see: cocaine, crack; methamphetamine HCl]
crop *low-quality heroin* [see: heroin]
cross tops [see: amphetamines]
crossroads [see: amphetamines]
crown crap [see: heroin]
crumbs *tiny pieces of crack* [see: cocaine, crack]
crunch and munch [see: cocaine, crack]
'cruz *opium from Veracruz, Mexico* [see: opium]
crying weed [see: marijuana]
crypto [see: methamphetamine HCl]
crystal [see: methamphetamine HCl; Desoxyn; amphetamines; PCP; cocaine]
crystal; krystal; crystal joint; krystal joint [see: PCP]
crystal joint [see: PCP]
crystal meth [see: methamphetamine HCl]
crystal tea; crystal T [see: LSD; PCP]
cube; cubes *morphine, LSD, marijuana tablets, or 1 oz. of any drug* [see: morphine; LSD; marijuana]
culican *high-potency marijuana from Mexico* [see: marijuana]
cupcakes [see: LSD]
cura (Spanish for "cure"; Italian for "care") [see: heroin]
cut-deck *heroin mixed with powdered milk* [see: heroin]
cycline; cyclones [see: PCP]
cyclones; cycline [see: PCP]
dagga [see: marijuana]
dama blanca (Spanish for "white lady") [see: cocaine]
dance fever [see: fentanyl citrate]
date rape drug *Rohypnol (flunitrazepam; not marketed in the U.S.)* [see: Rohypnol; flunitrazepam]
dawamesk [see: marijuana]
dead on arrival; DOA [see: heroin; PCP; cocaine, crack]

Street Slang

decadence [see: MDMA]

deck *1 to 15 g of heroin; also known as a "bag"* [see: heroin]

deeda [see: LSD]

demo *a sample-size piece of crack* [see: cocaine, crack]

demolish [see: cocaine, crack]

Detroit pink [see: PCP]

deuce *heroin or $2 worth of drugs* [see: heroin]

devil's dandruff; devilsmoke [see: cocaine, crack]

devil's dust [see: PCP]

dew; 'due *marijuana or the residue of oils left in a pipe after smoking crack* [see: marijuana; cocaine, crack]

dexies *Dexedrine (dextroamphetamine sulfate) or various other amphetamines, especially dextroamphetamine* [see: Dexedrine; dextroamphetamine sulfate; amphetamines]

diamba; djamba [see: marijuana]

diet pills [see: amphetamines]

dillys [see: Dilaudid; hydromorphone HCl]

dimba *marijuana from West Africa* [see: marijuana]

dime *$10 worth of crack* [see: cocaine, crack]

dime store high *glue sniffing* [see: petroleum distillate inhalants]

dime's worth *the amount of heroin needed to cause death* [see: heroin]

ding [see: marijuana]

dinkie dow [see: marijuana]

dip [see: cocaine, crack]

dipper [see: PCP]

dirt [see: heroin]

dirt grass *inferior-quality marijuana* [see: marijuana]

dirty basing [see: cocaine, crack]

disco biscuits *Quaalude (methaqualone; discontinued 1983) or other CNS depressants* [see: methaqualone]

ditch; ditch weed *inferior-quality marijuana from Mexico or any low-potency marijuana that grows wild* [see: marijuana]

djamba; diamba [see: marijuana]

do a joint *smoking marijuana* [see: marijuana]

do a line *inhaling (snorting) powdered cocaine* [see: cocaine]

DOA; dead on arrival [see: heroin; PCP; cocaine, crack]

doctor [see: MDMA]

dog food [see: heroin]

dogie; doojee [see: heroin]

dollies *methadone (from the brand name Dolophine)* [see: Dolophine HCl; methadone HCl]

dolls *various CNS depressants*

domes [see: LSD]

domestic *locally grown marijuana* [see: marijuana]

domex *a combination of PCP and MDMA* [see: PCP; MDMA]

dominoes [see: amphetamines]

don jem [see: marijuana]

Dona Juana; Dona Juanita [see: marijuana]

doobie [see: marijuana]

doojee; dogie [see: heroin]

dooley [see: heroin]

doors *Doriden (glutethimide; discontinued 1990)* [see: glutethimide]

doors and fours *Doriden (glutethimide; discontinued 1990) and codeine* [see: glutethimide; codeine]

dope *heroin, marijuana, or any other street drug* [see: heroin; marijuana]

dope smoke [see: marijuana]

dopium [see: opium]

doradilla [see: marijuana]

dots [see: LSD]

doub *a $20 piece of crack* [see: cocaine, crack]

double bubble [see: cocaine]

double cross [see: amphetamines]

double dome [see: LSD]

double rock *crack diluted with procaine* [see: cocaine, crack; procaine]

double trouble *Dexamyl (dextroamphetamine sulfate + amobarbital; discontinued 1980)* [see: dextroamphetamine sulfate; amobarbital]

double trouble *Tuinal (amobarbital sodium + secobarbital sodium) or other*

CNS *depressants* [see: Tuinal; amobarbital sodium; secobarbital sodium]
double yoke [see: cocaine, crack]
dove *a $35 piece of crack* [see: cocaine,
crack]
Dover's powder [see: opium]
down; downer; downies *various CNS
depressants*
down and dirty *Quaalude (methaqualone; discontinued 1983)* [see: metha-
qualone]
draf weed; drag weed [see: marijuana]
dream [see: cocaine]
dream gum; dream stick; dreams
[see: opium]
dreamer [see: morphine]
dreck [see: heroin]
drink [see: PCP]
drowsy high *various CNS depressants*
drug store dope [see: morphine]
dry high [see: marijuana]
duct [see: cocaine]
'due; dew *marijuana or the residue of
oils left in a pipe after smoking crack*
[see: marijuana; cocaine, crack]
duji [see: heroin]
dummy dust [see: PCP]
durog; duros [see: marijuana]
dust *heroin, cocaine, PCP, or marijuana
mixed with various other substances* [see:
heroin; cocaine; PCP; marijuana]
**dust joint; dust of angels; dusted
parsley** [see: PCP]
dusting *a combination of marijuana and
PCP, heroin, or other powdered street
drug* [see: marijuana; PCP; heroin]
dusty roads *a combination of cocaine and
PCP for smoking* [see: cocaine; PCP]
dynamite *a combination of heroin and
cocaine* [see: heroin; cocaine]
dyno; dyno-pure [see: heroin]
earth *a marijuana cigarette* [see: mari-
juana]
easing powder [see: opium]
eastside player [see: cocaine, crack]
easy lay; EZlay [see: gamma hydroxybutyrate (GHB)]
Eclipse *gamma butyrolactone (GBL), a
precursor to gamma hydroxybutyrate
(GHB)* [see: gamma butyrolactone

(GBL); gamma hydroxybutyrate
(GHB)]
ecstasy; ex; X [see: MDMA]
egg [see: cocaine, crack]
eight ball *heroin or 1/8 oz. of any drug*
[see: heroin]
eighth [see: heroin]
el diablillo (Spanish for "the little
devil") *a combination of marijuana,
cocaine, heroin, and PCP* [see: marijuana; cocaine; heroin; PCP]
el diablo (Spanish for "the devil") *a
combination of marijuana, cocaine,
and heroin* [see: marijuana; cocaine;
heroin]
electric Kool Aid [see: LSD]
elephant; elephant tranquilizer [see:
PCP]
embalming fluid [see: PCP]
emsel *a pronunciation of the brand name
MS/L (morphine sulfate liquid)* [see:
MS/L; morphine sulfate]
endo [see: marijuana]
energizer [see: PCP]
ephedrone [see: methcathinone]
esrar (Turkish for "secret prepara-
tion") *a mixture of marijuana and
tobacco* [see: marijuana; tobacco]
essence [see: MDMA]
estufa (Spanish for "stove") [see: heroin]
ET [see: alpha-ethyltryptamine]
Eve [see: MDMA]
ex; X; extasy *from "ecstasy"* [see:
MDMA]
eye opener [see: cocaine, crack;
amphetamines]
EZlay; easy lay [see: gamma hydroxybutyrate (GHB)]
fairy dust [see: heroin]
fake STP [see: PCP]
Fallbrook redhair *marijuana from
Fallbrook, California* [see: marijuana]
famous dimes [see: cocaine, crack]
fantasia [see: dimethyltryptamine]
fat bags [see: cocaine, crack]
fatty *a marijuana cigarette* [see: mari-
juana]
feenies [see: phenobarbital]
fennies; phennies [see: phenobarbital]
feno's; pheno's [see: phenobarbital]

fields [see: LSD]

fifty-one; one-fifty-one [see: cocaine, crack]

fine stuff [see: marijuana]

finger *a marijuana cigarette or a stick-shaped piece of hashish* [see: marijuana; hashish]

fir [see: marijuana]

fire *a combination of crack and methamphetamine* [see: cocaine, crack; methamphetamine HCl]

first line [see: morphine]

fish scales [see: cocaine, crack]

fives [see: amphetamine]

fizzies [see: methadone]

flake; flakes [see: cocaine; PCP]

flamethrowers *a cigarette laced with cocaine and heroin* [see: cocaine; heroin]

flash *glue (for sniffing) or LSD* [see: petroleum distillate inhalants; LSD]

flat blues [see: LSD]

flat chunks *crack cocaine cut (diluted) with benzocaine* [see: cocaine, crack]

flea powder *low-purity heroin* [see: heroin]

Florida snow *cocaine or a cocaine look-alike* [see: cocaine]

flower; flower tops [see: marijuana]

fly agaric [see: *Amanita muscaria* mushrooms]

Flying Saucers [see: morning glory seeds]

fo-do-nie [see: opium]

foo foo dust; foo foo stuff [see: cocaine; heroin]

foolish powder [see: cocaine; heroin]

footballs *Dilaudid (hydromorphone HCl) or Biphetamine (dextroamphetamine + amphetamine; discontinued 1979)* [see: Dilaudid; hydromorphone HCl; amphetamines]

forwards [see: amphetamines]

four doors *a combination of Doriden (glutethimide; discontinued 1990) and codeine* [see: glutethimide; codeine]

four ways *a combination of LSD, methamphetamine, strychnine, and STP* [see: LSD; methamphetamine HCl; strychnine; STP]

fours [see: Tylenol with Codeine No. 4; Empirin with Codeine No. 4; codeine]

fraho; frajo [see: marijuana]

freeze [see: cocaine]

French blue [see: amphetamine]

French fries; fries; fry [see: cocaine, crack]

fresh [see: PCP]

friend [see: fentanyl]

fries; French fries; fry [see: cocaine, crack]

frio *(Spanish for "cold") marijuana laced with PCP* [see: marijuana; PCP]

Frisco special; Frisco speedball *a combination of cocaine, heroin, and LSD* [see: cocaine; heroin; LSD]

Friskie powder [see: cocaine]

fry; fries; French fries [see: cocaine, crack]

fry daddy *a regular or marijuana cigarette laced with crack* [see: marijuana; cocaine, crack]

Fu [see: marijuana]

fuel *PCP or marijuana mixed with insecticides* [see: PCP; marijuana]

fumo d'Angola *(Spanish for "Angola smoke")* [see: marijuana]

fungus *a reference to the source (mushrooms)* [see: psilocybin]

funk [see: marijuana]

funny stuff [see: marijuana]

G; gee [see: paregoric; opium]

gaffel *fake cocaine* [see: cocaine]

gagers; gaggers [see: methcathinone]

galloping horse [see: heroin]

Gamma Ram *gamma butyrolactone (GBL), a precursor to gamma hydroxybutyrate (GHB)* [see: gamma butyrolactone (GBL); gamma hydroxybutyrate (GHB)]

gamot [see: heroin]

ganga; gange; ganja; Ghana; ghanja; gunga; gungeon [see: marijuana]

gangster [see: marijuana]

gank *fake crack* [see: cocaine, crack]

garbage rock [see: cocaine, crack]

gas [see: nitrous oxide]

gash [see: marijuana]

gasper; gasper stick *a marijuana ciga-rette* [see: marijuana]

gato (*Spanish for "cat"*) [see: heroin]

gauge; gauge butt [see: marijuana]

gee; G [see: paregoric; opium]

geek *a combination of crack and mari-juana* [see: cocaine, crack; marijuana]

George smack [see: heroin]

Georgia home boy [see: gamma hydroxybutyrate (GHB)]

get your own [see: cocaine]

GH Gold *gamma butyrolactone (GBL), a precursor to gamma hydroxybutyrate (GHB)* [see: gamma butyrolactone (GBL); gamma hydroxybutyrate (GHB)]

GH Revitalizer (GHR) *gamma buty-rolactone (GBL), a precursor to gamma hydroxybutyrate (GHB)* [see: gamma butyrolactone (GBL); gamma hydroxybutyrate (GHB)]

Ghana; ghanja; ganga; gange; ganja; gunga; gungeon [see: marijuana]

ghost [see: LSD]

GHR (GH Revitalizer) *gamma buty-rolactone (GBL), a precursor to gamma hydroxybutyrate (GHB)* [see: gamma butyrolactone (GBL); gamma hydroxybutyrate (GHB)]

GI gin *an elixir of terpin hydrate and codeine (disapproved in 1991)* [see: terpin hydrate; codeine]

gift of the sun [see: cocaine]

giggle weed; giggle smoke [see: mar-ijuana]

gimmie *a combination of crack and mari-juana* [see: cocaine, crack; marijuana]

gin [see: cocaine]

girl [see: cocaine; cocaine, crack; heroin]

girlfriend [see: cocaine]

glad stuff [see: cocaine]

glass [see: amphetamines]

glassines *from the type of translucent glazed paper in which heroin is sold* [see: heroin]

glo [see: cocaine, crack]

God's drug [see: morphine]

God's flesh [see: psilocybin; psilocin]

God's medicine [see: opium]

go-fast [see: methcathinone]

gold [see: marijuana; cocaine, crack]

gold dragon; green dragon; red dragon [see: LSD]

gold star [see: marijuana]

golden dragon [see: LSD]

golden girl [see: heroin]

golden leaf *very high quality marijuana* [see: marijuana]

golf ball [see: cocaine, crack]

golpe [see: heroin]

goma (*Spanish for "rubber"*) *morphine, opium, or black tar heroin* [see: mor-phine; opium; black tar heroin]

gondola [see: opium]

gong [see: marijuana; opium]

goob [see: methcathinone]

good [see: PCP]

good and plenty [see: heroin]

good butt *a marijuana cigarette* [see: marijuana]

good giggles [see: marijuana]

good H [see: heroin]

goodfellas [see: fentanyl]

goof butt *a marijuana cigarette* [see: marijuana]

goofball *barbiturates or a combination of cocaine and heroin* [see: barbiturates; cocaine; heroin]

goofers [see: barbiturates]

goofies [see: LSD]

goon; goon dust [see: PCP]

gooney birds [see: LSD]

'goric *from "paregoric"* [see: paregoric; opium]

gorilla biscuits; gorilla tabs [see: PCP]

gorilla pills *barbiturate sleeping pills* [see: barbiturates]

gram [see: hashish]

grape parfait [see: LSD]

grass; grass brownies [see: marijuana]

grata (*Spanish for "pleasing"*) [see: marijuana]

gravel [see: cocaine, crack]

gravy [see: heroin]

great bear [see: fentanyl]

great tobacco [see: opium]

green *inferior-quality marijuana, PCP, or ketamine* [see: marijuana; PCP; ketamine HCl]

Street Slang

green double domes; green single domes [see: LSD]

green dragon; gold dragon; red dragon [see: LSD]

green goddess [see: marijuana]

green gold [see: cocaine]

green leaves; green tea [see: PCP]

green single domes; green double domes [see: LSD]

green wedge [see: LSD]

greens and clears *Dexamyl (dextroamphetamine sulfate + amobarbital; discontinued 1980), named for the capsule color* [see: dextroamphetamine sulfate; amobarbital]

greeter [see: marijuana]

grefa; grifa; griff; griffa; griffo [see: marijuana]

Greta [see: marijuana]

grey shields [see: LSD]

grievous bodily harm [see: gamma hydroxybutyrate (GHB)]

grifa; grefa; griff; griffa; griffo [see: marijuana]

G-riffic [see: gamma hydroxybutyrate (GHB)]

grit [see: cocaine, crack]

groceries [see: cocaine, crack]

grocery store high [see: nitrous oxide]

g-rock *one gram of crack* [see: cocaine, crack]

groovy lemon *a yellow LSD tablet* [see: LSD]

gum; guma *opium refined for smoking* [see: opium]

gunga; gungeon; ganga; gange; ganja; Ghana; ghanja [see: marijuana]

gungeon; gungun *potent Jamaican marijuana* [see: marijuana]

gunny; gunnysack *a reference to sacks made with hemp fiber* [see: marijuana]

gutter glitter *cocaine or illegal drugs in general* [see: cocaine]

gyve *a marijuana cigarette* [see: marijuana]

hache [see: heroin]

hail [see: cocaine, crack]

hairy [see: heroin]

half moon [see: mescaline]

half track [see: cocaine, crack]

hamburger helper [see: cocaine, crack]

hanhich [see: marijuana]

hanyak *smokable speed* [see: amphetamines]

happy cigarette *a marijuana cigarette* [see: marijuana]

happy dust; happy powder; happy trails [see: cocaine]

hard candy [see: heroin]

hard line; hard rock [see: cocaine, crack]

hard on; heart on [see: amyl nitrite]

hard stuff [see: heroin; opium]

hardware [see: isobutyl nitrite]

Harry; Harry Jones [see: heroin]

hash [see: hashish; marijuana]

hats [see: LSD]

have a dust; haven dust [see: cocaine]

Hawaiian *very high potency marijuana* [see: marijuana]

Hawaiian sunshine [see: LSD]

hawk [see: LSD]

hay [see: marijuana]

hay butt *a marijuana cigarette* [see: marijuana]

haze [see: LSD]

Hazel [see: heroin]

H-caps [see: heroin]

head drugs [see: amphetamines]

headlights [see: LSD]

heart on; hard on [see: amyl nitrite]

hearts [see: amphetamines]

heaven and hell [see: PCP]

heaven dust [see: cocaine; heroin]

Heavenly Blue *LSD or a variety of psychedelic morning glory seeds* [see: LSD; morning glory seeds]

heavy stuff [see: cocaine; heroin]

Helen [see: heroin]

hell dust [see: heroin]

He-man [see: fentanyl; isobutyl nitrite]

hemp [see: marijuana]

Henry [see: heroin]

Henry VIII [see: cocaine]

Her [see: cocaine]

herb; herba ("herbaje" is Spanish for "grass") [see: marijuana]

Herb and Al *a combination of marijuana and alcohol* [see: alcohol; marijuana]

herms [see: PCP]

hero; heroina; heroine; hero of the underworld [see: heroin]

hessle [see: heroin]

hi speeds; high speed [see: amphetamines]

hikori [see: mescaline]

hikuli [see: mescaline]

Him [see: heroin]

Hinkley [see: PCP]

hiropon *smokable methamphetamine* [see: methamphetamine HCl]

hit *crack or a marijuana cigarette* [see: cocaine, crack; marijuana]

hocus [see: marijuana; opium]

hog [see: PCP]

hombre (Spanish for "man") [see: heroin]

hombrecitos (Spanish for "little men") [see: psilocybin]

homegrown [see: marijuana]

homer *freebase cocaine* [see: cocaine, crack]

honey blunts *marijuana cigars sealed with honey* [see: marijuana]

honey oil [see: ketamine HCl]

hong-yen *heroin in pill form* [see: heroin]

hooch [see: marijuana]

hooter [see: cocaine; marijuana]

hop; hops [see: opium]

horning *powdered cocaine or heroin* [see: cocaine; heroin]

horse [see: heroin]

horse heads [see: amphetamines]

horse tracks; horse tranquilizer [see: PCP]

hot dope [see: heroin]

hot heroin *poisoned heroin to give to a police informant* [see: heroin]

hot ice *smokable methamphetamine* [see: methamphetamine HCl]

hot stick *a marijuana cigarette* [see: marijuana]

hotcakes [see: cocaine, crack]

How do you like me now? [see: cocaine, crack]

hows [see: morphine]

hubba; hubbas; Hubba, I am back [see: cocaine, crack]

hug drug; huggers [see: MDMA]

hunter [see: cocaine]

hyatari [see: mescaline]

I am back [see: cocaine, crack]

ice [see: cocaine; amphetamines; MDMA; methamphetamine HCl; PCP]

ice cube [see: cocaine, crack]

icing [see: cocaine]

idiot pills [see: barbiturates]

in-betweens [see: amphetamines]

Inca message [see: cocaine]

incentive [see: cocaine]

Indian boy; Indian hay; Indian hemp [see: marijuana]

Indiana [see: mescaline]

Indiana ditchweed *low-potency wild marijuana that grows wild from seeds originally bred for hemp rope* [see: marijuana]

Indiana hay [see: marijuana]

Indica *a species of cannabis found in hot climates* [see: cannabis]

Indo; Indonesian bud [see: marijuana; opium]

instant Zen [see: LSD]

Invigorate *gamma butyrolactone (GBL), a precursor to gamma hydroxybutyrate (GHB)* [see: gamma butyrolactone (GBL); gamma hydroxybutyrate (GHB)]

Isda [see: heroin]

issues [see: cocaine, crack]

jackpot [see: fentanyl]

jam [see: amphetamine; cocaine]

Jam Cecil [see: amphetamine]

Jane [see: marijuana]

Jay; Jay smoke *a marijuana cigarette* [see: marijuana]

jee gee; jojee [see: heroin]

Jeff [see: methcathinone]

jellies [see: chloral hydrate]

jelly [see: cocaine]

jelly baby [see: amphetamines]

jelly beans [see: amphetamines; chloral hydrate; cocaine, crack]

jet [see: ketamine HCl]

jet fuel [see: PCP]

Jim Jones *marijuana laced with cocaine and PCP* [see: marijuana; cocaine; PCP]

jive [see: heroin; marijuana]

jive doo jee [see: heroin]

jive stick *a marijuana cigarette* [see: marijuana]

Joe Friday *Quaalude (methaqualone; discontinued 1983); the tablet ID# matches Sgt. Friday's badge number on Dragnet* [see: methaqualone]

Johnson [see: cocaine, crack]

Johnson grass *low-potency Texas marijuana (President Lyndon Johnson was from Texas)* [see: marijuana]

joint *a marijuana cigarette* [see: marijuana]

jojee; jee gee [see: heroin]

jolly bean [see: amphetamines]

jolly green [see: marijuana]

Jolt *gamma butyrolactone (GBL), a precursor to gamma hydroxybutyrate (GHB)* [see: gamma butyrolactone (GBL); gamma hydroxybutyrate (GHB)]

Jones [see: heroin]

joy flakes [see: heroin]

joy juice *chloral hydrate in an alcoholic beverage* [see: alcohol; chloral hydrate]

joy plant [see: opium]

joy powder [see: cocaine; heroin]

joy smoke [see: marijuana]

joy stick *a marijuana cigarette* [see: marijuana]

Juan Valdez [see: marijuana]

Juanita [see: marijuana]

Judas *a reference to Jesus' disciple ("the one who betrays")* [see: heroin]

jugs [see: amphetamines]

juice [see: PCP; anabolic steroids]

juice joint *a marijuana cigarette sprinkled with crack* [see: cocaine, crack; marijuana]

ju-ju *a marijuana cigarette* [see: marijuana]

junk [see: cocaine; heroin]

Kabayo [see: heroin]

Kaksonjae *smokable methamphetamine* [see: methamphetamine HCl]

Kali [see: marijuana]

kangaroo [see: cocaine, crack]

kaps [see: PCP]

Karachi *a reference to Karachi, Pakistan* [see: heroin]

kat; khat; q'at *leaves of the Catha edulis plant* [see: Catha edulis, cathinone]

kaya [see: marijuana]

K-blast [see: PCP]

Kentucky blue [see: marijuana]

keys to the kingdom [see: LSD]

KGB *"killer green bud"* [see: marijuana]

khat; kat; q'at *leaves of the Catha edulis plant* [see: Catha edulis, cathinone]

Kibbles and Bits *a combination of Talwin (pentazocine HCl) and Ritalin (methylphenidate HCl) or crumbs of crack* [see: Talwin; pentazocine HCl; Ritalin; methylphenidate HCl; cocaine, crack]

kick stick *a marijuana cigarette* [see: marijuana]

kif; kiff *potent Moroccan marijuana or hashish* [see: hashish; marijuana]

killer [see: marijuana; PCP]

killer weed *marijuana (1960s and 70s) or a combination of marijuana and PCP (1980s–)* [see: marijuana; PCP]

kilter [see: marijuana]

kind [see: marijuana]

king ivory [see: fentanyl]

King Kong pills *barbiturate sleeping pills or other CNS depressants* [see: barbiturates]

king's habit [see: cocaine]

Kleenex [see: MDMA]

knockout drops *chloral hydrate mixed in an alcoholic beverage* [see: alcohol; chloral hydrate]

Kokomo [see: cocaine, crack]

Kools [see: PCP]

Krypt Tonight *a brand-name soundalike to "kryptonite," the substance that makes Superman weak* [see: isobutyl nitrite]

kryptonite [see: cocaine, crack]

krystal; crystal; krystal joint; crystal joint [see: PCP]

kumbo [see: marijuana]

L.A. *a long-acting amphetamine* [see: amphetamines]

L.A. glass; L.A. ice *smokable methamphetamine* [see: methamphetamine HCl]

L.A. turnarounds *a reference to truckers' use of amphetamines for long-distance runs* [see: amphetamines]

lace *a combination of cocaine and marijuana* [see: cocaine; marijuana]

lady; lady caine; lady snow [see: cocaine]

Lakbay diva [see: marijuana]

lamb's bread [see: marijuana]

las mujercitas (Spanish for "the little women") [see: psilocybin]

lason sa daga [see: LSD]

laughing gas [see: nitrous oxide]

laughing grass; laughing weed [see: marijuana]

leaf [see: marijuana; cocaine]

leaky bolla; leaky leak [see: PCP]

leapers [see: amphetamines]

Lebanese *hashish from Lebanon* [see: hashish]

legal speed *Mini Thin (ephedrine HCl), an over-the-counter asthma drug* [see: Mini Thin; ephedrine HCl]

Lemmon 714; Lemmons *Quaalude (methaqualone; discontinued 1983), refers to the manufacturer (Lemmon) and tablet ID# (714)* [see: methaqualone]

lemonade *heroin or poor-quality street drugs in general* [see: heroin]

Lennons *Quaalude (methaqualone; discontinued 1983), probably a reference to musician John Lennon* [see: methaqualone]

lens [see: LSD]

lethal weapon [see: PCP]

Lib [see: Librium; chlordiazepoxide HCl]

lid poppers; lip poppers [see: amphetamines]

light stuff [see: marijuana]

lightning [see: amphetamines]

Lima [see: marijuana]

limbo [see: marijuana]

lime acid [see: LSD]

line [see: cocaine]

liquid ecstasy; liquid E; liquid ex; liquid X [see: gamma hydroxybutyrate (GHB)]

little bomb [see: amphetamines; heroin]

little ones [see: PCP]

little smoke [see: marijuana; psilocybin; psilocin]

live ones [see: PCP]

Llesca [see: marijuana]

loads *a combination of Doriden (glutethimide; discontinued 1990) and codeine* [see: glutethimide; codeine]

loaf [see: marijuana]

lobo (Spanish for "wolf") [see: marijuana]

locker room [see: isobutyl nitrite]

loco (Spanish for "crazy" or "insane") [see: marijuana]

locoweed [see: marijuana; jimsonweed]

log *a marijuana cigarette or PCP* [see: marijuana; PCP]

logor [see: LSD]

love [see: cocaine, crack]

love affair [see: cocaine]

love boat *PCP or marijuana dipped in formaldehyde* [see: marijuana; PCP]

love drug *Quaalude (methaqualone; discontinued 1983)* [see: methaqualone]

love drug of the '80s and '90s [see: MDMA]

love pearls; love pills [see: alpha-ethyltryptamine]

love trip *a combination of mescaline and MDMA* [see: mescaline; MDMA]

love weed [see: marijuana]

lovelies *marijuana laced with PCP* [see: marijuana; PCP]

lovely [see: PCP]

lovers *Quaalude (methaqualone; discontinued 1983)* [see: methaqualone]

lubage [see: marijuana]

Lucas [see: marijuana]

Lucy; Lucy in the sky with diamonds [see: LSD]

'ludes *Quaalude (methaqualone; discontinued 1983)* [see: methaqualone]

lumber *marijuana stems and waste* [see: marijuana]

machinery [see: marijuana]

Macon [see: marijuana]

mad dog *PCP or Mogen David 20/20 fortified wine* [see: PCP; alcohol]

madman [see: PCP]

magic; magic dust [see: PCP]

magic mushroom [see: psilocybin; psilocin]

magic smoke [see: marijuana]

Mama Coca [see: cocaine]

man [see: heroin]

Manhattan silver [see: marijuana]

marathons [see: amphetamines]

Marley [see: marijuana]

Mary; Mari [see: marijuana]

Mary and Johnny [see: marijuana]

Mary Ann; Mary Jane; Mary Warner [see: marijuana]

Matsakow [see: heroin]

Maui wowie; Maui waui *marijuana from Hawaii* [see: marijuana]

Max *GHB dissolved in water and mixed with amphetamine* [see: gamma hydroxybutyrate (GHB); amphetamines]

Mayo [see: cocaine; heroin]

mean green [see: PCP]

Meg; Megg; Meggie [see: marijuana]

mellow drug of America *MDA (methylenedioxyamphetamine), now called MDMA (methylenedioxymethamphetamine)* [see: MDMA]

mellow yellow *LSD or banana peels used for smoking* [see: LSD]

Merck *a reference to the manufacturer of pharmaceutical cocaine* [see: cocaine]

mesc'; mez [see: mescaline]

mescal *mescaline or an intoxicating distilled beverage from the same plant* [see: mescaline]

meserole *a marijuana cigarette* [see: marijuana]

meth [see: methamphetamine HCl]

Mexican brown [see: heroin; marijuana]

Mexican horse; Mexican mud [see: heroin]

Mexican mushrooms [see: psilocybin; psilocin]

Mexican red [see: marijuana]

Mexican Valium [see: Rohypnol; flunitrazepam]

mez; mesc' [see: mescaline]

Mickey Finn *chloral hydrate mixed in an alcoholic beverage* [see: chloral hydrate; alcohol]

microdot [see: LSD]

mic's; mikes *microdots of LSD* [see: LSD]

midnight oil [see: opium]

mighty mezz *a marijuana cigarette* [see: marijuana]

Mighty Quinn [see: LSD]

mikes; mic's *microdots of LSD* [see: LSD]

mind detergent [see: LSD]

minibennie [see: amphetamines]

mint leaf; mint weed [see: PCP]

45-minute psychosis [see: dimethyltryptamine]

mira (Spanish for "look" or "watch") [see: opium]

Miss Emma [see: morphine]

missile basing *a combination of crack liquid and PCP* [see: cocaine, crack; PCP]

mist *crack smoke or PCP* [see: cocaine, crack; PCP]

Mister Blue [see: morphine]

Mister Brownstone *hashish or brown heroin* [see: hashish; heroin]

Mister Natural [see: LSD]

M.O.; M.U. [see: marijuana]

modams [see: marijuana]

Mohasky [see: marijuana]

mojo [see: cocaine; heroin; morphine]

monkey *a cigarette made from cocaine paste and tobacco* [see: cocaine; tobacco]

monkey dust; monkey tranquilizer [see: PCP]

monos *cigarettes made from cocaine paste and tobacco* [see: cocaine; tobacco]

monte (Spanish for "mountain") *marijuana from South America* [see: marijuana]

mooca; moocah [see: marijuana]

moon [see: mescaline]

moonrock *a combination of crack and heroin* [see: cocaine, crack; heroin]

mooster [see: marijuana]

moota; mooters; mootie; mootos; muta; mutah *a marijuana cigarette* [see: marijuana]

mor a grifa [see: marijuana]

more [see: PCP]

morfina (Spanish for "morphine") [see: morphine]

morotgara [see: heroin]

morph; morphy [see: morphine]

mortal combat *high-potency heroin* [see: heroin]

mosquitos [see: cocaine]

mota; moto (Spanish for "speck") [see: marijuana]

mother [see: marijuana]

mother's little helper [see: Valium; diazepam]

movie star drug [see: cocaine]

M.U.; M.O. [see: marijuana]

mud [see: heroin; morphine; opium]

muggie; muggies; muggles *a marijuana cigarette* [see: marijuana]

mujer (Spanish for "woman" or "wife") [see: cocaine]

mulka [see: methcathinone]

murder 8 [see: fentanyl]

murder one *a combination of heroin and cocaine* [see: cocaine; heroin]

Murphy [see: morphine]

mushrooms [see: psilocybin; psilocin]

musk [see: psilocybin; psilocin]

muta; mutah; moota; mooters; mootie; mootos *a marijuana cigarette* [see: marijuana]

muzzle [see: heroin]

nail *a marijuana cigarette* [see: marijuana]

Nanoo [see: heroin]

nebbies [see: Nembutal Sodium; pentobarbital sodium]

nemish [see: Nembutal Sodium; pentobarbital sodium]

new acid [see: PCP]

New Jack Swing *a combination of heroin and morphine* [see: heroin; morphine]

new magic [see: PCP]

nice and easy [see: heroin]

nickel desk [see: heroin]

nie; nigh [see: nitrous oxide]

niebla (Spanish for "fog" or "haze") [see: PCP]

nimbies [see: Nembutal Sodium; pentobarbital sodium]

nitro; nitrogen [see: nitrous oxide]

Nixon *low-potency heroin* [see: heroin]

noise [see: heroin]

nose [see: heroin]

nose candy; nose powder; nose stuff [see: cocaine]

nose drops *liquefied heroin* [see: heroin]

NRG3 *gamma butyrolactone (GBL), a precursor to gamma hydroxybutyrate (GHB)* [see: gamma butyrolactone (GBL); gamma hydroxybutyrate (GHB)]

nubs [see: mescaline]

nuggets [see: amphetamines; cocaine, crack]

number *a marijuana cigarette* [see: marijuana]

number 3 [see: cocaine; heroin]

number 4; number 8 [see: heroin]

O; O.P. [see: opium]

octane *PCP laced with gasoline* [see: PCP; petroleum distillate inhalants]

ogoy [see: heroin]

oil *hashish oil, heroin, or PCP* [see: hashish; heroin; PCP]

O.J. [see: marijuana]

Old Steve [see: heroin]

one way [see: LSD]

one-fifty-one; fifty-one [see: cocaine, crack]

ope [see: opium]

O.P.P. [see: PCP]

optical illusions [see: LSD]

orange *Desoxyn (methamphetamine HCl), a reference to the capsule color* [see: Desoxyn; methamphetamine HCl]

orange barrels; orange cubes; orange haze; orange micro; orange wedges [see: LSD]

orange crystal [see: PCP]

orange cupcakes *a combination of LSD, methamphetamine, strychnine, and STP* [see: LSD; methamphetamine HCl; strychnine; STP]

oranges [see: amphetamines]

organic Quaalude [see: gamma hydroxybutyrate (GHB)]
outer limits *a combination of crack and LSD* [see: cocaine, crack; LSD]
Owsley; Owsley's acid; white Owsley [see: LSD]
ozone [see: PCP]
Ozzie's stuff *probably a reference to Ozzie Osborne* [see: LSD]
paca lolo; pakalolo *a Hawaiian term* [see: marijuana]
pack [see: heroin; marijuana]
pack of rocks *a marijuana cigarette* [see: marijuana]
Pakistani black [see: marijuana]
Panama cut; Panama gold; Panama red [see: marijuana]
panatella *a large cigar-shaped marijuana cigarette* [see: marijuana]
pancakes and syrup *a combination of glutethimide and codeine cough syrup* [see: glutethimide; codeine]
pane *a short form of "window pane," a reference to the glassine packaging* [see: LSD]
pangonadalot [see: heroin]
paper acid [see: LSD]
paper blunts *a marijuana cigarette rolled in cigarette paper rather than a tobacco leaf casing* [see: marijuana]
parachute *heroin or crack and PCP smoked together* [see: cocaine, crack; PCP; heroin]
paradise; paradise white [see: cocaine]
parlay [see: cocaine, crack]
parsley [see: marijuana; PCP]
paste [see: cocaine, crack]
Pat [see: marijuana]
'patico *from the Spanish "simpático," meaning "nice" or "pleasant"* [see: cocaine, crack]
paz [see: PCP]
PCPA [see: PCP]
P-dope *20-30% pure heroin* [see: heroin]
peace [see: LSD; PCP]
peace pill [see: PCP]
peace tablets [see: LSD]

peace weed *PCP or a combination of marijuana and PCP* [see: marijuana; PCP]
peaches *Benzedrine (amphetamine sulfate; discontinued 1982)* [see: amphetamine sulfate]
peanut butter *PCP mixed with peanut butter* [see: PCP]
peanuts *barbiturate sleeping pills* [see: barbiturates]
pearl [see: cocaine]
pearls [see: amyl nitrite]
pearly gates *LSD or a variety of psychedelic morning glory seeds* [see: LSD; morning glory seeds]
pebbles [see: cocaine, crack]
Pee Wee [see: cocaine, crack]
peep [see: PCP]
Peg [see: heroin]
pellets [see: LSD]
pen yan [see: opium]
pep pills [see: amphetamines]
perc's; perks [see: Percodan; oxycodone HCl]
perfect high [see: heroin]
perico *(Spanish for "parakeet")* [see: cocaine]
perp *fake crack made of candle wax and baking soda (to "perpetrate" a fraud)*
Peruvian; Peruvian flake; Peruvian lady [see: cocaine]
Peter [see: chloral hydrate]
Peter Pan [see: PCP]
peth *from "pethidine," the official British and International name for meperidine HCl* [see: Demerol HCl; meperidine HCl]
petrol *a British term for gasoline* [see: petroleum distillate inhalants]
peyote [see: mescaline]
P-funk *heroin or a combination of crack and PCP* [see: heroin; cocaine, crack; PCP]
phennies; fennies [see: phenobarbital]
pheno's; feno's [see: phenobarbital]
Phillies blunt *a cigar hollowed out and filled with marijuana* [see: marijuana]
piece [see: cocaine; cocaine, crack]
piedras *(Spanish for "stones")* [see: cocaine, crack]

pig killer [see: PCP]
piles [see: cocaine, crack]
pimp [see: cocaine]
pin; pinhead *a thinly rolled marijuana cigarette* [see: marijuana]
pin gun; pin yen [see: opium]
pineapple *a combination of heroin and Ritalin (methylphenidate HCl) or amphetamine* [see: heroin; Ritalin; methylphenidate HCl; amphetamines]
pink blotters [see: LSD]
pink hearts [see: amphetamines]
Pink Panther; pink robots; pink wedge; pink witches [see: LSD]
pink spoons [see: Percodan; oxycodone HCl]
pinks [see: Seconal Sodium; secobarbital sodium]
pit [see: PCP]
pixies [see: amphetamines]
platters [see: hashish]
pocket rocket [see: marijuana]
pod [see: marijuana]
poison [see: heroin; fentanyl]
poke [see: marijuana]
polvo (Spanish for "powder" or "dust") [see: heroin; PCP]
polvo blanco (Spanish for "white powder") [see: cocaine]
polvo de angel; polvo de estrellas (Spanish for "angel dust"; "star dust") [see: PCP]
pony [see: cocaine, crack]
poor man's speedball *a combination of heroin and methamphetamine* [see: heroin; methamphetamine HCl]
poppers [see: isobutyl nitrite; amyl nitrite]
poppy [see: heroin]
pot [see: marijuana]
pot liquor; pot likker *a tea brewed from marijuana waste* [see: marijuana]
potato [see: LSD]
potato chips *crack cocaine cut (diluted) with benzocaine* [see: cocaine, crack]
potten bush [see: marijuana]
powder [see: heroin; amphetamines]
powder diamonds [see: cocaine]
pox [see: opium]
P.R. (Panama Red) [see: marijuana]

preludes *Preludin (phenmetrazine HCl; discontinued 1992)* [see: phenmetrazine HCl]
prescription *a marijuana cigarette* [see: marijuana]
press [see: cocaine; cocaine, crack]
pretendica; pretendo (Spanish for "pretender") [see: marijuana]
primo (Spanish for "priority") *crack, marijuana and crack, or cigarettes with cocaine and heroin* [see: cocaine, crack; marijuana; cocaine; heroin]
Pro-G *1,4-butanediol, a precursor to gamma hydroxybutyrate (GHB)* [see: gamma hydroxybutyrate (GHB)]
pseudocaine *phenylpropanolamine, an adulterant for cutting crack*
puffy [see: PCP]
pulborn [see: heroin]
pure [see: heroin]
pure love [see: LSD]
purple [see: ketamine HCl]
purple barrels; purple flats; purple haze; purple ozoline [see: LSD]
purple hearts *Luminal Sodium (phenobarbital sodium), LSD, amphetamines, or various CNS depressants* [see: Luminal Sodium; phenobarbital sodium; LSD; amphetamines]
purple rain [see: PCP]
q'at; kat; khat *leaves of the Catha edulis plant* [see: Catha edulis, cathinone]
qua; quaa; quack; quad; quas *Quaalude (methaqualone; discontinued 1983)* [see: methaqualone]
quarter moon [see: hashish]
quartz *smokable speed* [see: amphetamines]
Queen Anne's lace [see: marijuana]
quicksilver [see: isobutyl nitrite]
quill [see: methamphetamine HCl; heroin; cocaine]
R and R *reds (Seconal Sodium; secobarbital sodium) and Ripple (wine)* [see: Seconal Sodium; secobarbital sodium; alcohol]
racehorse Charlie [see: cocaine; heroin]
ragweed *inferior-quality marijuana or heroin* [see: marijuana; heroin]

Street Slang

railroad weed [see: marijuana]

rainbows *Tuinal (amobarbital sodium + secobarbital sodium), which comes in multicolored striped capsules* [see: Tuinal; amobarbital sodium; secobarbital sodium]

rainy day woman *a marijuana cigarette* [see: marijuana]

Rambo [see: heroin]

Rane [see: cocaine; heroin]

rangood *marijuana grown wild* [see: marijuana]

Rasta weed [see: marijuana]

raw [see: cocaine, crack]

ReActive *gamma butyrolactone (GBL), a precursor to gamma hydroxybutyrate (GHB)* [see: gamma butyrolactone (GBL); gamma hydroxybutyrate (GHB)]

ready rock [see: cocaine; cocaine, crack; heroin]

recycle [see: LSD]

red and blues [see: Tuinal; amobarbital sodium; secobarbital sodium]

red birds; red bullets [see: secobarbital sodium]

red caps [see: cocaine, crack]

red chicken [see: heroin]

red chicken *Chinese heroin* [see: heroin]

red cross [see: marijuana]

red devil *PCP or Seconal Sodium (secobarbital sodium) capsules* [see: PCP; Seconal Sodium; secobarbital sodium]

red dirt [see: marijuana]

red dragon; gold dragon; green dragon [see: LSD]

red eagle [see: heroin]

red phosphorus *smokable speed* [see: amphetamines]

red rum *"murder" spelled backward; a potent form of heroin* [see: heroin]

reds [see: Seconal Sodium; secobarbital sodium]

reds and Ripple *a combination of Seconal Sodium (secobarbital sodium) and Ripple wine* [see: Seconal Sodium; secobarbital sodium; alcohol]

reefer [see: marijuana]

regular P [see: cocaine, crack]

reindeer dust [see: heroin]

Rejuv *1,4-butanediol, a precursor to gamma hydroxybutyrate (GHB)* [see: gamma hydroxybutyrate (GHB)]

Rem Force *gamma butyrolactone (GBL), a precursor to gamma hydroxybutyrate (GHB)* [see: gamma butyrolactone (GBL); gamma hydroxybutyrate (GHB)]

RenewTrient *gamma butyrolactone (GBL), a precursor to gamma hydroxybutyrate (GHB)* [see: gamma butyrolactone (GBL); gamma hydroxybutyrate (GHB)]

Revirarant *gamma butyrolactone (GBL), a precursor to gamma hydroxybutyrate (GHB)* [see: gamma butyrolactone (GBL); gamma hydroxybutyrate (GHB)]

Revitalize Plus *gamma butyraldehyde (GHB-aldehyde), a precursor to gamma hydroxybutyrate (GHB)* [see: gamma hydroxybutyrate (GHB)]

Rhine [see: heroin]

rhythm [see: amphetamines]

rib [see: Rohypnol; flunitrazepam]

rippers [see: amphetamines]

roach *the butt of a marijuana cigarette* [see: marijuana]

roach 2; roaches [see: Rohypnol; flunitrazepam]

road dope [see: amphetamines]

roca *(Spanish for "rock")* [see: cocaine, crack]

Roche [see: Rohypnol; flunitrazepam]

rock(s) [see: cocaine, crack]

rocket *a marijuana cigarette* [see: marijuana]

rocket fuel [see: PCP]

rocks; rox; rocks of hell [see: cocaine, crack]

Rocky III [see: cocaine, crack]

rolling [see: MDMA]

roofie; roofies [see: Rohypnol; flunitrazepam]

'rooms *Psilocybe mushrooms* [see: psilocybin]

roopies [see: Rohypnol; flunitrazepam]

rooster [see: cocaine, crack]

root *a marijuana cigarette* [see: marijuana]

rope [see: marijuana; Rohypnol; fluni-trazepam]

rophy; ropies; roples [see: Rohypnol; flunitrazepam]

Rosa (Spanish for "rose" or "pink") [see: amphetamines]

Rose Maria [see: marijuana]

roses *Benzedrine (amphetamine sulfate; discontinued 1982) tablets* [see: amphetamine sulfate]

rox; rocks; rocks of Hell [see: cocaine, crack]

Roxanne [see: cocaine; cocaine, crack]

royal blues [see: LSD]

Roz [see: cocaine, crack]

ruderalis *a species of cannabis found in Russia* [see: cannabis]

ruffies; ruffles [see: Rohypnol; flunitrazepam]

running [see: MDMA]

rush; rush snappers [see: isobutyl nitrite]

Russian sickles [see: LSD]

sack [see: heroin]

sacrament [see: LSD]

sacred mushrooms [see: psilocybin]

salt [see: heroin]

salt and pepper [see: marijuana]

salty water [see: gamma hydroxybutyrate (GHB)]

Sandoz *a reference to the manufacturer* [see: LSD]

sandwich *two layers of cocaine with a layer of heroin* [see: cocaine; heroin]

Santa Marta (Spanish for "Saint Marta") [see: marijuana]

sassafras [see: marijuana]

sativa *a species of cannabis found in cool, damp climates* [see: cannabis]

scaffle [see: PCP]

scag [see: heroin]

scat; scate [see: heroin]

schmack; smack; schmeck; shmeck [see: heroin]

schoolboy [see: cocaine; codeine]

schoolboy scotch *Scotch whiskey with codeine added* [see: codeine; alcohol]

Schoolcraft [see: cocaine, crack]

scissors [see: marijuana]

scoop [see: gamma hydroxybutyrate (GHB)]

scorpion [see: cocaine]

Scott [see: heroin]

Scottie; Scotty [see: cocaine; cocaine, crack]

scramble [see: cocaine, crack]

scrubwoman's kick *inhaled cleaning fluid, especially naphtha* [see: petroleum distillate inhalants]

scruples [see: cocaine, crack]

scuffle; skuffle [see: PCP]

seccy; seggy [see: Seconal Sodium; secobarbital sodium]

seeds [see: marijuana]

seggy; seccy [see: Seconal Sodium; secobarbital sodium]

sen [see: marijuana]

seni *peyote* [see: mescaline]

serenity; serenity, tranquility, and peace [see: STP]

Sernyl [see: PCP]

Serpico 21 [see: cocaine]

Sess [see: marijuana]

sets *a combination of Talwin (pentazo-cine HCl) and PBZ (pyribenzamine)* [see: Talwin; pentazocine HCl; tripe-lennamine]

seven fourteens *Quaalude (methaqua-lone; discontinued 1983), from ID# 714 on the tablets* [see: methaqualone]

Seven-up [see: cocaine; cocaine, crack]

sezz [see: marijuana]

shabu [see: cocaine; methamphet-amine HCl; amphetamines; MDMA; PCP]

shake [see: marijuana]

She [see: cocaine]

sheet rocking *a combination of crack and LSD* [see: cocaine, crack; LSD]

sheets [see: PCP]

Sherm(s); Sherman(s) *a tobacco ciga-rette laced with PCP* [see: PCP]

shmeck; schmeck; schmack; smack [see: heroin]

shoot the breeze [see: nitrous oxide]

'shrooms *from "mushrooms"* [see: psi-locybin; psilocin]

siddi [see: marijuana]

sightball [see: cocaine, crack]

Silly Putty [see: psilocybin; psilocin]

Simple Simon [see: psilocybin; psilocin]

sinse; sinsemilla *a potent variety of marijuana* [see: marijuana]

sixty-second trip [see: amyl nitrite]

skee [see: opium]

skid [see: heroin]

skunk [see: marijuana]

slab [see: cocaine, crack]

sleeper [see: heroin]

sleet [see: cocaine, crack]

slick superspeed [see: methcathinone]

slime [see: heroin]

smack; schmack; shmeck; schmeck [see: heroin]

smears [see: LSD]

smoke *marijuana, crack, or a combination of heroin and crack* [see: marijuana; cocaine, crack; heroin]

smoke Canada [see: marijuana]

smoking [see: PCP]

smoking gun [see: heroin; cocaine]

snap [see: amphetamines]

snappers [see: amyl nitrite; isobutyl nitrite]

sniff *methcathinone, an inhalant, or to inhale cocaine* [see: methcathinone; petroleum distillate inhalants; cocaine]

snop [see: marijuana]

snort *cocaine or inhalants* [see: cocaine; petroleum distillate inhalants]

snorts [see: PCP]

snot *the residue produced from smoking amphetamine* [see: amphetamines]

snot balls *rubber cement rolled into balls and burned* [see: petroleum distillate inhalants]

snow [see: cocaine; heroin; amphetamines]

snow bird [see: cocaine]

snow pallets [see: amphetamines]

snow seals *a combination of cocaine and amphetamine* [see: cocaine; amphetamines]

snow soke [see: cocaine, crack]

snow white [see: cocaine]

snowball *a combination of cocaine and heroin* [see: cocaine; heroin]

snowcones [see: cocaine]

soap [see: gamma hydroxybutyrate (GHB)]

soaper; Sopors *Sopor (methaqualone; discontinued 1981)* [see: methaqualone]

society high [see: cocaine]

soda *injectable cocaine* [see: cocaine]

soles [see: hashish]

soma (Italian for "burden" or "load") [see: PCP]

somatomax [see: gamma hydroxybutyrate (GHB)]

Somatopro *gamma butyrolactone (GBL), a precursor to gamma hydroxybutyrate (GHB)* [see: gamma butyrolactone (GBL); gamma hydroxybutyrate (GHB)]

Sopors; soaper *Sopor (methaqualone; discontinued 1981)* [see: methaqualone]

space base *crack dipped in PCP or a hollowed-out cigar refilled with PCP and crack* [see: cocaine, crack; PCP]

space cadet; space dust *crack dipped in PCP* [see: cocaine, crack; PCP]

sparkle plenty [see: amphetamines]

sparklers [see: amphetamines]

Special K [see: ketamine HCl]

special la coke [see: ketamine HCl]

speckled birds; speckled eggs [see: amphetamines]

specks [see: LSD]

speed [see: methamphetamine HCl; amphetamine; cocaine, crack; methcathinone]

speed boat *a combination of marijuana, PCP, and crack* [see: marijuana; PCP; cocaine, crack]

speed for lovers [see: MDMA]

speedball *amphetamine or a combination of heroin and cocaine* [see: amphetamines; heroin; cocaine]

spider blue [see: heroin]

splash [see: amphetamines]

spliff *a marijuana cigarette* [see: marijuana]

splim [see: marijuana]

splivins [see: amphetamines]

spores [see: PCP]

square mackerel *marijuana from Florida* [see: marijuana]

square time Bob [see: cocaine, crack]

squirrel *LSD or a combination of cocaine, marijuana, and PCP for smoking* [see: LSD; cocaine; marijuana; PCP]

stack [see: marijuana]

Stanley's stuff [see: LSD]

star *methcathinone or LSD blotter acid with star-shaped design* [see: methcathinone; LSD]

stardust [see: cocaine; PCP]

star-spangled powder [see: cocaine]

stat [see: methcathinone]

stems [see: marijuana]

stick [see: marijuana; PCP]

sticks *marijuana stems and waste* [see: marijuana]

stink weed [see: marijuana]

stones [see: cocaine, crack]

STP *the hallucinogen 2,5-dimethoxy-4-methylamphetamine (DOM), derived from amphetamine*

straw *a marijuana cigarette* [see: marijuana]

strawberry fields [see: LSD]

stuff [see: heroin]

stumblers [see: barbiturates]

sugar [see: cocaine; LSD; heroin]

sugar block [see: cocaine, crack]

sugar cubes; sugar lumps [see: LSD]

sugar weed [see: marijuana]

sunrise; sunshine *yellow LSD* [see: LSD]

super [see: PCP]

super acid; super C [see: ketamine HCl]

super cools; super kools *PCP-laced cigarettes* [see: PCP]

super grass; super weed *PCP or marijuana laced with PCP* [see: marijuana; PCP]

super ice *smokable methamphetamine* [see: methamphetamine HCl]

super joint [see: PCP]

super Sopors *Parest (methaqualone; discontinued 1983)* [see: methaqualone]

supers [see: methaqualone]

supper *Sopor (methaqualone; discontinued 1981)* [see: methaqualone]

surfer [see: PCP]

sweet Jesus [see: heroin]

sweet Lucy [see: marijuana]

sweet stuff [see: heroin; cocaine]

sweets [see: amphetamines]

swell up [see: cocaine, crack]

synthetic cocaine [see: PCP]

synthetic THT [see: PCP]

syrup and beans *a combination of Doriden (glutethimide; discontinued 1990) and codeine* [see: glutethimide; codeine]

tabs [see: LSD]

tac [see: PCP]

tail lights [see: LSD]

taima [see: marijuana]

taking a cruise [see: PCP]

Takkouri [see: marijuana]

tall [see: Talwin; pentazocine HCl]

Tango & Cash [see: fentanyl]

tar [see: opium; heroin]

tardust [see: cocaine]

taste *heroin or a small sample of drugs* [see: heroin]

T-birds [see: Tuinal; amobarbital sodium; secobarbital sodium]

T-buzz [see: PCP]

tea [see: marijuana; PCP]

tease and bees; T's and B's; tees and bees *a combination of Talwin (pentazocine HCl) and PBZ (pyribenzamine), used as a heroin substitute* [see: Talwin; pentazocine HCl; tripelennamine]

tease and blues; T's and blues; tees and blues *a combination of Talwin (pentazocine HCl) and PBZ (pyribenzamine), used as a heroin substitute* [see: Talwin; pentazocine HCl; tripelennamine]

tease and peas; T's and P's; tees and pees *a combination of Talwin (pentazocine HCl) and PBZ (pyribenzamine), used as a heroin substitute* [see: Talwin; pentazocine HCl; tripelennamine]

tecata; Tecate [see: heroin]

Teddies and Bettys *a combination of Talwin (pentazocine HCl) and PBZ (pyribenzamine), used as a heroin substitute* [see: Talwin; pentazocine HCl; tripelennamine]

tees and bees; T's and B's; tease and bees *a combination of Talwin (pentazocine HCl) and PBZ (pyribenzamine),*

Street Slang

used as a heroin substitute [see: Talwin; pentazocine HCl; tripelennamine]

tees and blues; T's and blues; tease and blues *a combination of Talwin (pentazocine HCl) and PBZ (pyribenzamine), used as a heroin substitute* [see: Talwin; pentazocine HCl; tripelennamine]

tees and pees; T's and P's; tease and peas *a combination of Talwin (pentazocine HCl) and PBZ (pyribenzamine), used as a heroin substitute* [see: Talwin; pentazocine HCl; tripelennamine]

teeth [see: cocaine; cocaine, crack]

temple balls [see: hashish]

ten-cent pistol *a heroin dose laced with poison* [see: heroin]

tens *10 mg amphetamine tablets* [see: amphetamines]

tension [see: cocaine, crack]

Texas pot; Texas tea; Tex-mex [see: marijuana]

Thai sticks *bundles of marijuana soaked in hashish oil or marijuana buds bound on short sections of bamboo* [see: marijuana; hashish]

The Beast [see: heroin]

The C [see: methcathinone]

the devil [see: cocaine, crack]

the witch [see: heroin]

Thing [see: heroin; cocaine]

thirteen [see: marijuana]

three hundreds *Quaaludes (methaqualone; discontinued 1983), a reference to 300 mg tablets* [see: methaqualone]

threes [see: Tylenol with Codeine No. 3; Empirin with Codeine No. 3]

thrust [see: isobutyl nitrite]

thrusters [see: amphetamines]

thumb *a marijuana cigarette* [see: marijuana]

Thunder *1,4-butanediol, a precursor to gamma hydroxybutyrate (GHB)* [see: gamma hydroxybutyrate (GHB)]

tic; tic tac [see: PCP]

ticket; ticket to ride [see: LSD]

Tijuana *a reference to a Mexican town on the U.S. border* [see: marijuana]

tish [see: PCP]

tissue [see: cocaine, crack]

titch [see: PCP]

toncho *an octane booster, which is inhaled* [see: petroleum distillate inhalants]

tooey; tuie; twoie [see: Tuinal; amobarbital sodium; secobarbital sodium]

tooly *toluene, which is inhaled* [see: petroleum distillate inhalants]

toot [see: cocaine]

Tootsie Roll [see: heroin]

top gun [see: cocaine, crack]

topi *peyote cactus* [see: mescaline]

tops *peyote* [see: mescaline]

tops and bottoms *a combination of Talwin (pentazocine HCl) and PBZ (pyribenzamine), used as a heroin substitute* [see: Talwin; pentazocine HCl; tripelennamine]

torch [see: marijuana]

torpedo *chloral hydrate in an alcoholic beverage or a combination of crack and marijuana* [see: chloral hydrate; cocaine, crack; marijuana]

toxy [see: opium]

toys [see: opium]

tragic magic *crack dipped in PCP* [see: cocaine, crack; PCP]

trank *from "tranquilizer"* [see: PCP]

trikes and bikes; tricycles and bicycles *a combination of Talwin (pentazocine HCl) and PBZ (pyribenzamine), used as a heroin substitute* [see: Talwin; pentazocine HCl; tripelennamine]

trip [see: LSD; alpha-ethyltryptamine]

trippers [see: LSD]

tropp [see: cocaine, crack]

truck drivers *a reference to their use of amphetamines during long-distance runs* [see: amphetamines]

T's and blues; tees and blues; tease and blues *a combination of Talwin (pentazocine HCl) and PBZ (pyribenzamine), used as a heroin substitute* [see: Talwin; pentazocine HCl; tripelennamine]

T's and B's; tees and bees; tease and bees *a combination of Talwin (pentazocine HCl) and PBZ (pyribenzamine), used as a heroin substitute* [see: Talwin; pentazocine HCl; tripelennamine]

T's and P's; tees and pees; tease and peas *a combination of Talwin (pentazocine HCl) and PBZ (pyribenzamine), used as a heroin substitute* [see: Talwin; pentazocine HCl; tripelennamine]

tuie; tooey; twoie [see: Tuinal; amobarbital sodium; secobarbital sodium]

turbo *a combination of crack and marijuana* [see: cocaine, crack; marijuana]

turkey [see: cocaine; amphetamines]

turnabout; turnarounds *a reference to truckers' use of amphetamines for long-distance runs* [see: amphetamines]

turp *an elixir of terpin hydrate and codeine (disapproved in 1991)* [see: terpin hydrate; codeine]

tutti-frutti *a flavored cocaine developed in Brazil* [see: cocaine]

tweek *a methamphetamine-like substance* [see: methamphetamine HCl; amphetamines]

tweeker [see: methcathinone]

twenty-five [see: LSD]

twist; twistum *a marijuana cigarette* [see: marijuana]

twoie; tuie; tooey [see: Tuinal; amobarbital sodium; secobarbital sodium]

ultimate [see: cocaine, crack]

Uncle Miltie; Uncle Milty [see: Miltown; meprobamate]

unkie [see: morphine]

uppers; uppies [see: amphetamines]

Utopiates *various hallucinogens*

Uzi [see: cocaine, crack]

video head cleaner [see: butyl nitrite]

vitamin Q *Quaalude (methaqualone; discontinued 1983)* [see: methaqualone]

vodka acid [see: LSD]

wac; wack *PCP or marijuana laced with PCP* [see: marijuana; PCP]

wacky dust [see: cocaine]

wacky terbacky; wacky weed [see: marijuana]

wafer [see: LSD]

wake-ups [see: amphetamines]

wallbangers *Quaalude (methaqualone; discontinued 1983)* [see: methaqualone]

water [see: methamphetamine HCl; PCP]

wave [see: cocaine, crack]

weasel dust [see: cocaine]

wedding bells [see: LSD]

wedge [see: LSD]

weed [see: marijuana; PCP]

weed tea *a tea made from marijuana waste* [see: marijuana]

West Coast turnaround *a reference to truckers' use of amphetamines for long-distance runs* [see: amphetamines]

whack *a combination of PCP and heroin* [see: PCP; heroin]

wheat [see: marijuana]

when-shee [see: opium]

whiffenpoppers [see: amyl nitrite]

whippets [see: nitrous oxide]

white [see: amphetamines]

white ball [see: cocaine, crack]

white boy [see: heroin]

white cross [see: methamphetamine HCl; amphetamines]

white dust [see: LSD]

white ghost [see: cocaine, crack]

white girl [see: cocaine; heroin]

white horizon [see: PCP]

white horse [see: cocaine]

white junk [see: heroin]

white lady [see: cocaine; heroin]

white lightning [see: LSD]

white mosquito [see: cocaine]

white nurse [see: heroin]

white Owsley; Owsley's acid; Owsley [see: LSD]

white powder [see: cocaine; PCP]

white stuff [see: heroin]

white sugar [see: cocaine, crack]

white tornado [see: cocaine, crack]

white-haired lady [see: marijuana]

whiteout [see: isobutyl nitrite]

whites *Benzedrine (amphetamine sulfate; discontinued 1982) or other amphetamines* [see: amphetamine sulfate; amphetamines]

whiz bang *a combination of cocaine and heroin* [see: cocaine; heroin]

whore pills *Quaalude (methaqualone; discontinued 1983)* [see: methaqualone]

wild cat *a combination of methcathinone and cocaine* [see: methcathinone; cocaine]

window glass; window pane [see: LSD]

wings [see: heroin; cocaine]

witch [see: heroin; cocaine]

witch hazel [see: heroin]

wobble weed [see: PCP]

wolf [see: PCP]

wollie *rocks of crack rolled into a marijuana cigarette* [see: cocaine, crack; marijuana]

wonder star [see: methcathinone]

woolah *a hollowed-out cigar refilled with marijuana and crack* [see: marijuana; cocaine, crack]

woolas *a cigarette laced with cocaine or a marijuana cigarette sprinkled with crack* [see: cocaine; cocaine, crack; marijuana]

woolies; wooly blunts *PCP or a combination of marijuana and crack* [see: PCP; marijuana; cocaine, crack]

worm [see: PCP]

wrecking crew [see: cocaine, crack]

X-ing *from "ecstasy"* [see: MDMA]

yahoo; yeaho [see: cocaine, crack]

Yale [see: cocaine, crack]

yeh [see: marijuana]

yellow [see: LSD]

yellow bam [see: methamphetamine HCl]

yellow dimples [see: LSD]

yellow fever [see: PCP]

yellow jackets *a reference to the capsule color* [see: Nembutal Sodium; pentobarbital sodium]

yellow submarine *a reference to the Beatles' song* [see: marijuana; Nembutal Sodium; pentobarbital sodium]

yellow sunshine [see: LSD]

yen pok *an opium pellet (for smoking)* [see: opium]

yen shen suey *opium wine* [see: opium]

yerba (Spanish for "herb" or "grass") [see: marijuana]

yerba mala (Spanish for "bad herb" or "bad grass") *a combination of PCP and marijuana* [see: PCP; marijuana]

yesca; yesco (Spanish for "tinder") [see: marijuana]

yeso (Spanish for "chalk") [see: cocaine]

yimyom [see: cocaine, crack]

yuppie psychedelic [see: MDMA]

Zacatecas purple ("zacate" is Spanish for "hay") *marijuana from Mexico* [see: marijuana]

zambi [see: marijuana]

zen [see: LSD]

zero [see: opium]

zigzag man [see: LSD; marijuana]

zip [see: cocaine]

zol *a marijuana cigarette* [see: marijuana]

zombie [see: PCP]

zombie weed *PCP or marijuana laced with PCP* [see: PCP; marijuana]

zoom *PCP or marijuana laced with PCP* [see: PCP; marijuana]

Hazardous Materials

Listed below are 3156 materials that pose a threat to human life and health. These industrial chemicals, poisons, flammable materials, radioactive substances, petroleum products, and biological agents produce a wide variety of adverse effects in the human body. Treatment for such hazardous material (HazMat) exposure also varies widely, depending on the nature of the specific material.

Each entry in this section is in the following format:

hazardous material [Hazard category] *Potential adverse effects.* ☑ sound-alike(s)

A HazMat will often fall into more than one hazard category. In such cases, multiple categories are shown, followed by the potential adverse effects associated with each category. Rarely, a HazMat is unique and therefore will have no category shown—only a list of potential adverse effects. [(n.o.s.) = not otherwise specified]

Abate [Organophosphate] *Pulmonary edema, respiratory muscle paralysis, respiratory failure, bradycardia, acetylcholinesterase inhibition, hypotension, pulmonary edema, overstimulation of parasympathetic nervous system, striated muscle, sympathetic ganglia, and CNS.*

accumulator, pressurized [Flammable gas] *Respiratory failure, cardiac arrest, arrhythmias.*

acenaphthene [Naphthalene] *Delayed-onset acute intravascular hemolysis.*

acenaphthylene [Naphthalene] *Delayed-onset acute intravascular hemolysis.*

acenocoumarol [Warfarin/hydroxycoumarin/indanedione] *Anticoagulation effect, internal hemorrhage.*

acephate [Organophosphate] *Pulmonary edema, respiratory muscle paralysis, respiratory failure, bradycardia, acetylcholinesterase inhibition, hypotension, pulmonary edema, overstimulation of parasympathetic nervous system, striated muscle, sympathetic ganglia, and CNS.*

acetaldehyde [Aldehyde] *Seizures, respiratory failure, pulmonary edema.*

acetaldehyde ammonia [Ammonia] *Pulmonary edema, hypotension.* [Aldehyde] *Seizures, respiratory failure, pulmonary edema.*

acetaldehyde oxime [Flammable/combustible liquid] *CNS depression, respiratory arrest, convulsions, arrhythmias, pulmonary edema.*

acetamide [Organic acid] *Pulmonary edema, circulatory collapse, laryngeal edema and spasm, severe chemical burns to skin, mucous membranes, and internal organs, GI tract perforation and hemorrhage, peritonitis.*

acetic acid [Organic acid] *Pulmonary edema, circulatory collapse, laryngeal edema and spasm, severe chemical burns to skin, mucous membranes, and internal organs, GI tract perforation and hemorrhage, peritonitis.*

acetic acid & boron trifluoride complex [Organic acid] *Pulmonary edema, circulatory collapse, laryngeal edema and spasm, severe chemical burns to skin, mucous membranes, and internal organs, GI tract perforation and hemorrhage, peritonitis.* [Boron] *Respiratory tract irritation, laryngeal*

HazMat

spasm and edema, pulmonary edema, severe chemical burns.

acetic anhydride [Organic acid] *Pulmonary edema, circulatory collapse, laryngeal edema and spasm, severe chemical burns to skin, mucous membranes, and internal organs, GI tract perforation and hemorrhage, peritonitis.*

acetone [Ketone] *Respiratory mucous membrane irritation, pulmonary edema, CNS depression.*

acetone cyanohydrin [Cyanide] *Impairment of cellular oxygenation and adenosine triphosphate production, hypoxia, death.*

acetone oil [Ketone] *Respiratory mucous membrane irritation, pulmonary edema, CNS depression.*

acetone thiosemicarbazide [Hydrazine] *Seizures, hemolysis of red blood cells, pulmonary edema.*

acetonitrile [Cyanide] *Impairment of cellular oxygenation and adenosine triphosphate production, hypoxia, death.*

acetophenone [Ketone] *Respiratory mucous membrane irritation, pulmonary edema, CNS depression.*

acetyl [Aldehyde] *Seizures, respiratory failure, pulmonary edema.*

acetyl acetone peroxide [Organic peroxide] *Pulmonary and laryngeal edema, circulatory arrest, hypovolemic shock, chemical burns to skin, mucous membranes, and internal organs.* [Ketone] *Respiratory mucous membrane irritation, pulmonary edema, CNS depression.* [Corrosive] *Upper airway burns and edema, circulatory collapse, severe chemical burns to skin, toxic systemic effects, GI tract perforation and hemorrhage, peritonitis.*

acetyl ammonia [Ammonia] *Pulmonary edema, hypotension.* [Aldehyde] *Seizures, respiratory failure, pulmonary edema.*

acetyl benzoyl peroxide [Organic peroxide] *Pulmonary and laryngeal edema, circulatory arrest, hypovolemic shock, chemical burns to skin, mucous membranes, and internal organs.*

acetyl bromide [Organic acid] *Pulmonary edema, circulatory collapse, laryngeal edema and spasm, severe chemical burns to skin, mucous membranes, and internal organs, GI tract perforation and hemorrhage, peritonitis.*

acetyl chloride [Organic acid] *Pulmonary edema, circulatory collapse, laryngeal edema and spasm, severe chemical burns to skin, mucous membranes, and internal organs, GI tract perforation and hemorrhage, peritonitis.*

acetyl cyclohexane sulfonyl peroxide [Organic peroxide] *Pulmonary and laryngeal edema, circulatory arrest, hypovolemic shock, chemical burns to skin, mucous membranes, and internal organs.*

acetyl iodide [Iodine] *Hypotension, circulatory collapse, pulmonary edema.*

acetyl methyl carbinol [Ketone] *Respiratory mucous membrane irritation, pulmonary edema, CNS depression.*

acetyl peroxide [Organic peroxide] *Pulmonary and laryngeal edema, circulatory arrest, hypovolemic shock, chemical burns to skin, mucous membranes, and internal organs.*

2-acetylaminofluorene [Poison] *Cardiovascular collapse, pulmonary edema, CNS depression, coma, seizures, nausea, vomiting, cardiopulmonary arrest.*

acetylene [Aliphatic hydrocarbon] *Arrhythmias, asphyxiation, anesthesia.* [Simple asphyxiant] *Asphyxiation.*

acetylene dichloride [Aliphatic hydrocarbon] *Arrhythmias, asphyxiation, anesthesia.* [Simple asphyxiant] *Asphyxiation.*

acetylene & propylene & ethylene mixture (cryogenic liquid) [Aliphatic hydrocarbon] *Arrhythmias, asphyxiation, anesthesia.* [Simple asphyxiant] *Asphyxiation.*

acetylene tetrabromide [Aliphatic hydrocarbon] *Arrhythmias, asphyxiation, anesthesia.* [Simple asphyxiant] *Asphyxiation.*

1-acetyl-2-thiourea [Nitrogen oxide] *Lower respiratory tract symptoms, pulmonary edema, laryngospasm, bronchospasm, asphyxiation.*

acid, liquid (n.o.s.) [Inorganic acid] *Pulmonary edema, bronchospasm, circulatory collapse, laryngeal spasm and edema, severe chemical burns to skin, mucous membranes, and internal organs, GI tract perforation and hemorrhage, peritonitis.* [Organic acid] *Pulmonary edema, circulatory collapse, laryngeal edema and spasm, severe chemical burns to skin, mucous membranes, and internal organs, GI tract perforation and hemorrhage, peritonitis.*

acid butyl phosphate [Organic acid] *Pulmonary edema, circulatory collapse, laryngeal edema and spasm, severe chemical burns to skin, mucous membranes, and internal organs, GI tract perforation and hemorrhage, peritonitis.*

acid mixture: hydrofluoric acid & sulfuric acid [Inorganic acid] *Pulmonary edema, bronchospasm, circulatory collapse, laryngeal spasm and edema, severe chemical burns to skin, mucous membranes, and internal organs, GI tract perforation and hemorrhage, peritonitis.* [Hydrofluoric acid] *Pulmonary and laryngeal edema, circulatory collapse, severe skin burns, GI tract perforation, systemic fluoride poisoning.*

acid mixture, nitrating [Inorganic acid] *Pulmonary edema, bronchospasm, circulatory collapse, laryngeal spasm and edema, severe chemical burns to skin, mucous membranes, and internal organs, GI tract perforation and hemorrhage, peritonitis.*

acid sludge [Inorganic acid] *Pulmonary edema, bronchospasm, circulatory collapse, laryngeal spasm and edema, severe chemical burns to skin, mucous membranes, and internal organs, GI tract perforation and hemorrhage, peritonitis.*

acridine [Aromatic hydrocarbon] *Arrhythmias, respiratory failure, pulmonary edema, paralysis, brain and kidney damage.*

acrolein; acrolein dimer [Acrolein] *Severe respiratory tract irritation, pulmonary edema, respiratory failure.*

acrylamide [Triorthocresyl phosphate] *Delayed-onset neurotoxicity, ascending paralysis of the extremities.*

acrylic acid [Organic acid] *Pulmonary edema, circulatory collapse, laryngeal edema and spasm, severe chemical burns to skin, mucous membranes, and internal organs, GI tract perforation and hemorrhage, peritonitis.*

acrylonitrile [Cyanide] *Impairment of cellular oxygenation and adenosine triphosphate production, hypoxia, death.*

acrylyl chloride [Irritant] *Severe immediate or delayed upper airway or respiratory tract irritation, pulmonary edema, glottic spasm, airway obstruction.*

activated carbon [Irritant] *Severe immediate or delayed upper airway or respiratory tract irritation, pulmonary edema, glottic spasm, airway obstruction.*

activated charcoal [Irritant] *Severe immediate or delayed upper airway or respiratory tract irritation, pulmonary edema, glottic spasm, airway obstruction.*

adhesive (n.o.s.) [Irritant] *Severe immediate or delayed upper airway or respiratory tract irritation, pulmonary edema, glottic spasm, airway obstruction.*

adhesive containing flammable liquid [Flammable/combustible liquid] *CNS depression, respiratory arrest, convulsions, arrhythmias, pulmonary edema.*

adipic acid [Organic acid] *Pulmonary edema, circulatory collapse, laryngeal edema and spasm, severe chemical burns to skin, mucous membranes, and internal organs, GI tract perforation and hemorrhage, peritonitis.*

adiponitrile [Cyanide] *Impairment of cellular oxygenation and adenosine triphosphate production, hypoxia, death.*

aerosol (n.o.s.) [Irritant] *Severe immediate or delayed upper airway or respiratory tract irritation, pulmonary edema, glottic spasm, airway obstruction.* [Poison] *Cardiovascular collapse, pulmonary edema, CNS depression,*

HazMat

coma, seizures, nausea, vomiting, cardiopulmonary arrest.

air (compressed gas or cryogenic liquid) [Nonflammable gas] *Pulmonary edema, respiratory failure, asphyxiation.*

aircraft M86 fuel [Hydrocarbon mixture] *CNS depression, respiratory arrest, seizures, arrhythmias, pulmonary edema.*

alcohol (n.o.s.) [Lower alcohol (1–3 carbons)] *CNS depression, coma, respiratory arrest, arrhythmias.* [Higher alcohol (4+ carbons)] *CNS depression, respiratory failure, arrhythmias.*

alcohol, beverage [Lower alcohol (1–3 carbons)] *CNS depression, coma, respiratory arrest, arrhythmias.*

alcohol, denatured [Methyl alcohol] *Respiratory failure, circulatory collapse.*

alcohol, ethyl [Lower alcohol (1–3 carbons)] *CNS depression, coma, respiratory arrest, arrhythmias.*

alcoholic beverage [Lower alcohol (1–3 carbons)] *CNS depression, coma, respiratory arrest, arrhythmias.*

aldehyde (n.o.s.) [Aldehyde] *Seizures, respiratory failure, pulmonary edema.*

aldicarb [Carbamate] *Acetylcholinesterase inhibition (reversible), bradycardia, hypotension, respiratory muscle paralysis, respiratory arrest, pulmonary edema.*

aldicarb & dichloromethane mixture [Halogenated aliphatic hydrocarbon] *CNS depression, respiratory arrest, circulatory collapse.* [Carbamate] *Acetylcholinesterase inhibition (reversible), bradycardia, hypotension, respiratory muscle paralysis, respiratory arrest, pulmonary edema.*

aldol [Aldehyde] *Seizures, respiratory failure, pulmonary edema.*

aldrin; aldrin mixture (n.o.s.) [Aldrin/dieldrin/endrin] *Seizures, respiratory failure.*

aliphatic hydrocarbon (n.o.s.) [Aliphatic hydrocarbon] *Arrhythmias, asphyxiation, anesthesia.*

aliphatic thiocyanate (n.o.s.) [Isocyanate/aliphatic thiocyanate] *CNS depression, respiratory arrest, respiratory paralysis, pulmonary edema, cyanide toxicity.*

alkali metal alloy (n.o.s.); alkaline earth metal alloy (n.o.s.) [Inorganic base/alkaline corrosive] *Upper airway burns and edema, pulmonary edema, skin burns, circulatory collapse, GI tract perforation and hemorrhage, peritonitis.*

alkali metal amalgam (n.o.s.); alkaline earth metal amalgam (n.o.s.) [Inorganic base/alkaline corrosive] *Upper airway burns and edema, pulmonary edema, skin burns, circulatory collapse, GI tract perforation and hemorrhage, peritonitis.*

alkali metal amide (n.o.s.) [Inorganic base/alkaline corrosive] *Upper airway burns and edema, pulmonary edema, skin burns, circulatory collapse, GI tract perforation and hemorrhage, peritonitis.*

alkali metal dispersion; alkali earth metal dispersion [Inorganic base/alkaline corrosive] *Upper airway burns and edema, pulmonary edema, skin burns, circulatory collapse, GI tract perforation and hemorrhage, peritonitis.*

alkaline corrosive liquid (n.o.s.) [Inorganic base/alkaline corrosive] *Upper airway burns and edema, pulmonary edema, skin burns, circulatory collapse, GI tract perforation and hemorrhage, peritonitis.*

alkaloid, poisonous (n.o.s.); alkaloid salt, poisonous (n.o.s.) [Organic base/amine] *Pulmonary edema, cardiac depression, seizures.*

alkane (C5–C8) [Aliphatic hydrocarbon] *Arrhythmias, asphyxiation, anesthesia.*

alkane sulfonic acid [Organic acid] *Pulmonary edema, circulatory collapse, laryngeal edema and spasm, severe chemical burns to skin, mucous membranes, and internal organs, GI tract perforation and hemorrhage, peritonitis.*

alkyl aluminum [Poison] *Cardiovascular collapse, pulmonary edema, CNS* depression, coma, seizures, nausea, vomiting, cardiopulmonary arrest.

alkyl mercuric chloride [Mercury] *Circulatory collapse, arrhythmias, respiratory failure, pulmonary edema, neurotoxic effects.*

alkyl phenol (n.o.s.) [Phenol] *Coma, hypotension, arrhythmias, pulmonary edema, respiratory arrest.*

alkyl sulfonic acid [Organic acid] *Pulmonary edema, circulatory collapse, laryngeal edema and spasm, severe chemical burns to skin, mucous membranes, and internal organs, GI tract perforation and hemorrhage, peritonitis.*

alkylamine (n.o.s.) [Organic base/amine] *Pulmonary edema, cardiac depression, seizures.*

allene [Aliphatic hydrocarbon] *Arrhythmias, asphyxiation, anesthesia.*

allethrin [Pyrethrin/pyrethroid] *Respiratory paralysis, convulsions.*

allyl acetate [Ester] *CNS depression, respiratory tract irritation, bronchitis, pneumonitis.*

allyl alcohol [Lower alcohol (1–3 carbons)] *CNS depression, coma, respiratory arrest, arrhythmias.*

allyl amine [Organic base/amine] *Pulmonary edema, cardiac depression, seizures.*

allyl bromide [Dichloropropane/dichloropropene] *Pulmonary edema, bronchospasm, alveolar hemorrhage.*

allyl chloride [Dichloropropane/dichloropropene] *Pulmonary edema, bronchospasm, alveolar hemorrhage.* [Chlorine] *Severe respiratory tract irritation, pulmonary edema, irritation of skin, eyes, and mucous membranes.*

allyl chlorocarbonate [Organic acid] *Pulmonary edema, circulatory collapse, laryngeal edema and spasm, severe chemical burns to skin, mucous membranes, and internal organs, GI tract perforation and hemorrhage, peritonitis.*

allyl chloroformate [Ester] *CNS depression, respiratory tract irritation, bronchitis, pneumonitis.*

allyl ethyl ether [Ether] *Anesthesia, respiratory arrest.*

allyl formate [Ester] *CNS depression, respiratory tract irritation, bronchitis, pneumonitis.*

allyl glycidyl ether [Ether] *Anesthesia, respiratory arrest.*

allyl iodide [Dichloropropane/dichloropropene] *Pulmonary edema, bronchospasm, alveolar hemorrhage.* [Iodine] *Hypotension, circulatory collapse, pulmonary edema.*

allyl isothiocyanate [Isocyanate/aliphatic thiocyanate] *CNS depression, respiratory arrest, respiratory paralysis, pulmonary edema, cyanide toxicity.*

allyl trichlorosilane [Silane/chlorosilane] *Respiratory tract irritation, pulmonary edema.*

alpha-benzene ethanamine; α-benzene ethanamine [Aniline] *Methemoglobinemia, hypoxia.*

alpha-dimethyl benzene ethanamine; α-dimethyl benzene ethanamine [Aniline] *Methemoglobinemia, hypoxia.*

alpha-endosulfan; α-endosulfan [Aldrin/dieldrin/endrin] *Seizures, respiratory failure.*

alpha-methylstyrene; α-methylstyrene [Aromatic hydrocarbon] *Arrhythmias, respiratory failure, pulmonary edema, paralysis, brain and kidney damage.*

alpha-naphthylthiourea (ANTU) [Naphthalene] *Delayed-onset acute intravascular hemolysis.*

alpha-pinene; α-pinene [Turpentine/terpene] *Respiratory failure, pulmonary edema, tachycardia.*

alum [Inorganic acid] *Pulmonary edema, bronchospasm, circulatory collapse, laryngeal spasm and edema, severe chemical burns to skin, mucous membranes, and internal organs, GI tract perforation and hemorrhage, peritonitis.*

aluminum [Poison] *Cardiovascular collapse, pulmonary edema, CNS depression, coma, seizures, nausea, vomiting, cardiopulmonary arrest.*

aluminum alkyl [Poison] *Cardiovascular collapse, pulmonary edema, CNS depression, coma, seizures, nausea, vomiting, cardiopulmonary arrest.*

aluminum alkyl chloride [Poison] *Cardiovascular collapse, pulmonary edema, CNS depression, coma, seizures, nausea, vomiting, cardiopulmonary arrest.* [Chlorine] *Severe respiratory tract irritation, pulmonary edema, irritation of skin, eyes, and mucous membranes.*

aluminum alkyl halide [Poison] *Cardiovascular collapse, pulmonary edema, CNS depression, coma, seizures, nausea, vomiting, cardiopulmonary arrest.*

aluminum alkyl hydride [Poison] *Cardiovascular collapse, pulmonary edema, CNS depression, coma, seizures, nausea, vomiting, cardiopulmonary arrest.*

aluminum borohydride [Boron] *Respiratory tract irritation, laryngeal spasm and edema, pulmonary edema, severe chemical burns.*

aluminum bromide [Bromine/methyl bromide] *Severe respiratory irritation, pulmonary edema, respiratory failure, coma, convulsions, death.*

aluminum carbide [Poison] *Cardiovascular collapse, pulmonary edema, CNS depression, coma, seizures, nausea, vomiting, cardiopulmonary arrest.*

aluminum chloride [Poison] *Cardiovascular collapse, pulmonary edema, CNS depression, coma, seizures, nausea, vomiting, cardiopulmonary arrest.* [Chlorine] *Severe respiratory tract irritation, pulmonary edema, irritation of skin, eyes, and mucous membranes.*

aluminum ferrosilicon [Iron] *Hypovolemic shock.*

aluminum hydride [Poison] *Cardiovascular collapse, pulmonary edema, CNS depression, coma, seizures, nausea, vomiting, cardiopulmonary arrest.*

aluminum nitrate [Nitrate/nitrite] *Methemoglobinemia, hypotension, circulatory collapse.*

aluminum oxide [Poison] *Cardiovascular collapse, pulmonary edema, CNS depression, coma, seizures, nausea, vomiting, cardiopulmonary arrest.*

aluminum phosphate [Inorganic acid] *Pulmonary edema, bronchospasm, circulatory collapse, laryngeal spasm and edema, severe chemical burns to skin, mucous membranes, and internal organs, GI tract perforation and hemorrhage, peritonitis.*

aluminum phosphide [Phosphine] *Severe pulmonary irritation, pulmonary edema.*

aluminum powder, pyrophoric [Flammable solid] *Shock, severe chemical and thermal burns, severe respiratory tract irritation, pulmonary edema, respiratory arrest, ECG changes, sudden death.*

aluminum resinate [Poison] *Cardiovascular collapse, pulmonary edema, CNS depression, coma, seizures, nausea, vomiting, cardiopulmonary arrest.*

aluminum silicon [Poison] *Cardiovascular collapse, pulmonary edema, CNS depression, coma, seizures, nausea, vomiting, cardiopulmonary arrest.*

aluminum sulfate [Inorganic acid] *Pulmonary edema, bronchospasm, circulatory collapse, laryngeal spasm and edema, severe chemical burns to skin, mucous membranes, and internal organs, GI tract perforation and hemorrhage, peritonitis.*

2-aminoanthraquinone [Poison] *Cardiovascular collapse, pulmonary edema, CNS depression, coma, seizures, nausea, vomiting, cardiopulmonary arrest.*

4-aminoazobenzene [Aniline] *Methemoglobinemia, hypoxia.*

4-aminobiphenyl [Nitrate/nitrite] *Methemoglobinemia, hypotension, circulatory collapse.*

Aminocarb [Carbamate] *Acetylcholinesterase inhibition (reversible), bradycardia, hypotension, respiratory muscle paralysis, respiratory arrest, pulmonary edema.*

aminochlorophenol [Phenol] *Coma, hypotension, arrhythmias, pulmonary edema, respiratory arrest.*

2-amino-5-diethylaminopentane [Organic base/amine] *Pulmonary edema, cardiac depression, seizures.* [Aliphatic hydrocarbon] *Arrhythmias, asphyxiation, anesthesia.*

aminodimethylbutyronitrile [Cyanide] *Impairment of cellular oxygenation and adenosine triphosphate production, hypoxia, death.*

aminoethoxyethanol [Organic base/amine] *Pulmonary edema, cardiac depression, seizures.* [Lower alcohol (1–3 carbons)] *CNS depression, coma, respiratory arrest, arrhythmias.*

2-aminoethylethanolamine [Organic base/amine] *Pulmonary edema, cardiac depression, seizures.* [Lower alcohol (1–3 carbons)] *CNS depression, coma, respiratory arrest, arrhythmias.*

aminoethylpiperazine [Organic base/amine] *Pulmonary edema, cardiac depression, seizures.*

1-amino-2-methylanthraquinone [Organic base/amine] *Pulmonary edema, cardiac depression, seizures.*

5-(aminomethyl)-3-isoxazolol [Poison] *Cardiovascular collapse, pulmonary edema, CNS depression, coma, seizures, nausea, vomiting, cardiopulmonary arrest.*

4-amino-2-nitrophenol [Aniline] *Methemoglobinemia, hypoxia.*

aminophenol [Aniline] *Methemoglobinemia, hypoxia.*

aminopropyldiethanolamine [Organic base/amine] *Pulmonary edema, cardiac depression, seizures.*

aminopropylmorpholine [Organic base/amine] *Pulmonary edema, cardiac depression, seizures.*

aminopropylpiperazine [Organic base/amine] *Pulmonary edema, cardiac depression, seizures.*

aminopterin [Poison] *Cardiovascular collapse, pulmonary edema, CNS depression, coma, seizures, nausea, vomiting, cardiopulmonary arrest.*

aminopyridine [Aromatic hydrocarbon] *Arrhythmias, respiratory failure, pulmonary edema, paralysis, brain and kidney damage.*

p-aminosalicylic acid [Organic acid] *Pulmonary edema, circulatory collapse, laryngeal edema and spasm, severe chemical burns to skin, mucous membranes, and internal organs, GI tract perforation and hemorrhage, peritonitis.*

Amiton [Organophosphate] *Pulmonary edema, respiratory muscle paralysis, respiratory failure, bradycardia, acetylcholinesterase inhibition, hypotension, pulmonary edema, overstimulation of parasympathetic nervous system, striated muscle, sympathetic ganglia, and CNS.*

Amiton Oxalate [Organophosphate] *Pulmonary edema, respiratory muscle paralysis, respiratory failure, bradycardia, acetylcholinesterase inhibition, hypotension, pulmonary edema, overstimulation of parasympathetic nervous system, striated muscle, sympathetic ganglia, and CNS.*

amitrole [Poison] *Cardiovascular collapse, pulmonary edema, CNS depression, coma, seizures, nausea, vomiting, cardiopulmonary arrest.*

ammonia; anhydrous ammonia; ammonium salt (n.o.s.) [Ammonia] *Pulmonary edema, hypotension.*

ammoniated cupric sulfate [Copper] *Respiratory tract irritation, respiratory arrest, hemorrhagic gastritis.*

ammoniated mercury [Mercury] *Circulatory collapse, arrhythmias, respiratory failure, pulmonary edema, neurotoxic effects.*

ammonium acetate [Ammonia] *Pulmonary edema, hypotension.*

ammonium arsenate [Arsenic] *Heavy metal toxicity, vomiting, GI bleeding, CNS depression, pulmonary edema, cardiac arrest.*

ammonium benzoate [Ammonia] *Pulmonary edema, hypotension.*

ammonium bicarbonate [Ammonia] *Pulmonary edema, hypotension.*

HazMat

ammonium bichromate [Ammonia] *Pulmonary edema, hypotension.*

ammonium bifluoride [Fluorine] *CNS depression, respiratory arrest, cardiovascular collapse, shock, arrhythmias.*

ammonium bisulfite [Ammonia] *Pulmonary edema, hypotension.* [Sulfur] *Respiratory tract irritation, pulmonary edema, anaphylaxis.*

ammonium bromide [Bromine/methyl bromide] *Severe respiratory irritation, pulmonary edema, respiratory failure, coma, convulsions, death.*

ammonium carbamate [Ammonia] *Pulmonary edema, hypotension.*

ammonium carbonate [Ammonia] *Pulmonary edema, hypotension.*

ammonium chloride [Ammonia] *Pulmonary edema, hypotension.*

ammonium chromate [Ammonia] *Pulmonary edema, hypotension.*

ammonium citrate [Ammonia] *Pulmonary edema, hypotension.*

ammonium dichromate [Ammonia] *Pulmonary edema, hypotension.*

ammonium dinitro-o-cresolate [Ammonia] *Pulmonary edema, hypotension.*

ammonium fluoride [Fluorine] *CNS depression, respiratory arrest, cardiovascular collapse, shock, arrhythmias.*

ammonium fluoroborate [Boron] *Respiratory tract irritation, laryngeal spasm and edema, pulmonary edema, severe chemical burns.*

ammonium fluororate [Boron] *Respiratory tract irritation, laryngeal spasm and edema, pulmonary edema, severe chemical burns.*

ammonium fluorosilicate [Fluorine] *CNS depression, respiratory arrest, cardiovascular collapse, shock, arrhythmias.*

ammonium hydrogen fluoride [Fluorine] *CNS depression, respiratory arrest, cardiovascular collapse, shock, arrhythmias.*

ammonium hydrogen sulfate [Inorganic acid] *Pulmonary edema, bronchospasm, circulatory collapse, laryngeal spasm and edema, severe chemical burns to skin, mucous membranes, and internal organs, GI tract perforation and hemorrhage, peritonitis.*

ammonium hydrosulfide [Ammonia] *Pulmonary edema, hypotension.*

ammonium hydroxide [Inorganic base/alkaline corrosive] *Upper airway burns and edema, pulmonary edema, skin burns, circulatory collapse, GI tract perforation and hemorrhage, peritonitis.*

ammonium metavanadate [Poison] *Cardiovascular collapse, pulmonary edema, CNS depression, coma, seizures, nausea, vomiting, cardiopulmonary arrest.*

ammonium nitrate [Nitrate/nitrite] *Methemoglobinemia, hypotension, circulatory collapse.*

ammonium nitrate & ammonium phosphate mixture [Nitrate/nitrite] *Methemoglobinemia, hypotension, circulatory collapse.*

ammonium nitrate & ammonium sulfate mixture [Ammonia] *Pulmonary edema, hypotension.* [Nitrate/nitrite] *Methemoglobinemia, hypotension, circulatory collapse.* [Sulfur] *Respiratory tract irritation, pulmonary edema, anaphylaxis.*

ammonium nitrate & calcium carbonate mixture [Nitrate/nitrite] *Methemoglobinemia, hypotension, circulatory collapse.*

ammonium nitrate & [diesel] fuel oil (ANFO) mixture [Explosive] *Multiple trauma, highly toxic chemical exposure.* [Nitrate/nitrite] *Methemoglobinemia, hypotension, circulatory collapse.*

ammonium nitrate & potassium carbonate mixture [Nitrate/nitrite] *Methemoglobinemia, hypotension, circulatory collapse.*

ammonium nitrate & potassium hydroxide mixture [Inorganic base/alkaline corrosive] *Upper airway burns and edema, pulmonary edema, skin burns, circulatory collapse, GI tract perforation and hemorrhage, peritonitis.* [Nitrate/nitrite] *Methemoglobinemia, hypotension, circulatory collapse.*

ammonium oxalate [Oxalate] *Cardiovascular collapse, arrhythmias, seizures.* [Ammonia] *Pulmonary edema, hypotension.*

ammonium perchlorate [Ammonia] *Pulmonary edema, hypotension.* [Chlorate] *Hemolysis, methemoglobinemia, hypoperfusion, CNS depression, delayed-onset renal failure.*

ammonium permanganate [Inorganic acid] *Pulmonary edema, bronchospasm, circulatory collapse, laryngeal spasm and edema, severe chemical burns to skin, mucous membranes, and internal organs, GI tract perforation and hemorrhage, peritonitis.*

ammonium persulfate [Inorganic acid] *Pulmonary edema, bronchospasm, circulatory collapse, laryngeal spasm and edema, severe chemical burns to skin, mucous membranes, and internal organs, GI tract perforation and hemorrhage, peritonitis.*

ammonium phosphate & ammonium nitrate mixture [Ammonia] *Pulmonary edema, hypotension.* [Nitrate/nitrite] *Methemoglobinemia, hypotension, circulatory collapse.*

ammonium picrate [Inorganic acid] *Pulmonary edema, bronchospasm, circulatory collapse, laryngeal spasm and edema, severe chemical burns to skin, mucous membranes, and internal organs, GI tract perforation and hemorrhage, peritonitis.*

ammonium polysulfide [Ammonia] *Pulmonary edema, hypotension.* [Sulfur] *Respiratory tract irritation, pulmonary edema, anaphylaxis.*

ammonium polyvanadate [Poison] *Cardiovascular collapse, pulmonary edema, CNS depression, coma, seizures, nausea, vomiting, cardiopulmonary arrest.*

ammonium salt (n.o.s.) [Ammonia] *Pulmonary edema, hypotension.*

ammonium silicofluoride [Fluorine] *CNS depression, respiratory arrest, cardiovascular collapse, shock, arrhythmias.*

ammonium sulfamate [Ammonia] *Pulmonary edema, hypotension.* [Sulfur] *Respiratory tract irritation, pulmonary edema, anaphylaxis.*

ammonium sulfate [Ammonia] *Pulmonary edema, hypotension.* [Sulfur] *Respiratory tract irritation, pulmonary edema, anaphylaxis.*

ammonium sulfate & ammonium nitrate mixture [Ammonia] *Pulmonary edema, hypotension.* [Nitrate/nitrite] *Methemoglobinemia, hypotension, circulatory collapse.* [Sulfur] *Respiratory tract irritation, pulmonary edema, anaphylaxis.*

ammonium sulfide [Ammonia] *Pulmonary edema, hypotension.* [Sulfur] *Respiratory tract irritation, pulmonary edema, anaphylaxis.*

ammonium sulfite [Ammonia] *Pulmonary edema, hypotension.* [Sulfur] *Respiratory tract irritation, pulmonary edema, anaphylaxis.*

ammonium tartrate [Organic acid] *Pulmonary edema, circulatory collapse, laryngeal edema and spasm, severe chemical burns to skin, mucous membranes, and internal organs, GI tract perforation and hemorrhage, peritonitis.*

ammonium thiocyanate [Isocyanate/aliphatic thiocyanate] *CNS depression, respiratory arrest, respiratory paralysis, pulmonary edema, cyanide toxicity.*

ammonium vanadate [Poison] *Cardiovascular collapse, pulmonary edema, CNS depression, coma, seizures, nausea, vomiting, cardiopulmonary arrest.*

ammosite; brown asbestos [Asbestos] *Asbestosis, lung cancer, malignant mesothelioma.*

ammunition, irritant nonexplosive [Irritant] *Severe immediate or delayed upper airway or respiratory tract irritation, pulmonary edema, glottic spasm, airway obstruction.*

ammunition, toxic nonexplosive [Poison] *Cardiovascular collapse, pulmonary edema, CNS depression,*

HazMat

coma, seizures, nausea, vomiting, cardiopulmonary arrest.

amphetamine [Poison] *Cardiovascular collapse, pulmonary edema, CNS depression, coma, seizures, nausea, vomiting, cardiopulmonary arrest.*

amygdalin [Cyanide] *Impairment of cellular oxygenation and adenosine triphosphate production, hypoxia, death.*

iso-amyl acetate; sec-amyl acetate; tert-amyl acetate; amyl acetate (n.o.s.) [Ester] *CNS depression, respiratory tract irritation, bronchitis, pneumonitis.*

amyl acid phosphate [Irritant] *Severe immediate or delayed upper airway or respiratory tract irritation, pulmonary edema, glottic spasm, airway obstruction.*

amyl alcohol [Higher alcohol (4+ carbons)] *CNS depression, respiratory failure, arrhythmias.*

amyl aldehyde [Aldehyde] *Seizures, respiratory failure, pulmonary edema.*

amyl butyrate [Organic acid] *Pulmonary edema, circulatory collapse, laryngeal edema and spasm, severe chemical burns to skin, mucous membranes, and internal organs, GI tract perforation and hemorrhage, peritonitis.*

amyl chloride [Halogenated aliphatic hydrocarbon] *CNS depression, respiratory arrest, circulatory collapse.*

amyl formate [Ester] *CNS depression, respiratory tract irritation, bronchitis, pneumonitis.*

tert-amyl hydroperoxide [Organic peroxide] *Pulmonary and laryngeal edema, circulatory arrest, hypovolemic shock, chemical burns to skin, mucous membranes, and internal organs.*

amyl mercaptan [Sulfur] *Respiratory tract irritation, pulmonary edema, anaphylaxis.*

amyl methyl ketone [Ketone] *Respiratory mucous membrane irritation, pulmonary edema, CNS depression.*

amyl nitrate [Nitrate/nitrite] *Methemoglobinemia, hypotension, circulatory collapse.*

amyl nitrite [Nitrate/nitrite] *Methemoglobinemia, hypotension, circulatory collapse.*

tert-amyl peroxybenzoate [Organic peroxide] *Pulmonary and laryngeal edema, circulatory arrest, hypovolemic shock, chemical burns to skin, mucous membranes, and internal organs.* [Organic acid] *Pulmonary edema, circulatory collapse, laryngeal edema and spasm, severe chemical burns to skin, mucous membranes, and internal organs, GI tract perforation and hemorrhage, peritonitis.*

tert-amyl peroxy-2-ethylhexanoate [Organic peroxide] *Pulmonary and laryngeal edema, circulatory arrest, hypovolemic shock, chemical burns to skin, mucous membranes, and internal organs.* [Organic acid] *Pulmonary edema, circulatory collapse, laryngeal edema and spasm, severe chemical burns to skin, mucous membranes, and internal organs, GI tract perforation and hemorrhage, peritonitis.*

tert-amyl peroxyneodecanoate [Organic peroxide] *Pulmonary and laryngeal edema, circulatory arrest, hypovolemic shock, chemical burns to skin, mucous membranes, and internal organs.* [Organic acid] *Pulmonary edema, circulatory collapse, laryngeal edema and spasm, severe chemical burns to skin, mucous membranes, and internal organs, GI tract perforation and hemorrhage, peritonitis.*

tert-amyl peroxypivalate [Organic peroxide] *Pulmonary and laryngeal edema, circulatory arrest, hypovolemic shock, chemical burns to skin, mucous membranes, and internal organs.* [Organic acid] *Pulmonary edema, circulatory collapse, laryngeal edema and spasm, severe chemical burns to skin, mucous membranes, and internal organs, GI tract perforation and hemorrhage, peritonitis.*

amyl phenol [Phenol] *Coma, hypotension, arrhythmias, pulmonary edema, respiratory arrest.*

amyl trichlorocyclane [Halogenated aliphatic hydrocarbon] *CNS depression, respiratory arrest, circulatory collapse.*

amyl trichlorosilane [Silane/chlorosilane] *Respiratory tract irritation, pulmonary edema.*

amylamine [Organic base/amine] *Pulmonary edema, cardiac depression, seizures.*

amylene [Simple asphyxiant] *Asphyxiation.*

anethole [Aromatic hydrocarbon] *Arrhythmias, respiratory failure, pulmonary edema, paralysis, brain and kidney damage.*

ANFO (ammonium nitrate & [diesel] fuel oil mixture) [Explosive] *Multiple trauma, highly toxic chemical exposure.* [Nitrate/nitrite] *Methemoglobinemia, hypotension, circulatory collapse.*

anhydrous ammonia [Ammonia] *Pulmonary edema, hypotension.*

aniline [Aniline] *Methemoglobinemia, hypoxia.*

aniline HCl [Aniline] *Methemoglobinemia, hypoxia.*

animal fabric with oil (n.o.s.) [Flammable/combustible liquid] *CNS depression, respiratory arrest, convulsions, arrhythmias, pulmonary edema.*

animal fiber, burnt (n.o.s.) [Irritant] *Severe immediate or delayed upper airway or respiratory tract irritation, pulmonary edema, glottic spasm, airway obstruction.*

animal fiber with oil (n.o.s.) [Flammable/combustible liquid] *CNS depression, respiratory arrest, convulsions, arrhythmias, pulmonary edema.*

anisidine; o-anisidine HCl [Benzene] *Arrhythmias, respiratory failure, pulmonary edema, CNS depression, liver and kidney damage.*

anisindione [Warfarin/hydroxycoumarin/indanedione] *Anticoagulation effect, internal hemorrhage.*

anisole [Aromatic hydrocarbon] *Arrhythmias, respiratory failure, pulmonary edema, paralysis, brain and kidney damage.*

anisoyl chloride [Organic acid] *Pulmonary edema, circulatory collapse, laryngeal edema and spasm, severe chemical burns to skin, mucous membranes, and internal organs, GI tract perforation and hemorrhage, peritonitis.*

anthophyllite [Asbestos] *Asbestosis, lung cancer, malignant mesothelioma.*

anthracene [Aromatic hydrocarbon] *Arrhythmias, respiratory failure, pulmonary edema, paralysis, brain and kidney damage.*

antifreeze [Ethylene glycol] *Respiratory failure, pulmonary edema, paralysis, cardiovascular collapse, severe acidosis.*

antiknock compound [Lead] *Circulatory collapse, coma, rare seizures.*

antimony; antimony mixture (n.o.s.); antimony salt (n.o.s.) [Poison] *Cardiovascular collapse, pulmonary edema, CNS depression, coma, seizures, nausea, vomiting, cardiopulmonary arrest.*

antimony chloride [Poison] *Cardiovascular collapse, pulmonary edema, CNS depression, coma, seizures, nausea, vomiting, cardiopulmonary arrest.*

antimony hydride [Poison] *Cardiovascular collapse, pulmonary edema, CNS depression, coma, seizures, nausea, vomiting, cardiopulmonary arrest.*

antimony lactate [Poison] *Cardiovascular collapse, pulmonary edema, CNS depression, coma, seizures, nausea, vomiting, cardiopulmonary arrest.*

antimony pentachloride [Poison] *Cardiovascular collapse, pulmonary edema, CNS depression, coma, seizures, nausea, vomiting, cardiopulmonary arrest.*

antimony pentafluoride [Fluorine] *CNS depression, respiratory arrest, cardiovascular collapse, shock, arrhythmias.*

antimony pentasulfide [Poison] *Cardiovascular collapse, pulmonary edema, CNS depression, coma, seizures, nausea, vomiting, cardiopulmonary arrest.*

HazMat

antimony potassium [Poison] *Cardiovascular collapse, pulmonary edema, CNS depression, coma, seizures, nausea, vomiting, cardiopulmonary arrest.*

antimony potassium tartrate [Poison] *Cardiovascular collapse, pulmonary edema, CNS depression, coma, seizures, nausea, vomiting, cardiopulmonary arrest.*

antimony tribromide [Bromine/methyl bromide] *Severe respiratory irritation, pulmonary edema, respiratory failure, coma, convulsions, death.*

antimony trichloride [Poison] *Cardiovascular collapse, pulmonary edema, CNS depression, coma, seizures, nausea, vomiting, cardiopulmonary arrest.*

antimony trifluoride [Fluorine] *CNS depression, respiratory arrest, cardiovascular collapse, shock, arrhythmias.*

antimony trioxide [Poison] *Cardiovascular collapse, pulmonary edema, CNS depression, coma, seizures, nausea, vomiting, cardiopulmonary arrest.*

ANTU (alpha-naphthylthiourea) [Naphthalene] *Delayed-onset acute intravascular hemolysis.*

Apl-Luster [Thiabendazole] *Cardiovascular collapse, respiratory tract irritation.*

Arbotect [Thiabendazole] *Cardiovascular collapse, respiratory tract irritation.*

argon (compressed gas or cryogenic liquid) [Simple asphyxiant] *Asphyxiation.*

aroclor 1016, 1221, 1232, 1242, 1248, 1254, or 1260 [Polychlorinated biphenyl/polybrominated biphenyl/polychlorinated dibenzofuran] *Liver and kidney damage.*

aromatic extract (n.o.s.) [Aromatic hydrocarbon] *Arrhythmias, respiratory failure, pulmonary edema, paralysis, brain and kidney damage.*

aromatic hydrocarbon, polynuclear (n.o.s.) [Poison] *Cardiovascular collapse, pulmonary edema, CNS depression, coma, seizures, nausea, vomiting, cardiopulmonary arrest.*

aromatic hydrocarbon solvent (n.o.s.) [Aromatic hydrocarbon] *Arrhythmias, respiratory failure, pulmonary edema, paralysis, brain and kidney damage.*

aromatic naphtha solvent [Naphthalene] *Delayed-onset acute intravascular hemolysis.*

aromatic nitrogen compound [Aniline] *Methemoglobinemia, hypoxia.*

arsanilic acid [Arsenic] *Heavy metal toxicity, vomiting, GI bleeding, CNS depression, pulmonary edema, cardiac arrest.*

arsenate (n.o.s.) [Arsenic] *Heavy metal toxicity, vomiting, GI bleeding, CNS depression, pulmonary edema, cardiac arrest.*

arsenic [Arsenic] *Heavy metal toxicity, vomiting, GI bleeding, CNS depression, pulmonary edema, cardiac arrest.*

arsenic acid [Arsenic] *Heavy metal toxicity, vomiting, GI bleeding, CNS depression, pulmonary edema, cardiac arrest.*

arsenic bromide [Arsenic] *Heavy metal toxicity, vomiting, GI bleeding, CNS depression, pulmonary edema, cardiac arrest.* [Bromine/methyl bromide] *Severe respiratory irritation, pulmonary edema, respiratory failure, coma, convulsions, death.*

arsenic chloride [Arsenic] *Heavy metal toxicity, vomiting, GI bleeding, CNS depression, pulmonary edema, cardiac arrest.* [Chlorine] *Severe respiratory tract irritation, pulmonary edema, irritation of skin, eyes, and mucous membranes.*

arsenic disulfide [Arsenic] *Heavy metal toxicity, vomiting, GI bleeding, CNS depression, pulmonary edema, cardiac arrest.*

arsenic iodide [Arsenic] *Heavy metal toxicity, vomiting, GI bleeding, CNS depression, pulmonary edema, cardiac arrest.*

arsenic mixture (n.o.s.) [Arsenic] *Heavy metal toxicity, vomiting, GI bleeding, CNS depression, pulmonary edema, cardiac arrest.*

arsenic pentoxide [Arsenic] *Heavy metal toxicity, vomiting, GI bleeding, CNS depression, pulmonary edema, cardiac arrest.*

arsenic trichloride [Arsenic] *Heavy metal toxicity, vomiting, GI bleeding, CNS depression, pulmonary edema, cardiac arrest.* [Chlorine] *Severe respiratory tract irritation, pulmonary edema, irritation of skin, eyes, and mucous membranes.*

arsenic trihydride [Arsenic] *Heavy metal toxicity, vomiting, GI bleeding, CNS depression, pulmonary edema, cardiac arrest.*

arsenic trioxide [Arsenic] *Heavy metal toxicity, vomiting, GI bleeding, CNS depression, pulmonary edema, cardiac arrest.*

arsenic trisulfide [Arsenic] *Heavy metal toxicity, vomiting, GI bleeding, CNS depression, pulmonary edema, cardiac arrest.*

arsenical flue dust [Arsenic] *Heavy metal toxicity, vomiting, GI bleeding, CNS depression, pulmonary edema, cardiac arrest.*

arsenical pesticide (n.o.s.) [Arsenic] *Heavy metal toxicity, vomiting, GI bleeding, CNS depression, pulmonary edema, cardiac arrest.*

arsenite (n.o.s.) [Arsenic] *Heavy metal toxicity, vomiting, GI bleeding, CNS depression, pulmonary edema, cardiac arrest.*

arsenite, bordeaux [Arsenic] *Heavy metal toxicity, vomiting, GI bleeding, CNS depression, pulmonary edema, cardiac arrest.* [Copper] *Respiratory tract irritation, respiratory arrest, hemorrhagic gastritis.*

arsenous oxide [Arsenic] *Heavy metal toxicity, vomiting, GI bleeding, CNS depression, pulmonary edema, cardiac arrest.*

arsenous trichloride [Arsenic] *Heavy metal toxicity, vomiting, GI bleeding, CNS depression, pulmonary edema, cardiac arrest.* [Chlorine] *Severe respiratory tract irritation, pulmonary edema, irritation of skin, eyes, and mucous membranes.*

arsine [Arsine] *Intravascular hemolysis, pulmonary edema, cardiac and respiratory arrest, delayed-onset jaundice, and acute or delayed-onset renal failure.*

aryl amine [Aniline] *Methemoglobinemia, hypoxia.*

aryl sulfonic acid [Organic acid] *Pulmonary edema, circulatory collapse, laryngeal edema and spasm, severe chemical burns to skin, mucous membranes, and internal organs, GI tract perforation and hemorrhage, peritonitis.*

asbestos [Asbestos] *Asbestosis, lung cancer, malignant mesothelioma.*

asphalt [Hydrocarbon mixture] *CNS depression, respiratory arrest, seizures, arrhythmias, pulmonary edema.*

auramine [Aniline] *Methemoglobinemia, hypoxia.*

aviation fuel [Hydrocarbon mixture] *CNS depression, respiratory arrest, seizures, arrhythmias, pulmonary edema.*

azaserine [Poison] *Cardiovascular collapse, pulmonary edema, CNS depression, coma, seizures, nausea, vomiting, cardiopulmonary arrest.*

azinphos-ethyl [Organophosphate] *Pulmonary edema, respiratory muscle paralysis, respiratory failure, bradycardia, acetylcholinesterase inhibition, hypotension, pulmonary edema, overstimulation of parasympathetic nervous system, striated muscle, sympathetic ganglia, and CNS.*

azinphos-methyl (Guthion) [Organophosphate] *Pulmonary edema, respiratory muscle paralysis, respiratory failure, bradycardia, acetylcholinesterase inhibition, hypotension, pulmonary edema, overstimulation of parasympathetic nervous system, striated muscle, sympathetic ganglia, and CNS.*

aziridine [Organic base/amine] *Pulmonary edema, cardiac depression, seizures.*

1-aziridinyl phosphine oxide (tris) [Poison] *Cardiovascular collapse, pulmonary edema, CNS depression,*

HazMat

coma, seizures, nausea, vomiting, cardiopulmonary arrest.

azobenzene [Aniline] *Methemoglobinemia, hypoxia.*

2,2'-azodi-(2,4-dimethyl-4-methoxyvaleronitrile) [Poison] *Cardiovascular collapse, pulmonary edema, CNS depression, coma, seizures, nausea, vomiting, cardiopulmonary arrest.*

2,2'-azodi-(2,4-dimethyl-valeronitrile) [Poison] *Cardiovascular collapse, pulmonary edema, CNS depression, coma, seizures, nausea, vomiting, cardiopulmonary arrest.*

1,1'-azodi-(hexahydrobenzonitrile) [Poison] *Cardiovascular collapse, pulmonary edema, CNS depression, coma, seizures, nausea, vomiting, cardiopulmonary arrest.*

azodiisobutyronitrile [Cyanide] *Impairment of cellular oxygenation and adenosine triphosphate production, hypoxia, death.*

2,2'-azodi-(2-methyl-butyronitrile) [Poison] *Cardiovascular collapse, pulmonary edema, CNS depression, coma, seizures, nausea, vomiting, cardiopulmonary arrest.*

Bandane [Chlordane] *Respiratory failure, seizures, exhaustion, death.*

barium; barium alloy (n.o.s.); barium metal; barium mixture (n.o.s.); barium salt (n.o.s.) [Barium] *Hypokalemia, muscle paralysis, arrhythmias, cardiac and respiratory arrest.*

barium azide [Barium] *Hypokalemia, muscle paralysis, arrhythmias, cardiac and respiratory arrest.*

barium bromate [Barium] *Hypokalemia, muscle paralysis, arrhythmias, cardiac and respiratory arrest.* [Bromate] *CNS and respiratory system depression, delayed-onset renal failure.*

barium chlorate [Barium] *Hypokalemia, muscle paralysis, arrhythmias, cardiac and respiratory arrest.* [Chlorate] *Hemolysis, methemoglobinemia, hypoperfusion, CNS depression, delayed-onset renal failure.*

barium cyanide [Barium] *Hypokalemia, muscle paralysis, arrhythmias, cardiac and respiratory arrest.* [Cyanide] *Impairment of cellular oxygenation and adenosine triphosphate production, hypoxia, death.*

barium fluosilicate [Rotenone] *Respiratory arrest, asphyxia.* [Barium] *Hypokalemia, muscle paralysis, arrhythmias, cardiac and respiratory arrest.*

barium hypochlorite [Hypochlorite] *Circulatory collapse, respiratory tract irritation, upper airway obstruction, pulmonary edema.* [Barium] *Hypokalemia, muscle paralysis, arrhythmias, cardiac and respiratory arrest.*

barium metaborate [Barium] *Hypokalemia, muscle paralysis, arrhythmias, cardiac and respiratory arrest.* [Boron] *Respiratory tract irritation, laryngeal spasm and edema, pulmonary edema, severe chemical burns.*

barium nitrate [Nitrate/nitrite] *Methemoglobinemia, hypotension, circulatory collapse.* [Barium] *Hypokalemia, muscle paralysis, arrhythmias, cardiac and respiratory arrest.*

barium oxide [Barium] *Hypokalemia, muscle paralysis, arrhythmias, cardiac and respiratory arrest.*

barium perchlorate [Barium] *Hypokalemia, muscle paralysis, arrhythmias, cardiac and respiratory arrest.* [Chlorate] *Hemolysis, methemoglobinemia, hypoperfusion, CNS depression, delayed-onset renal failure.*

barium permanganate [Inorganic acid] *Pulmonary edema, bronchospasm, circulatory collapse, laryngeal spasm and edema, severe chemical burns to skin, mucous membranes, and internal organs, GI tract perforation and hemorrhage, peritonitis.* [Barium] *Hypokalemia, muscle paralysis, arrhythmias, cardiac and respiratory arrest.*

barium peroxide [Barium] *Hypokalemia, muscle paralysis, arrhythmias, cardiac and respiratory arrest.*

barium selenate [Barium] *Hypokalemia, muscle paralysis, arrhythmias,* *cardiac and respiratory arrest.* [Selenium] *Arrhythmias, pulmonary edema, bronchospasm, seizures, vomiting, GI bleeding.*

barium selenite [Barium] *Hypokalemia, muscle paralysis, arrhythmias, cardiac and respiratory arrest.* [Selenium] *Arrhythmias, pulmonary edema, bronchospasm, seizures, vomiting, GI bleeding.*

barthrin [Pyrethrin/pyrethroid] *Respiratory paralysis, convulsions.*

battery (electric), acid-filled [Inorganic acid] *Pulmonary edema, bronchospasm, circulatory collapse, laryngeal spasm and edema, severe chemical burns to skin, mucous membranes, and internal organs, GI tract perforation and hemorrhage, peritonitis.*

battery (electric), alkali-filled [Inorganic base/alkaline corrosive] *Upper airway burns and edema, pulmonary edema, skin burns, circulatory collapse, GI tract perforation and hemorrhage, peritonitis.*

battery (electric) with potassium hydroxide [Inorganic base/alkaline corrosive] *Upper airway burns and edema, pulmonary edema, skin burns, circulatory collapse, GI tract perforation and hemorrhage, peritonitis.*

battery fluid, acid [Inorganic acid] *Pulmonary edema, bronchospasm, circulatory collapse, laryngeal spasm and edema, severe chemical burns to skin, mucous membranes, and internal organs, GI tract perforation and hemorrhage, peritonitis.*

battery fluid, alkali [Inorganic base/alkaline corrosive] *Upper airway burns and edema, pulmonary edema, skin burns, circulatory collapse, GI tract perforation and hemorrhage, peritonitis.*

Baygon [Carbamate] *Acetylcholinesterase inhibition (reversible), bradycardia, hypotension, respiratory muscle paralysis, respiratory arrest, pulmonary edema.*

bendiocarb [Carbamate] *Acetylcholinesterase inhibition (reversible), bradycardia,* *hypotension, respiratory muscle paralysis, respiratory arrest, pulmonary edema.*

benomyl [Dithiocarbamate] *Hypotension, respiratory failure.*

bensulfide [Organophosphate] *Pulmonary edema, respiratory muscle paralysis, respiratory failure, bradycardia, acetylcholinesterase inhibition, hypotension, pulmonary edema, overstimulation of parasympathetic nervous system, striated muscle, sympathetic ganglia, and CNS.*

benz[c]acridine [Poison] *Cardiovascular collapse, pulmonary edema, CNS depression, coma, seizures, nausea, vomiting, cardiopulmonary arrest.*

benzal chloride [Aromatic hydrocarbon] *Arrhythmias, respiratory failure, pulmonary edema, paralysis, brain and kidney damage.*

benzaldehyde [Aldehyde] *Seizures, respiratory failure, pulmonary edema.*

benzamide [Organic acid] *Pulmonary edema, circulatory collapse, laryngeal edema and spasm, severe chemical burns to skin, mucous membranes, and internal organs, GI tract perforation and hemorrhage, peritonitis.*

benz[a]anthracene [Naphthalene] *Delayed-onset acute intravascular hemolysis.*

benzenamine, 3-(trifluoromethyl) [Aniline] *Methemoglobinemia, hypoxia.*

benzene [Benzene] *Arrhythmias, respiratory failure, pulmonary edema, CNS depression, liver and kidney damage.* ☑ benzine

benzene, chlorinated [Lindane] *CNS stimulation, seizures, respiratory failure.*

α-benzene ethanamine; alpha-benzene ethanamine [Aniline] *Methemoglobinemia, hypoxia.*

benzene ethanamine, alpha-dimethyl [Aniline] *Methemoglobinemia, hypoxia.*

benzene hexachloride [Lindane] *CNS stimulation, seizures, respiratory failure.*

benzene phosphorus dichloride [Phosphorus] *Hypovolemic shock, severe tissue burns, severe respiratory* *irritation, pulmonary edema, respiratory arrest, arrhythmias, sudden death.*

benzene phosphorus thiodichloride [Phosphorus] *Hypovolemic shock, severe tissue burns, severe respiratory irritation, pulmonary edema, respiratory arrest, arrhythmias, sudden death.*

benzene sulfohydrazide [Organic acid] *Pulmonary edema, circulatory collapse, laryngeal edema and spasm, severe chemical burns to skin, mucous membranes, and internal organs, GI tract perforation and hemorrhage, peritonitis.*

benzene sulfonyl chloride [Organic acid] *Pulmonary edema, circulatory collapse, laryngeal edema and spasm, severe chemical burns to skin, mucous membranes, and internal organs, GI tract perforation and hemorrhage, peritonitis.*

benzenearsonic acid [Arsenic] *Heavy metal toxicity, vomiting, GI bleeding, CNS depression, pulmonary edema, cardiac arrest.*

benzene-1,3-disulfohydrazide [Aromatic hydrocarbon] *Arrhythmias, respiratory failure, pulmonary edema, paralysis, brain and kidney damage.*

benzenethiol [Aliphatic hydrocarbon] *Arrhythmias, asphyxiation, anesthesia.*

benzidine [Aliphatic hydrocarbon] *Arrhythmias, asphyxiation, anesthesia.*

benzimidazole, 4,5-dichloro-2-(trifluorome) [Aromatic hydrocarbon] *Arrhythmias, respiratory failure, pulmonary edema, paralysis, brain and kidney damage.*

benzine [Benzene] *Arrhythmias, respiratory failure, pulmonary edema, CNS depression, liver and kidney damage.* [Hydrocarbon mixture] *CNS depression, respiratory arrest, seizures, arrhythmias, pulmonary edema.* ② benzene

benzo[b]fluoranthene [Aromatic hydrocarbon] *Arrhythmias, respiratory failure, pulmonary edema, paralysis, brain and kidney damage.*

benzo[k]fluoranthene [Aromatic hydrocarbon] *Arrhythmias, respiratory failure, pulmonary edema, paralysis, brain and kidney damage.*

benzoic acid [Organic acid] *Pulmonary edema, circulatory collapse, laryngeal edema and spasm, severe chemical burns to skin, mucous membranes, and internal organs, GI tract perforation and hemorrhage, peritonitis.*

benzoic acid derivative pesticide (n.o.s.) [Organic acid] *Pulmonary edema, circulatory collapse, laryngeal edema and spasm, severe chemical burns to skin, mucous membranes, and internal organs, GI tract perforation and hemorrhage, peritonitis.*

benzoic trichloride [Organic acid] *Pulmonary edema, circulatory collapse, laryngeal edema and spasm, severe chemical burns to skin, mucous membranes, and internal organs, GI tract perforation and hemorrhage, peritonitis.*

benzol [Benzene] *Arrhythmias, respiratory failure, pulmonary edema, CNS depression, liver and kidney damage.*

benzonitrile [Cyanide] *Impairment of cellular oxygenation and adenosine triphosphate production, hypoxia, death.*

benzo[ghi]perylene [Aromatic hydrocarbon] *Arrhythmias, respiratory failure, pulmonary edema, paralysis, brain and kidney damage.*

benzo[a]pyrene [Aromatic hydrocarbon] *Arrhythmias, respiratory failure, pulmonary edema, paralysis, brain and kidney damage.*

benzoquinone [Aromatic hydrocarbon] *Arrhythmias, respiratory failure, pulmonary edema, paralysis, brain and kidney damage.*

benzotrichloride [Irritant] *Severe immediate or delayed upper airway or respiratory tract irritation, pulmonary edema, glottic spasm, airway obstruction.* [Aromatic hydrocarbon] *Arrhythmias, respiratory failure, pulmonary edema, paralysis, brain and kidney damage.*

benzotrifluoride [Irritant] *Severe immediate or delayed upper airway or respiratory tract irritation, pulmonary edema, glottic spasm, airway obstruction.* [Aromatic hydrocarbon]

Arrhythmias, respiratory failure, pulmonary edema, paralysis, brain and kidney damage.

benzoyl chloride [Irritant] *Severe immediate or delayed upper airway or respiratory tract irritation, pulmonary edema, glottic spasm, airway obstruction.* [Aromatic hydrocarbon] *Arrhythmias, respiratory failure, pulmonary edema, paralysis, brain and kidney damage.*

benzoyl peroxide [Organic peroxide] *Pulmonary and laryngeal edema, circulatory arrest, hypovolemic shock, chemical burns to skin, mucous membranes, and internal organs.*

benzyl bromide [Aromatic hydrocarbon] *Arrhythmias, respiratory failure, pulmonary edema, paralysis, brain and kidney damage.*

benzyl chloride [Aromatic hydrocarbon] *Arrhythmias, respiratory failure, pulmonary edema, paralysis, brain and kidney damage.*

benzyl chloroformate [Ester] *CNS depression, respiratory tract irritation, bronchitis, pneumonitis.*

benzyl cyanide [Cyanide] *Impairment of cellular oxygenation and adenosine triphosphate production, hypoxia, death.*

benzyl dimethylamine [Aniline] *Methemoglobinemia, hypoxia.*

benzyl iodide [Aromatic hydrocarbon] *Arrhythmias, respiratory failure, pulmonary edema, paralysis, brain and kidney damage.*

4-(benzyl(ethyl)amino)-3-ethoxy-benzenediazonium zinc chloride [Poison] *Cardiovascular collapse, pulmonary edema, CNS depression, coma, seizures, nausea, vomiting, cardiopulmonary arrest.* [Zinc] *Respiratory tract irritation, metal fume fever, pulmonary edema.*

benzylidene chloride [Aromatic hydrocarbon] *Arrhythmias, respiratory failure, pulmonary edema, paralysis, brain and kidney damage.*

4-(benzyl(methyl)amino)-3-ethoxy-benzenediazonium zinc chloride [Poison] *Cardiovascular collapse, pulmonary edema, CNS depression, coma, seizures, nausea, vomiting, cardiopulmonary arrest.* [Zinc] *Respiratory tract irritation, metal fume fever, pulmonary edema.*

o-benzyl-p-chlorophenol [Aromatic hydrocarbon] *Arrhythmias, respiratory failure, pulmonary edema, paralysis, brain and kidney damage.*

beryllium chloride [Beryllium] *Pneumonitis, pulmonary edema.*

beryllium fluoride [Beryllium] *Pneumonitis, pulmonary edema.*

beryllium mixture (n.o.s.) [Beryllium] *Pneumonitis, pulmonary edema.*

beryllium nitrate [Beryllium] *Pneumonitis, pulmonary edema.*

beryllium powder [Beryllium] *Pneumonitis, pulmonary edema.*

beta-endosulfan; β-endosulfan [Aldrin/dieldrin/endrin] *Seizures, respiratory failure.*

beta-naphthol; β-naphthol [Phenol] *Coma, hypotension, arrhythmias, pulmonary edema, respiratory arrest.*

beta-propiolactone; β-propiolactone; β-propionolactone [Ketone] *Respiratory mucous membrane irritation, pulmonary edema, CNS depression.*

BHC (alpha-, beta-, or delta-) [Lindane] *CNS stimulation, seizures, respiratory failure.*

bhusa [Poison] *Cardiovascular collapse, pulmonary edema, CNS depression, coma, seizures, nausea, vomiting, cardiopulmonary arrest.*

Bidrin [Organophosphate] *Pulmonary edema, respiratory muscle paralysis, respiratory failure, bradycardia, acetylcholinesterase inhibition, hypotension, pulmonary edema, overstimulation of parasympathetic nervous system, striated muscle, sympathetic ganglia, and CNS.*

bifluoride (n.o.s.) [Fluorine] *CNS depression, respiratory arrest, cardiovascular collapse, shock, arrhythmias.*

biological agent (n.o.s.) *No acute symptoms during incubation period.*

Physiologic response varies depending on strain of microorganism or toxin.

2,2'-bioxirane [Ether] *Anesthesia, respiratory arrest.*

biphenyl [Aromatic hydrocarbon] *Arrhythmias, respiratory failure, pulmonary edema, paralysis, brain and kidney damage.*

bipyridilium pesticide (n.o.s.) [Paraquat] *Pulmonary edema, cardiac damage, circulatory collapse, cerebral hemorrhage or infarcts, death. (Defoliant used in warfare.)*

bis(aminopropyl) amine [Organic base/amine] *Pulmonary edema, cardiac depression, seizures.*

bis(2-chloroethoxy) methane [Ether] *Anesthesia, respiratory arrest.*

bis(2-chloroethyl) ether [Ether] *Anesthesia, respiratory arrest.*

bis(2-chloroisopropyl) ether [Ether] *Anesthesia, respiratory arrest.*

bis(2-chloro-1-methyl(ethyl)) ether [Ether] *Anesthesia, respiratory arrest.*

bis(chloromethyl) ether; bis(2-chloromethyl) ether [Ether] *Anesthesia, respiratory arrest.*

bis(chloromethyl) ketone [Ketone] *Respiratory mucous membrane irritation, pulmonary edema, CNS depression.*

bis(dimethylamino) ethane [Aliphatic hydrocarbon] *Arrhythmias, asphyxiation, anesthesia.*

bis(2-ethyl(hexyl)) adipate [Organic acid] *Pulmonary edema, circulatory collapse, laryngeal edema and spasm, severe chemical burns to skin, mucous membranes, and internal organs, GI tract perforation and hemorrhage, peritonitis.*

bis(2-ethylhexyl) phthalate [Ester] *CNS depression, respiratory tract irritation, bronchitis, pneumonitis.*

bishydroxycoumarin [Warfarin/hydroxycoumarin/indanedione] *Anticoagulation effect, internal hemorrhage.*

bismuth subnitrate [Nitrate/nitrite] *Methemoglobinemia, hypotension, circulatory collapse.*

bisulfite mixture (n.o.s.) [Sulfur] *Respiratory tract irritation, pulmonary edema, anaphylaxis.*

bithionol [Sulfur] *Respiratory tract irritation, pulmonary edema, anaphylaxis.*

bitoscanate [Isocyanate/aliphatic thiocyanate] *CNS depression, respiratory arrest, respiratory paralysis, pulmonary edema, cyanide toxicity.*

blasting agent (n.o.s.) [Explosive] *Multiple trauma, highly toxic chemical exposure.*

bleaching powder [Hypochlorite] *Circulatory collapse, respiratory tract irritation, upper airway obstruction, pulmonary edema.*

blue asbestos [Asbestos] *Asbestosis, lung cancer, malignant mesothelioma.*

bomb, smoke [Irritant] *Severe immediate or delayed upper airway or respiratory tract irritation, pulmonary edema, glottic spasm, airway obstruction.* [Corrosive] *Upper airway burns and edema, circulatory collapse, severe chemical burns to skin, toxic systemic effects, GI tract perforation and hemorrhage, peritonitis.*

bomyl [Organophosphate] *Pulmonary edema, respiratory muscle paralysis, respiratory failure, bradycardia, acetylcholinesterase inhibition, hypotension, pulmonary edema, overstimulation of parasympathetic nervous system, striated muscle, sympathetic ganglia, and CNS.*

borate & chlorate mixture [Boron] *Respiratory tract irritation, laryngeal spasm and edema, pulmonary edema, severe chemical burns.* [Chlorate] *Hemolysis, methemoglobinemia, hypoperfusion, CNS depression, delayed-onset renal failure.*

bordeaux arsenite [Arsenic] *Heavy metal toxicity, vomiting, GI bleeding, CNS depression, pulmonary edema, cardiac arrest.* [Copper] *Respiratory tract irritation, respiratory arrest, hemorrhagic gastritis.*

Bordeaux mixture [Poison] *Cardiovascular collapse, pulmonary edema,*

CNS depression, coma, seizures, nausea, vomiting, cardiopulmonary arrest.

boric acid [Boron] Respiratory tract irritation, laryngeal spasm and edema, pulmonary edema, severe chemical burns.

borneol [Camphor] Status epilepticus, respiratory failure.

bornyl chloride [Camphor] Status epilepticus, respiratory failure.

boron; borate (n.o.s.) [Boron] Respiratory tract irritation, laryngeal spasm and edema, pulmonary edema, severe chemical burns.

boron oxide [Boron] Respiratory tract irritation, laryngeal spasm and edema, pulmonary edema, severe chemical burns.

boron tribromide [Boron] Respiratory tract irritation, laryngeal spasm and edema, pulmonary edema, severe chemical burns.

boron trichloride [Boron] Respiratory tract irritation, laryngeal spasm and edema, pulmonary edema, severe chemical burns.

boron trifluoride [Boron] Respiratory tract irritation, laryngeal spasm and edema, pulmonary edema, severe chemical burns.

boron trifluoride & acetic acid complex [Boron] Respiratory tract irritation, laryngeal spasm and edema, pulmonary edema, severe chemical burns.

boron trifluoride diethyl etherate [Boron] Respiratory tract irritation, laryngeal spasm and edema, pulmonary edema, severe chemical burns.

boron trifluoride dihydrate [Boron] Respiratory tract irritation, laryngeal spasm and edema, pulmonary edema, severe chemical burns.

boron trifluoride dimethyl etherate [Boron] Respiratory tract irritation, laryngeal spasm and edema, pulmonary edema, severe chemical burns.

boron trifluoride & propionic acid complex [Boron] Respiratory tract irritation, laryngeal spasm and edema, pulmonary edema, severe chemical burns.

Bovizole [Thiabendazole] Cardiovascular collapse, respiratory tract irritation.

BPMC [Carbamate] Acetylcholinesterase inhibition (reversible), bradycardia, hypotension, respiratory muscle paralysis, respiratory arrest, pulmonary edema.

brake fluid, hydraulic [Hydrocarbon mixture] CNS depression, respiratory arrest, seizures, arrhythmias, pulmonary edema.

bromadiolone [Warfarin/hydroxycoumarin/indanedione] Anticoagulation effect, internal hemorrhage.

bromate (n.o.s.) [Bromate] CNS and respiratory system depression, delayed-onset renal failure.

bromide, methyl [Bromine/methyl bromide] Severe respiratory irritation, pulmonary edema, respiratory failure, coma, convulsions, death.

bromine [Bromine/methyl bromide] Severe respiratory irritation, pulmonary edema, respiratory failure, coma, convulsions, death.

bromine chloride [Bromine/methyl bromide] Severe respiratory irritation, pulmonary edema, respiratory failure, coma, convulsions, death.

bromine pentafluoride [Bromine/methyl bromide] Severe respiratory irritation, pulmonary edema, respiratory failure, coma, convulsions, death.

bromine trifluoride [Bromine/methyl bromide] Severe respiratory irritation, pulmonary edema, respiratory failure, coma, convulsions, death.

bromoacetic acid [Bromine/methyl bromide] Severe respiratory irritation, pulmonary edema, respiratory failure, coma, convulsions, death.

bromoacetone [Ketone] Respiratory mucous membrane irritation, pulmonary edema, CNS depression. [Bromine/methyl bromide] Severe respiratory irritation, pulmonary edema, respiratory failure, coma, convulsions, death.

bromoacetyl bromide [Bromine/methyl bromide] Severe respiratory irritation, pulmonary edema, respiratory failure, coma, convulsions, death.

HazMat

bromobenzene [Halogenated aliphatic hydrocarbon] *CNS depression, respiratory arrest, circulatory collapse.*

bromobenzyl cyanide [Cyanide] *Impairment of cellular oxygenation and adenosine triphosphate production, hypoxia, death.*

2-bromobutane [Halogenated aliphatic hydrocarbon] *CNS depression, respiratory arrest, circulatory collapse.*

bromochlorodifluoromethane (Halon 1211) [Chlorinated fluorocarbon] *Asphyxiation, anesthesia, arrhythmias.*

1-bromo-2-chloroethane [Chlorinated fluorocarbon] *Asphyxiation, anesthesia, arrhythmias.*

bromochloromethane [Chlorinated fluorocarbon] *Asphyxiation, anesthesia, arrhythmias.*

bromoethyl ethyl ether [Ether] *Anesthesia, respiratory arrest.*

bromoethylbutane [Halogenated aliphatic hydrocarbon] *CNS depression, respiratory arrest, circulatory collapse.*

bromoethylpropane [Halogenated aliphatic hydrocarbon] *CNS depression, respiratory arrest, circulatory collapse.*

bromoform [Halogenated aliphatic hydrocarbon] *CNS depression, respiratory arrest, circulatory collapse.*

bromomethane [Halogenated aliphatic hydrocarbon] *CNS depression, respiratory arrest, circulatory collapse.*

bromomethylbutane [Halogenated aliphatic hydrocarbon] *CNS depression, respiratory arrest, circulatory collapse.*

bromomethylpropane [Halogenated aliphatic hydrocarbon] *CNS depression, respiratory arrest, circulatory collapse.*

bromopentane [Halogenated aliphatic hydrocarbon] *CNS depression, respiratory arrest, circulatory collapse.*

2-bromo-4-phenyl ether [Phenol] *Coma, hypotension, arrhythmias, pulmonary edema, respiratory arrest.*

4-bromophenyl phenyl ether [Ether] *Anesthesia, respiratory arrest.* [Phenol] *Coma, hypotension, arrhythmias, pulmonary edema, respiratory arrest.*

bromopropane [Halogenated aliphatic hydrocarbon] *CNS depression, respiratory arrest, circulatory collapse.*

bromopropylate [Poison] *Cardiovascular collapse, pulmonary edema, CNS depression, coma, seizures, nausea, vomiting, cardiopulmonary arrest.* [Organic acid] *Pulmonary edema, circulatory collapse, laryngeal edema and spasm, severe chemical burns to skin, mucous membranes, and internal organs, GI tract perforation and hemorrhage, peritonitis.*

bromopropyne [Halogenated aliphatic hydrocarbon] *CNS depression, respiratory arrest, circulatory collapse.*

bromotrifluoroethylene [Halogenated aliphatic hydrocarbon] *CNS depression, respiratory arrest, circulatory collapse.*

bromotrifluoromethane [Halogenated aliphatic hydrocarbon] *CNS depression, respiratory arrest, circulatory collapse.*

brown asbestos; amosite [Asbestos] *Asbestosis, lung cancer, malignant mesothelioma.*

brucine [Strychnine] *Convulsions, acidosis, diaphragmatic spasms, respiratory arrest.*

bufencarb [Carbamate] *Acetylcholinesterase inhibition (reversible), bradycardia, hypotension, respiratory muscle paralysis, respiratory arrest, pulmonary edema.*

Bulan [Lindane] *CNS stimulation, seizures, respiratory failure.*

butacarb [Carbamate] *Acetylcholinesterase inhibition (reversible), bradycardia, hypotension, respiratory muscle paralysis, respiratory arrest, pulmonary edema.*

1,3-butadiene [Aliphatic hydrocarbon] *Arrhythmias, asphyxiation, anesthesia.* ⊠ butylene

***n*-butane** [Aliphatic hydrocarbon] *Arrhythmias, asphyxiation, anesthesia.* ⊠ butene

1,3-butanediol [Higher alcohol (4+ carbons)] *CNS depression, respiratory failure, arrhythmias.*

butanedione [Ethylene oxide] *Respiratory tract irritation, pulmonary edema.*

butanethiol [Aliphatic hydrocarbon] *Arrhythmias, asphyxiation, anesthesia.* [Sulfur] *Respiratory tract irritation, pulmonary edema, anaphylaxis.*

butanol [Higher alcohol (4+ carbons)] *CNS depression, respiratory failure, arrhythmias.*

butene [Aliphatic hydrocarbon] *Arrhythmias, asphyxiation, anesthesia.* ⊡ butane

butonate [Organophosphate] *Pulmonary edema, respiratory muscle paralysis, respiratory failure, bradycardia, acetylcholinesterase inhibition, hypotension, pulmonary edema, overstimulation of parasympathetic nervous system, striated muscle, sympathetic ganglia, and CNS.*

butoxy polypropylene glycol [Ethylene glycol] *Respiratory failure, pulmonary edema, paralysis, cardiovascular collapse, severe acidosis.*

2-butoxyethanol; n-butoxyethanol [Ethylene glycol] *Respiratory failure, pulmonary edema, paralysis, cardiovascular collapse, severe acidosis.*

butoxyl [Ester] *CNS depression, respiratory tract irritation, bronchitis, pneumonitis.*

butyl acetate [Ester] *CNS depression, respiratory tract irritation, bronchitis, pneumonitis.*

butyl acid phosphate [Organic acid] *Pulmonary edema, circulatory collapse, laryngeal edema and spasm, severe chemical burns to skin, mucous membranes, and internal organs, GI tract perforation and hemorrhage, peritonitis.*

n-butyl acrylate [Ester] *CNS depression, respiratory tract irritation, bronchitis, pneumonitis.*

butyl alcohol [Higher alcohol (4+ carbons)] *CNS depression, respiratory failure, arrhythmias.*

butyl aldehyde [Aldehyde] *Seizures, respiratory failure, pulmonary edema.*

butyl benzene [Aromatic hydrocarbon] *Arrhythmias, respiratory failure, pulmonary edema, paralysis, brain and kidney damage.*

butyl benzyl phthalate [Ester] *CNS depression, respiratory tract irritation, bronchitis, pneumonitis.*

butyl bromide [Halogenated aliphatic hydrocarbon] *CNS depression, respiratory arrest, circulatory collapse.*

butyl carbitol [Ethylene glycol] *Respiratory failure, pulmonary edema, paralysis, cardiovascular collapse, severe acidosis.*

n-butyl chloride [Halogenated aliphatic hydrocarbon] *CNS depression, respiratory arrest, circulatory collapse.*

butyl chloroformate; sec-butyl chloroformate [Ester] *CNS depression, respiratory tract irritation, bronchitis, pneumonitis.*

tert-butyl cumene peroxide [Organic peroxide] *Pulmonary and laryngeal edema, circulatory arrest, hypovolemic shock, chemical burns to skin, mucous membranes, and internal organs.*

tert-butyl cumyl peroxide [Organic peroxide] *Pulmonary and laryngeal edema, circulatory arrest, hypovolemic shock, chemical burns to skin, mucous membranes, and internal organs.*

butyl ether [Ether] *Anesthesia, respiratory arrest.*

butyl formate [Ester] *CNS depression, respiratory tract irritation, bronchitis, pneumonitis.*

tert-butyl hydroperoxide [Organic peroxide] *Pulmonary and laryngeal edema, circulatory arrest, hypovolemic shock, chemical burns to skin, mucous membranes, and internal organs.*

butyl hydroxytoluene [Aromatic hydrocarbon] *Arrhythmias, respiratory failure, pulmonary edema, paralysis, brain and kidney damage.*

butyl imidazole [Aliphatic hydrocarbon] *Arrhythmias, asphyxiation, anesthesia.*

***n*-butyl isocyanate; *tert*-butyl isocyanate** [Isocyanate/aliphatic thiocyanate] *CNS depression, respiratory arrest, respiratory paralysis, pulmonary edema, cyanide toxicity.*

***tert*-butyl isopropyl benzene hydroperoxide** [Organic peroxide] *Pulmonary and laryngeal edema, circulatory arrest, hypovolemic shock, chemical burns to skin, mucous membranes, and internal organs.*

butyl lithium [Lithium] *Chemical burns to respiratory tract, pulmonary edema.*

butyl mercaptan [Sulfur] *Respiratory tract irritation, pulmonary edema, anaphylaxis.*

butyl methacrylate [Ester] *CNS depression, respiratory tract irritation, bronchitis, pneumonitis.*

butyl methyl ether [Ether] *Anesthesia, respiratory arrest.*

***tert*-butyl monoperoxy-maleate** [Organic peroxide] *Pulmonary and laryngeal edema, circulatory arrest, hypovolemic shock, chemical burns to skin, mucous membranes, and internal organs.* [Organic acid] *Pulmonary edema, circulatory collapse, laryngeal edema and spasm, severe chemical burns to skin, mucous membranes, and internal organs, GI tract perforation and hemorrhage, peritonitis.*

***tert*-butyl monoperoxy-phthalate** [Organic peroxide] *Pulmonary and laryngeal edema, circulatory arrest, hypovolemic shock, chemical burns to skin, mucous membranes, and internal organs.* [Organic acid] *Pulmonary edema, circulatory collapse, laryngeal edema and spasm, severe chemical burns to skin, mucous membranes, and internal organs, GI tract perforation and hemorrhage, peritonitis.*

butyl nitrite [Nitrate/nitrite] *Methemoglobinemia, hypotension, circulatory collapse.*

butyl perbenzoate [Organic peroxide] *Pulmonary and laryngeal edema, circulatory arrest, hypovolemic shock, chemical burns to skin, mucous membranes, and internal organs.* [Organic acid] *Pulmonary edema, circulatory collapse, laryngeal edema and spasm, severe chemical burns to skin, mucous membranes, and internal organs, GI tract perforation and hemorrhage, peritonitis.*

***tert*-butyl peroxide** [Organic peroxide] *Pulmonary and laryngeal edema, circulatory arrest, hypovolemic shock, chemical burns to skin, mucous membranes, and internal organs.*

2,2-DL-(*tert*-butyl peroxy) butane & *tert*-butyl peroxy-2-ethyl hexanoate mixture [Organic peroxide] *Pulmonary and laryngeal edema, circulatory arrest, hypovolemic shock, chemical burns to skin, mucous membranes, and internal organs.* [Organic acid] *Pulmonary edema, circulatory collapse, laryngeal edema and spasm, severe chemical burns to skin, mucous membranes, and internal organs, GI tract perforation and hemorrhage, peritonitis.*

***tert*-butyl peroxyacetate** [Organic peroxide] *Pulmonary and laryngeal edema, circulatory arrest, hypovolemic shock, chemical burns to skin, mucous membranes, and internal organs.* [Organic acid] *Pulmonary edema, circulatory collapse, laryngeal edema and spasm, severe chemical burns to skin, mucous membranes, and internal organs, GI tract perforation and hemorrhage, peritonitis.*

***tert*-butyl peroxybenzoate** [Organic peroxide] *Pulmonary and laryngeal edema, circulatory arrest, hypovolemic shock, chemical burns to skin, mucous membranes, and internal organs.* [Organic acid] *Pulmonary edema, circulatory collapse, laryngeal edema and spasm, severe chemical burns to skin, mucous membranes, and internal organs, GI tract perforation and hemorrhage, peritonitis.*

***tert*-butyl peroxybenzoate & *tert*-butyl peroxydiethylacetate mixture** [Organic peroxide] *Pulmonary and laryngeal edema, circulatory arrest, hypovolemic shock, chemical* burns to skin, *mucous membranes, and internal organs*. [Organic acid] *Pulmonary edema, circulatory collapse, laryngeal edema and spasm, severe chemical burns to skin, mucous membranes, and internal organs, GI tract perforation and hemorrhage, peritonitis.*

tert-butyl peroxycrotonate [Organic peroxide] *Pulmonary and laryngeal edema, circulatory arrest, hypovolemic shock, chemical burns to skin, mucous membranes, and internal organs.* [Organic acid] *Pulmonary edema, circulatory collapse, laryngeal edema and spasm, severe chemical burns to skin, mucous membranes, and internal organs, GI tract perforation and hemorrhage, peritonitis.*

butyl peroxydicarbonate [Organic peroxide] *Pulmonary and laryngeal edema, circulatory arrest, hypovolemic shock, chemical burns to skin, mucous membranes, and internal organs.* [Organic acid] *Pulmonary edema, circulatory collapse, laryngeal edema and spasm, severe chemical burns to skin, mucous membranes, and internal organs, GI tract perforation and hemorrhage, peritonitis.*

***tert*-butyl peroxydiethylacetate** [Organic peroxide] *Pulmonary and laryngeal edema, circulatory arrest, hypovolemic shock, chemical burns to skin, mucous membranes, and internal organs.* [Organic acid] *Pulmonary edema, circulatory collapse, laryngeal edema and spasm, severe chemical burns to skin, mucous membranes, and internal organs, GI tract perforation and hemorrhage, peritonitis.*

***tert*-butyl peroxydiethylacetate & *tert*-butyl peroxybenzoate mixture** [Organic peroxide] *Pulmonary and laryngeal edema, circulatory arrest, hypovolemic shock, chemical burns to skin, mucous membranes, and internal organs.* [Organic acid] *Pulmonary edema, circulatory collapse, laryngeal edema and spasm, severe chemical burns to skin, mucous mem-*

branes, and internal organs, GI tract perforation and hemorrhage, peritonitis.

***tert*-butyl peroxy-2-ethyl hexanoate** [Organic peroxide] *Pulmonary and laryngeal edema, circulatory arrest, hypovolemic shock, chemical burns to skin, mucous membranes, and internal organs.* [Organic acid] *Pulmonary edema, circulatory collapse, laryngeal edema and spasm, severe chemical burns to skin, mucous membranes, and internal organs, GI tract perforation and hemorrhage, peritonitis.*

***tert*-butyl peroxy-2-ethyl hexanoate & 2,2-DL-(*tert*-butylperoxy) butane mixture** [Organic peroxide] *Pulmonary and laryngeal edema, circulatory arrest, hypovolemic shock, chemical burns to skin, mucous membranes, and internal organs.* [Organic acid] *Pulmonary edema, circulatory collapse, laryngeal edema and spasm, severe chemical burns to skin, mucous membranes, and internal organs, GI tract perforation and hemorrhage, peritonitis.*

***tert*-butyl peroxyisobutyrate** [Organic peroxide] *Pulmonary and laryngeal edema, circulatory arrest, hypovolemic shock, chemical burns to skin, mucous membranes, and internal organs.* [Organic acid] *Pulmonary edema, circulatory collapse, laryngeal edema and spasm, severe chemical burns to skin, mucous membranes, and internal organs, GI tract perforation and hemorrhage, peritonitis.*

***tert*-butyl peroxyisononanoate** [Organic peroxide] *Pulmonary and laryngeal edema, circulatory arrest, hypovolemic shock, chemical burns to skin, mucous membranes, and internal organs.* [Organic acid] *Pulmonary edema, circulatory collapse, laryngeal edema and spasm, severe chemical burns to skin, mucous membranes, and internal organs, GI tract perforation and hemorrhage, peritonitis.*

***tert*-butyl peroxyisopropyl carbonate** [Organic peroxide] *Pulmonary and laryngeal edema, circulatory* *arrest, hypovolemic shock, chemical burns to skin, mucous membranes, and internal organs.* [Organic acid] *Pulmonary edema, circulatory collapse, laryngeal edema and spasm, severe chemical burns to skin, mucous membranes, and internal organs, GI tract perforation and hemorrhage, peritonitis.*

tert-butyl peroxymaleate [Organic peroxide] *Pulmonary and laryngeal edema, circulatory arrest, hypovolemic shock, chemical burns to skin, mucous membranes, and internal organs.* [Organic acid] *Pulmonary edema, circulatory collapse, laryngeal edema and spasm, severe chemical burns to skin, mucous membranes, and internal organs, GI tract perforation and hemorrhage, peritonitis.*

tert-butyl peroxy-neodecanoate [Organic peroxide] *Pulmonary and laryngeal edema, circulatory arrest, hypovolemic shock, chemical burns to skin, mucous membranes, and internal organs.* [Organic acid] *Pulmonary edema, circulatory collapse, laryngeal edema and spasm, severe chemical burns to skin, mucous membranes, and internal organs, GI tract perforation and hemorrhage, peritonitis.*

tert-butyl peroxy-3-phenylphthalide [Organic peroxide] *Pulmonary and laryngeal edema, circulatory arrest, hypovolemic shock, chemical burns to skin, mucous membranes, and internal organs.* [Organic acid] *Pulmonary edema, circulatory collapse, laryngeal edema and spasm, severe chemical burns to skin, mucous membranes, and internal organs, GI tract perforation and hemorrhage, peritonitis.*

tert-butyl peroxyphthalate [Organic peroxide] *Pulmonary and laryngeal edema, circulatory arrest, hypovolemic shock, chemical burns to skin, mucous membranes, and internal organs.* [Organic acid] *Pulmonary edema, circulatory collapse, laryngeal edema and spasm, severe chemical burns to skin, mucous membranes, and internal*

organs, GI tract perforation and hemorrhage, peritonitis.

tert-butyl peroxypivalate [Organic peroxide] *Pulmonary and laryngeal edema, circulatory arrest, hypovolemic shock, chemical burns to skin, mucous membranes, and internal organs.* [Organic acid] *Pulmonary edema, circulatory collapse, laryngeal edema and spasm, severe chemical burns to skin, mucous membranes, and internal organs, GI tract perforation and hemorrhage, peritonitis.*

tert-butyl peroxystearyl carbonate [Organic peroxide] *Pulmonary and laryngeal edema, circulatory arrest, hypovolemic shock, chemical burns to skin, mucous membranes, and internal organs.* [Organic acid] *Pulmonary edema, circulatory collapse, laryngeal edema and spasm, severe chemical burns to skin, mucous membranes, and internal organs, GI tract perforation and hemorrhage, peritonitis.*

tert-butyl peroxy-3,5,5-trimethylhexanoate [Organic peroxide] *Pulmonary and laryngeal edema, circulatory arrest, hypovolemic shock, chemical burns to skin, mucous membranes, and internal organs.* [Organic acid] *Pulmonary edema, circulatory collapse, laryngeal edema and spasm, severe chemical burns to skin, mucous membranes, and internal organs, GI tract perforation and hemorrhage, peritonitis.*

butyl phenol; o-sec-butyl phenol [Phenol] *Coma, hypotension, arrhythmias, pulmonary edema, respiratory arrest.*

butyl phosphoric acid [Organic acid] *Pulmonary edema, circulatory collapse, laryngeal edema and spasm, severe chemical burns to skin, mucous membranes, and internal organs, GI tract perforation and hemorrhage, peritonitis.*

n-butyl phthalate [Organic acid] *Pulmonary edema, circulatory collapse, laryngeal edema and spasm, severe chemical burns to skin, mucous mem-*

branes, and internal organs, GI tract perforation and hemorrhage, peritonitis.

butyl propionate [Ester] *CNS depression, respiratory tract irritation, bronchitis, pneumonitis.*

butyl toluene [Aromatic hydrocarbon] *Arrhythmias, respiratory failure, pulmonary edema, paralysis, brain and kidney damage.*

butyl trichlorosilane [Silane/chlorosilane] *Respiratory tract irritation, pulmonary edema.*

***tert*-butyl 2,4,6-trinitro-*m*-xylene** [Aromatic hydrocarbon] *Arrhythmias, respiratory failure, pulmonary edema, paralysis, brain and kidney damage.*

butyl vinyl ether [Ether] *Anesthesia, respiratory arrest.*

***n*-butylamine; *tert*-butylamine** [Organic base/amine] *Pulmonary edema, cardiac depression, seizures.*

butylaniline [Aniline] *Methemoglobinemia, hypoxia.*

***n*-butyl-4,4-*dl*(*tert*-butyl-peroxy valerate)** [Organic acid] *Pulmonary edema, circulatory collapse, laryngeal edema and spasm, severe chemical burns to skin, mucous membranes, and internal organs, GI tract perforation and hemorrhage, peritonitis.*

***tert*-butylcyclohexyl chloroformate** [Ester] *CNS depression, respiratory tract irritation, bronchitis, pneumonitis.*

butylene [Aliphatic hydrocarbon] *Arrhythmias, asphyxiation, anesthesia.* ⏵ butadiene

1,3-butylene glycol [Aliphatic hydrocarbon] *Arrhythmias, asphyxiation, anesthesia.*

butylene oxide; 1,2-butylene oxide [Ethylene oxide] *Respiratory tract irritation, pulmonary edema.*

butynediol [Higher alcohol (4+ carbons)] *CNS depression, respiratory failure, arrhythmias.*

butyraldehyde [Aldehyde] *Seizures, respiratory failure, pulmonary edema.*

butyraldoxime [Aldehyde] *Seizures, respiratory failure, pulmonary edema.*

butyric acid [Organic acid] *Pulmonary edema, circulatory collapse, laryngeal edema and spasm, severe chemical burns to skin, mucous membranes, and internal organs, GI tract perforation and hemorrhage, peritonitis.*

butyric anhydride [Organic acid] *Pulmonary edema, circulatory collapse, laryngeal edema and spasm, severe chemical burns to skin, mucous membranes, and internal organs, GI tract perforation and hemorrhage, peritonitis.*

butyrone [Ketone] *Respiratory mucous membrane irritation, pulmonary edema, CNS depression.*

***n*-butyronitrile** [Cyanide] *Impairment of cellular oxygenation and adenosine triphosphate production, hypoxia, death.*

butyryl chloride [Organic acid] *Pulmonary edema, circulatory collapse, laryngeal edema and spasm, severe chemical burns to skin, mucous membranes, and internal organs, GI tract perforation and hemorrhage, peritonitis.*

cacodylic acid [Arsenic] *Heavy metal toxicity, vomiting, GI bleeding, CNS depression, pulmonary edema, cardiac arrest.*

cadmium; cadmium mixture (n.o.s.) [Cadmium] *Respiratory tract irritation, pulmonary edema.*

cadmium acetate [Cadmium] *Respiratory tract irritation, pulmonary edema.*

cadmium bromide [Cadmium] *Respiratory tract irritation, pulmonary edema.*

cadmium chloride [Cadmium] *Respiratory tract irritation, pulmonary edema.*

cadmium oxide [Cadmium] *Respiratory tract irritation, pulmonary edema.*

cadmium stearate [Cadmium] *Respiratory tract irritation, pulmonary edema.*

calcium; calcium alloy (n.o.s.) [Poison] *Cardiovascular collapse, pulmonary edema, CNS depression, coma, seizures, nausea, vomiting, cardiopulmonary arrest.*

calcium, pyrophoric; calcium alloy, pyrophoric (n.o.s.) [Flammable solid] *Shock, severe chemical and thermal burns, severe respiratory tract irri-*

tation, *pulmonary edema, respiratory arrest, ECG changes, sudden death.* [Poison] *Cardiovascular collapse, pulmonary edema, CNS depression, coma, seizures, nausea, vomiting, cardiopulmonary arrest.*

calcium arsenate [Arsenic] *Heavy metal toxicity, vomiting, GI bleeding, CNS depression, pulmonary edema, cardiac arrest.*

calcium arsenite [Arsenic] *Heavy metal toxicity, vomiting, GI bleeding, CNS depression, pulmonary edema, cardiac arrest.*

calcium bisulfite [Sulfur] *Respiratory tract irritation, pulmonary edema, anaphylaxis.*

calcium carbide [Corrosive] *Upper airway burns and edema, circulatory collapse, severe chemical burns to skin, toxic systemic effects, GI tract perforation and hemorrhage, peritonitis.*

calcium carbonate & ammonium nitrate mixture [Nitrate/nitrite] *Methemoglobinemia, hypotension, circulatory collapse.*

calcium chlorate [Chlorate] *Hemolysis, methemoglobinemia, hypoperfusion, CNS depression, delayed-onset renal failure.*

calcium chlorite [Chlorine] *Severe respiratory tract irritation, pulmonary edema, irritation of skin, eyes, and mucous membranes.*

calcium chromate [Poison] *Cardiovascular collapse, pulmonary edema, CNS depression, coma, seizures, nausea, vomiting, cardiopulmonary arrest.*

calcium cyanamide [Poison] *Cardiovascular collapse, pulmonary edema, CNS depression, coma, seizures, nausea, vomiting, cardiopulmonary arrest.*

calcium cyanide [Cyanide] *Impairment of cellular oxygenation and adenosine triphosphate production, hypoxia, death.*

calcium dithionite [Sulfur] *Respiratory tract irritation, pulmonary edema, anaphylaxis.*

calcium dodecylbenzene sulfonate [Organic acid] *Pulmonary edema, cir-*

culatory collapse, laryngeal edema and spasm, severe chemical burns to skin, mucous membranes, and internal organs, GI tract perforation and hemorrhage, peritonitis.*

calcium hydride [Corrosive] *Upper airway burns and edema, circulatory collapse, severe chemical burns to skin, toxic systemic effects, GI tract perforation and hemorrhage, peritonitis.*

calcium hydrogen sulfite; calcium hydrosulfite [Sulfur] *Respiratory tract irritation, pulmonary edema, anaphylaxis.*

calcium hydroxide [Inorganic base/alkaline corrosive] *Upper airway burns and edema, pulmonary edema, skin burns, circulatory collapse, GI tract perforation and hemorrhage, peritonitis.*

calcium hypochlorite [Hypochlorite] *Circulatory collapse, respiratory tract irritation, upper airway obstruction, pulmonary edema.*

calcium manganese silicon [Manganese] *Respiratory tract irritation, pulmonary edema.*

calcium nitrate [Nitrate/nitrite] *Methemoglobinemia, hypotension, circulatory collapse.*

calcium oxide [Inorganic base/alkaline corrosive] *Upper airway burns and edema, pulmonary edema, skin burns, circulatory collapse, GI tract perforation and hemorrhage, peritonitis.*

calcium perchlorate [Chlorate] *Hemolysis, methemoglobinemia, hypoperfusion, CNS depression, delayed-onset renal failure.*

calcium permanganate [Inorganic acid] *Pulmonary edema, bronchospasm, circulatory collapse, laryngeal spasm and edema, severe chemical burns to skin, mucous membranes, and internal organs, GI tract perforation and hemorrhage, peritonitis.*

calcium peroxide [Organic peroxide] *Pulmonary and laryngeal edema, circulatory arrest, hypovolemic shock, chemical burns to skin, mucous membranes, and internal organs.*

calcium phosphide [Phosphine] *Severe pulmonary irritation, pulmonary edema.*

calcium polysulfide [Sulfur] *Respiratory tract irritation, pulmonary edema, anaphylaxis.*

calcium resinate [Flammable solid] *Shock, severe chemical and thermal burns, severe respiratory tract irritation, pulmonary edema, respiratory arrest, ECG changes, sudden death.*

calcium selenate [Selenium] *Arrhythmias, pulmonary edema, bronchospasm, seizures, vomiting, GI bleeding.*

calcium silicide [Flammable solid] *Shock, severe chemical and thermal burns, severe respiratory tract irritation, pulmonary edema, respiratory arrest, ECG changes, sudden death.*

calcium silicon [Flammable solid] *Shock, severe chemical and thermal burns, severe respiratory tract irritation, pulmonary edema, respiratory arrest, ECG changes, sudden death.*

camphechlor [Toxaphene] *Respiratory failure, seizures, exhaustion, death.*

camphene [Camphor] *Status epilepticus, respiratory failure.*

camphene, chlorinated [Toxaphene] *Respiratory failure, seizures, exhaustion, death.*

camphor [Camphor] *Status epilepticus, respiratory failure.*

camphor oil [Camphor] *Status epilepticus, respiratory failure.*

cantharidin [Irritant] *Severe immediate or delayed upper airway or respiratory tract irritation, pulmonary edema, glottic spasm, airway obstruction.*

caproic acid (hexanoic acid) [Organic acid] *Pulmonary edema, circulatory collapse, laryngeal edema and spasm, severe chemical burns to skin, mucous membranes, and internal organs, GI tract perforation and hemorrhage, peritonitis.*

caprolactam [Irritant] *Severe immediate or delayed upper airway or respiratory tract irritation, pulmonary edema, glottic spasm, airway obstruction.* [Poison] *Cardiovascular collapse, pulmonary edema, CNS depression, coma, seizures, nausea, vomiting, cardiopulmonary arrest.*

caprylic alcohol [Higher alcohol (4+ carbons)] *CNS depression, respiratory failure, arrhythmias.*

caprylyl peroxide [Organic peroxide] *Pulmonary and laryngeal edema, circulatory arrest, hypovolemic shock, chemical burns to skin, mucous membranes, and internal organs.*

captan [Dithiocarbamate] *Hypotension, respiratory failure.*

carbachol chloride [Carbamate] *Acetylcholinesterase inhibition (reversible), bradycardia, hypotension, respiratory muscle paralysis, respiratory arrest, pulmonary edema.*

carbamate pesticide (n.o.s.) [Carbamate] *Acetylcholinesterase inhibition (reversible), bradycardia, hypotension, respiratory muscle paralysis, respiratory arrest, pulmonary edema.*

carbamic acid, ethyl ester [Ester] *CNS depression, respiratory tract irritation, bronchitis, pneumonitis.*

carbamic acid, methyl-propoxur [Carbamate] *Acetylcholinesterase inhibition (reversible), bradycardia, hypotension, respiratory muscle paralysis, respiratory arrest, pulmonary edema.*

carbanolate [Carbamate] *Acetylcholinesterase inhibition (reversible), bradycardia, hypotension, respiratory muscle paralysis, respiratory arrest, pulmonary edema.*

carbaryl [Carbamate] *Acetylcholinesterase inhibition (reversible), bradycardia, hypotension, respiratory muscle paralysis, respiratory arrest, pulmonary edema.*

Carbitol [Ethylene glycol] *Respiratory failure, pulmonary edema, paralysis, cardiovascular collapse, severe acidosis.*

Carbitol ester [Ester] *CNS depression, respiratory tract irritation, bronchitis, pneumonitis.*

carbofuran [Carbamate] *Acetylcholinesterase inhibition (reversible), bradycardia, hypotension, respiratory muscle paralysis, respiratory arrest, pulmonary edema.*

HazMat

carbolic acid [Phenol] *Coma, hypotension, arrhythmias, pulmonary edema, respiratory arrest.*

carbon (animal or vegetable origin) [Flammable solid] *Shock, severe chemical and thermal burns, severe respiratory tract irritation, pulmonary edema, respiratory arrest, ECG changes, sudden death.* [Irritant] *Severe immediate or delayed upper airway or respiratory tract irritation, pulmonary edema, glottic spasm, airway obstruction.*

carbon, activated [Irritant] *Severe immediate or delayed upper airway or respiratory tract irritation, pulmonary edema, glottic spasm, airway obstruction.*

carbon bisulfide *CNS depression, respiratory paralysis and arrest.*

carbon dioxide (gas, cryogenic liquid, or Dry Ice) [Simple asphyxiant] *Asphyxiation.*

carbon dioxide & ethylene oxide mixture [Simple asphyxiant] *Asphyxiation.* [Ethylene oxide] *Respiratory tract irritation, pulmonary edema.*

carbon dioxide & nitrous oxide mixture [Simple asphyxiant] *Asphyxiation.*

carbon dioxide & oxygen mixture [Simple asphyxiant] *Asphyxiation.*

carbon disulfide *CNS depression, respiratory paralysis and arrest.*

carbon monoxide (gas or cryogenic liquid) [Carbon monoxide] *Impairment of cellular oxygenation, hypoxia, death.*

carbon monoxide from methylene chloride [Carbon monoxide] *Impairment of cellular oxygenation, hypoxia, death.* [Halogenated aliphatic hydrocarbon] *CNS depression, respiratory arrest, circulatory collapse.*

carbon monoxide & hydrogen mixture [Carbon monoxide] *Impairment of cellular oxygenation, hypoxia, death.*

carbon oxysulfide [Hydrogen sulfide] *Severe respiratory tract irritation, pulmonary edema, respiratory paralysis.*

carbon remover [Hydrocarbon mixture] *CNS depression, respiratory arrest, seizures, arrhythmias, pulmonary edema.*

carbon tetrabromide [Carbon tetrachloride] *CNS depression, respiratory arrest, circulatory collapse.*

carbon tetrachloride [Carbon tetrachloride] *CNS depression, respiratory arrest, circulatory collapse.*

carbon tetrachloride & sulfur chloride mixture [Carbon tetrachloride] *CNS depression, respiratory arrest, circulatory collapse.* [Sulfur] *Respiratory tract irritation, pulmonary edema, anaphylaxis.*

carbonic difluoride [Fluorine] *CNS depression, respiratory arrest, cardiovascular collapse, shock, arrhythmias.*

carbonyl chloride [Phosgene] *Severe respiratory irritation, alveolar damage, pulmonary edema.*

carbonyl fluoride [Hydrofluoric acid] *Pulmonary and laryngeal edema, circulatory collapse, severe skin burns, GI tract perforation, systemic fluoride poisoning.*

carbonyl sulfide [Hydrogen sulfide] *Severe respiratory tract irritation, pulmonary edema, respiratory paralysis.*

carbophenothion [Organophosphate] *Pulmonary edema, respiratory muscle paralysis, respiratory failure, bradycardia, acetylcholinesterase inhibition, hypotension, pulmonary edema, overstimulation of parasympathetic nervous system, striated muscle, sympathetic ganglia, and CNS.*

Carbowax [Ethylene glycol] *Respiratory failure, pulmonary edema, paralysis, cardiovascular collapse, severe acidosis.*

cartap [Ester] *CNS depression, respiratory tract irritation, bronchitis, pneumonitis.*

carvacrol [Phenol] *Coma, hypotension, arrhythmias, pulmonary edema, respiratory arrest.*

casinghead gasoline [Hydrocarbon mixture] *CNS depression, respiratory arrest, seizures, arrhythmias, pulmonary edema.*

castor beans [Poison] *Cardiovascular collapse, pulmonary edema, CNS depression, coma, seizures, nausea, vomiting, cardiopulmonary arrest.*

Castrix [Strychnine] *Convulsions, acidosis, diaphragmatic spasms, respiratory arrest.*

catechol [Phenol] *Coma, hypotension, arrhythmias, pulmonary edema, respiratory arrest.*

caustic alkali liquid (n.o.s.) [Inorganic base/alkaline corrosive] *Upper airway burns and edema, pulmonary edema, skin burns, circulatory collapse, GI tract perforation and hemorrhage, peritonitis.*

caustic potash [Inorganic base/alkaline corrosive] *Upper airway burns and edema, pulmonary edema, skin burns, circulatory collapse, GI tract perforation and hemorrhage, peritonitis.*

caustic soda [Inorganic base/alkaline corrosive] *Upper airway burns and edema, pulmonary edema, skin burns, circulatory collapse, GI tract perforation and hemorrhage, peritonitis.*

CBP [Dichloropropane/dichloropropene] *Pulmonary edema, bronchospasm, alveolar hemorrhage.*

Cellosolve; cellosolve sulfate [Ethylene glycol] *Respiratory failure, pulmonary edema, paralysis, cardiovascular collapse, severe acidosis.*

celluloid [Flammable solid] *Shock, severe chemical and thermal burns, severe respiratory tract irritation, pulmonary edema, respiratory arrest, ECG changes, sudden death.*

cement (n.o.s.) [Inorganic base/alkaline corrosive] *Upper airway burns and edema, pulmonary edema, skin burns, circulatory collapse, GI tract perforation and hemorrhage, peritonitis.*

cerium [Poison] *Cardiovascular collapse, pulmonary edema, CNS depression, coma, seizures, nausea, vomiting, cardiopulmonary arrest.*

cesium [Flammable solid] *Shock, severe chemical and thermal burns, severe respiratory tract irritation, pulmonary edema, respiratory arrest, ECG changes, sudden death.*

cesium hydroxide [Inorganic base/alkaline corrosive] *Upper airway burns and edema, pulmonary edema, skin burns, circulatory collapse, GI tract perforation and hemorrhage, peritonitis.*

cesium nitrate [Inorganic acid] *Pulmonary edema, bronchospasm, circulatory collapse, laryngeal spasm and edema, severe chemical burns to skin, mucous membranes, and internal organs, GI tract perforation and hemorrhage, peritonitis.* [Nitrate/nitrite] *Methemoglobinemia, hypotension, circulatory collapse.*

cetyl alcohol [Higher alcohol (4+ carbons)] *CNS depression, respiratory failure, arrhythmias.*

CFC (chlorofluorocarbon) (n.o.s.) [Chlorinated fluorocarbon] *Asphyxiation, anesthesia, arrhythmias.*

charcoal [Irritant] *Severe immediate or delayed upper airway or respiratory tract irritation, pulmonary edema, glottic spasm, airway obstruction.*

chemical ammunition, irritant [Irritant] *Severe immediate or delayed upper airway or respiratory tract irritation, pulmonary edema, glottic spasm, airway obstruction.*

chemical ammunition, toxic [Irritant] *Severe immediate or delayed upper airway or respiratory tract irritation, pulmonary edema, glottic spasm, airway obstruction.* [Poison] *Cardiovascular collapse, pulmonary edema, CNS depression, coma, seizures, nausea, vomiting, cardiopulmonary arrest.*

chemical kit [Poison] *Cardiovascular collapse, pulmonary edema, CNS depression, coma, seizures, nausea, vomiting, cardiopulmonary arrest.*

chloral [Halogenated aliphatic hydrocarbon] *CNS depression, respiratory arrest, circulatory collapse.*

chloramben [Organic acid] *Pulmonary edema, circulatory collapse, laryngeal edema and spasm, severe chemical burns to skin, mucous membranes, and*

HazMat

internal organs, GI tract perforation and hemorrhage, peritonitis.

chlorambucil [Poison] *Cardiovascular collapse, pulmonary edema, CNS depression, coma, seizures, nausea, vomiting, cardiopulmonary arrest.*

chloramine (n.o.s.) [Organic base/amine] *Pulmonary edema, cardiac depression, seizures.*

chloramine T [Hypochlorite] *Circulatory collapse, respiratory tract irritation, upper airway obstruction, pulmonary edema.*

chlorasol [Hypochlorite] *Circulatory collapse, respiratory tract irritation, upper airway obstruction, pulmonary edema.*

chlorate; chlorate salt (n.o.s.) [Chlorate] *Hemolysis, methemoglobinemia, hypoperfusion, CNS depression, delayed-onset renal failure.*

chlorate & borate mixture [Chlorate] *Hemolysis, methemoglobinemia, hypoperfusion, CNS depression, delayed-onset renal failure.* [Boron] *Respiratory tract irritation, laryngeal spasm and edema, pulmonary edema, severe chemical burns.*

chlorate & magnesium chloride mixture [Chlorate] *Hemolysis, methemoglobinemia, hypoperfusion, CNS depression, delayed-onset renal failure.* [Magnesium] *Cardiovascular collapse, respiratory depression.*

chlorate of potash [Chlorate] *Hemolysis, methemoglobinemia, hypoperfusion, CNS depression, delayed-onset renal failure.*

chlorate of soda [Chlorate] *Hemolysis, methemoglobinemia, hypoperfusion, CNS depression, delayed-onset renal failure.*

chlordane [Chlordane] *Respiratory failure, seizures, exhaustion, death.*

chlordecone [Lindane] *CNS stimulation, seizures, respiratory failure.*

chlordimeform [Aniline] *Methemoglobinemia, hypoxia.*

chlorfenvinphos [Organophosphate] *Pulmonary edema, respiratory muscle paralysis, respiratory failure, bradycar-dia, acetylcholinesterase inhibition, hypotension, pulmonary edema, over-stimulation of parasympathetic nervous system, striated muscle, sympathetic ganglia, and CNS.*

chloric acid [Inorganic acid] *Pulmonary edema, bronchospasm, circulatory collapse, laryngeal spasm and edema, severe chemical burns to skin, mucous membranes, and internal organs, GI tract perforation and hemorrhage, peritonitis.*

chloride of phosphorus [Chlorine] *Severe respiratory tract irritation, pulmonary edema, irritation of skin, eyes, and mucous membranes.* [Phosphorus] *Hypovolemic shock, severe tissue burns, severe respiratory irritation, pulmonary edema, respiratory arrest, arrhythmias, sudden death.*

chloride of sulfur [Sulfur] *Respiratory tract irritation, pulmonary edema, anaphylaxis.*

chlorinated benzene [Lindane] *CNS stimulation, seizures, respiratory failure.*

chlorinated camphene [Toxaphene] *Respiratory failure, seizures, exhaustion, death.*

chlorinated ethane [Halogenated aliphatic hydrocarbon] *CNS depression, respiratory arrest, circulatory collapse.*

chlorinated hydrocarbon [Halogenated aliphatic hydrocarbon] *CNS depression, respiratory arrest, circulatory collapse.*

chlorinated lime [Hypochlorite] *Circulatory collapse, respiratory tract irritation, upper airway obstruction, pulmonary edema.*

chlorinated naphthalene [Naphthalene] *Delayed-onset acute intravascular hemolysis.*

chlorinated phenol [Phenol] *Coma, hypotension, arrhythmias, pulmonary edema, respiratory arrest.*

chlorinated solvent (n.o.s.) [Halogenated aliphatic hydrocarbon] *CNS depression, respiratory arrest, circulatory collapse.*

chlorinated trisodium phosphate [Inorganic base/alkaline corrosive]

Upper airway burns and edema, pulmonary edema, skin burns, circulatory collapse, GI tract perforation and hemorrhage, peritonitis. [Hypochlorite] *Circulatory collapse, respiratory tract irritation, upper airway obstruction, pulmonary edema.*

chlorine [Chlorine] *Severe respiratory tract irritation, pulmonary edema, irritation of skin, eyes, and mucous membranes.*

chlorine dioxide [Chlorine] *Severe respiratory tract irritation, pulmonary edema, irritation of skin, eyes, and mucous membranes.*

chlorine dioxide hydrate [Chlorine] *Severe respiratory tract irritation, pulmonary edema, irritation of skin, eyes, and mucous membranes.*

chlorine pentafluoride [Chlorine] *Severe respiratory tract irritation, pulmonary edema, irritation of skin, eyes, and mucous membranes.* [Fluorine] *CNS depression, respiratory arrest, cardiovascular collapse, shock, arrhythmias.*

chlorine trifluoride [Hydrofluoric acid] *Pulmonary and laryngeal edema, circulatory collapse, severe skin burns, GI tract perforation, systemic fluoride poisoning.* [Chlorine] *Severe respiratory tract irritation, pulmonary edema, irritation of skin, eyes, and mucous membranes.*

chlorite (n.o.s.) [Chlorine] *Severe respiratory tract irritation, pulmonary edema, irritation of skin, eyes, and mucous membranes.*

chlormephos [Organophosphate] *Pulmonary edema, respiratory muscle paralysis, respiratory failure, bradycardia, acetylcholinesterase inhibition, hypotension, pulmonary edema, overstimulation of parasympathetic nervous system, striated muscle, sympathetic ganglia, and CNS.*

chlormequat chloride [Poison] *Cardiovascular collapse, pulmonary edema, CNS depression, coma, seizures, nausea, vomiting, cardiopulmonary arrest.*

chlornaphazine [Poison] *Cardiovascular collapse, pulmonary edema, CNS depression, coma, seizures, nausea, vomiting, cardiopulmonary arrest.*

chloroacetaldehyde [Aldehyde] *Seizures, respiratory failure, pulmonary edema.*

chloroacetic acid [Organic acid] *Pulmonary edema, circulatory collapse, laryngeal edema and spasm, severe chemical burns to skin, mucous membranes, and internal organs, GI tract perforation and hemorrhage, peritonitis.*

chloroacetone [Ketone] *Respiratory mucous membrane irritation, pulmonary edema, CNS depression.*

chloroacetonitrile [Cyanide] *Impairment of cellular oxygenation and adenosine triphosphate production, hypoxia, death.*

chloroacetophenone; 2-chloroacetophenone [Ketone] *Respiratory mucous membrane irritation, pulmonary edema, CNS depression.*

chloroacetyl chloride [Chlorine] *Severe respiratory tract irritation, pulmonary edema, irritation of skin, eyes, and mucous membranes.*

chloroaniline [Aniline] *Methemoglobinemia, hypoxia.*

chloroanisidine [Aromatic hydrocarbon] *Arrhythmias, respiratory failure, pulmonary edema, paralysis, brain and kidney damage.* [Nitrate/nitrite] *Methemoglobinemia, hypotension, circulatory collapse.*

chlorobenzene [Benzene] *Arrhythmias, respiratory failure, pulmonary edema, CNS depression, liver and kidney damage.*

chlorobenzilate [Lindane] *CNS stimulation, seizures, respiratory failure.*

3-chlorobenzoic acid & 3-chloroperoxybenzoic acid mixture [Organic acid] *Pulmonary edema, circulatory collapse, laryngeal edema and spasm, severe chemical burns to skin, mucous membranes, and internal organs, GI tract perforation and hemorrhage, peritonitis.*

HazMat

chlorobenzotrifluoride [Aromatic hydrocarbon] *Arrhythmias, respiratory failure, pulmonary edema, paralysis, brain and kidney damage.*

p-chlorobenzoyl peroxide [Organic peroxide] *Pulmonary and laryngeal edema, circulatory arrest, hypovolemic shock, chemical burns to skin, mucous membranes, and internal organs.*

chlorobenzyl chloride [Aromatic hydrocarbon] *Arrhythmias, respiratory failure, pulmonary edema, paralysis, brain and kidney damage.*

o-chlorobenzylidene malonitrile [Cyanide] *Impairment of cellular oxygenation and adenosine triphosphate production, hypoxia, death.*

chlorobromomethane [Halogenated aliphatic hydrocarbon] *CNS depression, respiratory arrest, circulatory collapse.*

chlorobromopropane [Chlorinated fluorocarbon] *Asphyxiation, anesthesia, arrhythmias.*

chlorobutane [Chlorinated fluorocarbon] *Asphyxiation, anesthesia, arrhythmias.*

p-chloro-m-cresol [Phenol] *Coma, hypotension, arrhythmias, pulmonary edema, respiratory arrest.*

4-chloro-2-cyclopentylphenol [Phenol] *Coma, hypotension, arrhythmias, pulmonary edema, respiratory arrest.*

chlorodibromomethane [Halogenated aliphatic hydrocarbon] *CNS depression, respiratory arrest, circulatory collapse.*

chlorodiethylaluminum [Flammable solid] *Shock, severe chemical and thermal burns, severe respiratory tract irritation, pulmonary edema, respiratory arrest, ECG changes, sudden death.* [Poison] *Cardiovascular collapse, pulmonary edema, CNS depression, coma, seizures, nausea, vomiting, cardiopulmonary arrest.*

3-chloro-4-diethylamino-benediazonium zinc chloride [Zinc] *Respiratory tract irritation, metal fume fever, pulmonary edema.*

chlorodifluorobromomethane [Chlorinated fluorocarbon] *Asphyxiation, anesthesia, arrhythmias.*

chlorodifluoroethane [Chlorinated fluorocarbon] *Asphyxiation, anesthesia, arrhythmias.*

chlorodifluoromethane [Chlorinated fluorocarbon] *Asphyxiation, anesthesia, arrhythmias.*

chlorodifluoromethane & chloropentafluoroethane mixture [Chlorinated fluorocarbon] *Asphyxiation, anesthesia, arrhythmias.*

chlorodifluoromethane & dichlorodifluoromethane mixture [Chlorinated fluorocarbon] *Asphyxiation, anesthesia, arrhythmias.*

chlorodifluoromethane & dichlorodifluoromethane & trichlorofluoromethane mixture [Chlorinated fluorocarbon] *Asphyxiation, anesthesia, arrhythmias.*

chlorodinitrobenzene; 1-chloro-2,4-dinitrobenzene [Aromatic hydrocarbon] *Arrhythmias, respiratory failure, pulmonary edema, paralysis, brain and kidney damage.* [Nitrate/nitrite] *Methemoglobinemia, hypotension, circulatory collapse.*

chlorodiphenyl [Polychlorinated biphenyl/polybrominated biphenyl/polychlorinated dibenzofuran] *Liver and kidney damage.*

chloroethane [Halogenated aliphatic hydrocarbon] *CNS depression, respiratory arrest, circulatory collapse.*

chloroethanol [Ether] *Anesthesia, respiratory arrest.*

chloroethyl chloroformate [Ester] *CNS depression, respiratory tract irritation, bronchitis, pneumonitis.*

2-chloroethyl vinyl ether [Chlorinated fluorocarbon] *Asphyxiation, anesthesia, arrhythmias.*

chlorofluorocarbon (CFC) (n.o.s.) [Chlorinated fluorocarbon] *Asphyxiation, anesthesia, arrhythmias.*

chloroform [Halogenated aliphatic hydrocarbon] *CNS depression, respiratory arrest, circulatory collapse.*

chloroformate (n.o.s.) [Ester] *CNS depression, respiratory tract irritation, bronchitis, pneumonitis.*

2-chloro-4-(hydroxymercuri)phenol [Mercury] *Circulatory collapse, arrhythmias, respiratory failure, pulmonary edema, neurotoxic effects.*

chloromethane [Halogenated aliphatic hydrocarbon] *CNS depression, respiratory arrest, circulatory collapse.*

chloromethyl ethyl ether [Ether] *Anesthesia, respiratory arrest.*

chloromethyl methyl ether [Ether] *Anesthesia, respiratory arrest.*

5-chloro-6-((((methylamino)carbonyl)oxy)imino)-bicyclo(2.2.1) heptane-2-carbonitrile [Carbamate] *Acetylcholinesterase inhibition (reversible), bradycardia, hypotension, respiratory muscle paralysis, respiratory arrest, pulmonary edema.*

3-chloro-4-methylaniline [Aniline] *Methemoglobinemia, hypoxia.*

chloromethylchloroformate [Ester] *CNS depression, respiratory tract irritation, bronchitis, pneumonitis.*

chloromethyloxypropylmercuric acetate [Ester] *CNS depression, respiratory tract irritation, bronchitis, pneumonitis.*

chloromethylphenylisocyanate [Isocyanate/aliphatic thiocyanate] *CNS depression, respiratory arrest, respiratory paralysis, pulmonary edema, cyanide toxicity.*

3-chloro-2-methyl-1-propene [Dichloropropane/dichloropropene] *Pulmonary edema, bronchospasm, alveolar hemorrhage.*

2-chloronaphthalene [Naphthalene] *Delayed-onset acute intravascular hemolysis.*

chloronitroaniline [Aniline] *Methemoglobinemia, hypoxia.*

chloronitrobenzenes [Aromatic hydrocarbon] *Arrhythmias, respiratory failure, pulmonary edema, paralysis, brain and kidney damage.* [Nitrate/nitrite] *Methemoglobinemia, hypotension, circulatory collapse.*

1-chloro-1-nitropropane [Halogenated aliphatic hydrocarbon] *CNS depression, respiratory arrest, circulatory collapse.* [Nitrate/nitrite] *Methemoglobinemia, hypotension, circulatory collapse.*

chloronitrotoluene [Aromatic hydrocarbon] *Arrhythmias, respiratory failure, pulmonary edema, paralysis, brain and kidney damage.*

chloropentafluoroethane [Chlorinated fluorocarbon] *Asphyxiation, anesthesia, arrhythmias.*

chloropentafluoroethane & chlorodifluoromethane mixture [Chlorinated fluorocarbon] *Asphyxiation, anesthesia, arrhythmias.*

3-chloroperoxybenzoic acid [Organic acid] *Pulmonary edema, circulatory collapse, laryngeal edema and spasm, severe chemical burns to skin, mucous membranes, and internal organs, GI tract perforation and hemorrhage, peritonitis.*

3-chloroperoxybenzoic acid & 3-chlorobenzoic acid mixture [Organic acid] *Pulmonary edema, circulatory collapse, laryngeal edema and spasm, severe chemical burns to skin, mucous membranes, and internal organs, GI tract perforation and hemorrhage, peritonitis.*

chlorophacinone [Warfarin/hydroxycoumarin/indanedione] *Anticoagulation effect, internal hemorrhage.*

chlorophenate [Phenol] *Coma, hypotension, arrhythmias, pulmonary edema, respiratory arrest.*

2-chlorophenol [Phenol] *Coma, hypotension, arrhythmias, pulmonary edema, respiratory arrest.*

chlorophenol (n.o.s.) [Phenol] *Coma, hypotension, arrhythmias, pulmonary edema, respiratory arrest.*

p-chlorophenoxyacetic acid [Chlorophenoxy herbicide] *CNS depression, CNS stimulation, respiratory failure, ventricular fibrillation, seizures.*

4-chlorophenyl phenyl ether [Ether] *Anesthesia, respiratory arrest.* [Phe-

HazMat

nol] *Coma, hypotension, arrhythmias, pulmonary edema, respiratory arrest.*

chlorophenyl trichlorosilane [Silane/chlorosilane] *Respiratory tract irritation, pulmonary edema.*

chloro-2-phenylphenol [Phenol] *Coma, hypotension, arrhythmias, pulmonary edema, respiratory arrest.*

chloropicrin [Irritant] *Severe immediate or delayed upper airway or respiratory tract irritation, pulmonary edema, glottic spasm, airway obstruction.* [Halogenated aliphatic hydrocarbon] *CNS depression, respiratory arrest, circulatory collapse.*

chloropicrin & methyl bromide mixture [Irritant] *Severe immediate or delayed upper airway or respiratory tract irritation, pulmonary edema, glottic spasm, airway obstruction.* [Halogenated aliphatic hydrocarbon] *CNS depression, respiratory arrest, circulatory collapse.* [Bromine/methyl bromide] *Severe respiratory irritation, pulmonary edema, respiratory failure, coma, convulsions, death.*

chloropicrin & methyl chloride mixture [Irritant] *Severe immediate or delayed upper airway or respiratory tract irritation, pulmonary edema, glottic spasm, airway obstruction.* [Halogenated aliphatic hydrocarbon] *CNS depression, respiratory arrest, circulatory collapse.*

chloropicrin mixture (n.o.s.) [Irritant] *Severe immediate or delayed upper airway or respiratory tract irritation, pulmonary edema, glottic spasm, airway obstruction.* [Halogenated aliphatic hydrocarbon] *CNS depression, respiratory arrest, circulatory collapse.*

chloropivaloyl chloride [Poison] *Cardiovascular collapse, pulmonary edema, CNS depression, coma, seizures, nausea, vomiting, cardiopulmonary arrest.*

chloroplatinic acid [Inorganic acid] *Pulmonary edema, bronchospasm, circulatory collapse, laryngeal spasm and edema, severe chemical burns to skin,*

mucous membranes, and internal organs, GI tract perforation and hemorrhage, peritonitis.

chloroprene [Irritant] *Severe immediate or delayed upper airway or respiratory tract irritation, pulmonary edema, glottic spasm, airway obstruction.* [Aliphatic hydrocarbon] *Arrhythmias, asphyxiation, anesthesia.*

chloropropane [Aliphatic hydrocarbon] *Arrhythmias, asphyxiation, anesthesia.* ⊇ chloropropene

chloropropanol; 2-chloro-1-propanol; 3-chloropropanol; 3-chloropropanol-1 [Higher alcohol (4+ carbons)] *CNS depression, respiratory failure, arrhythmias.*

chloropropene [Aliphatic hydrocarbon] *Arrhythmias, asphyxiation, anesthesia.* ⊇ chloropropane

chloropropionic acid [Organic acid] *Pulmonary edema, circulatory collapse, laryngeal edema and spasm, severe chemical burns to skin, mucous membranes, and internal organs, GI tract perforation and hemorrhage, peritonitis.*

3-chloropropionitrile [Cyanide] *Impairment of cellular oxygenation and adenosine triphosphate production, hypoxia, death.*

chloropyridine [Aromatic hydrocarbon] *Arrhythmias, respiratory failure, pulmonary edema, paralysis, brain and kidney damage.*

chlorosilane (n.o.s.) [Silane/chlorosilane] *Respiratory tract irritation, pulmonary edema.*

N-chlorosuccinimide [Phenol] *Coma, hypotension, arrhythmias, pulmonary edema, respiratory arrest.*

chlorosulfonic acid [Inorganic acid] *Pulmonary edema, bronchospasm, circulatory collapse, laryngeal spasm and edema, severe chemical burns to skin, mucous membranes, and internal organs, GI tract perforation and hemorrhage, peritonitis.*

chlorosulfonic acid & sulfur trioxide mixture [Inorganic acid] *Pulmonary edema, bronchospasm, circulatory* collapse, laryngeal spasm and edema, severe chemical burns to skin, mucous membranes, and internal organs, GI tract perforation and hemorrhage, peritonitis. [Sulfur] Respiratory tract irritation, pulmonary edema, anaphylaxis.

chlorotetrafluoroethane [Chlorinated fluorocarbon] Asphyxiation, anesthesia, arrhythmias.

chlorothalonil [Poison] Cardiovascular collapse, pulmonary edema, CNS depression, coma, seizures, nausea, vomiting, cardiopulmonary arrest.

Chlorothion [Organophosphate] Pulmonary edema, respiratory muscle paralysis, respiratory failure, bradycardia, acetylcholinesterase inhibition, hypotension, pulmonary edema, overstimulation of parasympathetic nervous system, striated muscle, sympathetic ganglia, and CNS.

chlorothymol [Phenol] Coma, hypotension, arrhythmias, pulmonary edema, respiratory arrest.

chlorotoluene; o-chlorotoluene [Aromatic hydrocarbon] Arrhythmias, respiratory failure, pulmonary edema, paralysis, brain and kidney damage.

chlorotoluidine [Organic base/amine] Pulmonary edema, cardiac depression, seizures.

4-chloro-o-toluidine HCl [Organic base/amine] Pulmonary edema, cardiac depression, seizures.

chlorotrifluoroethane [Chlorinated fluorocarbon] Asphyxiation, anesthesia, arrhythmias.

chlorotrifluoromethane [Chlorinated fluorocarbon] Asphyxiation, anesthesia, arrhythmias.

chlorotrifluoromethane & trifluoromethane mixture [Chlorinated fluorocarbon] Asphyxiation, anesthesia, arrhythmias.

chlorotrifluoropyridine [Aromatic hydrocarbon] Arrhythmias, respiratory failure, pulmonary edema, paralysis, brain and kidney damage.

chloroxuron [Poison] Cardiovascular collapse, pulmonary edema, CNS depression, coma, seizures, nausea, vomiting, cardiopulmonary arrest.

4-chloro-3,5-xylenol [Phenol] Coma, hypotension, arrhythmias, pulmonary edema, respiratory arrest.

chlorpyrifos [Organophosphate] Pulmonary edema, respiratory muscle paralysis, respiratory failure, bradycardia, acetylcholinesterase inhibition, hypotension, pulmonary edema, overstimulation of parasympathetic nervous system, striated muscle, sympathetic ganglia, and CNS.

chlorthiophos [Organophosphate] Pulmonary edema, respiratory muscle paralysis, respiratory failure, bradycardia, acetylcholinesterase inhibition, hypotension, pulmonary edema, overstimulation of parasympathetic nervous system, striated muscle, sympathetic ganglia, and CNS.

chromic acetate [Inorganic acid] Pulmonary edema, bronchospasm, circulatory collapse, laryngeal spasm and edema, severe chemical burns to skin, mucous membranes, and internal organs, GI tract perforation and hemorrhage, peritonitis.

chromic acid [Inorganic acid] Pulmonary edema, bronchospasm, circulatory collapse, laryngeal spasm and edema, severe chemical burns to skin, mucous membranes, and internal organs, GI tract perforation and hemorrhage, peritonitis.

chromic anhydride [Inorganic acid] Pulmonary edema, bronchospasm, circulatory collapse, laryngeal spasm and edema, severe chemical burns to skin, mucous membranes, and internal organs, GI tract perforation and hemorrhage, peritonitis.

chromic chloride; chromous chloride [Inorganic acid] Pulmonary edema, bronchospasm, circulatory collapse, laryngeal spasm and edema, severe chemical burns to skin, mucous membranes, and internal organs, GI tract perforation and hemorrhage, peritonitis.

HazMat

chromic fluoride [Fluorine] *CNS depression, respiratory arrest, cardiovascular collapse, shock, arrhythmias.*

chromic sulfate [Inorganic acid] *Pulmonary edema, bronchospasm, circulatory collapse, laryngeal spasm and edema, severe chemical burns to skin, mucous membranes, and internal organs, GI tract perforation and hemorrhage, peritonitis.*

chromium; chromate salt (n.o.s.) [Inorganic acid] *Pulmonary edema, bronchospasm, circulatory collapse, laryngeal spasm and edema, severe chemical burns to skin, mucous membranes, and internal organs, GI tract perforation and hemorrhage, peritonitis.*

chromium nitrate [Nitrate/nitrite] *Methemoglobinemia, hypotension, circulatory collapse.*

chromium oxychloride [Inorganic acid] *Pulmonary edema, bronchospasm, circulatory collapse, laryngeal spasm and edema, severe chemical burns to skin, mucous membranes, and internal organs, GI tract perforation and hemorrhage, peritonitis.*

chromium trioxide [Inorganic acid] *Pulmonary edema, bronchospasm, circulatory collapse, laryngeal spasm and edema, severe chemical burns to skin, mucous membranes, and internal organs, GI tract perforation and hemorrhage, peritonitis.*

chromosulfuric acid [Inorganic acid] *Pulmonary edema, bronchospasm, circulatory collapse, laryngeal spasm and edema, severe chemical burns to skin, mucous membranes, and internal organs, GI tract perforation and hemorrhage, peritonitis.*

chromous chloride; chromic chloride [Inorganic acid] *Pulmonary edema, bronchospasm, circulatory collapse, laryngeal spasm and edema, severe chemical burns to skin, mucous membranes, and internal organs, GI tract perforation and hemorrhage, peritonitis.*

chrysene [Naphthalene] *Delayed-onset acute intravascular hemolysis.*

chrysotile [Asbestos] *Asbestosis, lung cancer, malignant mesothelioma.*

cigarette, self-lighting [Nicotine] *Respiratory and cardiac arrest, CNS stimulation, CNS depression.*

cigarette lighter; cigarette lighter refills [Aliphatic hydrocarbon] *Arrhythmias, asphyxiation, anesthesia.*

cleaning compound [Inorganic base/alkaline corrosive] *Upper airway burns and edema, pulmonary edema, skin burns, circulatory collapse, GI tract perforation and hemorrhage, peritonitis.*

coal [Flammable solid] *Shock, severe chemical and thermal burns, severe respiratory tract irritation, pulmonary edema, respiratory arrest, ECG changes, sudden death.*

coal gas [Flammable gas] *Respiratory failure, cardiac arrest, arrhythmias.*

coal tar creosote [Aromatic hydrocarbon] *Arrhythmias, respiratory failure, pulmonary edema, paralysis, brain and kidney damage.* [Phenol] *Coma, hypotension, arrhythmias, pulmonary edema, respiratory arrest.*

coal tar distillate [Aromatic hydrocarbon] *Arrhythmias, respiratory failure, pulmonary edema, paralysis, brain and kidney damage.* [Benzene] *Arrhythmias, respiratory failure, pulmonary edema, CNS depression, liver and kidney damage.*

coal tar naphtha [Hydrocarbon mixture] *CNS depression, respiratory arrest, seizures, arrhythmias, pulmonary edema.* [Naphthalene] *Delayed-onset acute intravascular hemolysis.*

coal tar oil [Aromatic hydrocarbon] *Arrhythmias, respiratory failure, pulmonary edema, paralysis, brain and kidney damage.* [Benzene] *Arrhythmias, respiratory failure, pulmonary edema, CNS depression, liver and kidney damage.*

coating solution [Poison] *Cardiovascular collapse, pulmonary edema, CNS depression, coma, seizures, nausea, vomiting, cardiopulmonary arrest.*

cobalt carbonyl [Cobalt] *Respiratory tract irritation, possible pulmonary edema and fibrosis.*

cobalt hydrocarbonyl [Cobalt] *Respiratory tract irritation, possible pulmonary edema and fibrosis.*

cobalt naphthenate [Cobalt] *Respiratory tract irritation, possible pulmonary edema and fibrosis.*

cobalt resinate [Cobalt] *Respiratory tract irritation, possible pulmonary edema and fibrosis.*

cobalt salt (n.o.s.) [Cobalt] *Respiratory tract irritation, possible pulmonary edema and fibrosis.*

cobaltous bromide [Cobalt] *Respiratory tract irritation, possible pulmonary edema and fibrosis.* [Bromine/methyl bromide] *Severe respiratory irritation, pulmonary edema, respiratory failure, coma, convulsions, death.*

cobaltous formate [Cobalt] *Respiratory tract irritation, possible pulmonary edema and fibrosis.*

cobaltous sulfamate [Cobalt] *Respiratory tract irritation, possible pulmonary edema and fibrosis.*

cocculus [Poison] *Cardiovascular collapse, pulmonary edema, CNS depression, coma, seizures, nausea, vomiting, cardiopulmonary arrest.*

colchicine [Poison] *Cardiovascular collapse, pulmonary edema, CNS depression, coma, seizures, nausea, vomiting, cardiopulmonary arrest.*

collodion [Lower alcohol (1–3 carbons)] *CNS depression, coma, respiratory arrest, arrhythmias.* [Ether] *Anesthesia, respiratory arrest.*

combustible liquid (n.o.s.) [Flammable/combustible liquid] *CNS depression, respiratory arrest, convulsions, arrhythmias, pulmonary edema.*

compressed gas (n.o.s.) [Nonflammable gas] *Pulmonary edema, respiratory failure, asphyxiation.*

compressed gas, flammable (n.o.s.) [Flammable gas] *Respiratory failure, cardiac arrest, arrhythmias.*

compressed gas, flammable poison (n.o.s.) [Flammable gas] *Respiratory failure, cardiac arrest, arrhythmias.* [Poison] *Cardiovascular collapse, pulmonary edema, CNS depression, coma, seizures, nausea, vomiting, cardiopulmonary arrest.*

compressed gas, poisonous (n.o.s.) [Poison] *Cardiovascular collapse, pulmonary edema, CNS depression, coma, seizures, nausea, vomiting, cardiopulmonary arrest.*

copper; copper mixture (n.o.s.) [Copper] *Respiratory tract irritation, respiratory arrest, hemorrhagic gastritis.*

copper acetoarsenite; cupric acetoarsenite [Copper] *Respiratory tract irritation, respiratory arrest, hemorrhagic gastritis.*

copper arsenate [Arsenic] *Heavy metal toxicity, vomiting, GI bleeding, CNS depression, pulmonary edema, cardiac arrest.* [Copper] *Respiratory tract irritation, respiratory arrest, hemorrhagic gastritis.*

copper arsenite; cupric arsenite [Arsenic] *Heavy metal toxicity, vomiting, GI bleeding, CNS depression, pulmonary edema, cardiac arrest.* [Copper] *Respiratory tract irritation, respiratory arrest, hemorrhagic gastritis.*

copper chlorate [Copper] *Respiratory tract irritation, respiratory arrest, hemorrhagic gastritis.* [Chlorate] *Hemolysis, methemoglobinemia, hypoperfusion, CNS depression, delayed-onset renal failure.*

copper chloride; cupric chloride; cuprous chloride [Copper] *Respiratory tract irritation, respiratory arrest, hemorrhagic gastritis.*

copper cyanide [Copper] *Respiratory tract irritation, respiratory arrest, hemorrhagic gastritis.* [Cyanide] *Impairment of cellular oxygenation and adenosine triphosphate production, hypoxia, death.*

copper naphthenates [Naphthalene] *Delayed-onset acute intravascular hemolysis.* [Copper] *Respiratory tract*

HazMat

irritation, respiratory arrest, hemor-
rhagic gastritis.

copper oxychloride sulfate [Copper]
Respiratory tract irritation, respiratory
arrest, hemorrhagic gastritis.

copper 3-phenyl-salicylate [Copper]
Respiratory tract irritation, respiratory
arrest, hemorrhagic gastritis.

copper quinolinolate [Copper] *Respi-*
ratory tract irritation, respiratory
arrest, hemorrhagic gastritis.

copper selenate [Copper] *Respiratory*
tract irritation, respiratory arrest, hem-
orrhagic gastritis. [Selenium] *Arrhyth-*
mias, pulmonary edema, broncho-
spasm, seizures, vomiting, GI bleeding.

copper selenite [Copper] *Respiratory*
tract irritation, respiratory arrest, hem-
orrhagic gastritis. [Selenium] *Arrhyth-*
mias, pulmonary edema, broncho-
spasm, seizures, vomiting, GI bleeding.

copper sulfate, tribasic [Copper] *Res-*
piratory tract irritation, respiratory
arrest, hemorrhagic gastritis.

copper-based pesticide (n.o.s.)
[Copper] *Respiratory tract irritation,*
respiratory arrest, hemorrhagic gastritis.

copra [Flammable/combustible liquid]
CNS depression, respiratory arrest, con-
vulsions, arrhythmias, pulmonary edema.

corrosive: acid [Inorganic acid] *Pul-*
monary edema, bronchospasm, circula-
tory collapse, laryngeal spasm and
edema, severe chemical burns to skin,
mucous membranes, and internal
organs, GI tract perforation and hem-
orrhage, peritonitis. [Organic acid]
Pulmonary edema, circulatory collapse,
laryngeal edema and spasm, severe
chemical burns to skin, mucous mem-
branes, and internal organs, GI tract
perforation and hemorrhage, peritonitis.

corrosive: ammonia [Ammonia] *Pul-*
monary edema, hypotension.

corrosive: ammonium hydroxide
[Ammonia] *Pulmonary edema, hypo-*
tension.

corrosive liquid, flammable (n.o.s.)
[Flammable/combustible liquid]
CNS depression, respiratory arrest,

convulsions, arrhythmias, pulmonary
edema. [Corrosive] *Upper airway*
burns and edema, circulatory collapse,
severe chemical burns to skin, toxic
systemic effects, GI tract perforation
and hemorrhage, peritonitis.

corrosive solid, flammable (n.o.s.)
[Flammable solid] *Shock, severe*
chemical and thermal burns, severe res-
piratory tract irritation, pulmonary
edema, respiratory arrest, ECG
changes, sudden death. [Corrosive]
Upper airway burns and edema, circu-
latory collapse, severe chemical burns
to skin, toxic systemic effects, GI tract
perforation and hemorrhage, peritonitis.

corrosive solid, self-heating (n.o.s.)
[Corrosive] *Upper airway burns and*
edema, circulatory collapse, severe
chemical burns to skin, toxic systemic
effects, GI tract perforation and hem-
orrhage, peritonitis.

corrosive solid or liquid (n.o.s.)
[Corrosive] *Upper airway burns and*
edema, circulatory collapse, severe
chemical burns to skin, toxic systemic
effects, GI tract perforation and hem-
orrhage, peritonitis.

**corrosive solid or liquid, flammable
in contact with water (n.o.s.)**
[Flammable gas] *Respiratory failure,*
cardiac arrest, arrhythmias. [Corrosive]
Upper airway burns and edema, circu-
latory collapse, severe chemical burns to
skin, toxic systemic effects, GI tract
perforation and hemorrhage, peritonitis.

**corrosive solid or liquid, oxidizing
(n.o.s.)** [Oxidizer] *Pulmonary and*
laryngeal edema, circulatory arrest,
hypovolemic shock, chemical burns of
skin, mucous membranes, and internal
organs. [Corrosive] *Upper airway*
burns and edema, circulatory collapse,
severe chemical burns to skin, toxic
systemic effects, GI tract perforation
and hemorrhage, peritonitis.

**corrosive solid or liquid, poisonous
(n.o.s.)** [Poison] *Cardiovascular col-*
lapse, pulmonary edema, CNS depres-
sion, coma, seizures, nausea, vomiting,

cardiopulmonary arrest. [Corrosive] Upper airway burns and edema, circulatory collapse, severe chemical burns to skin, toxic systemic effects, GI tract perforation and hemorrhage, peritonitis.

cosmetic, corrosive (n.o.s.) [Corrosive] Upper airway burns and edema, circulatory collapse, severe chemical burns to skin, toxic systemic effects, GI tract perforation and hemorrhage, peritonitis.

cosmetic, flammable liquid (n.o.s.) [Flammable/combustible liquid] CNS depression, respiratory arrest, convulsions, arrhythmias, pulmonary edema.

cosmetic, flammable solid (n.o.s.) [Flammable solid] Shock, severe chemical and thermal burns, severe respiratory tract irritation, pulmonary edema, respiratory arrest, ECG changes, sudden death.

cosmetic, oxidizer (n.o.s.) [Oxidizer] Pulmonary and laryngeal edema, circulatory arrest, hypovolemic shock, chemical burns of skin, mucous membranes, and internal organs.

cotton [Irritant] Severe immediate or delayed upper airway or respiratory tract irritation, pulmonary edema, glottic spasm, airway obstruction.

coumachlor [Warfarin/hydroxycoumarin/indanedione] Anticoagulation effect, internal hemorrhage.

coumafuryl [Warfarin/hydroxycoumarin/indanedione] Anticoagulation effect, internal hemorrhage.

coumaphos [Organophosphate] Pulmonary edema, respiratory muscle paralysis, respiratory failure, bradycardia, acetylcholinesterase inhibition, hypotension, pulmonary edema, overstimulation of parasympathetic nervous system, striated muscle, sympathetic ganglia, and CNS.

coumarin derivative pesticide (n.o.s.) [Ketone] Respiratory mucous membrane irritation, pulmonary edema, CNS depression.

coumatetralyl [Warfarin/hydroxycoumarin/indanedione] Anticoagulation effect, internal hemorrhage.

Creolin [Acrolein] Severe respiratory tract irritation, pulmonary edema, respiratory failure.

creosol [Phenol] Coma, hypotension, arrhythmias, pulmonary edema, respiratory arrest.

creosote, coal tar [Aromatic hydrocarbon] Arrhythmias, respiratory failure, pulmonary edema, paralysis, brain and kidney damage. [Phenol] Coma, hypotension, arrhythmias, pulmonary edema, respiratory arrest.

creosote salt (n.o.s.) [Phenol] Coma, hypotension, arrhythmias, pulmonary edema, respiratory arrest.

***p*-cresidine** [Aromatic hydrocarbon] Arrhythmias, respiratory failure, pulmonary edema, paralysis, brain and kidney damage.

cresol; *m*-cresol; *o*-cresol; *p*-cresol [Phenol] Coma, hypotension, arrhythmias, pulmonary edema, respiratory arrest.

***m*-cresyl acetate** [Ester] CNS depression, respiratory tract irritation, bronchitis, pneumonitis.

cresylic acid [Phenol] Coma, hypotension, arrhythmias, pulmonary edema, respiratory arrest.

crimidine [Poison] Cardiovascular collapse, pulmonary edema, CNS depression, coma, seizures, nausea, vomiting, cardiopulmonary arrest.

crotonaldehyde [Acrolein] Severe respiratory tract irritation, pulmonary edema, respiratory failure.

crotonic acid [Organic acid] Pulmonary edema, circulatory collapse, laryngeal edema and spasm, severe chemical burns to skin, mucous membranes, and internal organs, GI tract perforation and hemorrhage, peritonitis.

crotonylene [Aliphatic hydrocarbon] Arrhythmias, asphyxiation, anesthesia.

crufomate [Organophosphate] Pulmonary edema, respiratory muscle paralysis, respiratory failure, bradycardia,

HazMat

acetylcholinesterase inhibition, hypotension, pulmonary edema, overstimulation of parasympathetic nervous system, striated muscle, sympathetic ganglia, and CNS.

cryolite [Fluorine] *CNS depression, respiratory arrest, cardiovascular collapse, shock, arrhythmias.*

cubé [Rotenone] *Respiratory arrest, asphyxia.*

cumene [Aromatic hydrocarbon] *Arrhythmias, respiratory failure, pulmonary edema, paralysis, brain and kidney damage.*

cumene hydroperoxide [Organic peroxide] *Pulmonary and laryngeal edema, circulatory arrest, hypovolemic shock, chemical burns to skin, mucous membranes, and internal organs.* [Aromatic hydrocarbon] *Arrhythmias, respiratory failure, pulmonary edema, paralysis, brain and kidney damage.*

cumyl hydroperoxide [Organic peroxide] *Pulmonary and laryngeal edema, circulatory arrest, hypovolemic shock, chemical burns to skin, mucous membranes, and internal organs.* [Aromatic hydrocarbon] *Arrhythmias, respiratory failure, pulmonary edema, paralysis, brain and kidney damage.*

cumyl peroxy-neo-decanoate [Organic peroxide] *Pulmonary and laryngeal edema, circulatory arrest, hypovolemic shock, chemical burns to skin, mucous membranes, and internal organs.* [Aromatic hydrocarbon] *Arrhythmias, respiratory failure, pulmonary edema, paralysis, brain and kidney damage.*

cumyl peroxypivalate [Organic peroxide] *Pulmonary and laryngeal edema, circulatory arrest, hypovolemic shock, chemical burns to skin, mucous membranes, and internal organs.* [Aromatic hydrocarbon] *Arrhythmias, respiratory failure, pulmonary edema, paralysis, brain and kidney damage.*

cupferron [Organic base/amine] *Pulmonary edema, cardiac depression, seizures.*

cupric acetate [Copper] *Respiratory tract irritation, respiratory arrest, hemorrhagic gastritis.*

cupric acetoarsenite; copper acetoarsenite [Copper] *Respiratory tract irritation, respiratory arrest, hemorrhagic gastritis.*

cupric arsenite; copper arsenite [Arsenic] *Heavy metal toxicity, vomiting, GI bleeding, CNS depression, pulmonary edema, cardiac arrest.* [Copper] *Respiratory tract irritation, respiratory arrest, hemorrhagic gastritis.*

cupric chloride; copper chloride; cuprous chloride [Copper] *Respiratory tract irritation, respiratory arrest, hemorrhagic gastritis.*

cupric nitrate [Copper] *Respiratory tract irritation, respiratory arrest, hemorrhagic gastritis.*

cupric oxalate [Copper] *Respiratory tract irritation, respiratory arrest, hemorrhagic gastritis.*

cupric sulfate [Copper] *Respiratory tract irritation, respiratory arrest, hemorrhagic gastritis.*

cupric tartrate [Copper] *Respiratory tract irritation, respiratory arrest, hemorrhagic gastritis.*

cupriethylenediamine [Organic base/amine] *Pulmonary edema, cardiac depression, seizures.* [Copper] *Respiratory tract irritation, respiratory arrest, hemorrhagic gastritis.*

cuprous chloride; copper chloride; cupric chloride [Copper] *Respiratory tract irritation, respiratory arrest, hemorrhagic gastritis.*

cuprous oxide [Copper] *Respiratory tract irritation, respiratory arrest, hemorrhagic gastritis.*

cyanic acid [Isocyanate/aliphatic thiocyanate] *CNS depression, respiratory arrest, respiratory paralysis, pulmonary edema, cyanide toxicity.*

cyanide; cyanide mixture (n.o.s.) [Cyanide] *Impairment of cellular oxygenation and adenosine triphosphate production, hypoxia, death.*

cyanide potassium; potassium cyanide [Cyanide] *Impairment of cellular oxygenation and adenosine triphosphate production, hypoxia, death.*

cyanide sodium [Cyanide] *Impairment of cellular oxygenation and adenosine triphosphate production, hypoxia, death.*

cyanogen [Cyanide] *Impairment of cellular oxygenation and adenosine triphosphate production, hypoxia, death.*

cyanogen bromide [Cyanide] *Impairment of cellular oxygenation and adenosine triphosphate production, hypoxia, death.*

cyanogen chloride [Cyanide] *Impairment of cellular oxygenation and adenosine triphosphate production, hypoxia, death.*

cyanogen iodide [Cyanide] *Impairment of cellular oxygenation and adenosine triphosphate production, hypoxia, death.*

cyano-organic mixture (n.o.s.) [Cyanide] *Impairment of cellular oxygenation and adenosine triphosphate production, hypoxia, death.*

cyanophos [Organophosphate] *Pulmonary edema, respiratory muscle paralysis, respiratory failure, bradycardia, acetylcholinesterase inhibition, hypotension, pulmonary edema, overstimulation of parasympathetic nervous system, striated muscle, sympathetic ganglia, and CNS.*

cyanuric chloride [Organic acid] *Pulmonary edema, circulatory collapse, laryngeal edema and spasm, severe chemical burns to skin, mucous membranes, and internal organs, GI tract perforation and hemorrhage, peritonitis.*

cyanuric fluoride [Hydrofluoric acid] *Pulmonary and laryngeal edema, circulatory collapse, severe skin burns, GI tract perforation, systemic fluoride poisoning.*

cyclethrin [Pyrethrin/pyrethroid] *Respiratory paralysis, convulsions.*

cyclobutane [Simple asphyxiant] *Asphyxiation.*

cyclobutylchloroformate [Ester] *CNS depression, respiratory tract irritation, bronchitis, pneumonitis.*

cyclocoumarol [Warfarin/hydroxycoumarin/indanedione] *Anticoagulation effect, internal hemorrhage.*

cyclododecatriene [Aliphatic hydrocarbon] *Arrhythmias, asphyxiation, anesthesia.*

cycloheptane [Aliphatic hydrocarbon] *Arrhythmias, asphyxiation, anesthesia.*

cycloheptatriene [Aliphatic hydrocarbon] *Arrhythmias, asphyxiation, anesthesia.*

cycloheptene [Aliphatic hydrocarbon] *Arrhythmias, asphyxiation, anesthesia.*

cyclohexane [Aliphatic hydrocarbon] *Arrhythmias, asphyxiation, anesthesia.*

cyclohexanol [Higher alcohol (4+ carbons)] *CNS depression, respiratory failure, arrhythmias.*

cyclohexanone [Ketone] *Respiratory mucous membrane irritation, pulmonary edema, CNS depression.*

cyclohexanone peroxide [Organic peroxide] *Pulmonary and laryngeal edema, circulatory arrest, hypovolemic shock, chemical burns to skin, mucous membranes, and internal organs.* [Ketone] *Respiratory mucous membrane irritation, pulmonary edema, CNS depression.* [Corrosive] *Upper airway burns and edema, circulatory collapse, severe chemical burns to skin, toxic systemic effects, GI tract perforation and hemorrhage, peritonitis.*

cyclohexene [Aliphatic hydrocarbon] *Arrhythmias, asphyxiation, anesthesia.*

cyclohexene & ozone mixture [Aliphatic hydrocarbon] *Arrhythmias, asphyxiation, anesthesia.* [Ozone] *Pulmonary edema, airway obstruction.*

cyclohexenyl trichlorosilane [Silane/chlorosilane] *Respiratory tract irritation, pulmonary edema.*

cycloheximide [Irritant] *Severe immediate or delayed upper airway or respiratory tract irritation, pulmonary edema, glottic spasm, airway obstruction.* [Poison] *Cardiovascular collapse, pulmonary edema, CNS depression, coma, seizures, nausea, vomiting, cardiopulmonary arrest.*

cyclohexyl acetate [Ester] *CNS depression, respiratory tract irritation, bronchitis, pneumonitis.*

cyclohexyl isocyanate [Isocyanate/aliphatic thiocyanate] *CNS depression, respiratory arrest, respiratory paralysis, pulmonary edema, cyanide toxicity.*

cyclohexyl mercaptan [Sulfur] *Respiratory tract irritation, pulmonary edema, anaphylaxis.*

cyclohexyl trichlorosilane [Silane/chlorosilane] *Respiratory tract irritation, pulmonary edema.*

cyclohexylamine [Organic base/amine] *Pulmonary edema, cardiac depression, seizures.*

2-cyclohexyl-4,6-dinitrophenol [Dinitrophenol] *Respiratory and circulatory collapse, pulmonary edema, hyperthermia.*

cyclonite (RDX, T4, or C4) [Explosive] *Multiple trauma, highly toxic chemical exposure.*

cyclooctadiene [Aliphatic hydrocarbon] *Arrhythmias, asphyxiation, anesthesia.*

cyclooctadiene phosphine [Phosphine] *Severe pulmonary irritation, pulmonary edema.*

cyclooctatetraene [Aliphatic hydrocarbon] *Arrhythmias, asphyxiation, anesthesia.*

cyclopentane [Aliphatic hydrocarbon] *Arrhythmias, asphyxiation, anesthesia.*

cyclopentanol [Higher alcohol (4+ carbons)] *CNS depression, respiratory failure, arrhythmias.*

cyclopentanone [Ketone] *Respiratory mucous membrane irritation, pulmonary edema, CNS depression.*

cyclopentene [Aliphatic hydrocarbon] *Arrhythmias, asphyxiation, anesthesia.*

cyclophosphamide [Poison] *Cardiovascular collapse, pulmonary edema, CNS depression, coma, seizures, nausea, vomiting, cardiopulmonary arrest.*

cyclopropane [Simple asphyxiant] *Asphyxiation.*

cymene [Aromatic hydrocarbon] *Arrhythmias, respiratory failure, pulmonary edema, paralysis, brain and kidney damage.*

2,4-D; 2,4-D ester (n.o.s.); 2,4-D salt (n.o.s.) [Chlorophenoxy herbicide] *CNS depression, CNS stimulation, respiratory failure, ventricular fibrillation, seizures.*

daunomycin [Poison] *Cardiovascular collapse, pulmonary edema, CNS depression, coma, seizures, nausea, vomiting, cardiopulmonary arrest.*

DBCP [Dichloropropane/dichloropropene] *Pulmonary edema, bronchospasm, alveolar hemorrhage.*

DD mixture [Dichloropropane/dichloropropene] *Pulmonary edema, bronchospasm, alveolar hemorrhage.*

DDD [DDT] *CNS disruption, respiratory control center paralysis, ventricular fibrillation, seizures, respiratory arrest.*

DDE [DDT] *CNS disruption, respiratory control center paralysis, ventricular fibrillation, seizures, respiratory arrest.*

DDT (dichlorodiphenyltrichloroethane) [DDT] *CNS disruption, respiratory control center paralysis, ventricular fibrillation, seizures, respiratory arrest.* [Lindane] *CNS stimulation, seizures, respiratory failure.*

decaborane [Boron] *Respiratory tract irritation, laryngeal spasm and edema, pulmonary edema, severe chemical burns.*

decabromodiphenyl oxide [Boron] *Respiratory tract irritation, laryngeal spasm and edema, pulmonary edema, severe chemical burns.*

decahydronaphthalene [Naphthalene] *Delayed-onset acute intravascular hemolysis.*

decane [Aliphatic hydrocarbon] *Arrhythmias, asphyxiation, anesthesia.*

decanoyl peroxide [Organic peroxide] *Pulmonary and laryngeal edema, circulatory arrest, hypovolemic shock, chemical burns to skin, mucous membranes, and internal organs.*

decyl alcohol [Higher alcohol (4+ carbons)] *CNS depression, respiratory failure, arrhythmias.*

degreaser [Hydrocarbon mixture] *CNS depression, respiratory arrest, seizures, arrhythmias, pulmonary edema.*

DEHP [Ester] *CNS depression, respiratory tract irritation, bronchitis, pneumonitis.*

dehydrorotenone [Rotenone] *Respiratory arrest, asphyxia.*

demeton [Organophosphate] *Pulmonary edema, respiratory muscle paralysis, respiratory failure, bradycardia, acetylcholinesterase inhibition, hypotension, pulmonary edema, overstimulation of parasympathetic nervous system, striated muscle, sympathetic ganglia, and CNS.*

demeton-methyl [Organophosphate] *Pulmonary edema, respiratory muscle paralysis, respiratory failure, bradycardia, acetylcholinesterase inhibition, hypotension, pulmonary edema, overstimulation of parasympathetic nervous system, striated muscle, sympathetic ganglia, and CNS.*

denatured alcohol [Methyl alcohol] *Respiratory failure, circulatory collapse.*

Deobase [Hydrocarbon mixture] *CNS depression, respiratory arrest, seizures, arrhythmias, pulmonary edema.*

Derris powder [Rotenone] *Respiratory arrest, asphyxia.*

desmedipham [Aniline] *Methemoglobinemia, hypoxia.* [Carbamate] *Acetylcholinesterase inhibition (reversible), bradycardia, hypotension, respiratory muscle paralysis, respiratory arrest, pulmonary edema.*

deuterium [Flammable gas] *Respiratory failure, cardiac arrest, arrhythmias.* [Simple asphyxiant] *Asphyxiation.*

DFDT [Simple asphyxiant] *Asphyxiation.*

DFP [Organophosphate] *Pulmonary edema, respiratory muscle paralysis, respiratory failure, bradycardia, acetylcholinesterase inhibition, hypotension, pulmonary edema, overstimulation of parasympathetic nervous system, striated muscle, sympathetic ganglia, and CNS.*

diacetone alcohol [Ketone] *Respiratory mucous membrane irritation, pulmonary edema, CNS depression.*

diacetone alcohol peroxide [Organic peroxide] *Pulmonary and laryngeal edema, circulatory arrest, hypovolemic shock, chemical burns to skin, mucous membranes, and internal organs.* [Ketone] *Respiratory mucous membrane irritation, pulmonary edema, CNS depression.* [Corrosive] *Upper airway burns and edema, circulatory collapse, severe chemical burns to skin, toxic systemic effects, GI tract perforation and hemorrhage, peritonitis.*

diacetyl [Ketone] *Respiratory mucous membrane irritation, pulmonary edema, CNS depression.*

diacetyl peroxide [Organic peroxide] *Pulmonary and laryngeal edema, circulatory arrest, hypovolemic shock, chemical burns to skin, mucous membranes, and internal organs.* [Ketone] *Respiratory mucous membrane irritation, pulmonary edema, CNS depression.* [Corrosive] *Upper airway burns and edema, circulatory collapse, severe chemical burns to skin, toxic systemic effects, GI tract perforation and hemorrhage, peritonitis.*

dialifor; dialiphor [Organophosphate] *Pulmonary edema, respiratory muscle paralysis, respiratory failure, bradycardia, acetylcholinesterase inhibition, hypotension, pulmonary edema, overstimulation of parasympathetic nervous system, striated muscle, sympathetic ganglia, and CNS.*

dialifos; dialiphos [Organophosphate] *Pulmonary edema, respiratory muscle paralysis, respiratory failure, bradycardia, acetylcholinesterase inhibition, hypotension, pulmonary edema, overstimulation of parasympathetic nervous system, striated muscle, sympathetic ganglia, and CNS.*

di-allate [Dithiocarbamate] *Hypotension, respiratory failure.*

diallylamine [Organic base/amine] *Pulmonary edema, cardiac depression, seizures.*

diallylether [Ether] *Anesthesia, respiratory arrest.*

HazMat

diamidafos [Organophosphate] *Pulmonary edema, respiratory muscle paralysis, respiratory failure, bradycardia, acetylcholinesterase inhibition, hypotension, pulmonary edema, overstimulation of parasympathetic nervous system, striated muscle, sympathetic ganglia, and CNS.*

2,4-diaminoanisole [Organic base/amine] *Pulmonary edema, cardiac depression, seizures.*

2,4-diaminoanisole sulfate [Organic base/amine] *Pulmonary edema, cardiac depression, seizures.*

4,4′-diaminodiphenoyl ether [Aniline] *Methemoglobinemia, hypoxia.*

diaminodiphenyl methane [Nitrate/nitrite] *Methemoglobinemia, hypotension, circulatory collapse.*

diaminotoluene; 2,4-diaminotoluene [Aniline] *Methemoglobinemia, hypoxia.*

diamylamine [Organic base/amine] *Pulmonary edema, cardiac depression, seizures.*

Diazinon [Organophosphate] *Pulmonary edema, respiratory muscle paralysis, respiratory failure, bradycardia, acetylcholinesterase inhibition, hypotension, pulmonary edema, overstimulation of parasympathetic nervous system, striated muscle, sympathetic ganglia, and CNS.*

diazomethane [Phosgene] *Severe respiratory irritation, alveolar damage, pulmonary edema.*

2-diazo-1-naphthol-4-sulfochloride; 2-diazo-1-naphthol-5-sulfochloride [Naphthalene] *Delayed-onset acute intravascular hemolysis.*

dibenz[*a,h*]anthracene [Aromatic hydrocarbon] *Arrhythmias, respiratory failure, pulmonary edema, paralysis, brain and kidney damage.*

dibenzofuran [Polychlorinated biphenyl/polybrominated biphenyl/polychlorinated dibenzofuran] *Liver and kidney damage.*

dibenzoyl peroxide [Organic peroxide] *Pulmonary and laryngeal edema, circulatory arrest, hypovolemic shock,* chemical burns to skin, mucous membranes, and internal organs.*

dibenz[*a,i*]pyrine [Aromatic hydrocarbon] *Arrhythmias, respiratory failure, pulmonary edema, paralysis, brain and kidney damage.*

dibenzyl peroxy-dicarbonate [Organic peroxide] *Pulmonary and laryngeal edema, circulatory arrest, hypovolemic shock, chemical burns to skin, mucous membranes, and internal organs.*

dibenzyldichlorosilane [Silane/chlorosilane] *Respiratory tract irritation, pulmonary edema.*

diborane; diborane mixture (n.o.s.) [Boron] *Respiratory tract irritation, laryngeal spasm and edema, pulmonary edema, severe chemical burns.*

dibromobenzene [Aromatic hydrocarbon] *Arrhythmias, respiratory failure, pulmonary edema, paralysis, brain and kidney damage.*

dibromobutanone [Ketone] *Respiratory mucous membrane irritation, pulmonary edema, CNS depression.*

dibromochloropropane; 1,2-dibromo-3-chloropropane [Dichloropropane/dichloropropene] *Pulmonary edema, bronchospasm, alveolar hemorrhage.*

dibromodifluoromethane [Chlorinated fluorocarbon] *Asphyxiation, anesthesia, arrhythmias.*

dibromoethane; 1,2-dibromoethane [Chlorinated fluorocarbon] *Asphyxiation, anesthesia, arrhythmias.*

dibromomethane [Chlorinated fluorocarbon] *Asphyxiation, anesthesia, arrhythmias.*

dibromotetrafluoroethane (Halon 2402) [Chlorinated fluorocarbon] *Asphyxiation, anesthesia, arrhythmias.*

dibutyl ether [Ether] *Anesthesia, respiratory arrest.*

dibutyl peroxide; di-*tert*-butyl peroxide [Organic peroxide] *Pulmonary and laryngeal edema, circulatory arrest, hypovolemic shock, chemical burns to skin, mucous membranes, and internal organs.*

dibutyl peroxy-dicarbonate; di-sec-butyl peroxy-dicarbonate [Organic peroxide] *Pulmonary and laryngeal edema, circulatory arrest, hypovolemic shock, chemical burns to skin, mucous membranes, and internal organs.*

dibutyl phthalate [Ester] *CNS depression, respiratory tract irritation, bronchitis, pneumonitis.*

dibutylamine [Organic base/amine] *Pulmonary edema, cardiac depression, seizures.*

dibutylaminoethanol [Higher alcohol (4+ carbons)] *CNS depression, respiratory failure, arrhythmias.*

di(4-tert-butylcyclohexyl) peroxy-dicarbonate [Organic peroxide] *Pulmonary and laryngeal edema, circulatory arrest, hypovolemic shock, chemical burns to skin, mucous membranes, and internal organs.*

2,2-di(tert-butylperoxy)-butane [Organic peroxide] *Pulmonary and laryngeal edema, circulatory arrest, hypovolemic shock, chemical burns to skin, mucous membranes, and internal organs.* [Aliphatic hydrocarbon] *Arrhythmias, asphyxiation, anesthesia.*

1,1-di(tert-butylperoxy)-cyclohexane; 1,2-di(tert-butylperoxy)-cyclohexane [Organic peroxide] *Pulmonary and laryngeal edema, circulatory arrest, hypovolemic shock, chemical burns to skin, mucous membranes, and internal organs.* [Aliphatic hydrocarbon] *Arrhythmias, asphyxiation, anesthesia.*

di-(2-tert-butylperoxy-isopropyl) benzene [Organic peroxide] *Pulmonary and laryngeal edema, circulatory arrest, hypovolemic shock, chemical burns to skin, mucous membranes, and internal organs.* [Aromatic hydrocarbon] *Arrhythmias, respiratory failure, pulmonary edema, paralysis, brain and kidney damage.*

1,3-di(2-tert-butylperoxy-isopropyl) benzene; 1,4-di(2-tert-butyl-peroxy-isopropyl) benzene [Organic peroxide] *Pulmonary and laryngeal edema, circulatory arrest, hypovolemic shock, chemical burns to skin, mucous membranes, and internal organs.* [Aromatic hydrocarbon] *Arrhythmias, respiratory failure, pulmonary edema, paralysis, brain and kidney damage.*

di-tert-butylperoxyphthalate [Ester] *CNS depression, respiratory tract irritation, bronchitis, pneumonitis.*

2,2-di(tert-butylperoxy)-propane [Organic peroxide] *Pulmonary and laryngeal edema, circulatory arrest, hypovolemic shock, chemical burns to skin, mucous membranes, and internal organs.* [Aliphatic hydrocarbon] *Arrhythmias, asphyxiation, anesthesia.*

1,1-di(tert-butylperoxy)-3,3,5-trimethylcyclohexane [Organic peroxide] *Pulmonary and laryngeal edema, circulatory arrest, hypovolemic shock, chemical burns to skin, mucous membranes, and internal organs.* [Aliphatic hydrocarbon] *Arrhythmias, asphyxiation, anesthesia.*

dicamba [Chlorophenoxy herbicide] *CNS depression, CNS stimulation, respiratory failure, ventricular fibrillation, seizures.*

dicetyl peroxydicarbonate [Organic peroxide] *Pulmonary and laryngeal edema, circulatory arrest, hypovolemic shock, chemical burns to skin, mucous membranes, and internal organs.*

dichlobenil [Poison] *Cardiovascular collapse, pulmonary edema, CNS depression, coma, seizures, nausea, vomiting, cardiopulmonary arrest.*

dichlofenthion [Organophosphate] *Pulmonary edema, respiratory muscle paralysis, respiratory failure, bradycardia, acetylcholinesterase inhibition, hypotension, pulmonary edema, overstimulation of parasympathetic nervous system, striated muscle, sympathetic ganglia, and CNS.*

dichlone [Poison] *Cardiovascular collapse, pulmonary edema, CNS depression, coma, seizures, nausea, vomiting, cardiopulmonary arrest.*

HazMat

Dichloran [Benzene] *Arrhythmias, respiratory failure, pulmonary edema, CNS depression, liver and kidney damage.*

dichloro acetylene [Aliphatic hydrocarbon] *Arrhythmias, asphyxiation, anesthesia.* [Simple asphyxiant] *Asphyxiation.*

dichloroacetic acid [Organic acid] *Pulmonary edema, circulatory collapse, laryngeal edema and spasm, severe chemical burns to skin, mucous membranes, and internal organs, GI tract perforation and hemorrhage, peritonitis.*

1,3-dichloroacetone [Ketone] *Respiratory mucous membrane irritation, pulmonary edema, CNS depression.*

dichloroacetyl chloride [Organic acid] *Pulmonary edema, circulatory collapse, laryngeal edema and spasm, severe chemical burns to skin, mucous membranes, and internal organs, GI tract perforation and hemorrhage, peritonitis.*

dichloroaniline [Aniline] *Methemoglobinemia, hypoxia.*

o-dichlorobenzene; p-dichlorobenzene [Lindane] *CNS stimulation, seizures, respiratory failure.*

dichlorobenzidine; 3,3′-dichlorobenzidine [Aniline] *Methemoglobinemia, hypoxia.*

di-(4-chlorobenzoyl) peroxide; 2,4-dichlorobenzoyl peroxide [Organic peroxide] *Pulmonary and laryngeal edema, circulatory arrest, hypovolemic shock, chemical burns to skin, mucous membranes, and internal organs.*

1,1-dichloro-2,2-bis(p-chlorophenyl) ethane [Lindane] *CNS stimulation, seizures, respiratory failure.*

dichlorobromomethane [Chlorinated fluorocarbon] *Asphyxiation, anesthesia, arrhythmias.*

dichlorobutene; trans-1,4-dichlorobutene [Chlorinated fluorocarbon] *Asphyxiation, anesthesia, arrhythmias.*

dichlorodiethyl ether [Ether] *Anesthesia, respiratory arrest.*

dichlorodifluoroethylene [Chlorinated fluorocarbon] *Asphyxiation, anesthesia, arrhythmias.*

dichlorodifluoromethane (Freon 12) [Chlorinated fluorocarbon] *Asphyxiation, anesthesia, arrhythmias.*

dichlorodifluoromethane & chlorodifluoromethane mixture [Chlorinated fluorocarbon] *Asphyxiation, anesthesia, arrhythmias.*

dichlorodifluoromethane & dichlorotetrafluoroethane mixture [Chlorinated fluorocarbon] *Asphyxiation, anesthesia, arrhythmias.*

dichlorodifluoromethane & difluoroethane mixture [Chlorinated fluorocarbon] *Asphyxiation, anesthesia, arrhythmias.*

dichlorodifluoromethane & ethylene oxide mixture [Chlorinated fluorocarbon] *Asphyxiation, anesthesia, arrhythmias.* [Ethylene oxide] *Respiratory tract irritation, pulmonary edema.*

dichlorodifluoromethane & trichlorofluoromethane mixture [Chlorinated fluorocarbon] *Asphyxiation, anesthesia, arrhythmias.*

dichlorodifluoromethane & trichlorofluoromethane & chlorodifluoromethane mixture [Chlorinated fluorocarbon] *Asphyxiation, anesthesia, arrhythmias.*

dichlorodifluoromethane & trichlorotrifluoroethane mixture [Chlorinated fluorocarbon] *Asphyxiation, anesthesia, arrhythmias.*

dichlorodimethyl ether [Ether] *Anesthesia, respiratory arrest.*

1,3-dichloro-5,5-dimethyl hydantoin [Poison] *Cardiovascular collapse, pulmonary edema, CNS depression, coma, seizures, nausea, vomiting, cardiopulmonary arrest.*

3,5-dichloro-N-(1,1-dimethyl-2-propynyl) benzamide [Lindane] *CNS stimulation, seizures, respiratory failure.*

dichlorodiphenyltrichloroethane (DDT) [DDT] *CNS disruption, respiratory control center paralysis, ventricular fibrillation, seizures, respiratory arrest.* [Lindane] *CNS stimulation, seizures, respiratory failure.*

1,1-dichloroethane; 1,2-dichloroethane [Chlorinated fluorocarbon] *Asphyxiation, anesthesia, arrhythmias.*

dichloroethyl ether [Ether] *Anesthesia, respiratory arrest.*

dichloroethylene; 1,1-dichloroethylene; 1,2-dichloroethylene [Chlorinated fluorocarbon] *Asphyxiation, anesthesia, arrhythmias.*

1,1-dichloro-1-fluoroethane [Chlorinated fluorocarbon] *Asphyxiation, anesthesia, arrhythmias.*

dichlorofluoromethane [Chlorinated fluorocarbon] *Asphyxiation, anesthesia, arrhythmias.*

dichloroisocyanuric acid; dichloroisocyanuric acid salt (n.o.s.) [Organic acid] *Pulmonary edema, circulatory collapse, laryngeal edema and spasm, severe chemical burns to skin, mucous membranes, and internal organs, GI tract perforation and hemorrhage, peritonitis.*

dichloroisopropyl ether [Ether] *Anesthesia, respiratory arrest.*

dichloromethane [Chlorinated fluorocarbon] *Asphyxiation, anesthesia, arrhythmias.*

dichloromethyl ether [Ether] *Anesthesia, respiratory arrest.*

dichloromonofluoromethane [Chlorinated fluorocarbon] *Asphyxiation, anesthesia, arrhythmias.*

dichloronitroethane; 1,1-dichloro-1-nitroethane [Chlorinated fluorocarbon] *Asphyxiation, anesthesia, arrhythmias.*

dichloropentane [Chlorinated fluorocarbon] *Asphyxiation, anesthesia, arrhythmias.*

dichlorophen; dichlorophene [Phenol] *Coma, hypotension, arrhythmias, pulmonary edema, respiratory arrest.*

2,4-dichlorophenol; 2,6-dichlorophenol [Phenol] *Coma, hypotension, arrhythmias, pulmonary edema, respiratory arrest.*

4-(2,4-dichlorophenoxy) butyric acid [Chlorophenoxy herbicide] *CNS depression, CNS stimulation,* *respiratory failure, ventricular fibrillation, seizures.*

2-(2,4-dichlorophenoxy) ethyl sulfate sodium salt (n.o.s.) [Chlorophenoxy herbicide] *CNS depression, CNS stimulation, respiratory failure, ventricular fibrillation, seizures.*

2-(2,4-dichlorophenoxy) propionic acid [Chlorophenoxy herbicide] *CNS depression, CNS stimulation, respiratory failure, ventricular fibrillation, seizures.*

2,4-dichlorophenoxyacetic acid [Chlorophenoxy herbicide] *CNS depression, CNS stimulation, respiratory failure, ventricular fibrillation, seizures.*

di-(p-chlorophenyl) methylcarbinol (DMC) [DDT] *CNS disruption, respiratory control center paralysis, ventricular fibrillation, seizures, respiratory arrest.*

dichlorophenylarsine [Arsine] *Intravascular hemolysis, pulmonary edema, cardiac and respiratory arrest, delayed-onset jaundice, and acute or delayed-onset renal failure.*

dichlorophenylisocyanate [Isocyanate/aliphatic thiocyanate] *CNS depression, respiratory arrest, respiratory paralysis, pulmonary edema, cyanide toxicity.*

dichlorophenylsilane [Silane/chlorosilane] *Respiratory tract irritation, pulmonary edema.*

dichlorophenyltrichlorosilane [Silane/chlorosilane] *Respiratory tract irritation, pulmonary edema.*

dichloropropane; 1,1-dichloropropane; 1,2-dichloropropane; 1,3-dichloropropane [Dichloropropane/dichloropropene] *Pulmonary edema, bronchospasm, alveolar hemorrhage.*

dichloropropanol; 1,3-dichloro-2-propanol [Higher alcohol (4+ carbons)] *CNS depression, respiratory failure, arrhythmias.*

dichloropropanone [Ketone] *Respiratory mucous membrane irritation, pulmonary edema, CNS depression.*

dichloropropene; 1,3-dichloropropene; 2,3-dichloropropene [Dichloropropane/dichloropropene] *Pulmonary edema, bronchospasm, alveolar hemorrhage.*

dichloropropene & propylene dichloride mixture [Dichloropropane/dichloropropene] *Pulmonary edema, bronchospasm, alveolar hemorrhage.*

dichloropropionic acid; 2,2-dichloropropionic acid [Organic acid] *Pulmonary edema, circulatory collapse, laryngeal edema and spasm, severe chemical burns to skin, mucous membranes, and internal organs, GI tract perforation and hemorrhage, peritonitis.*

1,3-dichloropropylene [Dichloropropane/dichloropropene] *Pulmonary edema, bronchospasm, alveolar hemorrhage.*

dichlorosilane [Silane/chlorosilane] *Respiratory tract irritation, pulmonary edema.*

dichlorotetrafluoroethane [Chlorinated fluorocarbon] *Asphyxiation, anesthesia, arrhythmias.*

dichlorotetrafluoroethane & dichlorodifluoromethane mixture [Chlorinated fluorocarbon] *Asphyxiation, anesthesia, arrhythmias.*

dichloro-S-triazinetrione; dichloro-S-triazinetrione salt (n.o.s.) [Irritant] *Severe immediate or delayed upper airway or respiratory tract irritation, pulmonary edema, glottic spasm, airway obstruction.*

4,5-dichloro-2-(trifluorome) benzimidazole [Aromatic hydrocarbon] *Arrhythmias, respiratory failure, pulmonary edema, paralysis, brain and kidney damage.*

3,5-dichloro-2,4,6-trifluoropyridine [Aromatic hydrocarbon] *Arrhythmias, respiratory failure, pulmonary edema, paralysis, brain and kidney damage.*

dichlorvos [Organophosphate] *Pulmonary edema, respiratory muscle paralysis, respiratory failure, bradycardia, acetylcholinesterase inhibition, hypoten-sion, pulmonary edema, overstimulation of parasympathetic nervous system, striated muscle, sympathetic ganglia, and CNS.*

dichromate salt (n.o.s.) [Poison] *Cardiovascular collapse, pulmonary edema, CNS depression, coma, seizures, nausea, vomiting, cardiopulmonary arrest.*

dicofol [Chlordane] *Respiratory failure, seizures, exhaustion, death.*

dicrotophos [Organophosphate] *Pulmonary edema, respiratory muscle paralysis, respiratory failure, bradycardia, acetylcholinesterase inhibition, hypotension, pulmonary edema, overstimulation of parasympathetic nervous system, striated muscle, sympathetic ganglia, and CNS.*

dicumyl peroxide [Organic peroxide] *Pulmonary and laryngeal edema, circulatory arrest, hypovolemic shock, chemical burns to skin, mucous membranes, and internal organs.*

dicycloheptadiene [Aliphatic hydrocarbon] *Arrhythmias, asphyxiation, anesthesia.*

dicyclohexyl peroxy-dicarbonate [Organic peroxide] *Pulmonary and laryngeal edema, circulatory arrest, hypovolemic shock, chemical burns to skin, mucous membranes, and internal organs.*

dicyclohexylamine [Dinitrophenol] *Respiratory and circulatory collapse, pulmonary edema, hyperthermia.*

dicyclohexylamine 4,6-dinitro-o-cyclohexylphenolate [Dinitrophenol] *Respiratory and circulatory collapse, pulmonary edema, hyperthermia.*

dicyclohexylamine nitrite [Nitrate/nitrite] *Methemoglobinemia, hypotension, circulatory collapse.* [Dinitrophenol] *Respiratory and circulatory collapse, pulmonary edema, hyperthermia.*

dicyclohexylammonium nitrite [Nitrate/nitrite] *Methemoglobinemia, hypotension, circulatory collapse.*

dicyclopentadiene [Aliphatic hydrocarbon] *Arrhythmias, asphyxiation, anesthesia.*

didecanoyl peroxide [Organic peroxide] *Pulmonary and laryngeal edema, circulatory arrest, hypovolemic shock, chemical burns to skin, mucous membranes, and internal organs.*

2,2-di(4,4-di-*tert*-butylperoxy cyclohexyl) propane [Organic peroxide] *Pulmonary and laryngeal edema, circulatory arrest, hypovolemic shock, chemical burns to skin, mucous membranes, and internal organs.*

di-2,4-dichlorobenzoyl peroxide [Organic peroxide] *Pulmonary and laryngeal edema, circulatory arrest, hypovolemic shock, chemical burns to skin, mucous membranes, and internal organs.*

1,2-di-(dimethylamino) ethane [Aniline] *Methemoglobinemia, hypoxia.* [Aliphatic hydrocarbon] *Arrhythmias, asphyxiation, anesthesia.*

didymium nitrate [Nitrate/nitrite] *Methemoglobinemia, hypotension, circulatory collapse.*

dieldrin [Aldrin/dieldrin/endrin] *Seizures, respiratory failure.*

dienochlor [Chlordane] *Respiratory failure, seizures, exhaustion, death.*

diepoxybutane [Ethylene oxide] *Respiratory tract irritation, pulmonary edema.*

diesel fuel; diesel oil [Hydrocarbon mixture] *CNS depression, respiratory arrest, seizures, arrhythmias, pulmonary edema.*

diesel fuel oil & ammonium nitrate (ANFO) mixture [Explosive] *Multiple trauma, highly toxic chemical exposure.* [Nitrate/nitrite] *Methemoglobinemia, hypotension, circulatory collapse.*

diethanolamine [Organic base/amine] *Pulmonary edema, cardiac depression, seizures.*

diethoxyethane [Ether] *Anesthesia, respiratory arrest.*

diethoxymentane [Ether] *Anesthesia, respiratory arrest.*

2,5-diethoxy-4-morpholinebenzenediazonium zinc chloride [Poison] *Cardiovascular collapse, pulmonary edema, CNS depression, coma, seizures, nausea, vomiting, cardiopulmonary arrest.*

diethoxypropene [Acrolein] *Severe respiratory tract irritation, pulmonary edema, respiratory failure.*

diethyl aniline [Aniline] *Methemoglobinemia, hypoxia.*

diethyl carbonate [Ester] *CNS depression, respiratory tract irritation, bronchitis, pneumonitis.*

diethyl cellosolve [Ethylene glycol] *Respiratory failure, pulmonary edema, paralysis, cardiovascular collapse, severe acidosis.*

diethyl chlorophosphate [Organophosphate] *Pulmonary edema, respiratory muscle paralysis, respiratory failure, bradycardia, acetylcholinesterase inhibition, hypotension, pulmonary edema, overstimulation of parasympathetic nervous system, striated muscle, sympathetic ganglia, and CNS.*

diethyl 2-chlorovinyl phosphate [Organophosphate] *Pulmonary edema, respiratory muscle paralysis, respiratory failure, bradycardia, acetylcholinesterase inhibition, hypotension, pulmonary edema, overstimulation of parasympathetic nervous system, striated muscle, sympathetic ganglia, and CNS.*

diethyl dichlorosilane [Silane/chlorosilane] *Respiratory tract irritation, pulmonary edema.*

diethyl ether [Ether] *Anesthesia, respiratory arrest.*

diethyl isopropylthiomethyl dithiophosphate [Organophosphate] *Pulmonary edema, respiratory muscle paralysis, respiratory failure, bradycardia, acetylcholinesterase inhibition, hypotension, pulmonary edema, overstimulation of parasympathetic nervous system, striated muscle, sympathetic ganglia, and CNS.*

diethyl ketone [Ketone] *Respiratory mucous membrane irritation, pulmonary edema, CNS depression.*

diethyl peroxydicarbonate [Organic peroxide] *Pulmonary and laryngeal edema, circulatory arrest, hypovolemic*

HazMat

shock, chemical burns to skin, mucous membranes, and internal organs.

diethyl phthalate [Ester] *CNS depression, respiratory tract irritation, bronchitis, pneumonitis.*

diethyl propylmethylpyrimidyl thiophosphate [Organophosphate] *Pulmonary edema, respiratory muscle paralysis, respiratory failure, bradycardia, acetylcholinesterase inhibition, hypotension, pulmonary edema, overstimulation of parasympathetic nervous system, striated muscle, sympathetic ganglia, and CNS.*

diethyl sulfate [Sulfur] *Respiratory tract irritation, pulmonary edema, anaphylaxis.*

diethyl sulfide [Sulfur] *Respiratory tract irritation, pulmonary edema, anaphylaxis.*

diethylamine [Organic base/amine] *Pulmonary edema, cardiac depression, seizures.*

diethylaminoethanol [Organic base/amine] *Pulmonary edema, cardiac depression, seizures.*

diethylaminopropylamine [Organic base/amine] *Pulmonary edema, cardiac depression, seizures.*

diethylarsine [Arsine] *Intravascular hemolysis, pulmonary edema, cardiac and respiratory arrest, delayed-onset jaundice, and acute or delayed-onset renal failure.*

diethylbenzene [Aromatic hydrocarbon] *Arrhythmias, respiratory failure, pulmonary edema, paralysis, brain and kidney damage.*

diethylcarbamazine citrate [Poison] *Cardiovascular collapse, pulmonary edema, CNS depression, coma, seizures, nausea, vomiting, cardiopulmonary arrest.*

diethylene glycol [Ethylene glycol] *Respiratory failure, pulmonary edema, paralysis, cardiovascular collapse, severe acidosis.*

diethylene glycol abietate [Ethylene glycol] *Respiratory failure, pulmonary edema, paralysis, cardiovascular collapse, severe acidosis.*

diethylene glycol diester; diethylene glycol monoester [Ethylene glycol] *Respiratory failure, pulmonary edema, paralysis, cardiovascular collapse, severe acidosis.*

diethylene triamine [Organic base/amine] *Pulmonary edema, cardiac depression, seizures.*

diethylethylene diamine [Organic base/amine] *Pulmonary edema, cardiac depression, seizures.*

di-(2-ethylhexyl) peroxy-dicarbonate [Organic peroxide] *Pulmonary and laryngeal edema, circulatory arrest, hypovolemic shock, chemical burns to skin, mucous membranes, and internal organs.*

di-(2-ethylhexyl) phosphoric acid [Organic acid] *Pulmonary edema, circulatory collapse, laryngeal edema and spasm, severe chemical burns to skin, mucous membranes, and internal organs, GI tract perforation and hemorrhage, peritonitis.*

di-(2-ethylhexyl) phthalate [Ester] *CNS depression, respiratory tract irritation, bronchitis, pneumonitis.*

diethylmagnesium [Magnesium] *Cardiovascular collapse, respiratory depression.*

diethyl-*p*-nitrophenyl phosphate [Organophosphate] *Pulmonary edema, respiratory muscle paralysis, respiratory failure, bradycardia, acetylcholinesterase inhibition, hypotension, pulmonary edema, overstimulation of parasympathetic nervous system, striated muscle, sympathetic ganglia, and CNS.*

O,O-diethyl-O-pyrazinyl phosphorothioate [Organophosphate] *Pulmonary edema, respiratory muscle paralysis, respiratory failure, bradycardia, acetylcholinesterase inhibition, hypotension, pulmonary edema, overstimulation of parasympathetic nervous system, striated muscle, sympathetic ganglia, and CNS.*

diethylstilbestrol [Poison] *Cardiovascular collapse, pulmonary edema, CNS depression, coma, seizures, nausea, vomiting, cardiopulmonary arrest.*

diethylthiophosphoryl chloride [Organophosphate] *Pulmonary edema, respiratory muscle paralysis, respiratory failure, bradycardia, acetylcholinesterase inhibition, hypotension, pulmonary edema, overstimulation of parasympathetic nervous system, striated muscle, sympathetic ganglia, and CNS.*

diethylzinc [Zinc] *Respiratory tract irritation, metal fume fever, pulmonary edema.*

difluorochloroethane [Chlorinated fluorocarbon] *Asphyxiation, anesthesia, arrhythmias.*

difluoroethane [Chlorinated fluorocarbon] *Asphyxiation, anesthesia, arrhythmias.*

difluoroethane & dichlorodifluoromethane mixture [Chlorinated fluorocarbon] *Asphyxiation, anesthesia, arrhythmias.*

difluoroethylene; 1,1-difluoroethylene [Chlorinated fluorocarbon] *Asphyxiation, anesthesia, arrhythmias.*

difluoromonochloroethane [Chlorinated fluorocarbon] *Asphyxiation, anesthesia, arrhythmias.*

difluorophosphoric acid [Inorganic acid] *Pulmonary edema, bronchospasm, circulatory collapse, laryngeal spasm and edema, severe chemical burns to skin, mucous membranes, and internal organs, GI tract perforation and hemorrhage, peritonitis.*

digitoxin [Poison] *Cardiovascular collapse, pulmonary edema, CNS depression, coma, seizures, nausea, vomiting, cardiopulmonary arrest.*

diglycidyl ether [Ether] *Anesthesia, respiratory arrest.*

digoxin [Poison] *Cardiovascular collapse, pulmonary edema, CNS depression, coma, seizures, nausea, vomiting, cardiopulmonary arrest.*

2,2-dihydroperoxy propane [Organic peroxide] *Pulmonary and laryngeal edema, circulatory arrest, hypovolemic shock, chemical burns to skin, mucous membranes, and internal organs.*

dihydropyran [Aromatic hydrocarbon] *Arrhythmias, respiratory failure, pulmonary edema, paralysis, brain and kidney damage.*

dihydrorotenone [Rotenone] *Respiratory arrest, asphyxia.*

dihydrosafrole [Phenol] *Coma, hypotension, arrhythmias, pulmonary edema, respiratory arrest.*

di-(1-hydroxycyclohexyl) peroxide [Organic peroxide] *Pulmonary and laryngeal edema, circulatory arrest, hypovolemic shock, chemical burns to skin, mucous membranes, and internal organs.*

2,6-diiodo-4-nitrophenol [Dinitrophenol] *Respiratory and circulatory collapse, pulmonary edema, hyperthermia.*

diisobutyl carbinol [Higher alcohol (4+ carbons)] *CNS depression, respiratory failure, arrhythmias.*

diisobutyl ketone [Ketone] *Respiratory mucous membrane irritation, pulmonary edema, CNS depression.*

diisobutylamine [Organic base/amine] *Pulmonary edema, cardiac depression, seizures.*

diisobutylene [Aliphatic hydrocarbon] *Arrhythmias, asphyxiation, anesthesia.*

diisobutyryl peroxide [Organic peroxide] *Pulmonary and laryngeal edema, circulatory arrest, hypovolemic shock, chemical burns to skin, mucous membranes, and internal organs.*

diisooctyl acid phosphate [Organic acid] *Pulmonary edema, circulatory collapse, laryngeal edema and spasm, severe chemical burns to skin, mucous membranes, and internal organs, GI tract perforation and hemorrhage, peritonitis.*

diisopropyl ether [Ether] *Anesthesia, respiratory arrest.*

diisopropyl fluorophosphate [Organophosphate] *Pulmonary edema, respiratory muscle paralysis, respiratory failure, bradycardia, acetylcholinesterase inhibition, hypotension, pulmonary edema, overstimulation of parasympa-*

HazMat

thetic nervous system, striated muscle, sympathetic ganglia, and CNS.

diisopropyl peroxydicarbonate [Organic peroxide] *Pulmonary and laryngeal edema, circulatory arrest, hypovolemic shock, chemical burns to skin, mucous membranes, and internal organs.*

diisopropylamine [Organic base/amine] *Pulmonary edema, cardiac depression, seizures.*

diisopropylbenzene hydroperoxide [Organic peroxide] *Pulmonary and laryngeal edema, circulatory arrest, hypovolemic shock, chemical burns to skin, mucous membranes, and internal organs.*

diisopropylethanolamine [Organic base/amine] *Pulmonary edema, cardiac depression, seizures.*

diisotridecylperoxydicarbonate [Organic peroxide] *Pulmonary and laryngeal edema, circulatory arrest, hypovolemic shock, chemical burns to skin, mucous membranes, and internal organs.*

diketene [Ketone] *Respiratory mucous membrane irritation, pulmonary edema, CNS depression.*

Dilan [DDT] *CNS disruption, respiratory control center paralysis, ventricular fibrillation, seizures, respiratory arrest.*

dilauroyl peroxide [Organic peroxide] *Pulmonary and laryngeal edema, circulatory arrest, hypovolemic shock, chemical burns to skin, mucous membranes, and internal organs.*

dimefox [Organophosphate] *Pulmonary edema, respiratory muscle paralysis, respiratory failure, bradycardia, acetylcholinesterase inhibition, hypotension, pulmonary edema, overstimulation of parasympathetic nervous system, striated muscle, sympathetic ganglia, and CNS.*

di-1-*p*-menthene [Turpentine/terpene] *Respiratory failure, pulmonary edema, tachycardia.*

Dimetan [Carbamate] *Acetylcholinesterase inhibition (reversible), bradycardia, hypotension, respiratory muscle paralysis, respiratory arrest, pulmonary edema.*

dimethoate [Organophosphate] *Pulmonary edema, respiratory muscle paralysis, respiratory failure, bradycardia, acetylcholinesterase inhibition, hypotension, pulmonary edema, overstimulation of parasympathetic nervous system, striated muscle, sympathetic ganglia, and CNS.*

3,3′-dimethoxybenzidine [Aniline] *Methemoglobinemia, hypoxia.*

dimethoxyethane; 1,1-dimethoxyethane; 1,2-dimethoxyethane [Ethylene glycol] *Respiratory failure, pulmonary edema, paralysis, cardiovascular collapse, severe acidosis.*

dimethrin [Pyrethrin/pyrethroid] *Respiratory paralysis, convulsions.*

α-dimethyl benzene ethanamine; alpha-dimethyl benzene ethanamine [Aniline] *Methemoglobinemia, hypoxia.*

dimethyl carbonate [Ester] *CNS depression, respiratory tract irritation, bronchitis, pneumonitis.*

dimethyl chlorothiophosphate [Organophosphate] *Pulmonary edema, respiratory muscle paralysis, respiratory failure, bradycardia, acetylcholinesterase inhibition, hypotension, pulmonary edema, overstimulation of parasympathetic nervous system, striated muscle, sympathetic ganglia, and CNS.*

dimethyl ether [Ether] *Anesthesia, respiratory arrest.*

dimethyl phosphorochloridothioate [Organophosphate] *Pulmonary edema, respiratory muscle paralysis, respiratory failure, bradycardia, acetylcholinesterase inhibition, hypotension, pulmonary edema, overstimulation of parasympathetic nervous system, striated muscle, sympathetic ganglia, and CNS.*

dimethyl phthalate [Ester] *CNS depression, respiratory tract irritation, bronchitis, pneumonitis.*

dimethyl sulfate [Sulfur] *Respiratory tract irritation, pulmonary edema, anaphylaxis.*

dimethyl sulfide [Sulfur] *Respiratory tract irritation, pulmonary edema, anaphylaxis.*

dimethyl thiophosphoryl chloride [Organophosphate] *Pulmonary edema, respiratory muscle paralysis, respiratory failure, bradycardia, acetylcholinesterase inhibition, hypotension, pulmonary edema, overstimulation of parasympathetic nervous system, striated muscle, sympathetic ganglia, and CNS.*

dimethylamine [Organic base/amine] *Pulmonary edema, cardiac depression, seizures.*

dimethylaminoacetonitrile [Cyanide] *Impairment of cellular oxygenation and adenosine triphosphate production, hypoxia, death.*

dimethylaminoazobenzene; 4-dimethylaminoazobenzene [Aniline] *Methemoglobinemia, hypoxia.*

4-dimethylamino-6-(2-di-methylaminoethoxy)toluene-2-diazonium zinc chloride [Zinc] *Respiratory tract irritation, metal fume fever, pulmonary edema.*

dimethylaminoethanol [Organic base/amine] *Pulmonary edema, cardiac depression, seizures.*

dimethylaminoethyl methacrylate [Ester] *CNS depression, respiratory tract irritation, bronchitis, pneumonitis.*

dimethylaniline; N,N-dimethylaniline [Aniline] *Methemoglobinemia, hypoxia.*

7,12-dimethylbenz[a]anthracene [Aromatic hydrocarbon] *Arrhythmias, respiratory failure, pulmonary edema, paralysis, brain and kidney damage.*

3,3'-dimethylbenzidine [Aniline] *Methemoglobinemia, hypoxia.*

di-(2-methylbenzoyl) peroxide [Organic peroxide] *Pulmonary and laryngeal edema, circulatory arrest, hypovolemic shock, chemical burns to skin, mucous membranes, and internal organs.*

dimethylbutane [Aliphatic hydrocarbon] *Arrhythmias, asphyxiation, anesthesia.*

dimethylbutylamine; 1,3-dimethylbutylamine [Organic base/amine] *Pulmonary edema, cardiac depression, seizures.*

dimethylcarbamoyl chloride [Poison] *Cardiovascular collapse, pulmonary edema, CNS depression, coma, seizures, nausea, vomiting, cardiopulmonary arrest.*

dimethylcyclohexane [Aliphatic hydrocarbon] *Arrhythmias, asphyxiation, anesthesia.*

2,3-dimethylcyclohexylamine [Poison] *Cardiovascular collapse, pulmonary edema, CNS depression, coma, seizures, nausea, vomiting, cardiopulmonary arrest.* [Organic base/amine] *Pulmonary edema, cardiac depression, seizures.*

2,5-dimethyl-2,5-di-(benzoylperoxy) hexane [Organic peroxide] *Pulmonary and laryngeal edema, circulatory arrest, hypovolemic shock, chemical burns to skin, mucous membranes, and internal organs.*

2,5-dimethyl-2,5-di(tert-butylperoxy) hexane [Organic peroxide] *Pulmonary and laryngeal edema, circulatory arrest, hypovolemic shock, chemical burns to skin, mucous membranes, and internal organs.*

2,5-dimethyl-2,5-di(tert-butylperoxy) hexyne-3 [Organic peroxide] *Pulmonary and laryngeal edema, circulatory arrest, hypovolemic shock, chemical burns to skin, mucous membranes, and internal organs.*

dimethyldichlorosilane [Silane/chlorosilane] *Respiratory tract irritation, pulmonary edema.*

dimethyldiethoxysilane [Silane/chlorosilane] *Respiratory tract irritation, pulmonary edema.*

2,5-dimethyl-2,5-di(2-ethyl-hexanoylperoxy) hexane [Organic peroxide] *Pulmonary and laryngeal edema, circulatory arrest, hypovolemic shock, chemical burns to skin, mucous membranes, and internal organs.*

2,5-dimethyl-2,5-dihydroperoxy hexane [Organic peroxide] *Pulmo-*

nary and laryngeal edema, circulatory arrest, hypovolemic shock, chemical burns to skin, mucous membranes, and internal organs.

3,5-dimethyl-3,5-dihydroxydioxolane-1,2 [Ethylene glycol] *Respiratory failure, pulmonary edema, paralysis, cardiovascular collapse, severe acidosis.*

2,5-dimethyl-2,5-di(iso-nonanopyl-peroxy) hexane [Organic peroxide] *Pulmonary and laryngeal edema, circulatory arrest, hypovolemic shock, chemical burns to skin, mucous membranes, and internal organs.*

dimethyldioxane [Dioxane] *Pulmonary irritation, respiratory failure, pulmonary edema, CNS depression.*

dimethyldisulfide [Sulfur] *Respiratory tract irritation, pulmonary edema, anaphylaxis.*

2,5-dimethyl-2,5-di(3,5,5-trimethyl-hexanoylperoxy) hexane [Organic peroxide] *Pulmonary and laryngeal edema, circulatory arrest, hypovolemic shock, chemical burns to skin, mucous membranes, and internal organs.*

dimethylethanolamine [Organic base/amine] *Pulmonary edema, cardiac depression, seizures.*

dimethylformamide [Poison] *Cardiovascular collapse, pulmonary edema, CNS depression, coma, seizures, nausea, vomiting, cardiopulmonary arrest.*

N,N-dimethylformamide [Poison] *Cardiovascular collapse, pulmonary edema, CNS depression, coma, seizures, nausea, vomiting, cardiopulmonary arrest.* [Organic acid] *Pulmonary edema, circulatory collapse, laryngeal edema and spasm, severe chemical burns to skin, mucous membranes, and internal organs, GI tract perforation and hemorrhage, peritonitis.*

dimethylhydrazine; 1,1-dimethylhydrazine [Hydrazine] *Seizures, hemolysis of red blood cells, pulmonary edema.*

dimethylmagnesium [Magnesium] *Cardiovascular collapse, respiratory depression.*

dimethyl-p-nitrosoaniline [Aniline] *Methemoglobinemia, hypoxia.*

2,4-dimethylphenol [Phenol] *Coma, hypotension, arrhythmias, pulmonary edema, respiratory arrest.*

dimethyl-p-phenylenediamine [Organic base/amine] *Pulmonary edema, cardiac depression, seizures.*

dimethylpropane [Aliphatic hydrocarbon] *Arrhythmias, asphyxiation, anesthesia.*

dimethyl-propylamine [Organic base/amine] *Pulmonary edema, cardiac depression, seizures.*

dimethylzinc [Zinc] *Respiratory tract irritation, metal fume fever, pulmonary edema.*

dimetilan [Carbamate] *Acetylcholinesterase inhibition (reversible), bradycardia, hypotension, respiratory muscle paralysis, respiratory arrest, pulmonary edema.*

dimyristyl peroxy-dicarbonate [Organic peroxide] *Pulmonary and laryngeal edema, circulatory arrest, hypovolemic shock, chemical burns to skin, mucous membranes, and internal organs.*

4,6-dinitro-o-amylphenol [Dinitrophenol] *Respiratory and circulatory collapse, pulmonary edema, hyperthermia.*

dinitroaniline [Aniline] *Methemoglobinemia, hypoxia.*

dinitrobenzene (n.o.s.) [Aniline] *Methemoglobinemia, hypoxia.*

dinitrochlorobenzene [Aniline] *Methemoglobinemia, hypoxia.*

dinitro-o-cresol; 4,6-dinitro-o-cresol [Phenol] *Coma, hypotension, arrhythmias, pulmonary edema, respiratory arrest.*

4,6-dinitro-o-cresol salt (n.o.s.) [Phenol] *Coma, hypotension, arrhythmias, pulmonary edema, respiratory arrest.*

dinitrocyclohexylphenol; 4,6 dinitro-o-cyclohexylphenol [Dinitrophenol] *Respiratory and circulatory collapse, pulmonary edema, hyperthermia.*

dinitrogen tetroxide [Nitrogen oxide] *Lower respiratory tract symptoms, pulmonary edema, laryngospasm, bronchospasm, asphyxiation.*

dinitrogen tetroxide & nitric oxide mixture [Nitrogen oxide] *Lower respiratory tract symptoms, pulmonary edema, laryngospasm, bronchospasm, asphyxiation.*

dinitrophenol; 2,4-dinitrophenol; 2,5-dinitrophenol; 2,6-dinitrophenol [Dinitrophenol] *Respiratory and circulatory collapse, pulmonary edema, hyperthermia.*

dinitrophenolate [Dinitrophenol] *Respiratory and circulatory collapse, pulmonary edema, hyperthermia.*

dinitroresorcinol [Dinitrophenol] *Respiratory and circulatory collapse, pulmonary edema, hyperthermia.*

dinitroso-dimethyl terephthalamide [Poison] *Cardiovascular collapse, pulmonary edema, CNS depression, coma, seizures, nausea, vomiting, cardiopulmonary arrest.*

dinitrosopentamethylene tetramine [Organic base/amine] *Pulmonary edema, cardiac depression, seizures.*

dinitrotoluene; 2,4-dinitrotoluene; 2,6-dinitrotoluene; 3,4-dinitrotoluene [Aniline] *Methemoglobinemia, hypoxia.*

dinocap [Dinitrophenol] *Respiratory and circulatory collapse, pulmonary edema, hyperthermia.*

dinonanoyl peroxide [Organic peroxide] *Pulmonary and laryngeal edema, circulatory arrest, hypovolemic shock, chemical burns to skin, mucous membranes, and internal organs.*

dinoseb [Dinitrophenol] *Respiratory and circulatory collapse, pulmonary edema, hyperthermia.*

dinoterb [Dinitrophenol] *Respiratory and circulatory collapse, pulmonary edema, hyperthermia.*

dioctanoyl peroxide [Organic peroxide] *Pulmonary and laryngeal edema, circulatory arrest, hypovolemic shock, chemical burns to skin, mucous membranes, and internal organs.*

dioctyl phthalate [Ester] *CNS depression, respiratory tract irritation, bronchitis, pneumonitis.*

n-dioctylphthalate [Ester] *CNS depression, respiratory tract irritation, bronchitis, pneumonitis.*

dioxacarb [Carbamate] *Acetylcholinesterase inhibition (reversible), bradycardia, hypotension, respiratory muscle paralysis, respiratory arrest, pulmonary edema.*

dioxane; 1,4-dioxane [Dioxane] *Pulmonary irritation, respiratory failure, pulmonary edema, CNS depression.*

dioxathion [Organophosphate] *Pulmonary edema, respiratory muscle paralysis, respiratory failure, bradycardia, acetylcholinesterase inhibition, hypotension, pulmonary edema, overstimulation of parasympathetic nervous system, striated muscle, sympathetic ganglia, and CNS.*

dioxolane [Ethylene glycol] *Respiratory failure, pulmonary edema, paralysis, cardiovascular collapse, severe acidosis.*

dipentene [Turpentine/terpene] *Respiratory failure, pulmonary edema, tachycardia.*

diperoxy azelaic acid [Organic peroxide] *Pulmonary and laryngeal edema, circulatory arrest, hypovolemic shock, chemical burns to skin, mucous membranes, and internal organs.*

diperoxydodecane diacid & sodium sulfate mixture [Organic peroxide] *Pulmonary and laryngeal edema, circulatory arrest, hypovolemic shock, chemical burns to skin, mucous membranes, and internal organs.* [Sulfur] *Respiratory tract irritation, pulmonary edema, anaphylaxis.*

diphacinone [Warfarin/hydroxycoumarin/indanedione] *Anticoagulation effect, internal hemorrhage.*

diphenadione [Warfarin/hydroxycoumarin/indanedione] *Anticoagulation effect, internal hemorrhage.*

di-(2-phenoxyethyl) peroxydicarbonate [Organic peroxide] *Pulmonary and laryngeal edema, circulatory arrest, hypovolemic shock, chemical burns to skin, mucous membranes, and internal organs.*

HazMat

diphenyl dichlorosilane [Silane/ chlorosilane] *Respiratory tract irritation, pulmonary edema.*

diphenylamine [Aniline] *Methemoglobinemia, hypoxia.*

diphenylaminechloroarsine [Arsenic] *Heavy metal toxicity, vomiting, GI bleeding, CNS depression, pulmonary edema, cardiac arrest.*

diphenylchloroarsine [Arsine] *Intravascular hemolysis, pulmonary edema, cardiac and respiratory arrest, delayed-onset jaundice, and acute or delayed-onset renal failure.*

1,2-diphenylhydrazine [Hydrazine] *Seizures, hemolysis of red blood cells, pulmonary edema.*

diphenylmethane-4,4'-diisocyanate (MDI) [Isocyanate/aliphatic thiocyanate] *CNS depression, respiratory arrest, respiratory paralysis, pulmonary edema, cyanide toxicity.*

diphenylmethyl bromide [Bromine/ methyl bromide] *Severe respiratory irritation, pulmonary edema, respiratory failure, coma, convulsions, death.*

diphenyloxide-4,4'-disulfohydrazide [Hydrazine] *Seizures, hemolysis of red blood cells, pulmonary edema.*

diphosphoramide, octamethyl [Organophosphate] *Pulmonary edema, respiratory muscle paralysis, respiratory failure, bradycardia, acetylcholinesterase inhibition, hypotension, pulmonary edema, overstimulation of parasympathetic nervous system, striated muscle, sympathetic ganglia, and CNS.*

dipicryl sulfide [Nitrate/nitrite] *Methemoglobinemia, hypotension, circulatory collapse.*

dipropionyl peroxide [Organic peroxide] *Pulmonary and laryngeal edema, circulatory arrest, hypovolemic shock, chemical burns to skin, mucous membranes, and internal organs.*

dipropyl ether [Ether] *Anesthesia, respiratory arrest.*

dipropyl ketone [Ketone] *Respiratory mucous membrane irritation, pulmonary edema, CNS depression.*

dipropyl peroxy-dicarbonate [Organic peroxide] *Pulmonary and laryngeal edema, circulatory arrest, hypovolemic shock, chemical burns to skin, mucous membranes, and internal organs.*

dipropylamine [Organic base/amine] *Pulmonary edema, cardiac depression, seizures.*

4-dipropylaminobenzene-diazonium zinc chloride [Zinc] *Respiratory tract irritation, metal fume fever, pulmonary edema.*

dipropylene glycol [Ethylene glycol] *Respiratory failure, pulmonary edema, paralysis, cardiovascular collapse, severe acidosis.*

dipropylene triamine [Organic base/ amine] *Pulmonary edema, cardiac depression, seizures.*

dipropylnitrosamine [Nitrate/nitrite] *Methemoglobinemia, hypotension, circulatory collapse.*

diquat [Paraquat] *Pulmonary edema, cardiac damage, circulatory collapse, cerebral hemorrhage or infarcts, death. (Defoliant used in warfare.)*

diquat dibromide [Paraquat] *Pulmonary edema, cardiac damage, circulatory collapse, cerebral hemorrhage or infarcts, death. (Defoliant used in warfare.)* [Bromine/methyl bromide] *Severe respiratory irritation, pulmonary edema, respiratory failure, coma, convulsions, death.*

disinfectant, corrosive (n.o.s.) [Corrosive] *Upper airway burns and edema, circulatory collapse, severe chemical burns to skin, toxic systemic effects, GI tract perforation and hemorrhage, peritonitis.*

disinfectant, poisonous (n.o.s.) [Poison] *Cardiovascular collapse, pulmonary edema, CNS depression, coma, seizures, nausea, vomiting, cardiopulmonary arrest.*

disodium methanearsonate [Arsenic] *Heavy metal toxicity, vomiting, GI bleeding, CNS depression, pulmonary edema, cardiac arrest.*

dispersant gas (n.o.s.) [Nonflammable gas] *Pulmonary edema, respiratory failure, asphyxiation.*

dispersant gas, flammable (n.o.s.) [Flammable gas] *Respiratory failure, cardiac arrest, arrhythmias.*

distearyl peroxy-dicarbonate [Organic peroxide] *Pulmonary and laryngeal edema, circulatory arrest, hypovolemic shock, chemical burns to skin, mucous membranes, and internal organs.*

disuccinic acid peroxide [Organic peroxide] *Pulmonary and laryngeal edema, circulatory arrest, hypovolemic shock, chemical burns to skin, mucous membranes, and internal organs.*

disulfoton [Organophosphate] *Pulmonary edema, respiratory muscle paralysis, respiratory failure, bradycardia, acetylcholinesterase inhibition, hypotension, pulmonary edema, overstimulation of parasympathetic nervous system, striated muscle, sympathetic ganglia, and CNS.*

dithiazanine iodide [Poison] *Cardiovascular collapse, pulmonary edema, CNS depression, coma, seizures, nausea, vomiting, cardiopulmonary arrest.*

dithiobiuret [Sulfur] *Respiratory tract irritation, pulmonary edema, anaphylaxis.*

dithiocarbamate pesticide (n.o.s.) [Dithiocarbamate] *Hypotension, respiratory failure.*

di(3,5,5-trimethyl-1,2-dioxolanul-3) peroxide [Organic peroxide] *Pulmonary and laryngeal edema, circulatory arrest, hypovolemic shock, chemical burns to skin, mucous membranes, and internal organs.*

di(3,5,5-trimethylhexanoyl) peroxide [Organic peroxide] *Pulmonary and laryngeal edema, circulatory arrest, hypovolemic shock, chemical burns to skin, mucous membranes, and internal organs.*

diuron [Poison] *Cardiovascular collapse, pulmonary edema, CNS depression, coma, seizures, nausea, vomiting, cardiopulmonary arrest.*

divinyl ether [Ether] *Anesthesia, respiratory arrest.*

DMC (di-(p-chlorophenyl) methylcarbinol) [DDT] *CNS disruption, respiratory control center paralysis, ventricular fibrillation, seizures, respiratory arrest.*

dodecyl trichlorosilane [Silane/chlorosilane] *Respiratory tract irritation, pulmonary edema.*

dodecylbenzene-sulfonic acid [Organic acid] *Pulmonary edema, circulatory collapse, laryngeal edema and spasm, severe chemical burns to skin, mucous membranes, and internal organs, GI tract perforation and hemorrhage, peritonitis.*

Donovan solution [Arsenic] *Heavy metal toxicity, vomiting, GI bleeding, CNS depression, pulmonary edema, cardiac arrest.* [Mercury] *Circulatory collapse, arrhythmias, respiratory failure, pulmonary edema, neurotoxic effects.*

Dowicide (n.o.s.) [Phenol] *Coma, hypotension, arrhythmias, pulmonary edema, respiratory arrest.*

drier, paint and varnish (n.o.s.) [Poison] *Cardiovascular collapse, pulmonary edema, CNS depression, coma, seizures, nausea, vomiting, cardiopulmonary arrest.*

drug (n.o.s.) [Poison] *Cardiovascular collapse, pulmonary edema, CNS depression, coma, seizures, nausea, vomiting, cardiopulmonary arrest.*

Dry Ice [Simple asphyxiant] *Asphyxiation.*

dye, corrosive (n.o.s.) [Corrosive] *Upper airway burns and edema, circulatory collapse, severe chemical burns to skin, toxic systemic effects, GI tract perforation and hemorrhage, peritonitis.*

dye, poisonous (n.o.s.) [Poison] *Cardiovascular collapse, pulmonary edema, CNS depression, coma, seizures, nausea, vomiting, cardiopulmonary arrest.*

EDE [Carbon tetrachloride] *CNS depression, respiratory arrest, circulatory collapse.*

HazMat

EDTA (ethylenediamine tetraacetic acid) [Organic base/amine] *Pulmonary edema, cardiac depression, seizures.*

electrolyte, acid [Inorganic acid] *Pulmonary edema, bronchospasm, circulatory collapse, laryngeal spasm and edema, severe chemical burns to skin, mucous membranes, and internal organs, GI tract perforation and hemorrhage, peritonitis.*

electrolyte, alkaline [Inorganic base/alkaline corrosive] *Upper airway burns and edema, pulmonary edema, skin burns, circulatory collapse, GI tract perforation and hemorrhage, peritonitis.*

electrolyte, battery fluid acid [Poison] *Cardiovascular collapse, pulmonary edema, CNS depression, coma, seizures, nausea, vomiting, cardiopulmonary arrest.* [Corrosive] *Upper airway burns and edema, circulatory collapse, severe chemical burns to skin, toxic systemic effects, GI tract perforation and hemorrhage, peritonitis.*

emetine dihydrochloride [Poison] *Cardiovascular collapse, pulmonary edema, CNS depression, coma, seizures, nausea, vomiting, cardiopulmonary arrest.*

EMMI [Mercury] *Circulatory collapse, arrhythmias, respiratory failure, pulmonary edema, neurotoxic effects.*

enamel [Poison] *Cardiovascular collapse, pulmonary edema, CNS depression, coma, seizures, nausea, vomiting, cardiopulmonary arrest.* [Hydrocarbon mixture] *CNS depression, respiratory arrest, seizures, arrhythmias, pulmonary edema.*

endosulfan; α-endosulfan (alpha-endosulfan); β-endosulfan (beta-endosulfan) [Aldrin/dieldrin/endrin] *Seizures, respiratory failure.*

endosulfan sulfate [Aldrin/dieldrin/endrin] *Seizures, respiratory failure.*

endothal; endothall [Dithiocarbamate] *Hypotension, respiratory failure.*

endothion [Organophosphate] *Pulmonary edema, respiratory muscle paralysis, respiratory failure, bradycardia, acetylcholinesterase inhibition, hypotension, pulmonary edema, overstimulation of parasympathetic nervous system, striated muscle, sympathetic ganglia, and CNS.*

endrin aldehyde [Aldrin/dieldrin/endrin] *Seizures, respiratory failure.*

endrin mixture (n.o.s.) [Aldrin/dieldrin/endrin] *Seizures, respiratory failure.*

engine-starting fluid [Hydrocarbon mixture] *CNS depression, respiratory arrest, seizures, arrhythmias, pulmonary edema.*

enviromentally hazardous substance (n.o.s.) [Poison] *Cardiovascular collapse, pulmonary edema, CNS depression, coma, seizures, nausea, vomiting, cardiopulmonary arrest.*

epibromohydrin [Dichloropropane/dichloropropene] *Pulmonary edema, bronchospasm, alveolar hemorrhage.*

epichlorohydrin [Dichloropropane/dichloropropene] *Pulmonary edema, bronchospasm, alveolar hemorrhage.*

epinephrine [Poison] *Cardiovascular collapse, pulmonary edema, CNS depression, coma, seizures, nausea, vomiting, cardiopulmonary arrest.*

EPN [Organophosphate] *Pulmonary edema, respiratory muscle paralysis, respiratory failure, bradycardia, acetylcholinesterase inhibition, hypotension, pulmonary edema, overstimulation of parasympathetic nervous system, striated muscle, sympathetic ganglia, and CNS.*

epoxyethane [Ethylene oxide] *Respiratory tract irritation, pulmonary edema.*

epoxyethoxypropane; 1,2-epoxy-3-ethoxypropane [Ether] *Anesthesia, respiratory arrest.*

1,2-epoxy-3-ethyloxypropane [Ether] *Anesthesia, respiratory arrest.*

EPTC [Dithiocarbamate] *Hypotension, respiratory failure.*

eradicator, paint and grease [Flammable/combustible liquid] *CNS depression, respiratory arrest, convulsions, arrhythmias, pulmonary edema.*

erbon [Chlorophenoxy herbicide] *CNS depression, CNS stimulation,* respiratory failure, ventricular fibrillation, seizures.

ergocalciferol [Poison] *Cardiovascular collapse, pulmonary edema, CNS depression, coma, seizures, nausea, vomiting, cardiopulmonary arrest.*

ergotamine tartrate [Poison] *Cardiovascular collapse, pulmonary edema, CNS depression, coma, seizures, nausea, vomiting, cardiopulmonary arrest.*

ET-15 [Organophosphate] *Pulmonary edema, respiratory muscle paralysis, respiratory failure, bradycardia, acetylcholinesterase inhibition, hypotension, pulmonary edema, overstimulation of parasympathetic nervous system, striated muscle, sympathetic ganglia, and CNS.*

etching acid [Inorganic acid] *Pulmonary edema, bronchospasm, circulatory collapse, laryngeal spasm and edema, severe chemical burns to skin, mucous membranes, and internal organs, GI tract perforation and hemorrhage, peritonitis.* [Hydrofluoric acid] *Pulmonary and laryngeal edema, circulatory collapse, severe skin burns, GI tract perforation, systemic fluoride poisoning.*

ethane (gas or cryogenic liquid) [Aliphatic hydrocarbon] *Arrhythmias, asphyxiation, anesthesia.*

ethane, chlorinated [Halogenated aliphatic hydrocarbon] *CNS depression, respiratory arrest, circulatory collapse.*

ethane & propane mixture (cryogenic liquid) [Aliphatic hydrocarbon] *Arrhythmias, asphyxiation, anesthesia.*

ethanesulfonyl chloride [Halogenated aliphatic hydrocarbon] *CNS depression, respiratory arrest, circulatory collapse.*

ethanol; ethanol mixture (n.o.s.) [Lower alcohol (1–3 carbons)] *CNS depression, coma, respiratory arrest, arrhythmias.*

ethanolamine; ethanolamine mixture (n.o.s.) [Organic base/amine] *Pulmonary edema, cardiac depression, seizures.*

ether [Ether] *Anesthesia, respiratory arrest.*

ethiofencarb [Carbamate] *Acetylcholinesterase inhibition (reversible), bradycardia, hypotension, respiratory muscle paralysis, respiratory arrest, pulmonary edema.*

ethion [Organophosphate] *Pulmonary edema, respiratory muscle paralysis, respiratory failure, bradycardia, acetylcholinesterase inhibition, hypotension, pulmonary edema, overstimulation of parasympathetic nervous system, striated muscle, sympathetic ganglia, and CNS.*

ethoxyethanol; 2-ethoxyethanol [Ethylene glycol] *Respiratory failure, pulmonary edema, paralysis, cardiovascular collapse, severe acidosis.*

ethoxyethyl acetate; 2-ethoxyethyl acetate [Ethylene glycol] *Respiratory failure, pulmonary edema, paralysis, cardiovascular collapse, severe acidosis.*

ethoxypropane [Ether] *Anesthesia, respiratory arrest.*

ethyl acetate [Ester] *CNS depression, respiratory tract irritation, bronchitis, pneumonitis.*

ethyl acetylene [Aliphatic hydrocarbon] *Arrhythmias, asphyxiation, anesthesia.* [Simple asphyxiant] *Asphyxiation.*

ethyl acrylate [Ester] *CNS depression, respiratory tract irritation, bronchitis, pneumonitis.*

ethyl alcohol [Lower alcohol (1–3 carbons)] *CNS depression, coma, respiratory arrest, arrhythmias.*

ethyl aluminum dichloride [Poison] *Cardiovascular collapse, pulmonary edema, CNS depression, coma, seizures, nausea, vomiting, cardiopulmonary arrest.*

ethyl aluminum sesquichloride [Poison] *Cardiovascular collapse, pulmonary edema, CNS depression, coma, seizures, nausea, vomiting, cardiopulmonary arrest.*

ethyl amyl ketone [Ketone] *Respiratory mucous membrane irritation, pulmonary edema, CNS depression.*

ethyl biscoumacetate [Warfarin/ hydroxycoumarin/indanedione] *Anticoagulation effect, internal hemorrhage.*

ethyl borate [Boron] *Respiratory tract irritation, laryngeal spasm and edema, pulmonary edema, severe chemical burns.*

ethyl bromide [Bromine/methyl bromide] *Severe respiratory irritation, pulmonary edema, respiratory failure, coma, convulsions, death.*

ethyl bromoacetate [Bromate] *CNS and respiratory system depression, delayed-onset renal failure.*

ethyl butyl ether [Ether] *Anesthesia, respiratory arrest.*

ethyl butyraldehyde [Aldehyde] *Seizures, respiratory failure, pulmonary edema.*

ethyl butyrate [Ester] *CNS depression, respiratory tract irritation, bronchitis, pneumonitis.*

ethyl chloride [Halogenated aliphatic hydrocarbon] *CNS depression, respiratory arrest, circulatory collapse.*

ethyl chloroacetate [Ester] *CNS depression, respiratory tract irritation, bronchitis, pneumonitis.*

ethyl chloroformate [Ester] *CNS depression, respiratory tract irritation, bronchitis, pneumonitis.*

ethyl chloropropionate [Ester] *CNS depression, respiratory tract irritation, bronchitis, pneumonitis.*

ethyl chlorothioformate [Ester] *CNS depression, respiratory tract irritation, bronchitis, pneumonitis.*

ethyl crotonate [Ester] *CNS depression, respiratory tract irritation, bronchitis, pneumonitis.*

ethyl cyanoacetate [Ester] *CNS depression, respiratory tract irritation, bronchitis, pneumonitis.*

ethyl 3,3-di(*tert*-butylperoxy) butyrate [Organic peroxide] *Pulmonary and laryngeal edema, circulatory arrest, hypovolemic shock, chemical burns to skin, mucous membranes, and internal organs.*

ethyl dichloroarsine [Arsine] *Intravascular hemolysis, pulmonary edema, cardiac and respiratory arrest, delayed-onset jaundice, and acute or delayed-onset renal failure.*

O-ethyl S,S-dipropyl phosphorodithioate [Organophosphate] *Pulmonary edema, respiratory muscle paralysis, respiratory failure, bradycardia, acetylcholinesterase inhibition, hypotension, pulmonary edema, overstimulation of parasympathetic nervous system, striated muscle, sympathetic ganglia, and CNS.*

ethyl ether [Ether] *Anesthesia, respiratory arrest.*

ethyl ether & methyl magnesium bromide mixture [Ether] *Anesthesia, respiratory arrest.* [Bromine/ methyl bromide] *Severe respiratory irritation, pulmonary edema, respiratory failure, coma, convulsions, death.*

ethyl fluid [Aliphatic hydrocarbon] *Arrhythmias, asphyxiation, anesthesia.*

ethyl fluoride [Chlorinated fluorocarbon] *Asphyxiation, anesthesia, arrhythmias.*

ethyl formate [Ester] *CNS depression, respiratory tract irritation, bronchitis, pneumonitis.*

ethyl hexaldehyde; 2-ethyl hexaldehyde [Aldehyde] *Seizures, respiratory failure, pulmonary edema.*

ethyl hexylamine [Organic base/ amine] *Pulmonary edema, cardiac depression, seizures.*

ethyl hexylchloroformate [Ester] *CNS depression, respiratory tract irritation, bronchitis, pneumonitis.*

ethyl isobutyrate [Ester] *CNS depression, respiratory tract irritation, bronchitis, pneumonitis.*

ethyl isocyanate [Isocyanate/aliphatic thiocyanate] *CNS depression, respiratory arrest, respiratory paralysis, pulmonary edema, cyanide toxicity.*

ethyl lactate [Ester] *CNS depression, respiratory tract irritation, bronchitis, pneumonitis.*

ethyl mercaptan [Sulfur] *Respiratory tract irritation, pulmonary edema, anaphylaxis.*

ethyl mercuric chloride [Mercury] *Circulatory collapse, arrhythmias, respiratory failure, pulmonary edema, neurotoxic effects.*

ethyl mercuri-2,3-dihydroxypropylmercaptide [Mercury] *Circulatory collapse, arrhythmias, respiratory failure, pulmonary edema, neurotoxic effects.*

N-ethyl mercuri-p-toluene sulfonanilide [Mercury] *Circulatory collapse, arrhythmias, respiratory failure, pulmonary edema, neurotoxic effects.*

ethyl mercury phosphate [Mercury] *Circulatory collapse, arrhythmias, respiratory failure, pulmonary edema, neurotoxic effects.*

ethyl methacrylate [Ester] *CNS depression, respiratory tract irritation, bronchitis, pneumonitis.*

ethyl methyl ether [Ether] *Anesthesia, respiratory arrest.*

ethyl methyl ketone [Ketone] *Respiratory mucous membrane irritation, pulmonary edema, CNS depression.*

ethyl methyl ketone peroxide [Organic peroxide] *Pulmonary and laryngeal edema, circulatory arrest, hypovolemic shock, chemical burns to skin, mucous membranes, and internal organs.* [Ketone] *Respiratory mucous membrane irritation, pulmonary edema, CNS depression.* [Corrosive] *Upper airway burns and edema, circulatory collapse, severe chemical burns to skin, toxic systemic effects, GI tract perforation and hemorrhage, peritonitis.*

ethyl nitrate; ethyl nitrate mixture (n.o.s.) [Nitrate/nitrite] *Methemoglobinemia, hypotension, circulatory collapse.*

ethyl orthoformate [Ester] *CNS depression, respiratory tract irritation, bronchitis, pneumonitis.*

ethyl oxalate [Oxalate] *Cardiovascular collapse, arrhythmias, seizures.*

ethyl phenyl dichlorosilane [Silane/chlorosilane] *Respiratory tract irritation, pulmonary edema.*

ethyl phosphonous dichloride [Phosphorus] *Hypovolemic shock, severe tissue burns, severe respiratory irritation, pulmonary edema, respiratory arrest, arrhythmias, sudden death.*

ethyl phosphorodichloridate [Corrosive] *Upper airway burns and edema, circulatory collapse, severe chemical burns to skin, toxic systemic effects, GI tract perforation and hemorrhage, peritonitis.*

ethyl piperidine [Organic base/amine] *Pulmonary edema, cardiac depression, seizures.*

ethyl propionate [Ester] *CNS depression, respiratory tract irritation, bronchitis, pneumonitis.*

ethyl propyl ether [Ether] *Anesthesia, respiratory arrest.*

ethyl silicate [Silane/chlorosilane] *Respiratory tract irritation, pulmonary edema.*

ethyl sulfate [Organic acid] *Pulmonary edema, circulatory collapse, laryngeal edema and spasm, severe chemical burns to skin, mucous membranes, and internal organs, GI tract perforation and hemorrhage, peritonitis.*

ethyl sulfuric acid [Organic acid] *Pulmonary edema, circulatory collapse, laryngeal edema and spasm, severe chemical burns to skin, mucous membranes, and internal organs, GI tract perforation and hemorrhage, peritonitis.*

ethyl toluidine [Aniline] *Methemoglobinemia, hypoxia.*

ethylamine; ethylamine mixture (n.o.s.) [Organic base/amine] *Pulmonary edema, cardiac depression, seizures.*

ethylaniline; 2-ethylaniline; N-ethylaniline [Aniline] *Methemoglobinemia, hypoxia.*

ethylbenzene [Aromatic hydrocarbon] *Arrhythmias, respiratory failure, pulmonary edema, paralysis, brain and kidney damage.*

HazMat

ethylbenzyl toluidine [Aniline] *Methemoglobinemia, hypoxia.*

ethylbenzylaniline [Aniline] *Methemoglobinemia, hypoxia.*

ethylbutanol [Higher alcohol (4+ carbons)] *CNS depression, respiratory failure, arrhythmias.*

ethylbutyl acetate [Ester] *CNS depression, respiratory tract irritation, bronchitis, pneumonitis.*

ethyldichlorosilane [Silane/chlorosilane] *Respiratory tract irritation, pulmonary edema.*

ethylene (gas or cryogenic liquid) [Aliphatic hydrocarbon] *Arrhythmias, asphyxiation, anesthesia.* [Simple asphyxiant] *Asphyxiation.*

ethylene & acetylene & propylene mixture (cryogenic liquid) [Aliphatic hydrocarbon] *Arrhythmias, asphyxiation, anesthesia.* [Simple asphyxiant] *Asphyxiation.*

ethylene chlorohydrin [Carbon tetrachloride] *CNS depression, respiratory arrest, circulatory collapse.* [Dichloropropane/dichloropropene] *Pulmonary edema, bronchospasm, alveolar hemorrhage.*

ethylene dibromide [Bromine/methyl bromide] *Severe respiratory irritation, pulmonary edema, respiratory failure, coma, convulsions, death.*

ethylene dibromide & methyl bromide mixture [Bromine/methyl bromide] *Severe respiratory irritation, pulmonary edema, respiratory failure, coma, convulsions, death.*

ethylene dichloride [Halogenated aliphatic hydrocarbon] *CNS depression, respiratory arrest, circulatory collapse.*

ethylene fluorohydrin [Monofluoroacetate] *Ventricular arrhythmias, seizures.*

ethylene glycol [Ethylene glycol] *Respiratory failure, pulmonary edema, paralysis, cardiovascular collapse, severe acidosis.*

ethylene glycol alkyl ester; ethylene glycol aryl ester [Ethylene glycol] *Respiratory failure, pulmonary edema, paralysis, cardiovascular collapse, severe acidosis.*

ethylene glycol diethyl ether [Ethylene glycol] *Respiratory failure, pulmonary edema, paralysis, cardiovascular collapse, severe acidosis.*

ethylene glycol dinitrate [Nitrate/nitrite] *Methemoglobinemia, hypotension, circulatory collapse.*

ethylene glycol monobutyl ether [Ethylene glycol] *Respiratory failure, pulmonary edema, paralysis, cardiovascular collapse, severe acidosis.*

ethylene glycol monoethyl ether [Ethylene glycol] *Respiratory failure, pulmonary edema, paralysis, cardiovascular collapse, severe acidosis.*

ethylene glycol monoethyl ether acetate [Ethylene glycol] *Respiratory failure, pulmonary edema, paralysis, cardiovascular collapse, severe acidosis.*

ethylene glycol monomethyl ether [Ethylene glycol] *Respiratory failure, pulmonary edema, paralysis, cardiovascular collapse, severe acidosis.*

ethylene glycol monomethyl ether & acetate mixture [Ethylene glycol] *Respiratory failure, pulmonary edema, paralysis, cardiovascular collapse, severe acidosis.*

ethylene oxide (ETO) [Ethylene oxide] *Respiratory tract irritation, pulmonary edema.*

ethylene oxide & carbon dioxide mixture [Ethylene oxide] *Respiratory tract irritation, pulmonary edema.* [Simple asphyxiant] *Asphyxiation.*

ethylene oxide & dichlorodifluoromethane mixture [Chlorinated fluorocarbon] *Asphyxiation, anesthesia, arrhythmias.* [Ethylene oxide] *Respiratory tract irritation, pulmonary edema.*

ethylene oxide & propylene oxide mixture [Ethylene oxide] *Respiratory tract irritation, pulmonary edema.*

ethylenediamine [Organic base/amine] *Pulmonary edema, cardiac depression, seizures.*

ethylenediamine & lithium acetylide mixture [Lithium] *Chem-*

ical burns to respiratory tract, pulmonary edema.

ethylenediamine tetraacetic acid (EDTA) [Organic base/amine] *Pulmonary edema, cardiac depression, seizures.*

ethyleneimine [Organic base/amine] *Pulmonary edema, cardiac depression, seizures.*

2-ethylhexyl alcohol [Higher alcohol (4+ carbons)] *CNS depression, respiratory failure, arrhythmias.*

DL-(2-ethylhexyl) phosphoric acid [Organic acid] *Pulmonary edema, circulatory collapse, laryngeal edema and spasm, severe chemical burns to skin, mucous membranes, and internal organs, GI tract perforation and hemorrhage, peritonitis.*

ethylphosphonothioic dichloride [Corrosive] *Upper airway burns and edema, circulatory collapse, severe chemical burns to skin, toxic systemic effects, GI tract perforation and hemorrhage, peritonitis.*

2-ethyl-3-propyl acrolein [Acrolein] *Severe respiratory tract irritation, pulmonary edema, respiratory failure.*

ethyltrichlorosilane [Silane/chlorosilane] *Respiratory tract irritation, pulmonary edema.*

etiologic agent (n.o.s.) *No acute symptoms during incubation period. Physiologic response varies depending on strain of microorganism or toxin.*

ETO (ethylene oxide) [Ethylene oxide] *Respiratory tract irritation, pulmonary edema.*

eucalyptol [Camphor] *Status epilepticus, respiratory failure.*

eugenol [Phenol] *Coma, hypotension, arrhythmias, pulmonary edema, respiratory arrest.*

explosive A, B, or C [Explosive] *Multiple trauma, highly toxic chemical exposure.*

extract, aromatic (n.o.s.) [Aromatic hydrocarbon] *Arrhythmias, respiratory failure, pulmonary edema, paralysis, brain and kidney damage.*

extract, flavoring (n.o.s.) [Flammable/combustible liquid] *CNS depression, respiratory arrest, convulsions, arrhythmias, pulmonary edema.*

fabric, animal or vegetable with oil (n.o.s.) [Flammable/combustible liquid] *CNS depression, respiratory arrest, convulsions, arrhythmias, pulmonary edema.*

Fenac [Chlorophenoxy herbicide] *CNS depression, CNS stimulation, respiratory failure, ventricular fibrillation, seizures.*

fenamiphos [Organophosphate] *Pulmonary edema, respiratory muscle paralysis, respiratory failure, bradycardia, acetylcholinesterase inhibition, hypotension, pulmonary edema, overstimulation of parasympathetic nervous system, striated muscle, sympathetic ganglia, and CNS.*

fenitrothion [Organophosphate] *Pulmonary edema, respiratory muscle paralysis, respiratory failure, bradycardia, acetylcholinesterase inhibition, hypotension, pulmonary edema, overstimulation of parasympathetic nervous system, striated muscle, sympathetic ganglia, and CNS.*

fensulfothion [Organophosphate] *Pulmonary edema, respiratory muscle paralysis, respiratory failure, bradycardia, acetylcholinesterase inhibition, hypotension, pulmonary edema, overstimulation of parasympathetic nervous system, striated muscle, sympathetic ganglia, and CNS.*

fenthion [Organophosphate] *Pulmonary edema, respiratory muscle paralysis, respiratory failure, bradycardia, acetylcholinesterase inhibition, hypotension, pulmonary edema, overstimulation of parasympathetic nervous system, striated muscle, sympathetic ganglia, and CNS.*

fenvalerate [Pyrethrin/pyrethroid] *Respiratory paralysis, convulsions.*

ferbam [Dithiocarbamate] *Hypotension, respiratory failure.*

HazMat

ferric ammonium citrate [Iron] *Hypovolemic shock.*

ferric arsenate; ferrous arsenate [Arsenic] *Heavy metal toxicity, vomiting, GI bleeding, CNS depression, pulmonary edema, cardiac arrest.* [Iron] *Hypovolemic shock.*

ferric arsenite [Arsenic] *Heavy metal toxicity, vomiting, GI bleeding, CNS depression, pulmonary edema, cardiac arrest.* [Iron] *Hypovolemic shock.*

ferric chloride; ferrous chloride; iron chloride [Iron] *Hypovolemic shock.*

ferric cyanide [Cyanide] *Impairment of cellular oxygenation and adenosine triphosphate production, hypoxia, death.*

ferric fluoride [Iron] *Hypovolemic shock.* [Fluorine] *CNS depression, respiratory arrest, cardiovascular collapse, shock, arrhythmias.*

ferric nitrate [Nitrate/nitrite] *Methemoglobinemia, hypotension, circulatory collapse.* [Iron] *Hypovolemic shock.*

ferric salt (n.o.s.); ferrous salt (n.o.s.) [Iron] *Hypovolemic shock.*

ferric subsulfate [Iron] *Hypovolemic shock.*

ferric sulfate; ferrous sulfate [Iron] *Hypovolemic shock.*

ferrocerium [Iron] *Hypovolemic shock.*

ferrocholinate [Iron] *Hypovolemic shock.*

ferrosilicon [Iron] *Hypovolemic shock.*

ferrous arsenate; ferric arsenate [Arsenic] *Heavy metal toxicity, vomiting, GI bleeding, CNS depression, pulmonary edema, cardiac arrest.* [Iron] *Hypovolemic shock.*

ferrous chloride; ferric chloride; iron chloride [Iron] *Hypovolemic shock.*

ferrous metal; ferrous salt (n.o.s.); ferric salt (n.o.s.) [Iron] *Hypovolemic shock.*

ferrous sulfate; ferric sulfate [Iron] *Hypovolemic shock.*

fertilizer, ammoniating [Ammonia] *Pulmonary edema, hypotension.* [Nitrate/nitrite] *Methemoglobinemia, hypotension, circulatory collapse.*

fiber, animal or vegetable, burnt (n.o.s.) [Irritant] *Severe immediate or delayed upper airway or respiratory tract irritation, pulmonary edema, glottic spasm, airway obstruction.*

fiber, animal or vegetable, with oil (n.o.s.) [Flammable/combustible liquid] *CNS depression, respiratory arrest, convulsions, arrhythmias, pulmonary edema.*

film, motion picture, nitrocellulose based [Flammable solid] *Shock, severe chemical and thermal burns, severe respiratory tract irritation, pulmonary edema, respiratory arrest, ECG changes, sudden death.*

fire extinguisher with compressed or liquefied gas [Simple asphyxiant] *Asphyxiation.*

fire extinguisher with corrosive liquid charge [Corrosive] *Upper airway burns and edema, circulatory collapse, severe chemical burns to skin, toxic systemic effects, GI tract perforation and hemorrhage, peritonitis.*

fire lighter, solid with flammable liquid [Aliphatic hydrocarbon] *Arrhythmias, asphyxiation, anesthesia.*

fish meal and scrap [Irritant] *Severe immediate or delayed upper airway or respiratory tract irritation, pulmonary edema, glottic spasm, airway obstruction.*

flammable gas (n.o.s.) [Flammable gas] *Respiratory failure, cardiac arrest, arrhythmias.*

flammable gas in cigarette lighter [Aliphatic hydrocarbon] *Arrhythmias, asphyxiation, anesthesia.*

flammable liquid (n.o.s.) [Flammable/combustible liquid] *CNS depression, respiratory arrest, convulsions, arrhythmias, pulmonary edema.*

flammable liquid, corrosive (n.o.s.) [Flammable/combustible liquid] *CNS depression, respiratory arrest, convulsions, arrhythmias, pulmonary edema.* [Corrosive] *Upper airway burns and edema, circulatory collapse, severe chemical burns to skin, toxic systemic effects, GI tract perforation and hemorrhage, peritonitis.*

flammable liquid, poisonous (n.o.s.) [Flammable/combustible liquid] *CNS depression, respiratory arrest, convulsions, arrhythmias, pulmonary edema.* [Poison] *Cardiovascular collapse, pulmonary edema, CNS depression, coma, seizures, nausea, vomiting, cardiopulmonary arrest.*

flammable solid (n.o.s.) [Flammable solid] *Shock, severe chemical and thermal burns, severe respiratory tract irritation, pulmonary edema, respiratory arrest, ECG changes, sudden death.*

flammable solid, corrosive (n.o.s.) [Flammable solid] *Shock, severe chemical and thermal burns, severe respiratory tract irritation, pulmonary edema, respiratory arrest, ECG changes, sudden death.* [Corrosive] *Upper airway burns and edema, circulatory collapse, severe chemical burns to skin, toxic systemic effects, GI tract perforation and hemorrhage, peritonitis.*

flammable solid, oxidizing (n.o.s.) [Flammable solid] *Shock, severe chemical and thermal burns, severe respiratory tract irritation, pulmonary edema, respiratory arrest, ECG changes, sudden death.* [Oxidizer] *Pulmonary and laryngeal edema, circulatory arrest, hypovolemic shock, chemical burns of skin, mucous membranes, and internal organs.*

flammable solid, poisonous (n.o.s.) [Flammable solid] *Shock, severe chemical and thermal burns, severe respiratory tract irritation, pulmonary edema, respiratory arrest, ECG changes, sudden death.* [Poison] *Cardiovascular collapse, pulmonary edema, CNS depression, coma, seizures, nausea, vomiting, cardiopulmonary arrest.*

flavoring extract (n.o.s.) [Flammable/combustible liquid] *CNS depression, respiratory arrest, convulsions, arrhythmias, pulmonary edema.*

flue dust, poisonous [Poison] *Cardiovascular collapse, pulmonary edema,* *CNS depression, coma, seizures, nausea, vomiting, cardiopulmonary arrest.*

fluoboric acid [Hydrofluoric acid] *Pulmonary and laryngeal edema, circulatory collapse, severe skin burns, GI tract perforation, systemic fluoride poisoning.* [Boron] *Respiratory tract irritation, laryngeal spasm and edema, pulmonary edema, severe chemical burns.*

fluoric acid [Hydrofluoric acid] *Pulmonary and laryngeal edema, circulatory collapse, severe skin burns, GI tract perforation, systemic fluoride poisoning.*

fluoride (n.o.s.) [Fluorine] *CNS depression, respiratory arrest, cardiovascular collapse, shock, arrhythmias.*

fluorine (gas or cryogenic liquid) [Fluorine] *CNS depression, respiratory arrest, cardiovascular collapse, shock, arrhythmias.*

fluoroacetamide [Monofluoroacetate] *Ventricular arrhythmias, seizures.*

fluoroacetate; fluroacetate-1080 [Monofluoroacetate] *Ventricular arrhythmias, seizures.*

fluoroacetic acid [Monofluoroacetate] *Ventricular arrhythmias, seizures.*

fluoroaniline [Aniline] *Methemoglobinemia, hypoxia.*

fluorobenzene [Benzene] *Arrhythmias, respiratory failure, pulmonary edema, CNS depression, liver and kidney damage.*

fluorophosphoric acid [Inorganic acid] *Pulmonary edema, bronchospasm, circulatory collapse, laryngeal spasm and edema, severe chemical burns to skin, mucous membranes, and internal organs, GI tract perforation and hemorrhage, peritonitis.*

fluorosilicate (n.o.s.) [Fluorine] *CNS depression, respiratory arrest, cardiovascular collapse, shock, arrhythmias.*

fluorosulfonic acid [Inorganic acid] *Pulmonary edema, bronchospasm, circulatory collapse, laryngeal spasm and edema, severe chemical burns to skin, mucous membranes, and internal organs, GI tract perforation and hemorrhage, peritonitis.*

HazMat

fluorotoluene [Aromatic hydrocarbon] *Arrhythmias, respiratory failure, pulmonary edema, paralysis, brain and kidney damage.*

fluosilicate salt (n.o.s.) [Fluorine] *CNS depression, respiratory arrest, cardiovascular collapse, shock, arrhythmias.*

fluosilicic acid [Hydrofluoric acid] *Pulmonary and laryngeal edema, circulatory collapse, severe skin burns, GI tract perforation, systemic fluoride poisoning.*

formaldehyde solution (formalin) [Aldehyde] *Seizures, respiratory failure, pulmonary edema.*

formetanate [Carbamate] *Acetylcholinesterase inhibition (reversible), bradycardia, hypotension, respiratory muscle paralysis, respiratory arrest, pulmonary edema.*

formic acid [Organic acid] *Pulmonary edema, circulatory collapse, laryngeal edema and spasm, severe chemical burns to skin, mucous membranes, and internal organs, GI tract perforation and hemorrhage, peritonitis.*

Fowler solution [Arsenic] *Heavy metal toxicity, vomiting, GI bleeding, CNS depression, pulmonary edema, cardiac arrest.*

Freon (all types) [Chlorinated fluorocarbon] *Asphyxiation, anesthesia, arrhythmias.*

fuel, aviation [Hydrocarbon mixture] *CNS depression, respiratory arrest, seizures, arrhythmias, pulmonary edema.*

fuel, pyrophoric (n.o.s.) [Flammable/combustible liquid] *CNS depression, respiratory arrest, convulsions, arrhythmias, pulmonary edema.*

fuel oil [Hydrocarbon mixture] *CNS depression, respiratory arrest, seizures, arrhythmias, pulmonary edema.*

fuel oil & ammonium nitrate (ANFO) mixture [Explosive] *Multiple trauma, highly toxic chemical exposure.* [Nitrate/nitrite] *Methemoglobinemia, hypotension, circulatory collapse.*

fumaric acid [Organic acid] *Pulmonary edema, circulatory collapse, laryngeal edema and spasm, severe chemical burns to skin, mucous membranes, and internal organs, GI tract perforation and hemorrhage, peritonitis.*

fumaryl chloride [Organic acid] *Pulmonary edema, circulatory collapse, laryngeal edema and spasm, severe chemical burns to skin, mucous membranes, and internal organs, GI tract perforation and hemorrhage, peritonitis.*

fumigant (n.o.s.) [Poison] *Cardiovascular collapse, pulmonary edema, CNS depression, coma, seizures, nausea, vomiting, cardiopulmonary arrest.*

fungicide, corrosive (n.o.s.) [Poison] *Cardiovascular collapse, pulmonary edema, CNS depression, coma, seizures, nausea, vomiting, cardiopulmonary arrest.* [Corrosive] *Upper airway burns and edema, circulatory collapse, severe chemical burns to skin, toxic systemic effects, GI tract perforation and hemorrhage, peritonitis.*

fungicide, poisonous (n.o.s.) [Poison] *Cardiovascular collapse, pulmonary edema, CNS depression, coma, seizures, nausea, vomiting, cardiopulmonary arrest.*

furan [Aliphatic hydrocarbon] *Arrhythmias, asphyxiation, anesthesia.*

furfural [Aldehyde] *Seizures, respiratory failure, pulmonary edema.*

furfuryl alcohol [Higher alcohol (4+ carbons)] *CNS depression, respiratory failure, arrhythmias.*

furfurylamine [Organic base/amine] *Pulmonary edema, cardiac depression, seizures.*

fusel oil [Higher alcohol (4+ carbons)] *CNS depression, respiratory failure, arrhythmias.*

gallic acid [Organic acid] *Pulmonary edema, circulatory collapse, laryngeal edema and spasm, severe chemical burns to skin, mucous membranes, and internal organs, GI tract perforation and hemorrhage, peritonitis.*

gallium [Poison] *Cardiovascular collapse, pulmonary edema, CNS depression, coma, seizures, nausea, vomiting, cardiopulmonary arrest.*

gas, liquefied [see: liquefied gas (various types)]

gas drip, hydrocarbon [Hydrocarbon mixture] *CNS depression, respiratory arrest, seizures, arrhythmias, pulmonary edema.*

gas oil [Hydrocarbon mixture] *CNS depression, respiratory arrest, seizures, arrhythmias, pulmonary edema.*

gasoline; gasohol [Hydrocarbon mixture] *CNS depression, respiratory arrest, seizures, arrhythmias, pulmonary edema.*

germane; germanium hydride [Arsine] *Intravascular hemolysis, pulmonary edema, cardiac and respiratory arrest, delayed-onset jaundice, and acute or delayed-onset renal failure.*

glifonox [Glyphosate] *Hypotension, arrhythmias, pulmonary edema.*

glutaraldehyde [Aldehyde] *Seizures, respiratory failure, pulmonary edema.*

glycerol-α-mono-chlorohydrin [Dichloropropane/dichloropropene] *Pulmonary edema, bronchospasm, alveolar hemorrhage.*

glyceryl trinitrate [Explosive] *Multiple trauma, highly toxic chemical exposure.* [Nitrate/nitrite] *Methemoglobinemia, hypotension, circulatory collapse.*

glycidaldehyde [Aldehyde] *Seizures, respiratory failure, pulmonary edema.*

glycofurol [Ethylene glycol] *Respiratory failure, pulmonary edema, paralysis, cardiovascular collapse, severe acidosis.*

glycolic acid [Organic acid] *Pulmonary edema, circulatory collapse, laryngeal edema and spasm, severe chemical burns to skin, mucous membranes, and internal organs, GI tract perforation and hemorrhage, peritonitis.*

glyphosate [Glyphosate] *Hypotension, arrhythmias, pulmonary edema.*

glyphosate isopropylamine salt (n.o.s.); glyphosate mono(isopropylamine) salt (n.o.s.) [Glyphosate] *Hypotension, arrhythmias, pulmonary edema.*

gold bronze powder [Copper] *Respiratory tract irritation, respiratory arrest, hemorrhagic gastritis.*

grease eradicator [Flammable/combustible liquid] *CNS depression, respiratory arrest, convulsions, arrhythmias, pulmonary edema.*

grenade, poisonous gas [Poison] *Cardiovascular collapse, pulmonary edema, CNS depression, coma, seizures, nausea, vomiting, cardiopulmonary arrest.*

grenade, tear gas [Irritant] *Severe immediate or delayed upper airway or respiratory tract irritation, pulmonary edema, glottic spasm, airway obstruction.*

guaiacol [Phenol] *Coma, hypotension, arrhythmias, pulmonary edema, respiratory arrest.*

guanidine nitrate [Organic base/amine] *Pulmonary edema, cardiac depression, seizures.*

Guthion (azinphos-methyl) [Organophosphate] *Pulmonary edema, respiratory muscle paralysis, respiratory failure, bradycardia, acetylcholinesterase inhibition, hypotension, pulmonary edema, overstimulation of parasympathetic nervous system, striated muscle, sympathetic ganglia, and CNS.*

gutta-percha [Turpentine/terpene] *Respiratory failure, pulmonary edema, tachycardia.*

hafnium; hafnium mixture (n.o.s.) [Flammable solid] *Shock, severe chemical and thermal burns, severe respiratory tract irritation, pulmonary edema, respiratory arrest, ECG changes, sudden death.*

halogenated solvent (n.o.s.) [Halogenated aliphatic hydrocarbon] *CNS depression, respiratory arrest, circulatory collapse.*

Halon (all types) [Chlorinated fluorocarbon] *Asphyxiation, anesthesia, arrhythmias.*

hay [Flammable solid] *Shock, severe chemical and thermal burns, severe respiratory tract irritation, pulmonary* *edema, respiratory arrest, ECG changes, sudden death.*

hazardous waste (n.o.s.) [Poison] *Cardiovascular collapse, pulmonary edema, CNS depression, coma, seizures, nausea, vomiting, cardiopulmonary arrest.*

helium (gas or cryogenic liquid) [Simple asphyxiant] *Asphyxiation.*

helium & oxygen mixture [Simple asphyxiant] *Asphyxiation.*

hendecane [Hydrocarbon mixture] *CNS depression, respiratory arrest, seizures, arrhythmias, pulmonary edema.*

heptachlor [Chlordane] *Respiratory failure, seizures, exhaustion, death.*

heptachlor epoxide [Chlordane] *Respiratory failure, seizures, exhaustion, death.*

n-heptaldehyde [Aldehyde] *Seizures, respiratory failure, pulmonary edema.*

heptane; n-heptane [Aliphatic hydrocarbon] *Arrhythmias, asphyxiation, anesthesia.* ▢ heptene

heptene [Aliphatic hydrocarbon] *Arrhythmias, asphyxiation, anesthesia.* ▢ heptane

hexachloroacetone [Ketone] *Respiratory mucous membrane irritation, pulmonary edema, CNS depression.*

hexachlorobenzene [Lindane] *CNS stimulation, seizures, respiratory failure.*

hexachlorobutadiene; hexachloro-1,3-butadiene [Halogenated aliphatic hydrocarbon] *CNS depression, respiratory arrest, circulatory collapse.*

hexachlorocyclohexane [Lindane] *CNS stimulation, seizures, respiratory failure.*

hexachlorocyclopentadiene [Halogenated aliphatic hydrocarbon] *CNS depression, respiratory arrest, circulatory collapse.*

hexachloro-epoxy-octahydro-dimethanonaphthalene [Aldrin/dieldrin/endrin] *Seizures, respiratory failure.*

hexachloroethane [Halogenated aliphatic hydrocarbon] *CNS depression, respiratory arrest, circulatory collapse.*

hexachloronaphthalene [Naphthalene] *Delayed-onset acute intravascular hemolysis.*

hexachlorophene [Halogenated aliphatic hydrocarbon] *CNS depression, respiratory arrest, circulatory collapse.* [Phenol] *Coma, hypotension, arrhythmias, pulmonary edema, respiratory arrest.*

hexachloropropene [Halogenated aliphatic hydrocarbon] *CNS depression, respiratory arrest, circulatory collapse.*

hexadecyl alcohol [Higher alcohol (4+ carbons)] *CNS depression, respiratory failure, arrhythmias.*

hexadecyl trichlorosilane [Silane/chlorosilane] *Respiratory tract irritation, pulmonary edema.*

hexadiene [Aliphatic hydrocarbon] *Arrhythmias, asphyxiation, anesthesia.*

hexaethyl tetraphosphate; hexaethyl tetraphosphate mixture (n.o.s.) [Organophosphate] *Pulmonary edema, respiratory muscle paralysis, respiratory failure, bradycardia, acetylcholinesterase inhibition, hypotension, pulmonary edema, overstimulation of parasympathetic nervous system, striated muscle, sympathetic ganglia, and CNS.*

hexafluoroacetone [Ketone] *Respiratory mucous membrane irritation, pulmonary edema, CNS depression.*

hexafluoroacetone hydrate [Ketone] *Respiratory mucous membrane irritation, pulmonary edema, CNS depression.*

hexafluoroethane [Halogenated aliphatic hydrocarbon] *CNS depression, respiratory arrest, circulatory collapse.*

hexafluorophosphoric acid [Inorganic acid] *Pulmonary edema, bronchospasm, circulatory collapse, laryngeal spasm and edema, severe chemical burns to skin, mucous membranes, and internal organs, GI tract perforation and hemorrhage, peritonitis.*

hexafluoropropylene [Halogenated aliphatic hydrocarbon] *CNS depression, respiratory arrest, circulatory collapse.*

hexafluoropropylene oxide [Halogenated aliphatic hydrocarbon] *CNS depression, respiratory arrest, circulatory collapse.* [Ether] *Anesthesia, respiratory arrest.*

hexahydrocresol [Phenol] *Coma, hypotension, arrhythmias, pulmonary edema, respiratory arrest.*

hexaldehyde [Aldehyde] *Seizures, respiratory failure, pulmonary edema.*

hexamethylene diamine [Organic base/amine] *Pulmonary edema, cardiac depression, seizures.*

hexamethylene diisocyanate [Isocyanate/aliphatic thiocyanate] *CNS depression, respiratory arrest, respiratory paralysis, pulmonary edema, cyanide toxicity.*

hexamethyleneimine [Organic base/amine] *Pulmonary edema, cardiac depression, seizures.*

hexamethylenetetramine [Organic base/amine] *Pulmonary edema, cardiac depression, seizures.*

hexamethylphosphoramide [Aliphatic hydrocarbon] *Arrhythmias, asphyxiation, anesthesia.*

3,3,6,6,9,9-hexamethyl-1,2,4,5-tetraoxocyclononane [Organic peroxide] *Pulmonary and laryngeal edema, circulatory arrest, hypovolemic shock, chemical burns to skin, mucous membranes, and internal organs.*

hexamine [Organic base/amine] *Pulmonary edema, cardiac depression, seizures.*

hexane; n-hexane [Aliphatic hydrocarbon] *Arrhythmias, asphyxiation, anesthesia.* ⑨ hexene

1,2,6-hexanetriol [Higher alcohol (4+ carbons)] *CNS depression, respiratory failure, arrhythmias.*

hexanoic acid (caproic acid) [Organic acid] *Pulmonary edema, circulatory collapse, laryngeal edema and spasm, severe chemical burns to skin, mucous membranes, and internal organs, GI tract perforation and hemorrhage, peritonitis.*

hexanol [Higher alcohol (4+ carbons)] *CNS depression, respiratory failure, arrhythmias.*

hexene; 1-hexene [Aliphatic hydrocarbon] *Arrhythmias, asphyxiation, anesthesia.* ⑨ hexane

hexyl alcohol [Higher alcohol (4+ carbons)] *CNS depression, respiratory failure, arrhythmias.*

hexyl trichorosilane [Silane/chlorosilane] *Respiratory tract irritation, pulmonary edema.*

hexylene glycol [Ethylene glycol] *Respiratory failure, pulmonary edema, paralysis, cardiovascular collapse, severe acidosis.*

hexylresorcinol [Phenol] *Coma, hypotension, arrhythmias, pulmonary edema, respiratory arrest.*

HF (hydrofluoric acid) [Hydrofluoric acid] *Pulmonary and laryngeal edema, circulatory collapse, severe skin burns, GI tract perforation, systemic fluoride poisoning.*

HFC 134A; R134A refrigerant (1,1,1,2-tetrafluoroethane) [Chlorinated fluorocarbon] *Asphyxiation, anesthesia, arrhythmias.*

hydrastine [Acrolein] *Severe respiratory tract irritation, pulmonary edema, respiratory failure.*

hydraulic fluids (n.o.s.) [Hydrocarbon mixture] *CNS depression, respiratory arrest, seizures, arrhythmias, pulmonary edema.*

hydrazine [Hydrazine] *Seizures, hemolysis of red blood cells, pulmonary edema.*

hydrazine hydrate [Hydrazine] *Seizures, hemolysis of red blood cells, pulmonary edema.*

hydrazine sulfate [Hydrazine] *Seizures, hemolysis of red blood cells, pulmonary edema.*

hydrazobenzene [Hydrazine] *Seizures, hemolysis of red blood cells, pulmonary edema.*

hydride, metal (n.o.s.) [Poison] *Cardiovascular collapse, pulmonary edema, CNS depression, coma, sei-*

zures, nausea, vomiting, cardiopulmonary arrest.

hydriodic acid; hydriodic acid mixture (n.o.s.) [Inorganic acid] *Pulmonary edema, bronchospasm, circulatory collapse, laryngeal spasm and edema, severe chemical burns to skin, mucous membranes, and internal organs, GI tract perforation and hemorrhage, peritonitis.* [Iodine] *Hypotension, circulatory collapse, pulmonary edema.*

hydrobromic acid; hydrobromic acid mixture (n.o.s.) [Bromine/methyl bromide] *Severe respiratory irritation, pulmonary edema, respiratory failure, coma, convulsions, death.*

hydrocarbon, aliphatic (n.o.s.) [Aliphatic hydrocarbon] *Arrhythmias, asphyxiation, anesthesia.*

hydrocarbon, chlorinated [Halogenated aliphatic hydrocarbon] *CNS depression, respiratory arrest, circulatory collapse.*

hydrocarbon gas (n.o.s.) [Flammable gas] *Respiratory failure, cardiac arrest, arrhythmias.* [Aliphatic hydrocarbon] *Arrhythmias, asphyxiation, anesthesia.*

hydrocarbon gas drip [Hydrocarbon mixture] *CNS depression, respiratory arrest, seizures, arrhythmias, pulmonary edema.*

hydrocarbon solvent (n.o.s.) [Hydrocarbon mixture] *CNS depression, respiratory arrest, seizures, arrhythmias, pulmonary edema.*

hydrocarbon solvent, aromatic (n.o.s.) [Aromatic hydrocarbon] *Arrhythmias, respiratory failure, pulmonary edema, paralysis, brain and kidney damage.*

hydrochloric acid [Inorganic acid] *Pulmonary edema, bronchospasm, circulatory collapse, laryngeal spasm and edema, severe chemical burns to skin, mucous membranes, and internal organs, GI tract perforation and hemorrhage, peritonitis.*

hydrocyanic acid [Cyanide] *Impairment of cellular oxygenation and adenosine triphosphate production, hypoxia, death.*

hydrofluoric acid (HF) [Hydrofluoric acid] *Pulmonary and laryngeal edema, circulatory collapse, severe skin burns, GI tract perforation, systemic fluoride poisoning.*

hydrofluoric acid & sulfuric acid mixture [Inorganic acid] *Pulmonary edema, bronchospasm, circulatory collapse, laryngeal spasm and edema, severe chemical burns to skin, mucous membranes, and internal organs, GI tract perforation and hemorrhage, peritonitis.* [Hydrofluoric acid] *Pulmonary and laryngeal edema, circulatory collapse, severe skin burns, GI tract perforation, systemic fluoride poisoning.*

hydrofluosilicic acid [Hydrofluoric acid] *Pulmonary and laryngeal edema, circulatory collapse, severe skin burns, GI tract perforation, systemic fluoride poisoning.*

hydrogen (gas or cryogenic liquid) [Flammable gas] *Respiratory failure, cardiac arrest, arrhythmias.* [Simple asphyxiant] *Asphyxiation.*

hydrogen arsenide [Arsenic] *Heavy metal toxicity, vomiting, GI bleeding, CNS depression, pulmonary edema, cardiac arrest.*

hydrogen bromide [Bromine/methyl bromide] *Severe respiratory irritation, pulmonary edema, respiratory failure, coma, convulsions, death.*

hydrogen & carbon monoxide mixture [Carbon monoxide] *Impairment of cellular oxygenation, hypoxia, death.*

hydrogen chloride [Inorganic acid] *Pulmonary edema, bronchospasm, circulatory collapse, laryngeal spasm and edema, severe chemical burns to skin, mucous membranes, and internal organs, GI tract perforation and hemorrhage, peritonitis.*

hydrogen cyanide [Cyanide] *Impairment of cellular oxygenation and adenosine triphosphate production, hypoxia, death.*

hydrogen fluoride [Hydrofluoric acid] *Pulmonary and laryngeal edema, circula-*

tory collapse, severe skin burns, GI tract perforation, systemic fluoride poisoning.

hydrogen iodide [Iodine] *Hypotension, circulatory collapse, pulmonary edema.*

hydrogen & methane mixture [Simple asphyxiant] *Asphyxiation.*

hydrogen peroxide [Oxidizer] *Pulmonary and laryngeal edema, circulatory arrest, hypovolemic shock, chemical burns of skin, mucous membranes, and internal organs.*

hydrogen peroxide & peroxyacetic acid mixture [Oxidizer] *Pulmonary and laryngeal edema, circulatory arrest, hypovolemic shock, chemical burns of skin, mucous membranes, and internal organs.*

hydrogen phosphide [Phosphine] *Severe pulmonary irritation, pulmonary edema.*

hydrogen selenide [Selenium] *Arrhythmias, pulmonary edema, bronchospasm, seizures, vomiting, GI bleeding.*

hydrogen sulfide [Hydrogen sulfide] *Severe respiratory tract irritation, pulmonary edema, respiratory paralysis.*

hydroperoxide [Oxidizer] *Pulmonary and laryngeal edema, circulatory arrest, hypovolemic shock, chemical burns of skin, mucous membranes, and internal organs.*

hydroquinone [Aniline] *Methemoglobinemia, hypoxia.* [Phenol] *Coma, hypotension, arrhythmias, pulmonary edema, respiratory arrest.*

hydroselenic acid [Inorganic acid] *Pulmonary edema, bronchospasm, circulatory collapse, laryngeal spasm and edema, severe chemical burns to skin, mucous membranes, and internal organs, GI tract perforation and hemorrhage, peritonitis.* [Selenium] *Arrhythmias, pulmonary edema, bronchospasm, seizures, vomiting, GI bleeding.*

hydrosilicofluoric acid [Hydrofluoric acid] *Pulmonary and laryngeal edema, circulatory collapse, severe skin burns, GI tract perforation, systemic fluoride poisoning.*

DL-(1-hydroxycyclohexyl) peroxide [Organic peroxide] *Pulmonary and laryngeal edema, circulatory arrest, hypovolemic shock, chemical burns to skin, mucous membranes, and internal organs.*

3-(2-hydroxyethoxy)-4-pyrrolidin-1-ylbenzene-diazonium zinc chloride [Zinc] *Respiratory tract irritation, metal fume fever, pulmonary edema.*

1-hydroxy-1′-hydroperoxy dicyclohexyl peroxide [Organic peroxide] *Pulmonary and laryngeal edema, circulatory arrest, hypovolemic shock, chemical burns to skin, mucous membranes, and internal organs.*

hydroxylamine [Organic base/amine] *Pulmonary edema, cardiac depression, seizures.*

hydroxylamine sulfate [Organic base/amine] *Pulmonary edema, cardiac depression, seizures.*

hydroxymercuricresol [Mercury] *Circulatory collapse, arrhythmias, respiratory failure, pulmonary edema, neurotoxic effects.*

hydroxymercurinitrophenol [Nitrate/nitrite] *Methemoglobinemia, hypotension, circulatory collapse.* [Mercury] *Circulatory collapse, arrhythmias, respiratory failure, pulmonary edema, neurotoxic effects.*

4-hydroxy-3-nitrophenylarsonic acid [Arsenic] *Heavy metal toxicity, vomiting, GI bleeding, CNS depression, pulmonary edema, cardiac arrest.*

hydroxyphenylmercurichloride [Mercury] *Circulatory collapse, arrhythmias, respiratory failure, pulmonary edema, neurotoxic effects.*

hypochlorite mixture (n.o.s.) [Hypochlorite] *Circulatory collapse, respiratory tract irritation, upper airway obstruction, pulmonary edema.*

ido methylpropane [Halogenated aliphatic hydrocarbon] *CNS depression, respiratory arrest, circulatory collapse.*

igniter for aircraft propulsion device [Flammable solid] *Shock, severe chemical and thermal burns, severe respiratory tract irritation, pul-*

HazMat

monary edema, respiratory arrest, ECG changes, sudden death.

Imidan [Organophosphate] *Pulmonary edema, respiratory muscle paralysis, respiratory failure, bradycardia, acetylcholinesterase inhibition, hypotension, pulmonary edema, overstimulation of parasympathetic nervous system, striated muscle, sympathetic ganglia, and CNS.*

iminobispropylamine [Organic base/amine] *Pulmonary edema, cardiac depression, seizures.*

iminodipropylamine [Organic base/amine] *Pulmonary edema, cardiac depression, seizures.*

indeno(1,2,3-cd)pyrene [Aromatic hydrocarbon] *Arrhythmias, respiratory failure, pulmonary edema, paralysis, brain and kidney damage.*

infectious substance (n.o.s.) *No acute symptoms during incubation period. Physiologic response varies depending on strain of microorganism or toxin.*

ink [Flammable/combustible liquid] *CNS depression, respiratory arrest, convulsions, arrhythmias, pulmonary edema.*

insecticide (n.o.s.) [Poison] *Cardiovascular collapse, pulmonary edema, CNS depression, coma, seizures, nausea, vomiting, cardiopulmonary arrest.*

insecticide gas (n.o.s.) [Poison] *Cardiovascular collapse, pulmonary edema, CNS depression, coma, seizures, nausea, vomiting, cardiopulmonary arrest.* [Organophosphate] *Pulmonary edema, respiratory muscle paralysis, respiratory failure, bradycardia, acetylcholinesterase inhibition, hypotension, pulmonary edema, overstimulation of parasympathetic nervous system, striated muscle, sympathetic ganglia, and CNS.*

iodine monochloride [Iodine] *Hypotension, circulatory collapse, pulmonary edema.*

iodine pentafluoride [Hydrofluoric acid] *Pulmonary and laryngeal edema, circulatory collapse, severe skin burns, GI tract perforation, systemic fluoride*

poisoning. [Iodine] *Hypotension, circulatory collapse, pulmonary edema.*

iodo butane [Halogenated aliphatic hydrocarbon] *CNS depression, respiratory arrest, circulatory collapse.*

iodo propane [Halogenated aliphatic hydrocarbon] *CNS depression, respiratory arrest, circulatory collapse.*

IPDI [Isocyanate/aliphatic thiocyanate] *CNS depression, respiratory arrest, respiratory paralysis, pulmonary edema, cyanide toxicity.*

iron carbonyl [Iron] *Hypovolemic shock.*

iron chloride; ferric chloride; ferrous chloride [Iron] *Hypovolemic shock.*

iron oxide [Iron] *Hypovolemic shock.*

iron pentacarbonyl [Iron] *Hypovolemic shock.*

iron sponge [Iron] *Hypovolemic shock.*

iron swarf [Iron] *Hypovolemic shock.*

irritating substance (n.o.s.) [Irritant] *Severe immediate or delayed upper airway or respiratory tract irritation, pulmonary edema, glottic spasm, airway obstruction.*

isoamyl acetate [Ester] *CNS depression, respiratory tract irritation, bronchitis, pneumonitis.*

isoamyl alcohol [Higher alcohol (4+ carbons)] *CNS depression, respiratory failure, arrhythmias.*

isobenzan [Lindane] *CNS stimulation, seizures, respiratory failure.*

isobutane; isobutane mixture (n.o.s.) [Simple asphyxiant] *Asphyxiation.*

isobutanol [Higher alcohol (4+ carbons)] *CNS depression, respiratory failure, arrhythmias.*

isobutyl acetate [Ester] *CNS depression, respiratory tract irritation, bronchitis, pneumonitis.*

isobutyl acrylate [Ester] *CNS depression, respiratory tract irritation, bronchitis, pneumonitis.*

isobutyl alcohol [Higher alcohol (4+ carbons)] *CNS depression, respiratory failure, arrhythmias.*

isobutyl aldehyde [Aldehyde] *Seizures, respiratory failure, pulmonary edema.*

isobutyl chloroformate [Organic acid] *Pulmonary edema, circulatory collapse, laryngeal edema and spasm, severe chemical burns to skin, mucous membranes, and internal organs, GI tract perforation and hemorrhage, peritonitis.*

isobutyl formate [Ester] *CNS depression, respiratory tract irritation, bronchitis, pneumonitis.*

isobutyl isobutyrate [Ester] *CNS depression, respiratory tract irritation, bronchitis, pneumonitis.*

isobutyl isocyanate [Isocyanate/aliphatic thiocyanate] *CNS depression, respiratory arrest, respiratory paralysis, pulmonary edema, cyanide toxicity.*

isobutyl methacrylate [Ester] *CNS depression, respiratory tract irritation, bronchitis, pneumonitis.*

isobutyl methyl ketone peroxide [Organic peroxide] *Pulmonary and laryngeal edema, circulatory arrest, hypovolemic shock, chemical burns to skin, mucous membranes, and internal organs.* [Ketone] *Respiratory mucous membrane irritation, pulmonary edema, CNS depression.* [Corrosive] *Upper airway burns and edema, circulatory collapse, severe chemical burns to skin, toxic systemic effects, GI tract perforation and hemorrhage, peritonitis.*

isobutyl propionate [Ester] *CNS depression, respiratory tract irritation, bronchitis, pneumonitis.*

isobutylamine; DL-isobutylamine [Organic base/amine] *Pulmonary edema, cardiac depression, seizures.*

isobutylene [Aliphatic hydrocarbon] *Arrhythmias, asphyxiation, anesthesia.*

DL-isobutylene [Simple asphyxiant] *Asphyxiation.*

isobutyraldehyde [Aldehyde] *Seizures, respiratory failure, pulmonary edema.*

isobutyric acid [Organic acid] *Pulmonary edema, circulatory collapse, laryngeal edema and spasm, severe chemical burns to skin, mucous membranes, and internal organs, GI tract perforation and hemorrhage, peritonitis.*

isobutyric anhydride [Organic acid] *Pulmonary edema, circulatory collapse, laryngeal edema and spasm, severe chemical burns to skin, mucous membranes, and internal organs, GI tract perforation and hemorrhage, peritonitis.*

isobutyronitrile [Cyanide] *Impairment of cellular oxygenation and adenosine triphosphate production, hypoxia, death.*

isobutyryl chloride [Halogenated aliphatic hydrocarbon] *CNS depression, respiratory arrest, circulatory collapse.*

isocyanate; isocyanate mixture (n.o.s.) [Isocyanate/aliphatic thiocyanate] *CNS depression, respiratory arrest, respiratory paralysis, pulmonary edema, cyanide toxicity.*

isocyanatobenzotrifluoride [Isocyanate/aliphatic thiocyanate] *CNS depression, respiratory arrest, respiratory paralysis, pulmonary edema, cyanide toxicity.* [Fluorine] *CNS depression, respiratory arrest, cardiovascular collapse, shock, arrhythmias.*

isocyanic acid [Isocyanate/aliphatic thiocyanate] *CNS depression, respiratory arrest, respiratory paralysis, pulmonary edema, cyanide toxicity.*

isocyanuric acid [Organic acid] *Pulmonary edema, circulatory collapse, laryngeal edema and spasm, severe chemical burns to skin, mucous membranes, and internal organs, GI tract perforation and hemorrhage, peritonitis.*

isododecane [Aliphatic hydrocarbon] *Arrhythmias, asphyxiation, anesthesia.*

isodrin [Aldrin/dieldrin/endrin] *Seizures, respiratory failure.*

isofluorphate [Organophosphate] *Pulmonary edema, respiratory muscle paralysis, respiratory failure, bradycardia, acetylcholinesterase inhibition, hypotension, pulmonary edema, overstimulation of parasympathetic nervous system, striated muscle, sympathetic ganglia, and CNS.*

isoheptene [Aliphatic hydrocarbon] *Arrhythmias, asphyxiation, anesthesia.*

isohexene [Aliphatic hydrocarbon] *Arrhythmias, asphyxiation, anesthesia.*

HazMat

Isolan [Carbamate] *Acetylcholinesterase inhibition (reversible), bradycardia, hypotension, respiratory muscle paralysis, respiratory arrest, pulmonary edema.*

isononanoyl peroxide [Organic peroxide] *Pulmonary and laryngeal edema, circulatory arrest, hypovolemic shock, chemical burns to skin, mucous membranes, and internal organs.*

isononyl alcohol [Higher alcohol (4+ carbons)] *CNS depression, respiratory failure, arrhythmias.*

isooctane [Aliphatic hydrocarbon] *Arrhythmias, asphyxiation, anesthesia.*

isooctene [Aliphatic hydrocarbon] *Arrhythmias, asphyxiation, anesthesia.*

isooctyl alcohol [Higher alcohol (4+ carbons)] *CNS depression, respiratory failure, arrhythmias.*

isopentane [Aliphatic hydrocarbon] *Arrhythmias, asphyxiation, anesthesia.* ⊡ isopentene

isopentanoic acid [Organic acid] *Pulmonary edema, circulatory collapse, laryngeal edema and spasm, severe chemical burns to skin, mucous membranes, and internal organs, GI tract perforation and hemorrhage, peritonitis.*

isopentene [Aliphatic hydrocarbon] *Arrhythmias, asphyxiation, anesthesia.* ⊡ isopentane

isophorone [Ketone] *Respiratory mucous membrane irritation, pulmonary edema, CNS depression.*

isophorone diisocyanate [Isocyanate/ aliphatic thiocyanate] *CNS depression, respiratory arrest, respiratory paralysis, pulmonary edema, cyanide toxicity.*

isophoronediamine [Organic base/ amine] *Pulmonary edema, cardiac depression, seizures.*

isoprene [Aliphatic hydrocarbon] *Arrhythmias, asphyxiation, anesthesia.*

isoprocarb [Carbamate] *Acetylcholinesterase inhibition (reversible), bradycardia, hypotension, respiratory muscle paralysis, respiratory arrest, pulmonary edema.*

isopropanol [Lower alcohol (1–3 carbons)] *CNS depression, coma, respiratory arrest, arrhythmias.*

isopropanolamine dodecylbenzene sulfonate [Poison] *Cardiovascular collapse, pulmonary edema, CNS depression, coma, seizures, nausea, vomiting, cardiopulmonary arrest.*

isopropenyl acetate [Ester] *CNS depression, respiratory tract irritation, bronchitis, pneumonitis.*

isopropenyl benzene [Aromatic hydrocarbon] *Arrhythmias, respiratory failure, pulmonary edema, paralysis, brain and kidney damage.*

isopropyl acetate [Ester] *CNS depression, respiratory tract irritation, bronchitis, pneumonitis.*

isopropyl acid phosphate [Ester] *CNS depression, respiratory tract irritation, bronchitis, pneumonitis.*

isopropyl alcohol [Lower alcohol (1– 3 carbons)] *CNS depression, coma, respiratory arrest, arrhythmias.*

isopropyl amine [Organic base/ amine] *Pulmonary edema, cardiac depression, seizures.*

isopropyl butyrate [Ester] *CNS depression, respiratory tract irritation, bronchitis, pneumonitis.*

isopropyl chloroacetate [Ester] *CNS depression, respiratory tract irritation, bronchitis, pneumonitis.*

isopropyl chloroformate [Ester] *CNS depression, respiratory tract irritation, bronchitis, pneumonitis.*

isopropyl chloropropionate [Ester] *CNS depression, respiratory tract irritation, bronchitis, pneumonitis.*

isopropyl ether; DL-isopropyl ether [Ether] *Anesthesia, respiratory arrest.*

isopropyl formate [Ester] *CNS depression, respiratory tract irritation, bronchitis, pneumonitis.*

isopropyl isobutyrate [Ester] *CNS depression, respiratory tract irritation, bronchitis, pneumonitis.*

isopropyl isocyanate [Isocyanate/aliphatic thiocyanate] *CNS depression, respiratory arrest, respiratory paralysis, pulmonary edema, cyanide toxicity.*

isopropyl mercaptan [Sulfur] *Respiratory tract irritation, pulmonary edema, anaphylaxis.*

isopropyl nitrate [Nitrate/nitrite] *Methemoglobinemia, hypotension, circulatory collapse.*

isopropyl peroxydicarbonate [Organic peroxide] *Pulmonary and laryngeal edema, circulatory arrest, hypovolemic shock, chemical burns to skin, mucous membranes, and internal organs.*

isopropyl propionate [Ester] *CNS depression, respiratory tract irritation, bronchitis, pneumonitis.*

isopropylbenzene [Aromatic hydrocarbon] *Arrhythmias, respiratory failure, pulmonary edema, paralysis, brain and kidney damage.*

isopropylcumyl hydroperoxide [Organic peroxide] *Pulmonary and laryngeal edema, circulatory arrest, hypovolemic shock, chemical burns to skin, mucous membranes, and internal organs.* [Aromatic hydrocarbon] *Arrhythmias, respiratory failure, pulmonary edema, paralysis, brain and kidney damage.*

4,4'-isopropylidene diphenol [Phenol] *Coma, hypotension, arrhythmias, pulmonary edema, respiratory arrest.*

isopropylmethylpyrazolyl dimethylcarbamate [Carbamate] *Acetylcholinesterase inhibition (reversible), bradycardia, hypotension, respiratory muscle paralysis, respiratory arrest, pulmonary edema.*

isosafrole [Phenol] *Coma, hypotension, arrhythmias, pulmonary edema, respiratory arrest.*

isosorbide dinitrate mixture (n.o.s.) [Nitrate/nitrite] *Methemoglobinemia, hypotension, circulatory collapse.*

jet fuel [Hydrocarbon mixture] *CNS depression, respiratory arrest, seizures, arrhythmias, pulmonary edema.*

kanechlor S [Polychlorinated biphenyl/polybrominated biphenyl/polychlorinated dibenzofuran] *Liver and kidney damage.*

Kelthane [Lindane] *CNS stimulation, seizures, respiratory failure.*

Kepone [Lindane] *CNS stimulation, seizures, respiratory failure.*

kerosene [Hydrocarbon mixture] *CNS depression, respiratory arrest, seizures, arrhythmias, pulmonary edema.*

ketene [Aldehyde] *Seizures, respiratory failure, pulmonary edema.*

ketone (n.o.s.) [Ketone] *Respiratory mucous membrane irritation, pulmonary edema, CNS depression.*

krypton (gas or cryogenic liquid) [Simple asphyxiant] *Asphyxiation.*

lacquer [Hydrocarbon mixture] *CNS depression, respiratory arrest, seizures, arrhythmias, pulmonary edema.*

lactic acid [Organic acid] *Pulmonary edema, circulatory collapse, laryngeal edema and spasm, severe chemical burns to skin, mucous membranes, and internal organs, GI tract perforation and hemorrhage, peritonitis.*

lactonitrile [Cyanide] *Impairment of cellular oxygenation and adenosine triphosphate production, hypoxia, death.*

landrin [Carbamate] *Acetylcholinesterase inhibition (reversible), bradycardia, hypotension, respiratory muscle paralysis, respiratory arrest, pulmonary edema.*

Lannate [Carbamate] *Acetylcholinesterase inhibition (reversible), bradycardia, hypotension, respiratory muscle paralysis, respiratory arrest, pulmonary edema.*

lasiocarpine [Poison] *Cardiovascular collapse, pulmonary edema, CNS depression, coma, seizures, nausea, vomiting, cardiopulmonary arrest.*

lauroyl peroxide [Organic peroxide] *Pulmonary and laryngeal edema, circulatory arrest, hypovolemic shock, chemical burns to skin, mucous membranes, and internal organs.*

lauryl alcohol [Higher alcohol (4+ carbons)] *CNS depression, respiratory failure, arrhythmias.*

lauryl thiocyanate [Isocyanate/aliphatic thiocyanate] *CNS depression, respiratory arrest, respiratory paralysis, pulmonary edema, cyanide toxicity.*

HazMat

lead; lead mixture (n.o.s.) [Lead] *Circulatory collapse, coma, rare seizures.*

lead acetate [Lead] *Circulatory collapse, coma, rare seizures.*

lead arsenate [Arsenic] *Heavy metal toxicity, vomiting, GI bleeding, CNS depression, pulmonary edema, cardiac arrest.* [Lead] *Circulatory collapse, coma, rare seizures.*

lead arsenite [Arsenic] *Heavy metal toxicity, vomiting, GI bleeding, CNS depression, pulmonary edema, cardiac arrest.* [Lead] *Circulatory collapse, coma, rare seizures.*

lead chloride [Lead] *Circulatory collapse, coma, rare seizures.*

lead chromate [Lead] *Circulatory collapse, coma, rare seizures.*

lead cyanide [Lead] *Circulatory collapse, coma, rare seizures.* [Cyanide] *Impairment of cellular oxygenation and adenosine triphosphate production, hypoxia, death.*

lead dioxide [Lead] *Circulatory collapse, coma, rare seizures.*

lead fluoborate [Lead] *Circulatory collapse, coma, rare seizures.* [Boron] *Respiratory tract irritation, laryngeal spasm and edema, pulmonary edema, severe chemical burns.*

lead fluoride [Lead] *Circulatory collapse, coma, rare seizures.* [Fluorine] *CNS depression, respiratory arrest, cardiovascular collapse, shock, arrhythmias.*

lead iodide [Lead] *Circulatory collapse, coma, rare seizures.* [Iodine] *Hypotension, circulatory collapse, pulmonary edema.*

lead nitrate [Nitrate/nitrite] *Methemoglobinemia, hypotension, circulatory collapse.* [Lead] *Circulatory collapse, coma, rare seizures.*

lead perchlorate [Lead] *Circulatory collapse, coma, rare seizures.*

lead peroxide [Lead] *Circulatory collapse, coma, rare seizures.*

lead phosphate [Lead] *Circulatory collapse, coma, rare seizures.*

lead phosphite [Lead] *Circulatory collapse, coma, rare seizures.*

lead stearate [Lead] *Circulatory collapse, coma, rare seizures.*

lead subacetate [Lead] *Circulatory collapse, coma, rare seizures.*

lead sulfate [Lead] *Circulatory collapse, coma, rare seizures.*

lead sulfide [Lead] *Circulatory collapse, coma, rare seizures.*

lead tetraethyl [Lead] *Circulatory collapse, coma, rare seizures.*

lead tetramethyl [Lead] *Circulatory collapse, coma, rare seizures.*

lead thiocyanate [Lead] *Circulatory collapse, coma, rare seizures.* [Isocyanate/aliphatic thiocyanate] *CNS depression, respiratory arrest, respiratory paralysis, pulmonary edema, cyanide toxicity.*

leptophos [Organophosphate] *Pulmonary edema, respiratory muscle paralysis, respiratory failure, bradycardia, acetylcholinesterase inhibition, hypotension, pulmonary edema, overstimulation of parasympathetic nervous system, striated muscle, sympathetic ganglia, and CNS.*

Lethane 60 [Isocyanate/aliphatic thiocyanate] *CNS depression, respiratory arrest, respiratory paralysis, pulmonary edema, cyanide toxicity.*

lewisite [Arsine] *Intravascular hemolysis, pulmonary edema, cardiac and respiratory arrest, delayed-onset jaundice, and acute or delayed-onset renal failure.*

lewisite (liquid arsenic compound) [Arsenic] *Heavy metal toxicity, vomiting, GI bleeding, CNS depression, pulmonary edema, cardiac arrest.*

lighter, cigarette, and refills [Aliphatic hydrocarbon] *Arrhythmias, asphyxiation, anesthesia.*

lighter fluid [Aliphatic hydrocarbon] *Arrhythmias, asphyxiation, anesthesia.*

lime [Inorganic base/alkaline corrosive] *Upper airway burns and edema, pulmonary edema, skin burns, circulatory collapse, GI tract perforation and hemorrhage, peritonitis.*

lime, chlorinated [Hypochlorite] *Circulatory collapse, respiratory tract irri-*

tation, upper airway obstruction, pulmonary edema.

limonene [Turpentine/terpene] *Respiratory failure, pulmonary edema, tachycardia.*

linamarin [Cyanide] *Impairment of cellular oxygenation and adenosine triphosphate production, hypoxia, death.*

lindane [Lindane] *CNS stimulation, seizures, respiratory failure.*

liquefied gas (n.o.s.) [Flammable gas] *Respiratory failure, cardiac arrest, arrhythmias.*

liquefied gas, flammable poison (n.o.s.) [Flammable gas] *Respiratory failure, cardiac arrest, arrhythmias.* [Poison] *Cardiovascular collapse, pulmonary edema, CNS depression, coma, seizures, nausea, vomiting, cardiopulmonary arrest.*

liquefied gas, nonflammable (nitrogen, carbon dioxide, or air) [Nonflammable gas] *Pulmonary edema, respiratory failure, asphyxiation.*

liquefied gas, poisonous (n.o.s.) [Flammable gas] *Respiratory failure, cardiac arrest, arrhythmias.* [Poison] *Cardiovascular collapse, pulmonary edema, CNS depression, coma, seizures, nausea, vomiting, cardiopulmonary arrest.*

liquefied natural gas (LNG) [Aliphatic hydrocarbon] *Arrhythmias, asphyxiation, anesthesia.* [Simple asphyxiant] *Asphyxiation.*

liquefied petroleum gas (LPG) [Flammable gas] *Respiratory failure, cardiac arrest, arrhythmias.* [Hydrocarbon mixture] *CNS depression, respiratory arrest, seizures, arrhythmias, pulmonary edema.*

lithium [Lithium] *Chemical burns to respiratory tract, pulmonary edema.*

lithium acetylide & ethylenediamine mixture [Lithium] *Chemical burns to respiratory tract, pulmonary edema.*

lithium alkyl [Lithium] *Chemical burns to respiratory tract, pulmonary edema.*

lithium aluminum hydride [Lithium] *Chemical burns to respiratory tract, pulmonary edema.*

lithium battery [Lithium] *Chemical burns to respiratory tract, pulmonary edema.*

lithium borohydride [Lithium] *Chemical burns to respiratory tract, pulmonary edema.* [Boron] *Respiratory tract irritation, laryngeal spasm and edema, pulmonary edema, severe chemical burns.*

lithium chromate [Lithium] *Chemical burns to respiratory tract, pulmonary edema.*

lithium ferrosilicon [Lithium] *Chemical burns to respiratory tract, pulmonary edema.*

lithium hydride [Lithium] *Chemical burns to respiratory tract, pulmonary edema.*

lithium hydroxide [Inorganic base/alkaline corrosive] *Upper airway burns and edema, pulmonary edema, skin burns, circulatory collapse, GI tract perforation and hemorrhage, peritonitis.* [Lithium] *Chemical burns to respiratory tract, pulmonary edema.*

lithium hypochlorite [Hypochlorite] *Circulatory collapse, respiratory tract irritation, upper airway obstruction, pulmonary edema.* [Lithium] *Chemical burns to respiratory tract, pulmonary edema.*

lithium nitrate [Nitrate/nitrite] *Methemoglobinemia, hypotension, circulatory collapse.* [Lithium] *Chemical burns to respiratory tract, pulmonary edema.*

lithium nitride [Nitrate/nitrite] *Methemoglobinemia, hypotension, circulatory collapse.* [Lithium] *Chemical burns to respiratory tract, pulmonary edema.*

lithium peroxide [Lithium] *Chemical burns to respiratory tract, pulmonary edema.*

lithium silicon [Lithium] *Chemical burns to respiratory tract, pulmonary edema.*

lithopone [Barium] *Hypokalemia, muscle paralysis, arrhythmias, cardiac and respiratory arrest.* [Zinc] *Respiratory* *tract irritation, metal fume fever, pulmonary edema.*

LNG (liquefied natural gas) [Aliphatic hydrocarbon] *Arrhythmias, asphyxiation, anesthesia.* [Simple asphyxiant] *Asphyxiation.*

London purple [Aniline] *Methemoglobinemia, hypoxia.* [Arsenic] *Heavy metal toxicity, vomiting, GI bleeding, CNS depression, pulmonary edema, cardiac arrest.*

LPG (liquefied petroleum gas) [Flammable gas] *Respiratory failure, cardiac arrest, arrhythmias.* [Hydrocarbon mixture] *CNS depression, respiratory arrest, seizures, arrhythmias, pulmonary edema.*

lye [Inorganic base/alkaline corrosive] *Upper airway burns and edema, pulmonary edema, skin burns, circulatory collapse, GI tract perforation and hemorrhage, peritonitis.*

magnesium; magnesium alloy (n.o.s.) [Magnesium] *Cardiovascular collapse, respiratory depression.*

magnesium alkyl [Magnesium] *Cardiovascular collapse, respiratory depression.*

magnesium aluminum phosphide [Magnesium] *Cardiovascular collapse, respiratory depression.* [Phosphine] *Severe pulmonary irritation, pulmonary edema.*

magnesium arsenate [Arsenic] *Heavy metal toxicity, vomiting, GI bleeding, CNS depression, pulmonary edema, cardiac arrest.* [Magnesium] *Cardiovascular collapse, respiratory depression.*

magnesium bisulfite [Magnesium] *Cardiovascular collapse, respiratory depression.* [Sulfur] *Respiratory tract irritation, pulmonary edema, anaphylaxis.*

magnesium bromate [Magnesium] *Cardiovascular collapse, respiratory depression.* [Bromate] *CNS and respiratory system depression, delayed-onset renal failure.*

magnesium chlorate [Magnesium] *Cardiovascular collapse, respiratory depression.* [Chlorate] *Hemolysis, met-*

hemoglobinemia, hypoperfusion, CNS depression, delayed-onset renal failure.

magnesium chloride & chlorate mixture [Magnesium] *Cardiovascular collapse, respiratory depression.* [Chlorate] *Hemolysis, methemoglobinemia, hypoperfusion, CNS depression, delayed-onset renal failure.*

magnesium diamide [Magnesium] *Cardiovascular collapse, respiratory depression.*

magnesium diphenyl [Magnesium] *Cardiovascular collapse, respiratory depression.*

magnesium fluorosilicate [Magnesium] *Cardiovascular collapse, respiratory depression.* [Fluorine] *CNS depression, respiratory arrest, cardiovascular collapse, shock, arrhythmias.*

magnesium hydride [Magnesium] *Cardiovascular collapse, respiratory depression.*

magnesium nitrate [Nitrate/nitrite] *Methemoglobinemia, hypotension, circulatory collapse.* [Magnesium] *Cardiovascular collapse, respiratory depression.*

magnesium perchlorate [Magnesium] *Cardiovascular collapse, respiratory depression.* [Chlorate] *Hemolysis, methemoglobinemia, hypoperfusion, CNS depression, delayed-onset renal failure.*

magnesium peroxide [Magnesium] *Cardiovascular collapse, respiratory depression.*

magnesium phosphide [Magnesium] *Cardiovascular collapse, respiratory depression.* [Phosphine] *Severe pulmonary irritation, pulmonary edema.*

magnesium silicide [Magnesium] *Cardiovascular collapse, respiratory depression.*

magnesium silicofluoride [Magnesium] *Cardiovascular collapse, respiratory depression.* [Fluorine] *CNS depression, respiratory arrest, cardiovascular collapse, shock, arrhythmias.*

malathion [Organophosphate] *Pulmonary edema, respiratory muscle paralysis, respiratory failure, bradycardia, acetylcholinesterase inhibition, hypoten-*

sion, *pulmonary edema, overstimulation of parasympathetic nervous system, striated muscle, sympathetic ganglia, and CNS.*

maleic acid [Organic acid] *Pulmonary edema, circulatory collapse, laryngeal edema and spasm, severe chemical burns to skin, mucous membranes, and internal organs, GI tract perforation and hemorrhage, peritonitis.*

maleic anhydride [Organic acid] *Pulmonary edema, circulatory collapse, laryngeal edema and spasm, severe chemical burns to skin, mucous membranes, and internal organs, GI tract perforation and hemorrhage, peritonitis.*

maleic hydrazide [Organic acid] *Pulmonary edema, circulatory collapse, laryngeal edema and spasm, severe chemical burns to skin, mucous membranes, and internal organs, GI tract perforation and hemorrhage, peritonitis.*

malonic dinitrile [Cyanide] *Impairment of cellular oxygenation and adenosine triphosphate production, hypoxia, death.*

malonic ethyl ester nitrile [Cyanide] *Impairment of cellular oxygenation and adenosine triphosphate production, hypoxia, death.*

malononitrile [Cyanide] *Impairment of cellular oxygenation and adenosine triphosphate production, hypoxia, death.*

mancozeb [Carbamate] *Acetylcholinesterase inhibition (reversible), bradycardia, hypotension, respiratory muscle paralysis, respiratory arrest, pulmonary edema.*

maneb; maneb mixture (n.o.s.) [Dithiocarbamate] *Hypotension, respiratory failure.*

manganese nitrate [Nitrate/nitrite] *Methemoglobinemia, hypotension, circulatory collapse.* [Manganese] *Respiratory tract irritation, pulmonary edema.*

manganese resinate [Manganese] *Respiratory tract irritation, pulmonary edema.*

manganese tricarbonyl methylcyclopentadine [Manganese] *Respiratory tract irritation, pulmonary edema.*

matches [Chlorate] *Hemolysis, methemoglobinemia, hypoperfusion, CNS depression, delayed-onset renal failure.*

MBOCA [Aniline] *Methemoglobinemia, hypoxia.*

MCPA [Chlorophenoxy herbicide] *CNS depression, CNS stimulation, respiratory failure, ventricular fibrillation, seizures.*

MDI (diphenylmethane-4,4'-diisocyanate) [Isocyanate/aliphatic thiocyanate] *CNS depression, respiratory arrest, respiratory paralysis, pulmonary edema, cyanide toxicity.*

MDI (methylene bis(4-phenyl isocyanate)) [Isocyanate/aliphatic thiocyanate] *CNS depression, respiratory arrest, respiratory paralysis, pulmonary edema, cyanide toxicity.*

mechlorethamine [Poison] *Cardiovascular collapse, pulmonary edema, CNS depression, coma, seizures, nausea, vomiting, cardiopulmonary arrest.*

mecoprop [Chlorophenoxy herbicide] *CNS depression, CNS stimulation, respiratory failure, ventricular fibrillation, seizures.*

medication (n.o.s.) [Poison] *Cardiovascular collapse, pulmonary edema, CNS depression, coma, seizures, nausea, vomiting, cardiopulmonary arrest.*

melphalan [Poison] *Cardiovascular collapse, pulmonary edema, CNS depression, coma, seizures, nausea, vomiting, cardiopulmonary arrest.*

***p*-menthane hydroperoxide** [Organic peroxide] *Pulmonary and laryngeal edema, circulatory arrest, hypovolemic shock, chemical burns to skin, mucous membranes, and internal organs.*

menthol [Aromatic hydrocarbon] *Arrhythmias, respiratory failure, pulmonary edema, paralysis, brain and kidney damage.*

***p*-menthyl hydroperoxide** [Organic peroxide] *Pulmonary and laryngeal edema, circulatory arrest, hypovolemic shock, chemical burns to skin, mucous membranes, and internal organs.*

HazMat

mercaptan; mercaptan mixture (n.o.s.) [Sulfur] *Respiratory tract irritation, pulmonary edema, anaphylaxis.*

mercaptodimethur [Carbamate] *Acetylcholinesterase inhibition (reversible), bradycardia, hypotension, respiratory muscle paralysis, respiratory arrest, pulmonary edema.*

mercuric acetate; mercurous acetate; mercury acetate [Mercury] *Circulatory collapse, arrhythmias, respiratory failure, pulmonary edema, neurotoxic effects.*

mercuric arsenate [Arsenic] *Heavy metal toxicity, vomiting, GI bleeding, CNS depression, pulmonary edema, cardiac arrest.* [Mercury] *Circulatory collapse, arrhythmias, respiratory failure, pulmonary edema, neurotoxic effects.*

mercuric bromide; mercurous bromide; mercury bromide [Mercury] *Circulatory collapse, arrhythmias, respiratory failure, pulmonary edema, neurotoxic effects.* [Bromine/methyl bromide] *Severe respiratory irritation, pulmonary edema, respiratory failure, coma, convulsions, death.*

mercuric chloride; mercurous chloride [Mercury] *Circulatory collapse, arrhythmias, respiratory failure, pulmonary edema, neurotoxic effects.*

mercuric cyanide; mercury cyanide [Mercury] *Circulatory collapse, arrhythmias, respiratory failure, pulmonary edema, neurotoxic effects.* [Cyanide] *Impairment of cellular oxygenation and adenosine triphosphate production, hypoxia, death.*

mercuric nitrate; mercurous nitrate [Nitrate/nitrite] *Methemoglobinemia, hypotension, circulatory collapse.* [Mercury] *Circulatory collapse, arrhythmias, respiratory failure, pulmonary edema, neurotoxic effects.*

mercuric oxide; mercury oxide [Mercury] *Circulatory collapse, arrhythmias, respiratory failure, pulmonary edema, neurotoxic effects.*

mercuric oxycyanide; mercury oxycyanide [Mercury] *Circulatory collapse, arrhythmias, respiratory failure, pulmonary edema, neurotoxic effects.* [Cyanide] *Impairment of cellular oxygenation and adenosine triphosphate production, hypoxia, death.*

mercuric potassium cyanide [Mercury] *Circulatory collapse, arrhythmias, respiratory failure, pulmonary edema, neurotoxic effects.* [Cyanide] *Impairment of cellular oxygenation and adenosine triphosphate production, hypoxia, death.*

mercuric sulfate; mercurous sulfate; mercury sulfate [Mercury] *Circulatory collapse, arrhythmias, respiratory failure, pulmonary edema, neurotoxic effects.*

mercuric thiocyanate; mercury thiocyanate [Mercury] *Circulatory collapse, arrhythmias, respiratory failure, pulmonary edema, neurotoxic effects.* [Isocyanate/aliphatic thiocyanate] *CNS depression, respiratory arrest, respiratory paralysis, pulmonary edema, cyanide toxicity.*

mercurol [Mercury] *Circulatory collapse, arrhythmias, respiratory failure, pulmonary edema, neurotoxic effects.*

mercurous acetate; mercuric acetate; mercury acetate [Mercury] *Circulatory collapse, arrhythmias, respiratory failure, pulmonary edema, neurotoxic effects.*

mercurous bromide; mercuric bromide; mercury bromide [Mercury] *Circulatory collapse, arrhythmias, respiratory failure, pulmonary edema, neurotoxic effects.* [Bromine/methyl bromide] *Severe respiratory irritation, pulmonary edema, respiratory failure, coma, convulsions, death.*

mercurous chloride; mercuric chloride [Mercury] *Circulatory collapse, arrhythmias, respiratory failure, pulmonary edema, neurotoxic effects.*

mercurous nitrate; mercuric nitrate [Nitrate/nitrite] *Methemoglobinemia, hypotension, circulatory collapse.* [Mercury] *Circulatory collapse,* arrhythmias, respiratory failure, pulmonary edema, neurotoxic effects.

mercurous sulfate; mercuric sulfate; mercury sulfate [Mercury] Circulatory collapse, arrhythmias, respiratory failure, pulmonary edema, neurotoxic effects.

mercury; mercury mixture (n.o.s.) [Mercury] Circulatory collapse, arrhythmias, respiratory failure, pulmonary edema, neurotoxic effects.

mercury acetate; mercuric acetate; mercurous acetate [Mercury] Circulatory collapse, arrhythmias, respiratory failure, pulmonary edema, neurotoxic effects.

mercury ammonium chloride [Mercury] Circulatory collapse, arrhythmias, respiratory failure, pulmonary edema, neurotoxic effects.

mercury benzoate [Mercury] Circulatory collapse, arrhythmias, respiratory failure, pulmonary edema, neurotoxic effects.

mercury bisulfate [Mercury] Circulatory collapse, arrhythmias, respiratory failure, pulmonary edema, neurotoxic effects.

mercury bromide; mercuric bromide; mercurous bromide [Mercury] Circulatory collapse, arrhythmias, respiratory failure, pulmonary edema, neurotoxic effects. [Bromine/methyl bromide] Severe respiratory irritation, pulmonary edema, respiratory failure, coma, convulsions, death.

mercury cyanide; mercuric cyanide [Mercury] Circulatory collapse, arrhythmias, respiratory failure, pulmonary edema, neurotoxic effects. [Cyanide] Impairment of cellular oxygenation and adenosine triphosphate production, hypoxia, death.

mercury fulminate [Mercury] Circulatory collapse, arrhythmias, respiratory failure, pulmonary edema, neurotoxic effects.

mercury gluconate [Mercury] Circulatory collapse, arrhythmias, respiratory failure, pulmonary edema, neurotoxic effects.

mercury iodide [Mercury] Circulatory collapse, arrhythmias, respiratory failure, pulmonary edema, neurotoxic effects. [Iodine] Hypotension, circulatory collapse, pulmonary edema.

mercury nucleate [Mercury] Circulatory collapse, arrhythmias, respiratory failure, pulmonary edema, neurotoxic effects.

mercury oleate [Mercury] Circulatory collapse, arrhythmias, respiratory failure, pulmonary edema, neurotoxic effects.

mercury oxide; mercuric oxide [Mercury] Circulatory collapse, arrhythmias, respiratory failure, pulmonary edema, neurotoxic effects.

mercury oxycyanide; mercuric oxycyanide [Mercury] Circulatory collapse, arrhythmias, respiratory failure, pulmonary edema, neurotoxic effects. [Cyanide] Impairment of cellular oxygenation and adenosine triphosphate production, hypoxia, death.

mercury potassium iodide [Mercury] Circulatory collapse, arrhythmias, respiratory failure, pulmonary edema, neurotoxic effects. [Iodine] Hypotension, circulatory collapse, pulmonary edema.

mercury salicylate [Mercury] Circulatory collapse, arrhythmias, respiratory failure, pulmonary edema, neurotoxic effects.

mercury sulfate; mercuric sulfate; mercurous sulfate [Mercury] Circulatory collapse, arrhythmias, respiratory failure, pulmonary edema, neurotoxic effects.

mercury thiocyanate; mercuric thiocyanate [Mercury] Circulatory collapse, arrhythmias, respiratory failure, pulmonary edema, neurotoxic effects. [Isocyanate/aliphatic thiocyanate] CNS depression, respiratory arrest, respiratory paralysis, pulmonary edema, cyanide toxicity.

mercury-based pesticide (n.o.s.) [Mercury] Circulatory collapse, arrhythmias, respiratory failure, pulmonary edema, neurotoxic effects.

HazMat

Merodicein [Mercury] *Circulatory collapse, arrhythmias, respiratory failure, pulmonary edema, neurotoxic effects.*

Mertect; Mertect 160 [Thiabendazole] *Cardiovascular collapse, respiratory tract irritation.*

mesityl oxide [Ketone] *Respiratory mucous membrane irritation, pulmonary edema, CNS depression.*

mesitylene [Aromatic hydrocarbon] *Arrhythmias, respiratory failure, pulmonary edema, paralysis, brain and kidney damage.*

metal alkyl; metal alkyl halide (n.o.s.); metal alkyl hydride (n.o.s.) [Poison] *Cardiovascular collapse, pulmonary edema, CNS depression, coma, seizures, nausea, vomiting, cardiopulmonary arrest.*

metal catalyst [Poison] *Cardiovascular collapse, pulmonary edema, CNS depression, coma, seizures, nausea, vomiting, cardiopulmonary arrest.*

metal hydride (n.o.s.) [Poison] *Cardiovascular collapse, pulmonary edema, CNS depression, coma, seizures, nausea, vomiting, cardiopulmonary arrest.*

metal powder, flammable (n.o.s.) [Flammable solid] *Shock, severe chemical and thermal burns, severe respiratory tract irritation, pulmonary edema, respiratory arrest, ECG changes, sudden death.* [Poison] *Cardiovascular collapse, pulmonary edema, CNS depression, coma, seizures, nausea, vomiting, cardiopulmonary arrest.*

metaldehyde [Aldehyde] *Seizures, respiratory failure, pulmonary edema.*

Meta-Systox [Organophosphate] *Pulmonary edema, respiratory muscle paralysis, respiratory failure, bradycardia, acetylcholinesterase inhibition, hypotension, pulmonary edema, overstimulation of parasympathetic nervous system, striated muscle, sympathetic ganglia, and CNS.*

methacrolein diacetate [Poison] *Cardiovascular collapse, pulmonary edema, CNS depression, coma, seizures, nausea, vomiting, cardiopulmonary arrest.*

methacrylaldehyde [Aldehyde] *Seizures, respiratory failure, pulmonary edema.*

methacrylic acid [Organic acid] *Pulmonary edema, circulatory collapse, laryngeal edema and spasm, severe chemical burns to skin, mucous membranes, and internal organs, GI tract perforation and hemorrhage, peritonitis.*

methacrylic anhydride [Organic acid] *Pulmonary edema, circulatory collapse, laryngeal edema and spasm, severe chemical burns to skin, mucous membranes, and internal organs, GI tract perforation and hemorrhage, peritonitis.*

methacrylonitrile [Cyanide] *Impairment of cellular oxygenation and adenosine triphosphate production, hypoxia, death.*

methacryloyl chloride [Poison] *Cardiovascular collapse, pulmonary edema, CNS depression, coma, seizures, nausea, vomiting, cardiopulmonary arrest.*

methacryloyloxyethyl isocyanate [Isocyanate/aliphatic thiocyanate] *CNS depression, respiratory arrest, respiratory paralysis, pulmonary edema, cyanide toxicity.*

methallyl alcohol [Higher alcohol (4+ carbons)] *CNS depression, respiratory failure, arrhythmias.*

methamidophos [Organophosphate] *Pulmonary edema, respiratory muscle paralysis, respiratory failure, bradycardia, acetylcholinesterase inhibition, hypotension, pulmonary edema, overstimulation of parasympathetic nervous system, striated muscle, sympathetic ganglia, and CNS.*

methanamine [Organic base/amine] *Pulmonary edema, cardiac depression, seizures.* ⬚ methenamine

methane (gas or cryogenic liquid) [Aliphatic hydrocarbon] *Arrhythmias, asphyxiation, anesthesia.* [Simple asphyxiant] *Asphyxiation.*

methane & hydrogen mixture
[Simple asphyxiant] *Asphyxiation.*

methanesulfonyl chloride [Organo-
phosphate] *Pulmonary edema, respiratory muscle paralysis, respiratory failure, bradycardia, acetylcholinesterase
inhibition, hypotension, pulmonary
edema, overstimulation of parasympathetic nervous system, striated muscle,
sympathetic ganglia, and CNS.*

methanesulfonyl fluoride [Organo-
phosphate] *Pulmonary edema, respiratory muscle paralysis, respiratory failure, bradycardia, acetylcholinesterase
inhibition, hypotension, pulmonary
edema, overstimulation of parasympathetic nervous system, striated muscle,
sympathetic ganglia, and CNS.*

methanol [Methyl alcohol] *Respiratory
failure, circulatory collapse.*

methapyrilene [Poison] *Cardiovascular collapse, pulmonary edema, CNS
depression, coma, seizures, nausea,
vomiting, cardiopulmonary arrest.*

methenamine [Aldehyde] *Seizures,
respiratory failure, pulmonary edema.*

methidathion [Organophosphate] *Pulmonary edema, respiratory muscle
paralysis, respiratory failure, bradycardia, acetylcholinesterase inhibition,
hypotension, pulmonary edema, overstimulation of parasympathetic nervous
system, striated muscle, sympathetic
ganglia, and CNS.*

methiocarb [Carbamate] *Acetylcholinesterase inhibition (reversible), bradycardia,
hypotension, respiratory muscle paralysis, respiratory arrest, pulmonary edema.*

methomyl [Carbamate] *Acetylcholinesterase inhibition (reversible), bradycardia,
hypotension, respiratory muscle paralysis, respiratory arrest, pulmonary edema.*

methoxychlor [Aldrin/dieldrin/
endrin] *Seizures, respiratory failure.*

2-methoxyethanol [Ethylene glycol]
*Respiratory failure, pulmonary edema,
paralysis, cardiovascular collapse,
severe acidosis.*

methoxyethylmercuric acetate
[Mercury] *Circulatory collapse,*
*arrhythmias, respiratory failure, pulmo-
nary edema, neurotoxic effects.*

methoxyethylmercuric chloride
[Mercury] *Circulatory collapse,
arrhythmias, respiratory failure, pulmonary edema, neurotoxic effects.*

methoxymethyl isocyanate [Isocya-
nate/aliphatic thiocyanate] *CNS
depression, respiratory arrest, respiratory paralysis, pulmonary edema, cyanide toxicity.*

methoxymethylpentanone [Ali-
phatic hydrocarbon] *Arrhythmias,
asphyxiation, anesthesia.* [Simple
asphyxiant] *Asphyxiation.*

4-methoxyphenol [Phenol] *Coma,
hypotension, arrhythmias, pulmonary
edema, respiratory arrest.*

1-methoxy-2-propanol [Ethylene
glycol] *Respiratory failure, pulmonary
edema, paralysis, cardiovascular collapse, severe acidosis.*

methyl acetate [Methyl alcohol] *Respiratory failure, circulatory collapse.*

methyl acetone [Ketone] *Respiratory
mucous membrane irritation, pulmonary edema, CNS depression.*

**methyl acetylene & propadiene
mixture** [Hydrocarbon mixture]
*CNS depression, respiratory arrest, sei-
zures, arrhythmias, pulmonary edema.*

methyl acrylonitrile [Cyanide]
*Impairment of cellular oxygenation and
adenosine triphosphate production,
hypoxia, death.*

methyl alcohol [Methyl alcohol] *Respiratory failure, circulatory collapse.*

methyl allyl chloride [Dichloropro-
pane/dichloropropene] *Pulmonary
edema, bronchospasm, alveolar hemorrhage.*

methyl aluminum sesquibromide
[Bromine/methyl bromide] *Severe
respiratory irritation, pulmonary
edema, respiratory failure, coma, convulsions, death.*

methyl aluminum sesquichloride
[Chlorine] *Severe respiratory tract irritation, pulmonary edema, irritation of
skin, eyes, and mucous membranes.*

HazMat

methyl amyl acetate [Ester] *CNS depression, respiratory tract irritation, bronchitis, pneumonitis.*

methyl amyl alcohol [Higher alcohol (4+ carbons)] *CNS depression, respiratory failure, arrhythmias.*

methyl amyl ketone [Ketone] *Respiratory mucous membrane irritation, pulmonary edema, CNS depression.*

2-methyl aziridine [Organic base/amine] *Pulmonary edema, cardiac depression, seizures.*

methyl benzoate [Organic acid] *Pulmonary edema, circulatory collapse, laryngeal edema and spasm, severe chemical burns to skin, mucous membranes, and internal organs, GI tract perforation and hemorrhage, peritonitis.*

methyl bromide [Bromine/methyl bromide] *Severe respiratory irritation, pulmonary edema, respiratory failure, coma, convulsions, death.*

methyl bromide & chloropicrin mixture [Halogenated aliphatic hydrocarbon] *CNS depression, respiratory arrest, circulatory collapse.* [Bromine/methyl bromide] *Severe respiratory irritation, pulmonary edema, respiratory failure, coma, convulsions, death.*

methyl bromide & ethylene dibromide mixture [Bromine/methyl bromide] *Severe respiratory irritation, pulmonary edema, respiratory failure, coma, convulsions, death.*

methyl bromide & nonflammable compressed gas mixture [Bromine/methyl bromide] *Severe respiratory irritation, pulmonary edema, respiratory failure, coma, convulsions, death.*

methyl bromoacetate [Bromine/methyl bromide] *Severe respiratory irritation, pulmonary edema, respiratory failure, coma, convulsions, death.*

methyl butanone [Ketone] *Respiratory mucous membrane irritation, pulmonary edema, CNS depression.*

methyl tert-butyl ether (MTBE) [Ether] *Anesthesia, respiratory arrest.*

methyl n-butyl ketone [Ketone] *Respiratory mucous membrane irritation, pulmonary edema, CNS depression.*

methyl butyrate [Ester] *CNS depression, respiratory tract irritation, bronchitis, pneumonitis.*

Methyl Cellosolve Acetate [Ethylene glycol] *Respiratory failure, pulmonary edema, paralysis, cardiovascular collapse, severe acidosis.*

methyl chloride [Halogenated aliphatic hydrocarbon] *CNS depression, respiratory arrest, circulatory collapse.*

methyl chloride & chloropicrin mixture [Irritant] *Severe immediate or delayed upper airway or respiratory tract irritation, pulmonary edema, glottic spasm, airway obstruction.* [Halogenated aliphatic hydrocarbon] *CNS depression, respiratory arrest, circulatory collapse.*

methyl chloride & methylene chloride mixture [Halogenated aliphatic hydrocarbon] *CNS depression, respiratory arrest, circulatory collapse.* [Carbon monoxide] *Impairment of cellular oxygenation, hypoxia, death.*

methyl chloroacetate [Ester] *CNS depression, respiratory tract irritation, bronchitis, pneumonitis.*

methyl 2-chloroacrylate [Ester] *CNS depression, respiratory tract irritation, bronchitis, pneumonitis.*

methyl chlorocarbonate [Halogenated aliphatic hydrocarbon] *CNS depression, respiratory arrest, circulatory collapse.*

methyl chloroform [Halogenated aliphatic hydrocarbon] *CNS depression, respiratory arrest, circulatory collapse.*

methyl chloroformate [Halogenated aliphatic hydrocarbon] *CNS depression, respiratory arrest, circulatory collapse.*

methyl chloromethyl ether [Halogenated aliphatic hydrocarbon] *CNS depression, respiratory arrest, circulatory collapse.* [Ether] *Anesthesia, respiratory arrest.*

methyl chloropropionate [Halogenated aliphatic hydrocarbon] *CNS depression, respiratory arrest, circulatory collapse.*

methyl cyanide [Cyanide] *Impairment of cellular oxygenation and adenosine triphosphate production, hypoxia, death.*

methyl cyclohexanone peroxide [Organic peroxide] *Pulmonary and laryngeal edema, circulatory arrest, hypovolemic shock, chemical burns to skin, mucous membranes, and internal organs.* [Ketone] *Respiratory mucous membrane irritation, pulmonary edema, CNS depression.* [Corrosive] *Upper airway burns and edema, circulatory collapse, severe chemical burns to skin, toxic systemic effects, GI tract perforation and hemorrhage, peritonitis.*

methyl cyclopentane [Aliphatic hydrocarbon] *Arrhythmias, asphyxiation, anesthesia.*

methyl demeton [Organophosphate] *Pulmonary edema, respiratory muscle paralysis, respiratory failure, bradycardia, acetylcholinesterase inhibition, hypotension, pulmonary edema, overstimulation of parasympathetic nervous system, striated muscle, sympathetic ganglia, and CNS.*

methyl dichloroacetate [Ester] *CNS depression, respiratory tract irritation, bronchitis, pneumonitis.*

methyl dichloroarsine [Arsine] *Intravascular hemolysis, pulmonary edema, cardiac and respiratory arrest, delayed-onset jaundice, and acute or delayed-onset renal failure.*

methyl dichlorosilane [Silane/chlorosilane] *Respiratory tract irritation, pulmonary edema.*

methyl ethyl ether [Ether] *Anesthesia, respiratory arrest.*

methyl ethyl ketone [Ketone] *Respiratory mucous membrane irritation, pulmonary edema, CNS depression.*

methyl ethyl ketone peroxide [Organic peroxide] *Pulmonary and laryngeal edema, circulatory arrest, hypovolemic shock, chemical burns to skin, mucous membranes, and internal organs.* [Ketone] *Respiratory mucous membrane irritation, pulmonary edema, CNS depression.* [Corrosive] *Upper airway burns and edema, circulatory collapse, severe chemical burns to skin, toxic systemic effects, GI tract perforation and hemorrhage, peritonitis.*

methyl ethyl pyridine; 2-methyl-5-ethyl pyridine [Aromatic hydrocarbon] *Arrhythmias, respiratory failure, pulmonary edema, paralysis, brain and kidney damage.*

methyl fluoride [Chlorinated fluorocarbon] *Asphyxiation, anesthesia, arrhythmias.*

methyl fluoroacetete [Monofluoroacetate] *Ventricular arrhythmias, seizures.*

methyl fluorosulfate [Halogenated aliphatic hydrocarbon] *CNS depression, respiratory arrest, circulatory collapse.*

methyl formate [Methyl alcohol] *Respiratory failure, circulatory collapse.*

methyl iodide [Pyrethrin/pyrethroid] *Respiratory paralysis, convulsions.*

methyl isoamyl ketone [Ketone] *Respiratory mucous membrane irritation, pulmonary edema, CNS depression.*

methyl isobutyl carbinol [Higher alcohol (4+ carbons)] *CNS depression, respiratory failure, arrhythmias.*

methyl isobutyl ketone [Ketone] *Respiratory mucous membrane irritation, pulmonary edema, CNS depression.*

methyl isobutyl ketone peroxide [Organic peroxide] *Pulmonary and laryngeal edema, circulatory arrest, hypovolemic shock, chemical burns to skin, mucous membranes, and internal organs.* [Ketone] *Respiratory mucous membrane irritation, pulmonary edema, CNS depression.* [Corrosive] *Upper airway burns and edema, circulatory collapse, severe chemical burns to skin, toxic systemic effects, GI tract perforation and hemorrhage, peritonitis.*

methyl isocyanate [Isocyanate/aliphatic thiocyanate] *CNS depression, respiratory arrest, respiratory paralysis, pulmonary edema, cyanide toxicity.*

HazMat

methyl isopropenyl ketone [Ketone] *Respiratory mucous membrane irritation, pulmonary edema, CNS depression.*

methyl isopropyl ketone [Ketone] *Respiratory mucous membrane irritation, pulmonary edema, CNS depression.*

methyl isothiocyanate [Isocyanate/aliphatic thiocyanate] *CNS depression, respiratory arrest, respiratory paralysis, pulmonary edema, cyanide toxicity.*

methyl isovalerate [Ester] *CNS depression, respiratory tract irritation, bronchitis, pneumonitis.*

methyl magnesium bromide & ethyl ether mixture [Ether] *Anesthesia, respiratory arrest.* [Bromine/methyl bromide] *Severe respiratory irritation, pulmonary edema, respiratory failure, coma, convulsions, death.*

methyl mercaptan [Sulfur] *Respiratory tract irritation, pulmonary edema, anaphylaxis.*

methyl methacrylate [Ester] *CNS depression, respiratory tract irritation, bronchitis, pneumonitis.*

methyl naphthalene [Naphthalene] *Delayed-onset acute intravascular hemolysis.*

methyl nitrite [Nitrate/nitrite] *Methemoglobinemia, hypotension, circulatory collapse.*

methyl orthosilicate [Silane/chlorosilane] *Respiratory tract irritation, pulmonary edema.*

methyl parathion [Organophosphate] *Pulmonary edema, respiratory muscle paralysis, respiratory failure, bradycardia, acetylcholinesterase inhibition, hypotension, pulmonary edema, overstimulation of parasympathetic nervous system, striated muscle, sympathetic ganglia, and CNS.*

methyl parathion & compressed gas mixture [Organophosphate] *Pulmonary edema, respiratory muscle paralysis, respiratory failure, bradycardia, acetylcholinesterase inhibition, hypotension, pulmonary edema, overstimulation of parasympathetic nervous system, striated muscle, sympathetic ganglia, and CNS.*

methyl phenkapton [Organophosphate] *Pulmonary edema, respiratory muscle paralysis, respiratory failure, bradycardia, acetylcholinesterase inhibition, hypotension, pulmonary edema, overstimulation of parasympathetic nervous system, striated muscle, sympathetic ganglia, and CNS.*

methyl phosphonic dichloride [Phosphorus] *Hypovolemic shock, severe tissue burns, severe respiratory irritation, pulmonary edema, respiratory arrest, arrhythmias, sudden death.*

methyl phosphonothioic dichloride [Phosphorus] *Hypovolemic shock, severe tissue burns, severe respiratory irritation, pulmonary edema, respiratory arrest, arrhythmias, sudden death.*

methyl phosphonous dichloride [Phosphorus] *Hypovolemic shock, severe tissue burns, severe respiratory irritation, pulmonary edema, respiratory arrest, arrhythmias, sudden death.*

methyl propionate [Ester] *CNS depression, respiratory tract irritation, bronchitis, pneumonitis.*

methyl propyl benzene [Aromatic hydrocarbon] *Arrhythmias, respiratory failure, pulmonary edema, paralysis, brain and kidney damage.*

methyl propyl ether [Ether] *Anesthesia, respiratory arrest.*

methyl propyl ketone [Ketone] *Respiratory mucous membrane irritation, pulmonary edema, CNS depression.*

methyl silicate [Silane/chlorosilane] *Respiratory tract irritation, pulmonary edema.*

methyl styrene [Aromatic hydrocarbon] *Arrhythmias, respiratory failure, pulmonary edema, paralysis, brain and kidney damage.*

methyl sulfate [Sulfur] *Respiratory tract irritation, pulmonary edema, anaphylaxis.*

methyl sulfide [Sulfur] *Respiratory tract irritation, pulmonary edema, anaphylaxis.*

methyl tetrahydrofuran [Ether] *Anesthesia, respiratory arrest.*

methyl thiocyanate [Isocyanate/aliphatic thiocyanate] *CNS depression, respiratory arrest, respiratory paralysis, pulmonary edema, cyanide toxicity.*

methyl trichloroacetate [Ester] *CNS depression, respiratory tract irritation, bronchitis, pneumonitis.*

methyl trichlorosilane [Silane/chlorosilane] *Respiratory tract irritation, pulmonary edema.*

Methyl Trithion [Organophosphate] *Pulmonary edema, respiratory muscle paralysis, respiratory failure, bradycardia, acetylcholinesterase inhibition, hypotension, pulmonary edema, overstimulation of parasympathetic nervous system, striated muscle, sympathetic ganglia, and CNS.*

methyl valeraldehyde [Organophosphate] *Pulmonary edema, respiratory muscle paralysis, respiratory failure, bradycardia, acetylcholinesterase inhibition, hypotension, pulmonary edema, overstimulation of parasympathetic nervous system, striated muscle, sympathetic ganglia, and CNS.*

methyl vinyl ketone [Ketone] *Respiratory mucous membrane irritation, pulmonary edema, CNS depression.*

methylacrylate [Ester] *CNS depression, respiratory tract irritation, bronchitis, pneumonitis.*

methylal [Ether] *Anesthesia, respiratory arrest.*

methylamine [Organic base/amine] *Pulmonary edema, cardiac depression, seizures.*

p-methylaminophenol sulfate [Aniline] *Methemoglobinemia, hypoxia.* [Phenol] *Coma, hypotension, arrhythmias, pulmonary edema, respiratory arrest.*

methylaniline [Aniline] *Methemoglobinemia, hypoxia.*

methylbenzyl alcohol [Higher alcohol (4+ carbons)] *CNS depression, respiratory failure, arrhythmias.*

methylbutene; 2-methyl-1-butene; 2-methyl-2-butene; 3-methyl-1-butene [Aliphatic hydrocarbon] *Arrhythmias, asphyxiation, anesthesia.*

methyl-*tert*-butyl ether [Ether] *Anesthesia, respiratory arrest.*

methylbutylamine [Organic base/amine] *Pulmonary edema, cardiac depression, seizures.*

4-(2-methyl-4-chlorophenoxy) butyric acid [Chlorophenoxy herbicide] *CNS depression, CNS stimulation, respiratory failure, ventricular fibrillation, seizures.*

methylchlorosilane [Silane/chlorosilane] *Respiratory tract irritation, pulmonary edema.*

3-methylcholanthrene [Aromatic hydrocarbon] *Arrhythmias, respiratory failure, pulmonary edema, paralysis, brain and kidney damage.*

methylcyclohexane [Aliphatic hydrocarbon] *Arrhythmias, asphyxiation, anesthesia.*

methylcyclohexanol [Higher alcohol (4+ carbons)] *CNS depression, respiratory failure, arrhythmias.*

2-methylcyclohexanone [Ketone] *Respiratory mucous membrane irritation, pulmonary edema, CNS depression.*

4,4′-methylene bis(2-chloroaniline) [Aniline] *Methemoglobinemia, hypoxia.*

4,4′-methylene bis(N,N-dimethyl) benzenamine [Poison] *Cardiovascular collapse, pulmonary edema, CNS depression, coma, seizures, nausea, vomiting, cardiopulmonary arrest.*

methylene bis(4-phenyl isocyanate) (MDI) [Isocyanate/aliphatic thiocyanate] *CNS depression, respiratory arrest, respiratory paralysis, pulmonary edema, cyanide toxicity.*

methylene bromide [Bromine/methyl bromide] *Severe respiratory irritation, pulmonary edema, respiratory failure, coma, convulsions, death.*

methylene chloride [Halogenated aliphatic hydrocarbon] *CNS depression, respiratory arrest, circulatory col-*

lapse. [Carbon monoxide] *Impairment of cellular oxygenation, hypoxia, death.*

methylene chloride & methyl chloride mixture [Halogenated aliphatic hydrocarbon] *CNS depression, respiratory arrest, circulatory collapse.* [Carbon monoxide] *Impairment of cellular oxygenation, hypoxia, death.*

methylene iodide [Iodine] *Hypotension, circulatory collapse, pulmonary edema.*

4,4′-methylenedianiline [Aniline] *Methemoglobinemia, hypoxia.*

methylfuran [Aliphatic hydrocarbon] *Arrhythmias, asphyxiation, anesthesia.*

5-methyl-3-heptanone [Ketone] *Respiratory mucous membrane irritation, pulmonary edema, CNS depression.*

methylhexanone [Ketone] *Respiratory mucous membrane irritation, pulmonary edema, CNS depression.*

methylhydrazine [Hydrazine] *Seizures, hemolysis of red blood cells, pulmonary edema.*

methylmercuric dicyanamide [Mercury] *Circulatory collapse, arrhythmias, respiratory failure, pulmonary edema, neurotoxic effects.*

methylmorpholine [Organic base/amine] *Pulmonary edema, cardiac depression, seizures.*

methylpentadiene [Aliphatic hydrocarbon] *Arrhythmias, asphyxiation, anesthesia.*

methylpentane [Aliphatic hydrocarbon] *Arrhythmias, asphyxiation, anesthesia.*

methylpentanol [Higher alcohol (4+ carbons)] *CNS depression, respiratory failure, arrhythmias.*

methylphenyldichlorosilane [Silane/chlorosilane] *Respiratory tract irritation, pulmonary edema.*

methylphosphonic difluoride [Phosphorus] *Hypovolemic shock, severe tissue burns, severe respiratory irritation, pulmonary edema, respiratory arrest, arrhythmias, sudden death.*

methylpiperidine [Organic base/amine] *Pulmonary edema, cardiac depression, seizures.*

α-methylstyrene; alpha-methylstyrene [Aromatic hydrocarbon] *Arrhythmias, respiratory failure, pulmonary edema, paralysis, brain and kidney damage.*

methylthiouracil [Poison] *Cardiovascular collapse, pulmonary edema, CNS depression, coma, seizures, nausea, vomiting, cardiopulmonary arrest.*

metolcarb [Carbamate] *Acetylcholinesterase inhibition (reversible), bradycardia, hypotension, respiratory muscle paralysis, respiratory arrest, pulmonary edema.*

mevinphos [Organophosphate] *Pulmonary edema, respiratory muscle paralysis, respiratory failure, bradycardia, acetylcholinesterase inhibition, hypotension, pulmonary edema, overstimulation of parasympathetic nervous system, striated muscle, sympathetic ganglia, and CNS.*

mexacarbate [Carbamate] *Acetylcholinesterase inhibition (reversible), bradycardia, hypotension, respiratory muscle paralysis, respiratory arrest, pulmonary edema.*

MGK 264 [Poison] *Cardiovascular collapse, pulmonary edema, CNS depression, coma, seizures, nausea, vomiting, cardiopulmonary arrest.*

MIBC [Higher alcohol (4+ carbons)] *CNS depression, respiratory failure, arrhythmias.*

Michler's ketone [Ketone] *Respiratory mucous membrane irritation, pulmonary edema, CNS depression.*

mineral seal oil [Hydrocarbon mixture] *CNS depression, respiratory arrest, seizures, arrhythmias, pulmonary edema.*

mineral spirits [Hydrocarbon mixture] *CNS depression, respiratory arrest, seizures, arrhythmias, pulmonary edema.*

mining reagent [Hydrocarbon mixture] *CNS depression, respiratory arrest, seizures, arrhythmias, pulmonary edema.*

mintezol [Thiabendazole] *Cardiovascular collapse, respiratory tract irritation.*

mipafox [Organophosphate] *Pulmonary edema, respiratory muscle paralysis, respiratory failure, bradycardia, acetylcholinesterase inhibition, hypotension, pulmonary edema, overstimulation of parasympathetic nervous system, striated muscle, sympathetic ganglia, and CNS.*

mirex [Lindane] *CNS stimulation, seizures, respiratory failure.*

misch metal (powder) [Flammable solid] *Shock, severe chemical and thermal burns, severe respiratory tract irritation, pulmonary edema, respiratory arrest, ECG changes, sudden death.* [Poison] *Cardiovascular collapse, pulmonary edema, CNS depression, coma, seizures, nausea, vomiting, cardiopulmonary arrest.*

mitomycin C [Poison] *Cardiovascular collapse, pulmonary edema, CNS depression, coma, seizures, nausea, vomiting, cardiopulmonary arrest.*

mixed acids (n.o.s.) [Inorganic acid] *Pulmonary edema, bronchospasm, circulatory collapse, laryngeal spasm and edema, severe chemical burns to skin, mucous membranes, and internal organs, GI tract perforation and hemorrhage, peritonitis.*

Moban [Carbamate] *Acetylcholinesterase inhibition (reversible), bradycardia, hypotension, respiratory muscle paralysis, respiratory arrest, pulmonary edema.*

MOCA [Aniline] *Methemoglobinemia, hypoxia.*

molybdenum disulfide [Poison] *Cardiovascular collapse, pulmonary edema, CNS depression, coma, seizures, nausea, vomiting, cardiopulmonary arrest.*

molybdenum pentachloride [Poison] *Cardiovascular collapse, pulmonary edema, CNS depression, coma, seizures, nausea, vomiting, cardiopulmonary arrest.*

molybdenum trioxide [Poison] *Cardiovascular collapse, pulmonary edema, CNS depression, coma, sei-zures, nausea, vomiting, cardiopulmonary arrest.*

Monitor [Organophosphate] *Pulmonary edema, respiratory muscle paralysis, respiratory failure, bradycardia, acetylcholinesterase inhibition, hypotension, pulmonary edema, overstimulation of parasympathetic nervous system, striated muscle, sympathetic ganglia, and CNS.*

monobromotrifluoromethane [Chlorinated fluorocarbon] *Asphyxiation, anesthesia, arrhythmias.*

monochloroacetic acid [Organic acid] *Pulmonary edema, circulatory collapse, laryngeal edema and spasm, severe chemical burns to skin, mucous membranes, and internal organs, GI tract perforation and hemorrhage, peritonitis.*

monochloroacetone [Ketone] *Respiratory mucous membrane irritation, pulmonary edema, CNS depression.*

monochloroethylene [Halogenated aliphatic hydrocarbon] *CNS depression, respiratory arrest, circulatory collapse.*

monochloropentafluorethane [Chlorinated fluorocarbon] *Asphyxiation, anesthesia, arrhythmias.*

monochlorotetrafluoroethane [Chlorinated fluorocarbon] *Asphyxiation, anesthesia, arrhythmias.*

monochlorotrifluoromethane [Chlorinated fluorocarbon] *Asphyxiation, anesthesia, arrhythmias.*

monocrotophos [Organophosphate] *Pulmonary edema, respiratory muscle paralysis, respiratory failure, bradycardia, acetylcholinesterase inhibition, hypotension, pulmonary edema, overstimulation of parasympathetic nervous system, striated muscle, sympathetic ganglia, and CNS.*

monoethanolamine [Organic base/amine] *Pulmonary edema, cardiac depression, seizures.*

monoethylamine [Organic base/amine] *Pulmonary edema, cardiac depression, seizures.*

HazMat

monofluorophosphoric acid [Inorganic acid] *Pulmonary edema, bronchospasm, circulatory collapse, laryngeal spasm and edema, severe chemical burns to skin, mucous membranes, and internal organs, GI tract perforation and hemorrhage, peritonitis.*

monomethylamine [Organic base/amine] *Pulmonary edema, cardiac depression, seizures.*

monomethylhydrazine [Hydrazine] *Seizures, hemolysis of red blood cells, pulmonary edema.*

monopropylamine [Organic base/amine] *Pulmonary edema, cardiac depression, seizures.*

mono-(trichloro)-tetra-(monopotassium dichloro)-penta-S-triazetrione [Irritant] *Severe immediate or delayed upper airway or respiratory tract irritation, pulmonary edema, glottic spasm, airway obstruction.*

morpholine; morpholine mixture (n.o.s.) [Organic base/amine] *Pulmonary edema, cardiac depression, seizures.*

motion picture film, nitrocellulose-based [Flammable solid] *Shock, severe chemical and thermal burns, severe respiratory tract irritation, pulmonary edema, respiratory arrest, ECG changes, sudden death.*

motor fuel (n.o.s.) [Hydrocarbon mixture] *CNS depression, respiratory arrest, seizures, arrhythmias, pulmonary edema.*

motor fuel anti-knock compound [Hydrocarbon mixture] *CNS depression, respiratory arrest, seizures, arrhythmias, pulmonary edema.* [Lead] *Circulatory collapse, coma, rare seizures.*

motor spirit [Hydrocarbon mixture] *CNS depression, respiratory arrest, seizures, arrhythmias, pulmonary edema.*

MPMC [Carbamate] *Acetylcholinesterase inhibition (reversible), bradycardia, hypotension, respiratory muscle paralysis, respiratory arrest, pulmonary edema.*

MTBE (methyl *tert*-butyl ether) [Ether] *Anesthesia, respiratory arrest.*

muriatic acid [Inorganic acid] *Pulmonary edema, bronchospasm, circulatory collapse, laryngeal spasm and edema, severe chemical burns to skin, mucous membranes, and internal organs, GI tract perforation and hemorrhage, peritonitis.*

muscimol [Poison] *Cardiovascular collapse, pulmonary edema, CNS depression, coma, seizures, nausea, vomiting, cardiopulmonary arrest.*

musk xylene [Aromatic hydrocarbon] *Arrhythmias, respiratory failure, pulmonary edema, paralysis, brain and kidney damage.*

mustard gas [Sulfur] *Respiratory tract irritation, pulmonary edema, anaphylaxis.*

nabam [Dithiocarbamate] *Hypotension, respiratory failure.*

naled [Organophosphate] *Pulmonary edema, respiratory muscle paralysis, respiratory failure, bradycardia, acetylcholinesterase inhibition, hypotension, pulmonary edema, overstimulation of parasympathetic nervous system, striated muscle, sympathetic ganglia, and CNS.*

naphtha [Hydrocarbon mixture] *CNS depression, respiratory arrest, seizures, arrhythmias, pulmonary edema.* [Naphthalene] *Delayed-onset acute intravascular hemolysis.*

naphtha solvent, aromatic [Naphthalene] *Delayed-onset acute intravascular hemolysis.*

naphthalene [Naphthalene] *Delayed-onset acute intravascular hemolysis.*

naphthalene, chlorinated [Naphthalene] *Delayed-onset acute intravascular hemolysis.*

naphthenic acid [Organic acid] *Pulmonary edema, circulatory collapse, laryngeal edema and spasm, severe chemical burns to skin, mucous membranes, and internal organs, GI tract perforation and hemorrhage, peritonitis.*

β-naphthol; beta-naphthol [Phenol] *Coma, hypotension, arrhythmias, pulmonary edema, respiratory arrest.*

1,4-naphthoquinone [Phenol] *Coma, hypotension, arrhythmias, pulmonary edema, respiratory arrest.*

naphthylamine (alpha or beta) [Organic base/amine] *Pulmonary edema, cardiac depression, seizures.*

α-naphthylthiourea [Naphthalene] *Delayed-onset acute intravascular hemolysis.*

naphthylurea [Naphthalene] *Delayed-onset acute intravascular hemolysis.*

natural gas (gas or cryogenic liquid) [Aliphatic hydrocarbon] *Arrhythmias, asphyxiation, anesthesia.* [Simple asphyxiant] *Asphyxiation.*

natural gasoline [Hydrocarbon mixture] *CNS depression, respiratory arrest, seizures, arrhythmias, pulmonary edema.*

Navadel [Organophosphate] *Pulmonary edema, respiratory muscle paralysis, respiratory failure, bradycardia, acetylcholinesterase inhibition, hypotension, pulmonary edema, overstimulation of parasympathetic nervous system, striated muscle, sympathetic ganglia, and CNS.*

neohexane [Aliphatic hydrocarbon] *Arrhythmias, asphyxiation, anesthesia.*

neon (gas or cryogenic liquid) [Simple asphyxiant] *Asphyxiation.*

neopentane [Aliphatic hydrocarbon] *Arrhythmias, asphyxiation, anesthesia.*

Neotran [Chlorophenoxy herbicide] *CNS depression, CNS stimulation, respiratory failure, ventricular fibrillation, seizures.*

nickel; soluble nickel mixture (n.o.s.) [Nickel] *Respiratory failure, cerebral edema, allergic reactions.*

nickel ammonium sulfate [Nickel] *Respiratory failure, cerebral edema, allergic reactions.*

nickel carbonyl [Nickel] *Respiratory failure, cerebral edema, allergic reactions.*

nickel catalyst [Nickel] *Respiratory failure, cerebral edema, allergic reactions.*

nickel chloride [Nickel] *Respiratory failure, cerebral edema, allergic reactions.*

nickel cyanide [Nickel] *Respiratory failure, cerebral edema, allergic reactions.* [Cyanide] *Impairment of cellular oxygenation and adenosine triphosphate production, hypoxia, death.*

nickel hydroxide [Nickel] *Respiratory failure, cerebral edema, allergic reactions.*

nickel nitrate [Nitrate/nitrite] *Methemoglobinemia, hypotension, circulatory collapse.* [Nickel] *Respiratory failure, cerebral edema, allergic reactions.*

nickel nitrite [Nitrate/nitrite] *Methemoglobinemia, hypotension, circulatory collapse.* [Nickel] *Respiratory failure, cerebral edema, allergic reactions.*

nickel sulfate [Nickel] *Respiratory failure, cerebral edema, allergic reactions.*

nicotine; nicotine mixture (n.o.s.) [Nicotine] *Respiratory and cardiac arrest, CNS stimulation, CNS depression.*

nicotine HCl; nicotine HCl mixture (n.o.s.) [Nicotine] *Respiratory and cardiac arrest, CNS stimulation, CNS depression.*

nicotine salicylate [Nicotine] *Respiratory and cardiac arrest, CNS stimulation, CNS depression.*

nicotine sulfate [Nicotine] *Respiratory and cardiac arrest, CNS stimulation, CNS depression.*

nicotine tartrate [Nicotine] *Respiratory and cardiac arrest, CNS stimulation, CNS depression.*

nitrate (n.o.s.); nitrate salt (n.o.s.) [Nitrate/nitrite] *Methemoglobinemia, hypotension, circulatory collapse.*

nitrate of sodium & potash mixture [Nitrate/nitrite] *Methemoglobinemia, hypotension, circulatory collapse.*

nitrating acid; nitrating acid mixture (n.o.s.) [Nitrate/nitrite] *Methemoglobinemia, hypotension, circulatory collapse.*

nitric acid [Inorganic acid] *Pulmonary edema, bronchospasm, circulatory collapse, laryngeal spasm and edema, severe chemical burns to skin, mucous membranes, and internal organs, GI tract perforation and hemorrhage, peritonitis.*

nitric oxide [Nitrogen oxide] *Lower respiratory tract symptoms, pulmonary edema, laryngospasm, bronchospasm, asphyxiation.*

nitric oxide & dinitrogen tetroxide mixture [Nitrogen oxide] *Lower respiratory tract symptoms, pulmonary edema, laryngospasm, bronchospasm, asphyxiation.*

nitric oxide & nitrogen dioxide mixture [Nitrogen oxide] *Lower respiratory tract symptoms, pulmonary edema, laryngospasm, bronchospasm, asphyxiation.*

nitric oxide & nitrogen tetroxide mixture [Nitrogen oxide] *Lower respiratory tract symptoms, pulmonary edema, laryngospasm, bronchospasm, asphyxiation.*

nitrilotriacetic acid [Organic acid] *Pulmonary edema, circulatory collapse, laryngeal edema and spasm, severe chemical burns to skin, mucous membranes, and internal organs, GI tract perforation and hemorrhage, peritonitis.*

nitrite (n.o.s.) [Nitrate/nitrite] *Methemoglobinemia, hypotension, circulatory collapse.*

nitro mixture (n.o.s.) [Nitrate/nitrite] *Methemoglobinemia, hypotension, circulatory collapse.*

***p*-nitroaniline** [Aniline] *Methemoglobinemia, hypoxia.*

nitroanisole [Aromatic hydrocarbon] *Arrhythmias, respiratory failure, pulmonary edema, paralysis, brain and kidney damage.* [Nitrate/nitrite] *Methemoglobinemia, hypotension, circulatory collapse.*

nitrobenzene [Aromatic hydrocarbon] *Arrhythmias, respiratory failure, pulmonary edema, paralysis, brain and kidney damage.* [Nitrate/nitrite] *Methemoglobinemia, hypotension, circulatory collapse.*

nitrobenzenesulfonic acid [Organic acid] *Pulmonary edema, circulatory collapse, laryngeal edema and spasm, severe chemical burns to skin, mucous membranes, and internal organs, GI tract perforation and hemorrhage, peritonitis.*

nitrobenzotrifluoride [Aromatic hydrocarbon] *Arrhythmias, respiratory failure, pulmonary edema, paralysis, brain and kidney damage.* [Nitrate/nitrite] *Methemoglobinemia, hypotension, circulatory collapse.*

4-nitrobiphenyl [Phenol] *Coma, hypotension, arrhythmias, pulmonary edema, respiratory arrest.* [Nitrate/nitrite] *Methemoglobinemia, hypotension, circulatory collapse.*

nitrobromobenzene [Nitrate/nitrite] *Methemoglobinemia, hypotension, circulatory collapse.* [Bromine/methyl bromide] *Severe respiratory irritation, pulmonary edema, respiratory failure, coma, convulsions, death.*

nitrocellulose [Flammable/combustible liquid] *CNS depression, respiratory arrest, convulsions, arrhythmias, pulmonary edema.*

nitrocellulose, with plasticizing substance [Flammable solid] *Shock, severe chemical and thermal burns, severe respiratory tract irritation, pulmonary edema, respiratory arrest, ECG changes, sudden death.* [Poison] *Cardiovascular collapse, pulmonary edema, CNS depression, coma, seizures, nausea, vomiting, cardiopulmonary arrest.*

nitrocellulose, with 20%+ water [Flammable solid] *Shock, severe chemical and thermal burns, severe respiratory tract irritation, pulmonary edema, respiratory arrest, ECG changes, sudden death.*

nitrochlorobenzene; O-nitrochlorobenzene; *p*-nitrochlorobenzene [Aromatic hydrocarbon] *Arrhythmias, respiratory failure, pulmonary edema, paralysis, brain and kidney damage.* [Nitrate/nitrite] *Methemoglobinemia, hypotension, circulatory collapse.*

nitrochlorobenzotrifluoride [Aromatic hydrocarbon] *Arrhythmias, respiratory failure, pulmonary edema, paralysis, brain and kidney damage.*

[Nitrate/nitrite] *Methemoglobinemia, hypotension, circulatory collapse.*

nitrocresol [Phenol] *Coma, hypotension, arrhythmias, pulmonary edema, respiratory arrest.* [Nitrate/nitrite] *Methemoglobinemia, hypotension, circulatory collapse.*

nitrocyclohexane [Aliphatic hydrocarbon] *Arrhythmias, asphyxiation, anesthesia.* [Nitrate/nitrite] *Methemoglobinemia, hypotension, circulatory collapse.*

nitroethane [Aliphatic hydrocarbon] *Arrhythmias, asphyxiation, anesthesia.* [Nitrate/nitrite] *Methemoglobinemia, hypotension, circulatory collapse.*

nitrofen [Aromatic hydrocarbon] *Arrhythmias, respiratory failure, pulmonary edema, paralysis, brain and kidney damage.* [Nitrate/nitrite] *Methemoglobinemia, hypotension, circulatory collapse.*

nitrogen (gas or cryogenic liquid) [Simple asphyxiant] *Asphyxiation.*

nitrogen compound, aromatic [Aniline] *Methemoglobinemia, hypoxia.*

nitrogen dioxide [Nitrogen oxide] *Lower respiratory tract symptoms, pulmonary edema, laryngospasm, bronchospasm, asphyxiation.*

nitrogen dioxide & nitric oxide mixture [Nitrogen oxide] *Lower respiratory tract symptoms, pulmonary edema, laryngospasm, bronchospasm, asphyxiation.*

nitrogen fluoride oxide [Nitrogen oxide] *Lower respiratory tract symptoms, pulmonary edema, laryngospasm, bronchospasm, asphyxiation.* [Fluorine] *CNS depression, respiratory arrest, cardiovascular collapse, shock, arrhythmias.*

nitrogen mustard [Organic base/amine] *Pulmonary edema, cardiac depression, seizures.*

nitrogen oxide (n.o.s.) [Nitrogen oxide] *Lower respiratory tract symptoms, pulmonary edema, laryngospasm, bronchospasm, asphyxiation.*

nitrogen oxide & ozone mixture [Nitrogen oxide] *Lower respiratory tract symptoms, pulmonary edema, laryngospasm, bronchospasm, asphyxiation.* [Ozone] *Pulmonary edema, airway obstruction.*

nitrogen peroxide [Nitrogen oxide] *Lower respiratory tract symptoms, pulmonary edema, laryngospasm, bronchospasm, asphyxiation.*

nitrogen & rare gas mixture [Poison] *Cardiovascular collapse, pulmonary edema, CNS depression, coma, seizures, nausea, vomiting, cardiopulmonary arrest.* [Simple asphyxiant] *Asphyxiation.*

nitrogen tetroxide [Nitrogen oxide] *Lower respiratory tract symptoms, pulmonary edema, laryngospasm, bronchospasm, asphyxiation.*

nitrogen tetroxide & nitric oxide mixture [Nitrogen oxide] *Lower respiratory tract symptoms, pulmonary edema, laryngospasm, bronchospasm, asphyxiation.*

nitrogen trifluoride [Fluorine] *CNS depression, respiratory arrest, cardiovascular collapse, shock, arrhythmias.*

nitrogen trioxide [Nitrogen oxide] *Lower respiratory tract symptoms, pulmonary edema, laryngospasm, bronchospasm, asphyxiation.*

nitroglycerin [Nitrate/nitrite] *Methemoglobinemia, hypotension, circulatory collapse.*

nitroglycerin in alcohol [Lower alcohol (1–3 carbons)] *CNS depression, coma, respiratory arrest, arrhythmias.* [Nitrate/nitrite] *Methemoglobinemia, hypotension, circulatory collapse.*

nitroguanidine [Dinitrophenol] *Respiratory and circulatory collapse, pulmonary edema, hyperthermia.*

nitrohydrochloric acid [Inorganic acid] *Pulmonary edema, bronchospasm, circulatory collapse, laryngeal spasm and edema, severe chemical burns to skin, mucous membranes, and internal organs, GI tract perforation and hemorrhage, peritonitis.*

nitroludine [Aromatic hydrocarbon] *Arrhythmias, respiratory failure, pul-*

monary edema, paralysis, brain and
kidney damage. [Nitrate/nitrite] Methemoglobinemia, hypotension, circulatory collapse.

nitromethane [Nitrate/nitrite] Methemoglobinemia, hypotension, circulatory
collapse.

nitromuriatic acid [Inorganic acid]
Pulmonary edema, bronchospasm, circulatory collapse, laryngeal spasm and
edema, severe chemical burns to skin,
mucous membranes, and internal
organs, GI tract perforation and hemorrhage, peritonitis.

nitronaphthalene [Naphthalene]
Delayed-onset acute intravascular
hemolysis.

N-nitro-N-methylurethane [Nitrate/
nitrite] Methemoglobinemia, hypotension, circulatory collapse. [Isocyanate/
aliphatic thiocyanate] CNS depression, respiratory arrest, respiratory paralysis, pulmonary edema, cyanide toxicity.

nitrophenol; p-nitrophenol [Dinitro-
phenol] Respiratory and circulatory collapse, pulmonary edema, hyperthermia.

nitropropane; 2-nitropropane
[Nitrate/nitrite] Methemoglobinemia,
hypotension, circulatory collapse.

nitroprusside salt (n.o.s.) [Cyanide]
Impairment of cellular oxygenation and
adenosine triphosphate production,
hypoxia, death.

N-nitrosodibutylamine [Organic
base/amine] Pulmonary edema, cardiac depression, seizures. [Nitrate/
nitrite] Methemoglobinemia, hypotension, circulatory collapse.

N-nitrosodiethanolamine [Organic
base/amine] Pulmonary edema, cardiac depression, seizures. [Nitrate/
nitrite] Methemoglobinemia, hypotension, circulatory collapse.

N-nitrosodiethylamine [Organic
base/amine] Pulmonary edema, cardiac depression, seizures. [Nitrate/
nitrite] Methemoglobinemia, hypotension, circulatory collapse.

**nitrosodimethylamine; N-nitrosodi-
methylamine** [Organic base/amine]

Pulmonary edema, cardiac depression,
seizures. [Nitrate/nitrite] Methemoglobinemia, hypotension, circulatory
collapse.

nitrosodimethylaniline [Aniline]
Methemoglobinemia, hypoxia.

**N-nitrosodiphenylamine; p-nitroso-
diphenylamine** [Organic base/
amine] Pulmonary edema, cardiac
depression, seizures. [Nitrate/nitrite]
Methemoglobinemia, hypotension, circulatory collapse.

N-nitrosodipropylamine [Organic
base/amine] Pulmonary edema, cardiac depression, seizures. [Nitrate/
nitrite] Methemoglobinemia, hypotension, circulatory collapse.

N-nitrosomethylvinylamine
[Organic base/amine] Pulmonary
edema, cardiac depression, seizures.
[Nitrate/nitrite] Methemoglobinemia,
hypotension, circulatory collapse.

N-nitrosomorpholine [Organic base/
amine] Pulmonary edema, cardiac
depression, seizures. [Nitrate/nitrite]
Methemoglobinemia, hypotension, circulatory collapse.

N-nitroso-N-ethylurea [Nitrate/
nitrite] Methemoglobinemia, hypotension, circulatory collapse. [Nitrogen
oxide] Lower respiratory tract symptoms, pulmonary edema, laryngospasm, bronchospasm, asphyxiation.

N-nitroso-N-methylurea [Nitrate/
nitrite] Methemoglobinemia, hypotension, circulatory collapse. [Nitrogen
oxide] Lower respiratory tract symptoms, pulmonary edema, laryngospasm, bronchospasm, asphyxiation.

N-nitrosonornicotine [Nicotine] Respiratory and cardiac arrest, CNS stimulation, CNS depression.

N-nitrosopiperidine [Nitrate/nitrite]
Methemoglobinemia, hypotension, circulatory collapse.

N-nitrosopyrrolidine [Nitrate/nitrite]
Methemoglobinemia, hypotension, circulatory collapse.

nitrostarch [Nitrate/nitrite] *Methemo-globinemia, hypotension, circulatory collapse.*

nitrosyl chloride [Inorganic acid] *Pulmonary edema, bronchospasm, circulatory collapse, laryngeal spasm and edema, severe chemical burns to skin, mucous membranes, and internal organs, GI tract perforation and hemorrhage, peritonitis.*

nitrosylsulfuric acid [Inorganic acid] *Pulmonary edema, bronchospasm, circulatory collapse, laryngeal spasm and edema, severe chemical burns to skin, mucous membranes, and internal organs, GI tract perforation and hemorrhage, peritonitis.*

nitrotoluene [Aromatic hydrocarbon] *Arrhythmias, respiratory failure, pulmonary edema, paralysis, brain and kidney damage.* [Nitrate/nitrite] *Methemoglobinemia, hypotension, circulatory collapse.*

nitrous oxide (gas or cryogenic liquid) [Nitrogen oxide] *Lower respiratory tract symptoms, pulmonary edema, laryngospasm, bronchospasm, asphyxiation.*

nitrous oxide & carbon dioxide mixture [Simple asphyxiant] *Asphyxiation.*

nitroxylene [Aromatic hydrocarbon] *Arrhythmias, respiratory failure, pulmonary edema, paralysis, brain and kidney damage.* [Nitrate/nitrite] *Methemoglobinemia, hypotension, circulatory collapse.*

nitroxylol [Phenol] *Coma, hypotension, arrhythmias, pulmonary edema, respiratory arrest.* [Nitrate/nitrite] *Methemoglobinemia, hypotension, circulatory collapse.*

nonane [Aliphatic hydrocarbon] *Arrhythmias, asphyxiation, anesthesia.*

nonflammable gas (n.o.s.) [Non-flammable gas] *Pulmonary edema, respiratory failure, asphyxiation.*

nonyl trichlorosilane [Silane/chlorosilane] *Respiratory tract irritation, pulmonary edema.*

norbornadiene [Aliphatic hydrocarbon] *Arrhythmias, asphyxiation, anesthesia.*

norbromide [Poison] *Cardiovascular collapse, pulmonary edema, CNS depression, coma, seizures, nausea, vomiting, cardiopulmonary arrest.*

normal propyl alcohol [Lower alcohol (1–3 carbons)] *CNS depression, coma, respiratory arrest, arrhythmias.*

nux vomica [Strychnine] *Convulsions, acidosis, diaphragmatic spasms, respiratory arrest.*

octachloronaphthalene [Naphthalene] *Delayed-onset acute intravascular hemolysis.*

octadecyl trichlorosilane [Silane/chlorosilane] *Respiratory tract irritation, pulmonary edema.*

octadiene [Aliphatic hydrocarbon] *Arrhythmias, asphyxiation, anesthesia.*

octafluorobutene [Halogenated aliphatic hydrocarbon] *CNS depression, respiratory arrest, circulatory collapse.*

octafluorocyclobutane [Halogenated aliphatic hydrocarbon] *CNS depression, respiratory arrest, circulatory collapse.*

octafluoropropane [Halogenated aliphatic hydrocarbon] *CNS depression, respiratory arrest, circulatory collapse.*

octamethyl diphosphoramide [Organophosphate] *Pulmonary edema, respiratory muscle paralysis, respiratory failure, bradycardia, acetylcholinesterase inhibition, hypotension, pulmonary edema, overstimulation of parasympathetic nervous system, striated muscle, sympathetic ganglia, and CNS.*

octamethyl pyrophosphoramide [Organophosphate] *Pulmonary edema, respiratory muscle paralysis, respiratory failure, bradycardia, acetylcholinesterase inhibition, hypotension, pulmonary edema, overstimulation of parasympathetic nervous system, striated muscle, sympathetic ganglia, and CNS.*

octane [Aliphatic hydrocarbon] *Arrhythmias, asphyxiation, anesthesia.*

HazMat

1-octanol [Higher alcohol (4+ carbons)] *CNS depression, respiratory failure, arrhythmias.*

octanoyl peroxide [Organic peroxide] *Pulmonary and laryngeal edema, circulatory arrest, hypovolemic shock, chemical burns to skin, mucous membranes, and internal organs.*

octyl aldehyde [Aldehyde] *Seizures, respiratory failure, pulmonary edema.*

octyl ammonium metharsonate [Arsenic] *Heavy metal toxicity, vomiting, GI bleeding, CNS depression, pulmonary edema, cardiac arrest.*

octyl cresols (n.o.s.) [Phenol] *Coma, hypotension, arrhythmias, pulmonary edema, respiratory arrest.*

***tert*-octyl hydroperoxide** [Organic peroxide] *Pulmonary and laryngeal edema, circulatory arrest, hypovolemic shock, chemical burns to skin, mucous membranes, and internal organs.*

***tert*-octyl mercaptan** [Sulfur] *Respiratory tract irritation, pulmonary edema, anaphylaxis.*

***tert*-octyl peroxy-2-ethylhexanoate** [Organic peroxide] *Pulmonary and laryngeal edema, circulatory arrest, hypovolemic shock, chemical burns to skin, mucous membranes, and internal organs.* [Organic acid] *Pulmonary edema, circulatory collapse, laryngeal edema and spasm, severe chemical burns to skin, mucous membranes, and internal organs, GI tract perforation and hemorrhage, peritonitis.*

octyl trichlorosilane [Silane/chlorosilane] *Respiratory tract irritation, pulmonary edema.*

oil, petroleum (n.o.s.) [Hydrocarbon mixture] *CNS depression, respiratory arrest, seizures, arrhythmias, pulmonary edema.*

oil gas [Hydrocarbon mixture] *CNS depression, respiratory arrest, seizures, arrhythmias, pulmonary edema.*

oleum [Inorganic acid] *Pulmonary edema, bronchospasm, circulatory collapse, laryngeal spasm and edema, severe chemical burns to skin, mucous membranes, and internal organs, GI tract perforation and hemorrhage, peritonitis.*

organic peroxide (n.o.s.); organic peroxide mixture (n.o.s.) [Organic peroxide] *Pulmonary and laryngeal edema, circulatory arrest, hypovolemic shock, chemical burns to skin, mucous membranes, and internal organs.*

organic peroxide, types B, C, D, E, and F [Organic peroxide] *Pulmonary and laryngeal edema, circulatory arrest, hypovolemic shock, chemical burns to skin, mucous membranes, and internal organs.*

organic phosphate compound (poison B) [Organophosphate] *Pulmonary edema, respiratory muscle paralysis, respiratory failure, bradycardia, acetylcholinesterase inhibition, hypotension, pulmonary edema, overstimulation of parasympathetic nervous system, striated muscle, sympathetic ganglia, and CNS.*

organic phosphorus compound & compressed gas mixture [Organophosphate] *Pulmonary edema, respiratory muscle paralysis, respiratory failure, bradycardia, acetylcholinesterase inhibition, hypotension, pulmonary edema, overstimulation of parasympathetic nervous system, striated muscle, sympathetic ganglia, and CNS.*

organic phosphorus pesticide (n.o.s.) [Organophosphate] *Pulmonary edema, respiratory muscle paralysis, respiratory failure, bradycardia, acetylcholinesterase inhibition, hypotension, pulmonary edema, overstimulation of parasympathetic nervous system, striated muscle, sympathetic ganglia, and CNS.*

organochlorine pesticide, liquid (n.o.s.) [Chlordane] *Respiratory failure, seizures, exhaustion, death.*

organochlorine pesticide, solid (n.o.s.) [Aldrin/dieldrin/endrin] *Seizures, respiratory failure.*

organomercury mixture (n.o.s.) [Mercury] *Circulatory collapse,* arrhythmias, *respiratory failure, pulmonary edema, neurotoxic effects.*

organophosphate (n.o.s.) [Organophosphate] *Pulmonary edema, respiratory muscle paralysis, respiratory failure, bradycardia, acetylcholinesterase inhibition, hypotension, pulmonary edema, overstimulation of parasympathetic nervous system, striated muscle, sympathetic ganglia, and CNS.*

organophosphorus pesticide (n.o.s.) [Organophosphate] *Pulmonary edema, respiratory muscle paralysis, respiratory failure, bradycardia, acetylcholinesterase inhibition, hypotension, pulmonary edema, overstimulation of parasympathetic nervous system, striated muscle, sympathetic ganglia, and CNS.*

organotin mixture (n.o.s.) [Organotin] *Respiratory failure, pulmonary edema, cerebral edema.*

organotin pesticide (n.o.s.) [Organotin] *Respiratory failure, pulmonary edema, cerebral edema.*

ORM-A (n.o.s.); ORM-B (n.o.s.); ORM-E (n.o.s.) [Poison] *Cardiovascular collapse, pulmonary edema, CNS depression, coma, seizures, nausea, vomiting, cardiopulmonary arrest.*

osmic acid [Inorganic acid] *Pulmonary edema, bronchospasm, circulatory collapse, laryngeal spasm and edema, severe chemical burns to skin, mucous membranes, and internal organs, GI tract perforation and hemorrhage, peritonitis.*

osmium; osmium mixture (n.o.s.) [Poison] *Cardiovascular collapse, pulmonary edema, CNS depression, coma, seizures, nausea, vomiting, cardiopulmonary arrest.*

osmium oxide [Poison] *Cardiovascular collapse, pulmonary edema, CNS depression, coma, seizures, nausea, vomiting, cardiopulmonary arrest.*

osmium tetroxide [Poison] *Cardiovascular collapse, pulmonary edema, CNS depression, coma, seizures, nausea, vomiting, cardiopulmonary arrest.*

ouabain [Poison] *Cardiovascular collapse, pulmonary edema, CNS depression, coma, seizures, nausea, vomiting, cardiopulmonary arrest.*

oxalate (n.o.s.) [Oxalate] *Cardiovascular collapse, arrhythmias, seizures.*

oxalic acid [Oxalate] *Cardiovascular collapse, arrhythmias, seizures.*

oxamyl [Carbamate] *Acetylcholinesterase inhibition (reversible), bradycardia, hypotension, respiratory muscle paralysis, respiratory arrest, pulmonary edema.*

oxetane [Ether] *Anesthesia, respiratory arrest.*

oxidizer (n.o.s.) [Oxidizer] *Pulmonary and laryngeal edema, circulatory arrest, hypovolemic shock, chemical burns of skin, mucous membranes, and internal organs.*

oxidizer, corrosive (n.o.s.) [Oxidizer] *Pulmonary and laryngeal edema, circulatory arrest, hypovolemic shock, chemical burns of skin, mucous membranes, and internal organs.* [Corrosive] *Upper airway burns and edema, circulatory collapse, severe chemical burns to skin, toxic systemic effects, GI tract perforation and hemorrhage, peritonitis.*

oxidizer, flammable solid (n.o.s.) [Flammable solid] *Shock, severe chemical and thermal burns, severe respiratory tract irritation, pulmonary edema, respiratory arrest, ECG changes, sudden death.* [Oxidizer] *Pulmonary and laryngeal edema, circulatory arrest, hypovolemic shock, chemical burns of skin, mucous membranes, and internal organs.*

oxidizer, poisonous (n.o.s.) [Oxidizer] *Pulmonary and laryngeal edema, circulatory arrest, hypovolemic shock, chemical burns of skin, mucous membranes, and internal organs.* [Poison] *Cardiovascular collapse, pulmonary edema, CNS depression, coma, seizures, nausea, vomiting, cardiopulmonary arrest.*

oxirane [Ethylene oxide] *Respiratory tract irritation, pulmonary edema.*

HazMat

oxydisulfoton [Organophosphate] *Pulmonary edema, respiratory muscle paralysis, respiratory failure, bradycardia, acetylcholinesterase inhibition, hypotension, pulmonary edema, overstimulation of parasympathetic nervous system, striated muscle, sympathetic ganglia, and CNS.*

oxygen (gas or cryogenic liquid) [Oxidizer] *Pulmonary and laryngeal edema, circulatory arrest, hypovolemic shock, chemical burns of skin, mucous membranes, and internal organs.*

oxygen & carbon dioxide mixture [Simple asphyxiant] *Asphyxiation.*

oxygen difluoride [Fluorine] *CNS depression, respiratory arrest, cardiovascular collapse, shock, arrhythmias.* [Ozone] *Pulmonary edema, airway obstruction.*

oxygen & helium mixture [Simple asphyxiant] *Asphyxiation.*

oxygen & rare gas mixture [Poison] *Cardiovascular collapse, pulmonary edema, CNS depression, coma, seizures, nausea, vomiting, cardiopulmonary arrest.* [Simple asphyxiant] *Asphyxiation.*

ozone (O₃) [Ozone] *Pulmonary edema, airway obstruction.*

ozone & cyclohexene mixture [Aliphatic hydrocarbon] *Arrhythmias, asphyxiation, anesthesia.* [Ozone] *Pulmonary edema, airway obstruction.*

ozone & nitrogen oxide mixture [Nitrogen oxide] *Lower respiratory tract symptoms, pulmonary edema, laryngospasm, bronchospasm, asphyxiation.* [Ozone] *Pulmonary edema, airway obstruction.*

ozone & sulfur dioxide mixture [Ozone] *Pulmonary edema, airway obstruction.* [Sulfur] *Respiratory tract irritation, pulmonary edema, anaphylaxis.*

paint and paint-related material, corrosive [Corrosive] *Upper airway burns and edema, circulatory collapse, severe chemical burns to skin, toxic systemic effects, GI tract perforation and hemorrhage, peritonitis.*

paint and paint-related material, flammable [Flammable/combustible liquid] *CNS depression, respiratory arrest, convulsions, arrhythmias, pulmonary edema.*

paint drier (n.o.s.) [Poison] *Cardiovascular collapse, pulmonary edema, CNS depression, coma, seizures, nausea, vomiting, cardiopulmonary arrest.*

paint eradicator [Flammable/combustible liquid] *CNS depression, respiratory arrest, convulsions, arrhythmias, pulmonary edema.*

paint stripper [Hydrocarbon mixture] *CNS depression, respiratory arrest, seizures, arrhythmias, pulmonary edema.*

painters' naphtha [Hydrocarbon mixture] *CNS depression, respiratory arrest, seizures, arrhythmias, pulmonary edema.*

paper, unsaturated oil–treated [Flammable solid] *Shock, severe chemical and thermal burns, severe respiratory tract irritation, pulmonary edema, respiratory arrest, ECG changes, sudden death.*

paradiaminobenzene [Aniline] *Methemoglobinemia, hypoxia.*

paradichlorobenzene [Lindane] *CNS stimulation, seizures, respiratory failure.*

paraffin [Aliphatic hydrocarbon] *Arrhythmias, asphyxiation, anesthesia.*

paraformaldehyde [Aldehyde] *Seizures, respiratory failure, pulmonary edema.*

paraldehyde [Aldehyde] *Seizures, respiratory failure, pulmonary edema.*

paramethane hydroperoxide [Organic peroxide] *Pulmonary and laryngeal edema, circulatory arrest, hypovolemic shock, chemical burns to skin, mucous membranes, and internal organs.*

Paraoxon (diethyl-*p*-nitrophenyl phosphate) [Organophosphate] *Pulmonary edema, respiratory muscle paralysis, respiratory failure, bradycardia, acetylcholinesterase inhibition, hypotension, pulmonary edema, overstimulation of parasympathetic nervous* system, striated muscle, sympathetic ganglia, and CNS.

paraquat [Paraquat] *Pulmonary edema, cardiac damage, circulatory collapse, cerebral hemorrhage or infarcts, death. (Defoliant used in warfare.)*

paraquat methosulfate [Paraquat] *Pulmonary edema, cardiac damage, circulatory collapse, cerebral hemorrhage or infarcts, death. (Defoliant used in warfare.)*

parathion; parathion mixture (n.o.s.) [Organophosphate] *Pulmonary edema, respiratory muscle paralysis, respiratory failure, bradycardia, acetylcholinesterase inhibition, hypotension, pulmonary edema, overstimulation of parasympathetic nervous system, striated muscle, sympathetic ganglia, and CNS.*

parathion & compressed gas mixture [Organophosphate] *Pulmonary edema, respiratory muscle paralysis, respiratory failure, bradycardia, acetylcholinesterase inhibition, hypotension, pulmonary edema, overstimulation of parasympathetic nervous system, striated muscle, sympathetic ganglia, and CNS.*

parathion-methyl [Organophosphate] *Pulmonary edema, respiratory muscle paralysis, respiratory failure, bradycardia, acetylcholinesterase inhibition, hypotension, pulmonary edema, overstimulation of parasympathetic nervous system, striated muscle, sympathetic ganglia, and CNS.*

Paris green [Arsenic] *Heavy metal toxicity, vomiting, GI bleeding, CNS depression, pulmonary edema, cardiac arrest.* [Copper] *Respiratory tract irritation, respiratory arrest, hemorrhagic gastritis.*

PBB (polybrominated biphenyl) [Polychlorinated biphenyl/polybrominated biphenyl/polychlorinated dibenzofuran] *Liver and kidney damage.*

PCB (polychlorinated biphenyl) [Polychlorinated biphenyl/polybrominated biphenyl/polychlorinated dibenzofuran] *Liver and kidney damage.*

PCDF (polychlorinated dibenzofuran) [Polychlorinated biphenyl/polybrominated biphenyl/polychlorinated dibenzofuran] *Liver and kidney damage.*

PCNB [Pentachlorophenol] *Respiratory and circulatory collapse, severe hyperthermia.*

PCP (pentachlorophenol) [Pentachlorophenol] *Respiratory and circulatory collapse, severe hyperthermia.*

pelargonyl peroxide [Organic peroxide] *Pulmonary and laryngeal edema, circulatory arrest, hypovolemic shock, chemical burns to skin, mucous membranes, and internal organs.*

pentaborane [Boron] *Respiratory tract irritation, laryngeal spasm and edema, pulmonary edema, severe chemical burns.*

pentachlorobenzene [Aromatic hydrocarbon] *Arrhythmias, respiratory failure, pulmonary edema, paralysis, brain and kidney damage.*

pentachloroethane [Halogenated aliphatic hydrocarbon] *CNS depression, respiratory arrest, circulatory collapse.*

pentachloronitrobenzene [Pentachlorophenol] *Respiratory and circulatory collapse, severe hyperthermia.*

pentachlorophenol (PCP) [Pentachlorophenol] *Respiratory and circulatory collapse, severe hyperthermia.*

pentadecylamine [Organic base/amine] *Pulmonary edema, cardiac depression, seizures.*

1,3-pentadiene [Aliphatic hydrocarbon] *Arrhythmias, asphyxiation, anesthesia.*

pentaerythritol [Ethylene glycol] *Respiratory failure, pulmonary edema, paralysis, cardiovascular collapse, severe acidosis.*

pentamethyl heptane [Aliphatic hydrocarbon] *Arrhythmias, asphyxiation, anesthesia.*

pentane [Aliphatic hydrocarbon] *Arrhythmias, asphyxiation, anesthesia.*

pentane-2,4-dione [Ketone] *Respiratory mucous membrane irritation, pulmonary edema, CNS depression.*

pentanoic acid; *n*-pentanoic acid (valeric acid) [Organic acid] *Pulmonary edema, circulatory collapse, laryngeal edema and spasm, severe chemical burns to skin, mucous membranes, and internal organs, GI tract perforation and hemorrhage, peritonitis.*

2-pentanone [Ketone] *Respiratory mucous membrane irritation, pulmonary edema, CNS depression.*

1-pentene [Aliphatic hydrocarbon] *Arrhythmias, asphyxiation, anesthesia.*

pentol [Higher alcohol (4+ carbons)] *CNS depression, respiratory failure, arrhythmias.*

peracetic acid [Organic peroxide] *Pulmonary and laryngeal edema, circulatory arrest, hypovolemic shock, chemical burns to skin, mucous membranes, and internal organs.* [Organic acid] *Pulmonary edema, circulatory collapse, laryngeal edema and spasm, severe chemical burns to skin, mucous membranes, and internal organs, GI tract perforation and hemorrhage, peritonitis.*

perc [Halogenated aliphatic hydrocarbon] *CNS depression, respiratory arrest, circulatory collapse.*

perchlorate (n.o.s.) [Chlorate] *Hemolysis, methemoglobinemia, hypoperfusion, CNS depression, delayed-onset renal failure.*

perchloric acid [Oxidizer] *Pulmonary and laryngeal edema, circulatory arrest, hypovolemic shock, chemical burns of skin, mucous membranes, and internal organs.* [Inorganic acid] *Pulmonary edema, bronchospasm, circulatory collapse, laryngeal spasm and edema, severe chemical burns to skin, mucous membranes, and internal organs, GI tract perforation and hemorrhage, peritonitis.*

perchloroethylene [Halogenated aliphatic hydrocarbon] *CNS depression, respiratory arrest, circulatory collapse.*

perchloromethyl mercaptan [Sulfur] *Respiratory tract irritation, pulmonary edema, anaphylaxis.*

perchloryl fluoride [Oxidizer] *Pulmonary and laryngeal edema, circulatory arrest, hypovolemic shock, chemical burns of skin, mucous membranes, and internal organs.* [Fluorine] *CNS depression, respiratory arrest, cardiovascular collapse, shock, arrhythmias.*

perfluoroethylvinyl ether [Ether] *Anesthesia, respiratory arrest.*

perfluoromethylvinyl ether [Ether] *Anesthesia, respiratory arrest.*

perfluoropropane [Halogenated aliphatic hydrocarbon] *CNS depression, respiratory arrest, circulatory collapse.*

perfume, flammable [Hydrocarbon mixture] *CNS depression, respiratory arrest, seizures, arrhythmias, pulmonary edema.*

permanganate (n.o.s.) [Inorganic acid] *Pulmonary edema, bronchospasm, circulatory collapse, laryngeal spasm and edema, severe chemical burns to skin, mucous membranes, and internal organs, GI tract perforation and hemorrhage, peritonitis.*

permethrin [Pyrethrin/pyrethroid] *Respiratory paralysis, convulsions.*

peroxide (n.o.s.) [Oxidizer] *Pulmonary and laryngeal edema, circulatory arrest, hypovolemic shock, chemical burns of skin, mucous membranes, and internal organs.*

peroxyacetic acid [Organic peroxide] *Pulmonary and laryngeal edema, circulatory arrest, hypovolemic shock, chemical burns to skin, mucous membranes, and internal organs.* [Organic acid] *Pulmonary edema, circulatory collapse, laryngeal edema and spasm, severe chemical burns to skin, mucous membranes, and internal organs, GI tract perforation and hemorrhage, peritonitis.*

peroxyacetic acid & hydrogen peroxide mixture [Oxidizer] *Pulmonary and laryngeal edema, circulatory arrest, hypovolemic shock, chemical burns of skin, mucous membranes, and internal organs.*

persulfate salt (n.o.s.) [Sulfur] *Respiratory tract irritation, pulmonary edema, anaphylaxis.*

Perthane [DDT] *CNS disruption, respiratory control center paralysis, ventricular fibrillation, seizures, respiratory arrest.*

pesticide, benzoic derivative (n.o.s.) [Organic acid] *Pulmonary edema, circulatory collapse, laryngeal edema and spasm, severe chemical burns to skin, mucous membranes, and internal organs, GI tract perforation and hemorrhage, peritonitis.*

pesticide, bipyridilium (n.o.s.) [Paraquat] *Pulmonary edema, cardiac damage, circulatory collapse, cerebral hemorrhage or infarcts, death. (Defoliant used in warfare.)*

pesticide, carbamate (n.o.s.) [Carbamate] *Acetylcholinesterase inhibition (reversible), bradycardia, hypotension, respiratory muscle paralysis, respiratory arrest, pulmonary edema.*

pesticide, copper-based (n.o.s.) [Copper] *Respiratory tract irritation, respiratory arrest, hemorrhagic gastritis.*

pesticide, coumarin derivative (n.o.s.) [Ketone] *Respiratory mucous membrane irritation, pulmonary edema, CNS depression.*

pesticide, dithiocarbamate (n.o.s.) [Dithiocarbamate] *Hypotension, respiratory failure.*

pesticide, flammable poison (n.o.s.) [Flammable/combustible liquid] *CNS depression, respiratory arrest, convulsions, arrhythmias, pulmonary edema.* [Poison] *Cardiovascular collapse, pulmonary edema, CNS depression, coma, seizures, nausea, vomiting, cardiopulmonary arrest.*

pesticide, maneb-containing [Dithiocarbamate] *Hypotension, respiratory failure.*

pesticide, mercury-based (n.o.s.) [Mercury] *Circulatory collapse, arrhythmias, respiratory failure, pulmonary edema, neurotoxic effects.*

pesticide, organophosphate (n.o.s.) [Organophosphate] *Pulmonary edema, respiratory muscle paralysis, respiratory failure, bradycardia, acetylcholinesterase inhibition, hypotension, pulmonary edema, overstimulation of parasympathetic nervous system, striated muscle, sympathetic ganglia, and CNS.*

pesticide, phenoxy (n.o.s.) [Chlorophenoxy herbicide] *CNS depression, CNS stimulation, respiratory failure, ventricular fibrillation, seizures.*

pesticide, phenylurea (n.o.s.) [Naphthalene] *Delayed-onset acute intravascular hemolysis.*

pesticide, phthalimide derivative (n.o.s.) [Irritant] *Severe immediate or delayed upper airway or respiratory tract irritation, pulmonary edema, glottic spasm, airway obstruction.*

pesticide, poisonous (n.o.s.) [Poison] *Cardiovascular collapse, pulmonary edema, CNS depression, coma, seizures, nausea, vomiting, cardiopulmonary arrest.*

pesticide, substituted nitrophenol (n.o.s.) [Dinitrophenol] *Respiratory and circulatory collapse, pulmonary edema, hyperthermia.*

pesticide, triazine (n.o.s.) [Irritant] *Severe immediate or delayed upper airway or respiratory tract irritation, pulmonary edema, glottic spasm, airway obstruction.*

petrol [Hydrocarbon mixture] *CNS depression, respiratory arrest, seizures, arrhythmias, pulmonary edema.*

petroleum crude oil [Hydrocarbon mixture] *CNS depression, respiratory arrest, seizures, arrhythmias, pulmonary edema.*

petroleum distillate (n.o.s.) [Hydrocarbon mixture] *CNS depression, respiratory arrest, seizures, arrhythmias, pulmonary edema.*

petroleum ether [Ether] *Anesthesia, respiratory arrest.*

petroleum gas, liquefied (LPG) [Flammable gas] *Respiratory failure, cardiac arrest, arrhythmias.* [Hydrocarbon mixture] *CNS depression, res-*

HazMat

piratory arrest, seizures, arrhythmias, pulmonary edema.

petroleum naphtha [Hydrocarbon mixture] *CNS depression, respiratory arrest, seizures, arrhythmias, pulmonary edema.*

petroleum oil [Hydrocarbon mixture] *CNS depression, respiratory arrest, seizures, arrhythmias, pulmonary edema.*

petroleum spirit [Hydrocarbon mixture] *CNS depression, respiratory arrest, seizures, arrhythmias, pulmonary edema.*

phenacetin [Aniline] *Methemoglobinemia, hypoxia.*

phenacyl bromide [Bromine/methyl bromide] *Severe respiratory irritation, pulmonary edema, respiratory failure, coma, convulsions, death.*

phenamiphos [Organophosphate] *Pulmonary edema, respiratory muscle paralysis, respiratory failure, bradycardia, acetylcholinesterase inhibition, hypotension, pulmonary edema, overstimulation of parasympathetic nervous system, striated muscle, sympathetic ganglia, and CNS.*

phenanthrene [Aromatic hydrocarbon] *Arrhythmias, respiratory failure, pulmonary edema, paralysis, brain and kidney damage.*

phenazopyridine HCl [Aniline] *Methemoglobinemia, hypoxia.* [Naphthalene] *Delayed-onset acute intravascular hemolysis.*

phenetidine [Aniline] *Methemoglobinemia, hypoxia.*

phenindione [Warfarin/hydroxycoumarin/indanedione] *Anticoagulation effect, internal hemorrhage.*

phenol [Phenol] *Coma, hypotension, arrhythmias, pulmonary edema, respiratory arrest.*

phenol, chlorinated [Phenol] *Coma, hypotension, arrhythmias, pulmonary edema, respiratory arrest.*

phenolsulfonic acid [Organic acid] *Pulmonary edema, circulatory collapse, laryngeal edema and spasm, severe chemical burns to skin, mucous membranes,*

and internal organs, GI tract perforation and hemorrhage, peritonitis. [Phenol] *Coma, hypotension, arrhythmias, pulmonary edema, respiratory arrest.*

phenoxarsine [Arsine] *Intravascular hemolysis, pulmonary edema, cardiac and respiratory arrest, delayed-onset jaundice, and acute or delayed-onset renal failure.*

phenoxy pesticide (n.o.s.) [Chlorophenoxy herbicide] *CNS depression, CNS stimulation, respiratory failure, ventricular fibrillation, seizures.*

phenprocoumon [Warfarin/hydroxycoumarin/indanedione] *Anticoagulation effect, internal hemorrhage.*

Phenyl Cellosolve [Ethylene glycol] *Respiratory failure, pulmonary edema, paralysis, cardiovascular collapse, severe acidosis.*

phenyl chloroformate [Halogenated aliphatic hydrocarbon] *CNS depression, respiratory arrest, circulatory collapse.*

phenyl isocyanate [Isocyanate/aliphatic thiocyanate] *CNS depression, respiratory arrest, respiratory paralysis, pulmonary edema, cyanide toxicity.*

phenyl mercaptan [Sulfur] *Respiratory tract irritation, pulmonary edema, anaphylaxis.*

phenyl phosphorous dichloride [Phosphorus] *Hypovolemic shock, severe tissue burns, severe respiratory irritation, pulmonary edema, respiratory arrest, arrhythmias, sudden death.*

phenyl phosphorous thiodichloride [Phosphorus] *Hypovolemic shock, severe tissue burns, severe respiratory irritation, pulmonary edema, respiratory arrest, arrhythmias, sudden death.*

phenylacetonitrile [Cyanide] *Impairment of cellular oxygenation and adenosine triphosphate production, hypoxia, death.*

phenylacetyl chloride [Aromatic hydrocarbon] *Arrhythmias, respiratory failure, pulmonary edema, paralysis, brain and kidney damage.*

phenylcarbylamine chloride [Aniline] *Methemoglobinemia, hypoxia.*

phenyldichloroarsine [Arsenic] *Heavy metal toxicity, vomiting, GI bleeding, CNS depression, pulmonary edema, cardiac arrest.* [Arsine] *Intravascular hemolysis, pulmonary edema, cardiac and respiratory arrest, delayed-onset jaundice, and acute or delayed-onset renal failure.*

phenylenediamine [Organic base/amine] *Pulmonary edema, cardiac depression, seizures.*

phenylhydrazine [Hydrazine] *Seizures, hemolysis of red blood cells, pulmonary edema.*

phenylhydrazine HCl [Hydrazine] *Seizures, hemolysis of red blood cells, pulmonary edema.*

phenylmercuric acetate [Mercury] *Circulatory collapse, arrhythmias, respiratory failure, pulmonary edema, neurotoxic effects.*

phenylmercuric acid salt (n.o.s.) [Mercury] *Circulatory collapse, arrhythmias, respiratory failure, pulmonary edema, neurotoxic effects.*

phenylmercuric hydroxide [Mercury] *Circulatory collapse, arrhythmias, respiratory failure, pulmonary edema, neurotoxic effects.*

phenylmercuric mixture (n.o.s.) [Mercury] *Circulatory collapse, arrhythmias, respiratory failure, pulmonary edema, neurotoxic effects.*

phenylmercuric nitrate [Nitrate/nitrite] *Methemoglobinemia, hypotension, circulatory collapse.* [Mercury] *Circulatory collapse, arrhythmias, respiratory failure, pulmonary edema, neurotoxic effects.*

phenylmercuric triethanol ammonium lactate [Mercury] *Circulatory collapse, arrhythmias, respiratory failure, pulmonary edema, neurotoxic effects.*

phenylmercury acetate [Mercury] *Circulatory collapse, arrhythmias, respiratory failure, pulmonary edema, neurotoxic effects.*

phenylphenol [Phenol] *Coma, hypotension, arrhythmias, pulmonary edema, respiratory arrest.*

phenylphosphine [Phosphine] *Severe pulmonary irritation, pulmonary edema.*

phenylsilatrane [Poison] *Cardiovascular collapse, pulmonary edema, CNS depression, coma, seizures, nausea, vomiting, cardiopulmonary arrest.*

phenylthiourea [Naphthalene] *Delayed-onset acute intravascular hemolysis.*

phenyltrichlorosilane [Silane/chlorosilane] *Respiratory tract irritation, pulmonary edema.*

phenylurea pesticide (n.o.s.) [Naphthalene] *Delayed-onset acute intravascular hemolysis.*

phorate [Organophosphate] *Pulmonary edema, respiratory muscle paralysis, respiratory failure, bradycardia, acetylcholinesterase inhibition, hypotension, pulmonary edema, overstimulation of parasympathetic nervous system, striated muscle, sympathetic ganglia, and CNS.*

phosacetim [Organophosphate] *Pulmonary edema, respiratory muscle paralysis, respiratory failure, bradycardia, acetylcholinesterase inhibition, hypotension, pulmonary edema, overstimulation of parasympathetic nervous system, striated muscle, sympathetic ganglia, and CNS.*

Phosdrin [Organophosphate] *Pulmonary edema, respiratory muscle paralysis, respiratory failure, bradycardia, acetylcholinesterase inhibition, hypotension, pulmonary edema, overstimulation of parasympathetic nervous system, striated muscle, sympathetic ganglia, and CNS.*

phosfolan [Organophosphate] *Pulmonary edema, respiratory muscle paralysis, respiratory failure, bradycardia, acetylcholinesterase inhibition, hypotension, pulmonary edema, overstimulation of parasympathetic nervous system, striated muscle, sympathetic ganglia, and CNS.*

phosgene [Phosgene] *Severe respiratory irritation, alveolar damage, pulmonary edema.*

phosmet [Organophosphate] *Pulmonary edema, respiratory muscle paralysis, respiratory failure, bradycardia, acetylcholinesterase inhibition, hypotension, pulmonary edema, overstimulation of parasympathetic nervous system, striated muscle, sympathetic ganglia, and CNS.*

phosphabicyclononane [Poison] *Cardiovascular collapse, pulmonary edema, CNS depression, coma, seizures, nausea, vomiting, cardiopulmonary arrest.*

phosphamidon [Organophosphate] *Pulmonary edema, respiratory muscle paralysis, respiratory failure, bradycardia, acetylcholinesterase inhibition, hypotension, pulmonary edema, overstimulation of parasympathetic nervous system, striated muscle, sympathetic ganglia, and CNS.*

phosphine [Phosphine] *Severe pulmonary irritation, pulmonary edema.*

phosphonothioic acid [Organophosphate] *Pulmonary edema, respiratory muscle paralysis, respiratory failure, bradycardia, acetylcholinesterase inhibition, hypotension, pulmonary edema, overstimulation of parasympathetic nervous system, striated muscle, sympathetic ganglia, and CNS.*

phosphoric acid [Inorganic acid] *Pulmonary edema, bronchospasm, circulatory collapse, laryngeal spasm and edema, severe chemical burns to skin, mucous membranes, and internal organs, GI tract perforation and hemorrhage, peritonitis.*

phosphoric acid triethyleneimine [Poison] *Cardiovascular collapse, pulmonary edema, CNS depression, coma, seizures, nausea, vomiting, cardiopulmonary arrest.*

phosphoric anhydride [Inorganic acid] *Pulmonary edema, bronchospasm, circulatory collapse, laryngeal spasm and edema, severe chemical*
burns to skin, mucous membranes, and internal organs, GI tract perforation and hemorrhage, peritonitis.

phosphorous acid [Inorganic acid] *Pulmonary edema, bronchospasm, circulatory collapse, laryngeal spasm and edema, severe chemical burns to skin, mucous membranes, and internal organs, GI tract perforation and hemorrhage, peritonitis.*

phosphorus (red, white, or yellow) [Phosphorus] *Hypovolemic shock, severe tissue burns, severe respiratory irritation, pulmonary edema, respiratory arrest, arrhythmias, sudden death.*

phosphorus heptasulfide [Sulfur] *Respiratory tract irritation, pulmonary edema, anaphylaxis.* [Phosphorus] *Hypovolemic shock, severe tissue burns, severe respiratory irritation, pulmonary edema, respiratory arrest, arrhythmias, sudden death.*

phosphorus oxybromide [Bromine/ methyl bromide] *Severe respiratory irritation, pulmonary edema, respiratory failure, coma, convulsions, death.* [Phosphorus] *Hypovolemic shock, severe tissue burns, severe respiratory irritation, pulmonary edema, respiratory arrest, arrhythmias, sudden death.*

phosphorus oxychloride [Chlorine] *Severe respiratory tract irritation, pulmonary edema, irritation of skin, eyes, and mucous membranes.* [Phosphorus] *Hypovolemic shock, severe tissue burns, severe respiratory irritation, pulmonary edema, respiratory arrest, arrhythmias, sudden death.*

phosphorus pentabromide [Bromine/ methyl bromide] *Severe respiratory irritation, pulmonary edema, respiratory failure, coma, convulsions, death.* [Phosphorus] *Hypovolemic shock, severe tissue burns, severe respiratory irritation, pulmonary edema, respiratory arrest, arrhythmias, sudden death.*

phosphorus pentachloride [Chlorine] *Severe respiratory tract irritation, pulmonary edema, irritation of skin, eyes, and mucous membranes.* [Phosphorus] *Hypovolemic shock, severe tissue burns, severe respiratory irritation, pulmonary edema, respiratory arrest, arrhythmias, sudden death.*

phosphorus pentafluoride [Fluorine] *CNS depression, respiratory arrest, cardiovascular collapse, shock, arrhythmias.* [Phosphorus] *Hypovolemic shock, severe tissue burns, severe respiratory irritation, pulmonary edema, respiratory arrest, arrhythmias, sudden death.*

phosphorus pentasulfide [Sulfur] *Respiratory tract irritation, pulmonary edema, anaphylaxis.* [Phosphorus] *Hypovolemic shock, severe tissue burns, severe respiratory irritation, pulmonary edema, respiratory arrest, arrhythmias, sudden death.*

phosphorus pentoxide [Phosphorus] *Hypovolemic shock, severe tissue burns, severe respiratory irritation, pulmonary edema, respiratory arrest, arrhythmias, sudden death.*

phosphorus sesquisulfide [Sulfur] *Respiratory tract irritation, pulmonary edema, anaphylaxis.* [Phosphorus] *Hypovolemic shock, severe tissue burns, severe respiratory irritation, pulmonary edema, respiratory arrest, arrhythmias, sudden death.*

phosphorus tribromide [Bromine/methyl bromide] *Severe respiratory irritation, pulmonary edema, respiratory failure, coma, convulsions, death.* [Phosphorus] *Hypovolemic shock, severe tissue burns, severe respiratory irritation, pulmonary edema, respiratory arrest, arrhythmias, sudden death.*

phosphorus trichloride [Chlorine] *Severe respiratory tract irritation, pulmonary edema, irritation of skin, eyes, and mucous membranes.* [Phosphorus] *Hypovolemic shock, severe tissue burns, severe respiratory irritation, pulmonary edema, respiratory arrest, arrhythmias, sudden death.*

phosphorus trifluoride [Fluorine] *CNS depression, respiratory arrest, cardiovascular collapse, shock, arrhythmias.* [Phosphorus] *Hypovolemic shock,*

severe tissue burns, severe respiratory irritation, pulmonary edema, respiratory arrest, arrhythmias, sudden death.

phosphorus trioxide [Phosphorus] *Hypovolemic shock, severe tissue burns, severe respiratory irritation, pulmonary edema, respiratory arrest, arrhythmias, sudden death.*

phosphorus trisulfide [Sulfur] *Respiratory tract irritation, pulmonary edema, anaphylaxis.* [Phosphorus] *Hypovolemic shock, severe tissue burns, severe respiratory irritation, pulmonary edema, respiratory arrest, arrhythmias, sudden death.*

phosphoryl chloride [Chlorine] *Severe respiratory tract irritation, pulmonary edema, irritation of skin, eyes, and mucous membranes.* [Phosphorus] *Hypovolemic shock, severe tissue burns, severe respiratory irritation, pulmonary edema, respiratory arrest, arrhythmias, sudden death.*

phostex [Organophosphate] *Pulmonary edema, respiratory muscle paralysis, respiratory failure, bradycardia, acetylcholinesterase inhibition, hypotension, pulmonary edema, overstimulation of parasympathetic nervous system, striated muscle, sympathetic ganglia, and CNS.*

phthalic anhydride [Organic acid] *Pulmonary edema, circulatory collapse, laryngeal edema and spasm, severe chemical burns to skin, mucous membranes, and internal organs, GI tract perforation and hemorrhage, peritonitis.*

phthalimide derivative pesticide (n.o.s.) [Irritant] *Severe immediate or delayed upper airway or respiratory tract irritation, pulmonary edema, glottic spasm, airway obstruction.*

phthalonitrile [Cyanide] *Impairment of cellular oxygenation and adenosine triphosphate production, hypoxia, death.*

physostigmine [Poison] *Cardiovascular collapse, pulmonary edema, CNS depression, coma, seizures, nausea, vomiting, cardiopulmonary arrest.*

picoline [Aromatic hydrocarbon] *Arrhythmias, respiratory failure, pul-*

monary edema, paralysis, brain and kidney damage.

picrate [Dinitrophenol] *Respiratory and circulatory collapse, pulmonary edema, hyperthermia.*

picric acid [Dinitrophenol] *Respiratory and circulatory collapse, pulmonary edema, hyperthermia.*

picrotoxin [Poison] *Cardiovascular collapse, pulmonary edema, CNS depression, coma, seizures, nausea, vomiting, cardiopulmonary arrest.*

pinane hydroperoxide [Organic peroxide] *Pulmonary and laryngeal edema, circulatory arrest, hypovolemic shock, chemical burns to skin, mucous membranes, and internal organs.*

pinayl hydroperoxide [Organic peroxide] *Pulmonary and laryngeal edema, circulatory arrest, hypovolemic shock, chemical burns to skin, mucous membranes, and internal organs.*

pindone [Warfarin/hydroxycoumarin/indanedione] *Anticoagulation effect, internal hemorrhage.*

pine oil [Turpentine/terpene] *Respiratory failure, pulmonary edema, tachycardia.*

α-pinene; alpha-pinene [Turpentine/terpene] *Respiratory failure, pulmonary edema, tachycardia.*

piperazine [Organic base/amine] *Pulmonary edema, cardiac depression, seizures.*

piperidine [Organic base/amine] *Pulmonary edema, cardiac depression, seizures.*

piperonyl butoxide [Poison] *Cardiovascular collapse, pulmonary edema, CNS depression, coma, seizures, nausea, vomiting, cardiopulmonary arrest.*

piperonyl cyclonene [Poison] *Cardiovascular collapse, pulmonary edema, CNS depression, coma, seizures, nausea, vomiting, cardiopulmonary arrest.*

pirimicarb [Carbamate] *Acetylcholinesterase inhibition (reversible), bradycardia, hypotension, respiratory muscle paralysis, respiratory arrest, pulmonary edema.*

pivaloyl chloride [Halogenated aliphatic hydrocarbon] *CNS depression, respiratory arrest, circulatory collapse.*

2-pivalyl-1,3-indandione [Warfarin/hydroxycoumarin/indanedione] *Anticoagulation effect, internal hemorrhage.*

plastic, nitrocellulose-based, spontaneously combustible (n.o.s.) [Flammable solid] *Shock, severe chemical and thermal burns, severe respiratory tract irritation, pulmonary edema, respiratory arrest, ECG changes, sudden death.*

plastic that evolves a flammable vapor (n.o.s.) [Flammable solid] *Shock, severe chemical and thermal burns, severe respiratory tract irritation, pulmonary edema, respiratory arrest, ECG changes, sudden death.*

poison B liquid (n.o.s.) [Poison] *Cardiovascular collapse, pulmonary edema, CNS depression, coma, seizures, nausea, vomiting, cardiopulmonary arrest.*

poisonous gas, flammable (n.o.s.) [Flammable gas] *Respiratory failure, cardiac arrest, arrhythmias.* [Poison] *Cardiovascular collapse, pulmonary edema, CNS depression, coma, seizures, nausea, vomiting, cardiopulmonary arrest.*

poisonous liquid, flammable (n.o.s.) [Flammable/combustible liquid] *CNS depression, respiratory arrest, convulsions, arrhythmias, pulmonary edema.* [Poison] *Cardiovascular collapse, pulmonary edema, CNS depression, coma, seizures, nausea, vomiting, cardiopulmonary arrest.*

poisonous solid, flammable (n.o.s.) [Flammable solid] *Shock, severe chemical and thermal burns, severe respiratory tract irritation, pulmonary edema, respiratory arrest, ECG changes, sudden death.* [Poison] *Cardiovascular collapse, pulmonary edema, CNS depression, coma, seizures, nausea, vomiting, cardiopulmonary arrest.*

poisonous solid, liquid, or gas (n.o.s.) [Poison] *Cardiovascular collapse, pulmonary edema, CNS depres-*

sion, coma, seizures, nausea, vomiting, cardiopulmonary arrest.

poisonous solid, self-heating (n.o.s.) [Poison] *Cardiovascular collapse, pulmonary edema, CNS depression, coma, seizures, nausea, vomiting, cardiopulmonary arrest.*

poisonous solid or liquid, corrosive (n.o.s.) [Poison] *Cardiovascular collapse, pulmonary edema, CNS depression, coma, seizures, nausea, vomiting, cardiopulmonary arrest.* [Corrosive] *Upper airway burns and edema, circulatory collapse, severe chemical burns to skin, toxic systemic effects, GI tract perforation and hemorrhage, peritonitis.*

poisonous solid or liquid, oxidizing (n.o.s.) [Oxidizer] *Pulmonary and laryngeal edema, circulatory arrest, hypovolemic shock, chemical burns of skin, mucous membranes, and internal organs.* [Poison] *Cardiovascular collapse, pulmonary edema, CNS depression, coma, seizures, nausea, vomiting, cardiopulmonary arrest.*

poisonous solid or liquid that evolves a flammable vapor (n.o.s.) [Flammable gas] *Respiratory failure, cardiac arrest, arrhythmias.* [Poison] *Cardiovascular collapse, pulmonary edema, CNS depression, coma, seizures, nausea, vomiting, cardiopulmonary arrest.*

polishing compound [Poison] *Cardiovascular collapse, pulmonary edema, CNS depression, coma, seizures, nausea, vomiting, cardiopulmonary arrest.*

polyalkylamine, corrosive (n.o.s.) [Organic base/amine] *Pulmonary edema, cardiac depression, seizures.*

polyalkylamine, flammable corrosive (n.o.s.) [Flammable/combustible liquid] *CNS depression, respiratory arrest, convulsions, arrhythmias, pulmonary edema.* [Organic base/amine] *Pulmonary edema, cardiac depression, seizures.*

polybrominated biphenyl (PBB) [Polychlorinated biphenyl/polybromi-nated biphenyl/polychlorinated dibenzofuran] *Liver and kidney damage.*

polychlorinated biphenyl (PCB) [Polychlorinated biphenyl/polybromi-nated biphenyl/polychlorinated dibenzofuran] *Liver and kidney damage.*

polychlorinated dibenzofuran (PCDF) [Polychlorinated biphenyl/polybrominated biphenyl/polychlorinated dibenzofuran] *Liver and kidney damage.*

polyester resin kit [Poison] *Cardiovascular collapse, pulmonary edema, CNS depression, coma, seizures, nausea, vomiting, cardiopulmonary arrest.*

polyethylene glycol [Ethylene glycol] *Respiratory failure, pulmonary edema, paralysis, cardiovascular collapse, severe acidosis.*

polyhalogenated biphenyl [Polychlorinated biphenyl/polybrominated biphenyl/polychlorinated dibenzofuran] *Liver and kidney damage.*

polyhalogenated terphenyl [Polychlorinated biphenyl/polybrominated biphenyl/polychlorinated dibenzofuran] *Liver and kidney damage.*

polynuclear aromatic hydrocarbon (n.o.s.) [Poison] *Cardiovascular collapse, pulmonary edema, CNS depression, coma, seizures, nausea, vomiting, cardiopulmonary arrest.*

polyol [Ethylene glycol] *Respiratory failure, pulmonary edema, paralysis, cardiovascular collapse, severe acidosis.*

polystyrene, expandable, that evolves a flammable vapor [Flammable/combustible liquid] *CNS depression, respiratory arrest, convulsions, arrhythmias, pulmonary edema.*

polytetrafluoroethylene [Halogenated aliphatic hydrocarbon] *CNS depression, respiratory arrest, circulatory collapse.*

Portland cement [Inorganic base/alkaline corrosive] *Upper airway burns and edema, pulmonary edema, skin burns, circulatory collapse, GI tract perforation and hemorrhage, peritonitis.*

HazMat

potash liquor [Inorganic base/alkaline corrosive] *Upper airway burns and edema, pulmonary edema, skin burns, circulatory collapse, GI tract perforation and hemorrhage, peritonitis.*

potash & sodium nitrate mixture [Nitrate/nitrite] *Methemoglobinemia, hypotension, circulatory collapse.*

potassium; potassium alloy (n.o.s.) [Poison] *Cardiovascular collapse, pulmonary edema, CNS depression, coma, seizures, nausea, vomiting, cardiopulmonary arrest.*

potassium arsenate [Arsenic] *Heavy metal toxicity, vomiting, GI bleeding, CNS depression, pulmonary edema, cardiac arrest.*

potassium arsenite [Arsenic] *Heavy metal toxicity, vomiting, GI bleeding, CNS depression, pulmonary edema, cardiac arrest.*

potassium bichromate [Inorganic acid] *Pulmonary edema, bronchospasm, circulatory collapse, laryngeal spasm and edema, severe chemical burns to skin, mucous membranes, and internal organs, GI tract perforation and hemorrhage, peritonitis.*

potassium bifluoride [Hydrofluoric acid] *Pulmonary and laryngeal edema, circulatory collapse, severe skin burns, GI tract perforation, systemic fluoride poisoning.*

potassium biosulfite [Sulfur] *Respiratory tract irritation, pulmonary edema, anaphylaxis.*

potassium bisulfate [Inorganic acid] *Pulmonary edema, bronchospasm, circulatory collapse, laryngeal spasm and edema, severe chemical burns to skin, mucous membranes, and internal organs, GI tract perforation and hemorrhage, peritonitis.*

potassium borohydride [Boron] *Respiratory tract irritation, laryngeal spasm and edema, pulmonary edema, severe chemical burns.*

potassium bromate [Bromate] *CNS and respiratory system depression, delayed-onset renal failure.*

potassium carbonate & ammonium nitrate mixture [Nitrate/nitrite] *Methemoglobinemia, hypotension, circulatory collapse.*

potassium chlorate [Chlorate] *Hemolysis, methemoglobinemia, hypoperfusion, CNS depression, delayed-onset renal failure.*

potassium chromate [Inorganic acid] *Pulmonary edema, bronchospasm, circulatory collapse, laryngeal spasm and edema, severe chemical burns to skin, mucous membranes, and internal organs, GI tract perforation and hemorrhage, peritonitis.*

potassium cuprocyanide [Cyanide] *Impairment of cellular oxygenation and adenosine triphosphate production, hypoxia, death.*

potassium cyanide; cyanide potassium [Cyanide] *Impairment of cellular oxygenation and adenosine triphosphate production, hypoxia, death.*

potassium dichloroisocyanurate [Hypochlorite] *Circulatory collapse, respiratory tract irritation, upper airway obstruction, pulmonary edema.*

potassium dichloro-S-triazinetrione [Hypochlorite] *Circulatory collapse, respiratory tract irritation, upper airway obstruction, pulmonary edema.*

potassium dichromate [Inorganic acid] *Pulmonary edema, bronchospasm, circulatory collapse, laryngeal spasm and edema, severe chemical burns to skin, mucous membranes, and internal organs, GI tract perforation and hemorrhage, peritonitis.*

potassium dithionite [Sulfur] *Respiratory tract irritation, pulmonary edema, anaphylaxis.*

potassium fluoborate [Fluorine] *CNS depression, respiratory arrest, cardiovascular collapse, shock, arrhythmias.* [Boron] *Respiratory tract irritation, laryngeal spasm and edema, pulmonary edema, severe chemical burns.*

potassium fluoride [Hydrofluoric acid] *Pulmonary and laryngeal edema, circula-*

tory collapse, severe skin burns, GI tract perforation, systemic fluoride poisoning.

potassium fluoroacetate [Monofluoroacetate] *Ventricular arrhythmias, seizures.*

potassium fluorosilicate [Fluorine] *CNS depression, respiratory arrest, cardiovascular collapse, shock, arrhythmias.*

potassium hydrogen fluoride [Hydrofluoric acid] *Pulmonary and laryngeal edema, circulatory collapse, severe skin burns, GI tract perforation, systemic fluoride poisoning.*

potassium hydrogen sulfate [Inorganic acid] *Pulmonary edema, bronchospasm, circulatory collapse, laryngeal spasm and edema, severe chemical burns to skin, mucous membranes, and internal organs, GI tract perforation and hemorrhage, peritonitis.*

potassium hydrosulfite [Sulfur] *Respiratory tract irritation, pulmonary edema, anaphylaxis.*

potassium hydroxide [Inorganic base/alkaline corrosive] *Upper airway burns and edema, pulmonary edema, skin burns, circulatory collapse, GI tract perforation and hemorrhage, peritonitis.*

potassium hydroxide & ammonium nitrate mixture [Inorganic base/alkaline corrosive] *Upper airway burns and edema, pulmonary edema, skin burns, circulatory collapse, GI tract perforation and hemorrhage, peritonitis.* [Nitrate/nitrite] *Methemoglobinemia, hypotension, circulatory collapse.*

potassium hypochlorite [Hypochlorite] *Circulatory collapse, respiratory tract irritation, upper airway obstruction, pulmonary edema.*

potassium metavanadate [Poison] *Cardiovascular collapse, pulmonary edema, CNS depression, coma, seizures, nausea, vomiting, cardiopulmonary arrest.*

potassium monopersulfate [Irritant] *Severe immediate or delayed upper airway or respiratory tract irritation, pulmonary edema, glottic spasm, airway obstruction.*

potassium monoxide [Inorganic base/alkaline corrosive] *Upper airway burns and edema, pulmonary edema, skin burns, circulatory collapse, GI tract perforation and hemorrhage, peritonitis.*

potassium nitrate [Nitrate/nitrite] *Methemoglobinemia, hypotension, circulatory collapse.*

potassium nitrate & sodium nitrate mixture [Nitrate/nitrite] *Methemoglobinemia, hypotension, circulatory collapse.*

potassium nitrate & sodium nitrite mixture [Nitrate/nitrite] *Methemoglobinemia, hypotension, circulatory collapse.*

potassium nitrite [Nitrate/nitrite] *Methemoglobinemia, hypotension, circulatory collapse.*

potassium oxide [Inorganic base/alkaline corrosive] *Upper airway burns and edema, pulmonary edema, skin burns, circulatory collapse, GI tract perforation and hemorrhage, peritonitis.*

potassium perchlorate [Chlorate] *Hemolysis, methemoglobinemia, hypoperfusion, CNS depression, delayed-onset renal failure.*

potassium permanganate [Inorganic acid] *Pulmonary edema, bronchospasm, circulatory collapse, laryngeal spasm and edema, severe chemical burns to skin, mucous membranes, and internal organs, GI tract perforation and hemorrhage, peritonitis.*

potassium peroxide [Oxidizer] *Pulmonary and laryngeal edema, circulatory arrest, hypovolemic shock, chemical burns of skin, mucous membranes, and internal organs.*

potassium persulfate [Irritant] *Severe immediate or delayed upper airway or respiratory tract irritation, pulmonary edema, glottic spasm, airway obstruction.*

potassium phosphate [Inorganic base/alkaline corrosive] *Upper airway burns and edema, pulmonary edema, skin burns, circulatory collapse, GI tract perforation and hemorrhage, peritonitis.*

HazMat

potassium phosphide [Phosphine] *Severe pulmonary irritation, pulmonary edema.*

potassium selenate [Selenium] *Arrhythmias, pulmonary edema, bronchospasm, seizures, vomiting, GI bleeding.*

potassium selenite [Selenium] *Arrhythmias, pulmonary edema, bronchospasm, seizures, vomiting, GI bleeding.*

potassium silicofluoride [Fluorine] *CNS depression, respiratory arrest, cardiovascular collapse, shock, arrhythmias.*

potassium silver cyanide [Cyanide] *Impairment of cellular oxygenation and adenosine triphosphate production, hypoxia, death.*

potassium sodium alloy (n.o.s.) [Flammable solid] *Shock, severe chemical and thermal burns, severe respiratory tract irritation, pulmonary edema, respiratory arrest, ECG changes, sudden death.*

potassium sulfide [Inorganic base/ alkaline corrosive] *Upper airway burns and edema, pulmonary edema, skin burns, circulatory collapse, GI tract perforation and hemorrhage, peritonitis.*

potassium superoxide [Poison] *Cardiovascular collapse, pulmonary edema, CNS depression, coma, seizures, nausea, vomiting, cardiopulmonary arrest.*

pressurized accumulator [Flammable gas] *Respiratory failure, cardiac arrest, arrhythmias.*

primifos-ethyl [Organophosphate] *Pulmonary edema, respiratory muscle paralysis, respiratory failure, bradycardia, acetylcholinesterase inhibition, hypotension, pulmonary edema, overstimulation of parasympathetic nervous system, striated muscle, sympathetic ganglia, and CNS.*

Prolan [Lindane] *CNS stimulation, seizures, respiratory failure.*

promecarb [Carbamate] *Acetylcholinesterase inhibition (reversible), bradycardia, hypotension, respiratory muscle paralysis, respiratory arrest, pulmonary edema.*

propadiene [Aliphatic hydrocarbon] *Arrhythmias, asphyxiation, anesthesia.*

propadiene & methyl acetylene mixture [Hydrocarbon mixture] *CNS depression, respiratory arrest, seizures, arrhythmias, pulmonary edema.*

propane [Aliphatic hydrocarbon] *Arrhythmias, asphyxiation, anesthesia.*

propane & ethane mixture (cryogenic liquid) [Aliphatic hydrocarbon] *Arrhythmias, asphyxiation, anesthesia.*

propane sulfone [Organic acid] *Pulmonary edema, circulatory collapse, laryngeal edema and spasm, severe chemical burns to skin, mucous membranes, and internal organs, GI tract perforation and hemorrhage, peritonitis.*

propanethiol [Sulfur] *Respiratory tract irritation, pulmonary edema, anaphylaxis.*

propanil [Aniline] *Methemoglobinemia, hypoxia.*

propanoic acid [Organic acid] *Pulmonary edema, circulatory collapse, laryngeal edema and spasm, severe chemical burns to skin, mucous membranes, and internal organs, GI tract perforation and hemorrhage, peritonitis.*

propanol [Lower alcohol (1–3 carbons)] *CNS depression, coma, respiratory arrest, arrhythmias.*

propargite [Poison] *Cardiovascular collapse, pulmonary edema, CNS depression, coma, seizures, nausea, vomiting, cardiopulmonary arrest.*

propargyl alcohol [Higher alcohol (4+ carbons)] *CNS depression, respiratory failure, arrhythmias.*

propargyl bromide [Bromine/methyl bromide] *Severe respiratory irritation, pulmonary edema, respiratory failure, coma, convulsions, death.*

β-propiolactone; beta-propiolactone; β-propionolactone [Ketone] *Respiratory mucous membrane irritation, pulmonary edema, CNS depression.*

propionaldehyde [Aldehyde] *Seizures, respiratory failure, pulmonary edema.*

propionic acid [Organic acid] *Pulmonary edema, circulatory collapse, laryngeal edema and spasm, severe chemical burns to skin, mucous membranes, and internal organs, GI tract perforation and hemorrhage, peritonitis.*

propionic acid & boron trifluoride complex [Boron] *Respiratory tract irritation, laryngeal spasm and edema, pulmonary edema, severe chemical burns.*

propionic anhydride [Organic acid] *Pulmonary edema, circulatory collapse, laryngeal edema and spasm, severe chemical burns to skin, mucous membranes, and internal organs, GI tract perforation and hemorrhage, peritonitis.*

propionitrile [Cyanide] *Impairment of cellular oxygenation and adenosine triphosphate production, hypoxia, death.*

propionyl chloride [Halogenated aliphatic hydrocarbon] *CNS depression, respiratory arrest, circulatory collapse.*

propionyl peroxide [Organic peroxide] *Pulmonary and laryngeal edema, circulatory arrest, hypovolemic shock, chemical burns to skin, mucous membranes, and internal organs.*

propiophenone [Phenol] *Coma, hypotension, arrhythmias, pulmonary edema, respiratory arrest.*

propoxur [Carbamate] *Acetylcholinesterase inhibition (reversible), bradycardia, hypotension, respiratory muscle paralysis, respiratory arrest, pulmonary edema.*

propyl acetate [Ester] *CNS depression, respiratory tract irritation, bronchitis, pneumonitis.*

propyl alcohol [Lower alcohol (1–3 carbons)] *CNS depression, coma, respiratory arrest, arrhythmias.*

propyl benzene [Aromatic hydrocarbon] *Arrhythmias, respiratory failure, pulmonary edema, paralysis, brain and kidney damage.*

propyl chloroformate; n-propyl chloroformate [Halogenated aliphatic hydrocarbon] *CNS depression, respiratory arrest, circulatory collapse.*

propyl formate [Ester] *CNS depression, respiratory tract irritation, bronchitis, pneumonitis.*

n-propyl gallate [Phenol] *Coma, hypotension, arrhythmias, pulmonary edema, respiratory arrest.*

propyl isocyanate [Isocyanate/aliphatic thiocyanate] *CNS depression, respiratory arrest, respiratory paralysis, pulmonary edema, cyanide toxicity.*

n-propyl isomer [Naphthalene] *Delayed-onset acute intravascular hemolysis.*

propyl mercaptan [Sulfur] *Respiratory tract irritation, pulmonary edema, anaphylaxis.*

propyl nitrate [Nitrate/nitrite] *Methemoglobinemia, hypotension, circulatory collapse.*

propyl peroxydicarbonate [Organic peroxide] *Pulmonary and laryngeal edema, circulatory arrest, hypovolemic shock, chemical burns to skin, mucous membranes, and internal organs.*

propyl trichlorosilane [Silane/chlorosilane] *Respiratory tract irritation, pulmonary edema.*

propylamine [Organic base/amine] *Pulmonary edema, cardiac depression, seizures.*

propylene [Aliphatic hydrocarbon] *Arrhythmias, asphyxiation, anesthesia.*

propylene chlorohydrin [Dichloropropane/dichloropropene] *Pulmonary edema, bronchospasm, alveolar hemorrhage.*

propylene dichloride [Dichloropropane/dichloropropene] *Pulmonary edema, bronchospasm, alveolar hemorrhage.*

propylene dichloride & dichloropropene mixture [Dichloropropane/dichloropropene] *Pulmonary edema, bronchospasm, alveolar hemorrhage.*

propylene & ethylene & acetylene mixture (cryogenic liquid) [Aliphatic hydrocarbon] *Arrhythmias, asphyxiation, anesthesia.* [Simple asphyxiant] *Asphyxiation.*

HazMat

propylene glycol [Ethylene glycol] *Respiratory failure, pulmonary edema, paralysis, cardiovascular collapse, severe acidosis.*

propylene glycol monomethyl ether [Ethylene glycol] *Respiratory failure, pulmonary edema, paralysis, cardiovascular collapse, severe acidosis.*

propylene glycol monostearate [Ethylene glycol] *Respiratory failure, pulmonary edema, paralysis, cardiovascular collapse, severe acidosis.*

propylene oxide [Ether] *Anesthesia, respiratory arrest.*

propylene oxide & ethylene oxide mixture [Ethylene oxide] *Respiratory tract irritation, pulmonary edema.*

propylene tetramer [Aliphatic hydrocarbon] *Arrhythmias, asphyxiation, anesthesia.*

propylenediamine [Organic base/amine] *Pulmonary edema, cardiac depression, seizures.*

propyleneimine [Organic base/amine] *Pulmonary edema, cardiac depression, seizures.*

prothoate [Organophosphate] *Pulmonary edema, respiratory muscle paralysis, respiratory failure, bradycardia, acetylcholinesterase inhibition, hypotension, pulmonary edema, overstimulation of parasympathetic nervous system, striated muscle, sympathetic ganglia, and CNS.*

pyramat [Carbamate] *Acetylcholinesterase inhibition (reversible), bradycardia, hypotension, respiratory muscle paralysis, respiratory arrest, pulmonary edema.*

pyrazothion [Organophosphate] *Pulmonary edema, respiratory muscle paralysis, respiratory failure, bradycardia, acetylcholinesterase inhibition, hypotension, pulmonary edema, overstimulation of parasympathetic nervous system, striated muscle, sympathetic ganglia, and CNS.*

Pyrazoxon [Organophosphate] *Pulmonary edema, respiratory muscle paralysis, respiratory failure, bradycardia, acetylcholinesterase inhibition, hypoten-*

sion, pulmonary edema, overstimulation of parasympathetic nervous system, striated muscle, sympathetic ganglia, and CNS.

pyrene [Aromatic hydrocarbon] *Arrhythmias, respiratory failure, pulmonary edema, paralysis, brain and kidney damage.*

pyrenone [Pyrethrin/pyrethroid] *Respiratory paralysis, convulsions.*

pyrethrin; pyrethrum [Pyrethrin/pyrethroid] *Respiratory paralysis, convulsions.*

pyrethroid (n.o.s.) [Pyrethrin/pyrethroid] *Respiratory paralysis, convulsions.*

pyridine [Aromatic hydrocarbon] *Arrhythmias, respiratory failure, pulmonary edema, paralysis, brain and kidney damage.*

pyriminil [Poison] *Cardiovascular collapse, pulmonary edema, CNS depression, coma, seizures, nausea, vomiting, cardiopulmonary arrest.*

pyrocatechol [Phenol] *Coma, hypotension, arrhythmias, pulmonary edema, respiratory arrest.*

pyrogallol [Phenol] *Coma, hypotension, arrhythmias, pulmonary edema, respiratory arrest.*

pyrolan [Carbamate] *Acetylcholinesterase inhibition (reversible), bradycardia, hypotension, respiratory muscle paralysis, respiratory arrest, pulmonary edema.*

pyrolysis products [Poison] *Cardiovascular collapse, pulmonary edema, CNS depression, coma, seizures, nausea, vomiting, cardiopulmonary arrest.*

pyrophoric fuel (n.o.s.); pyrophoric liquid (n.o.s.) [Flammable/combustible liquid] *CNS depression, respiratory arrest, convulsions, arrhythmias, pulmonary edema.*

pyrophoric metal (n.o.s.); pyrophoric metal alloy (n.o.s.); pyrophoric solid (n.o.s.) [Flammable solid] *Shock, severe chemical and thermal burns, severe respiratory tract irritation, pulmonary edema, respiratory arrest, ECG changes, sudden death.*

pyrosulfuric acid [Inorganic acid] *Pulmonary edema, bronchospasm, circulatory collapse, laryngeal spasm and edema, severe chemical burns to skin, mucous membranes, and internal organs, GI tract perforation and hemorrhage, peritonitis.*

pyrosulfuryl chloride [Inorganic acid] *Pulmonary edema, bronchospasm, circulatory collapse, laryngeal spasm and edema, severe chemical burns to skin, mucous membranes, and internal organs, GI tract perforation and hemorrhage, peritonitis.*

pyroxylin [Ether] *Anesthesia, respiratory arrest.*

pyrrolidine [Organic base/amine] *Pulmonary edema, cardiac depression, seizures.*

quinoline [Aromatic hydrocarbon] *Arrhythmias, respiratory failure, pulmonary edema, paralysis, brain and kidney damage.*

quinone [Ketone] *Respiratory mucous membrane irritation, pulmonary edema, CNS depression.*

quintozene [Pentachlorophenol] *Respiratory and circulatory collapse, severe hyperthermia.*

R134A refrigerant (1,1,1,2-tetrafluoroethane) [Chlorinated fluorocarbon] *Asphyxiation, anesthesia, arrhythmias.*

radioactive material (n.o.s.) [Radioactive] *DNA or RNA damage, severe GI or hematologic damage, loss of bone marrow function, immunocompromise, systemic infection, carcinoma.*

rare gas mixture (n.o.s.) [Poison] *Cardiovascular collapse, pulmonary edema, CNS depression, coma, seizures, nausea, vomiting, cardiopulmonary arrest.* [Simple asphyxiant] *Asphyxiation.*

rare gas & nitrogen mixture [Poison] *Cardiovascular collapse, pulmonary edema, CNS depression, coma, seizures, nausea, vomiting, cardiopulmonary arrest.* [Simple asphyxiant] *Asphyxiation.*

rare gas & oxygen mixture [Poison] *Cardiovascular collapse, pulmonary edema, CNS depression, coma, seizures, nausea, vomiting, cardiopulmonary arrest.* [Simple asphyxiant] *Asphyxiation.*

red phosphorus [Phosphorus] *Hypovolemic shock, severe tissue burns, severe respiratory irritation, pulmonary edema, respiratory arrest, arrhythmias, sudden death.*

reducing liquid [Poison] *Cardiovascular collapse, pulmonary edema, CNS depression, coma, seizures, nausea, vomiting, cardiopulmonary arrest.*

refrigerant gas (n.o.s.) [Chlorinated fluorocarbon] *Asphyxiation, anesthesia, arrhythmias.*

refrigerant gas, flammable (n.o.s.) [Flammable gas] *Respiratory failure, cardiac arrest, arrhythmias.*

refrigerant R134A (1,1,1,2-tetrafluoroethane) [Chlorinated fluorocarbon] *Asphyxiation, anesthesia, arrhythmias.*

refrigerator with flammable liquefied gas [Flammable gas] *Respiratory failure, cardiac arrest, arrhythmias.* [Simple asphyxiant] *Asphyxiation.*

refrigerator with nonflammable liquefied gas [Nonflammable gas] *Pulmonary edema, respiratory failure, asphyxiation.* [Simple asphyxiant] *Asphyxiation.*

removing liquid [Poison] *Cardiovascular collapse, pulmonary edema, CNS depression, coma, seizures, nausea, vomiting, cardiopulmonary arrest.*

reserpine [Poison] *Cardiovascular collapse, pulmonary edema, CNS depression, coma, seizures, nausea, vomiting, cardiopulmonary arrest.*

residual oil [Hydrocarbon mixture] *CNS depression, respiratory arrest, seizures, arrhythmias, pulmonary edema.*

resin compound, flammable [Flammable/combustible liquid] *CNS depression, respiratory arrest, convulsions, arrhythmias, pulmonary edema.*

HazMat

resin compound, poisonous [Poison] *Cardiovascular collapse, pulmonary edema, CNS depression, coma, seizures, nausea, vomiting, cardiopulmonary arrest.*

resmethrin [Pyrethrin/pyrethroid] *Respiratory paralysis, convulsions.*

resorcinol [Phenol] *Coma, hypotension, arrhythmias, pulmonary edema, respiratory arrest.*

road asphalt [Hydrocarbon mixture] *CNS depression, respiratory arrest, seizures, arrhythmias, pulmonary edema.*

road oil [Hydrocarbon mixture] *CNS depression, respiratory arrest, seizures, arrhythmias, pulmonary edema.*

rodenticide (n.o.s.) [Poison] *Cardiovascular collapse, pulmonary edema, CNS depression, coma, seizures, nausea, vomiting, cardiopulmonary arrest.*

ronnel [Organophosphate] *Pulmonary edema, respiratory muscle paralysis, respiratory failure, bradycardia, acetylcholinesterase inhibition, hypotension, pulmonary edema, overstimulation of parasympathetic nervous system, striated muscle, sympathetic ganglia, and CNS.*

rosin oil [Poison] *Cardiovascular collapse, pulmonary edema, CNS depression, coma, seizures, nausea, vomiting, cardiopulmonary arrest.*

rotenoid (n.o.s.) [Rotenone] *Respiratory arrest, asphyxia.*

rotenone [Rotenone] *Respiratory arrest, asphyxia.*

Roundup [Glyphosate] *Hypotension, arrhythmias, pulmonary edema.*

rubber scrap, powder, granules, or solution [Poison] *Cardiovascular collapse, pulmonary edema, CNS depression, coma, seizures, nausea, vomiting, cardiopulmonary arrest.*

rubber solvent (naphtha) [Hydrocarbon mixture] *CNS depression, respiratory arrest, seizures, arrhythmias, pulmonary edema.*

rubidium [Poison] *Cardiovascular collapse, pulmonary edema, CNS depression, coma, seizures, nausea, vomiting, cardiopulmonary arrest.*

rubidium hydroxide [Poison] *Cardiovascular collapse, pulmonary edema, CNS depression, coma, seizures, nausea, vomiting, cardiopulmonary arrest.*

Ruelene [Organophosphate] *Pulmonary edema, respiratory muscle paralysis, respiratory failure, bradycardia, acetylcholinesterase inhibition, hypotension, pulmonary edema, overstimulation of parasympathetic nervous system, striated muscle, sympathetic ganglia, and CNS.*

saccharin; saccharin salt (n.o.s.) [Poison] *Cardiovascular collapse, pulmonary edema, CNS depression, coma, seizures, nausea, vomiting, cardiopulmonary arrest.*

safrole [Phenol] *Coma, hypotension, arrhythmias, pulmonary edema, respiratory arrest.*

salcomine [Poison] *Cardiovascular collapse, pulmonary edema, CNS depression, coma, seizures, nausea, vomiting, cardiopulmonary arrest.*

saltpeter [Nitrate/nitrite] *Methemoglobinemia, hypotension, circulatory collapse.*

saprol [Phenol] *Coma, hypotension, arrhythmias, pulmonary edema, respiratory arrest.*

sarin [Organophosphate] *Pulmonary edema, respiratory muscle paralysis, respiratory failure, bradycardia, acetylcholinesterase inhibition, hypotension, pulmonary edema, overstimulation of parasympathetic nervous system, striated muscle, sympathetic ganglia, and CNS.*

sea coal [Flammable solid] *Shock, severe chemical and thermal burns, severe respiratory tract irritation, pulmonary edema, respiratory arrest, ECG changes, sudden death.*

selenate (n.o.s.) [Selenium] *Arrhythmias, pulmonary edema, bronchospasm, seizures, vomiting, GI bleeding.*

selenic acid [Inorganic acid] *Pulmonary edema, bronchospasm, circulatory collapse, laryngeal spasm and edema, severe chemical burns to skin, mucous membranes, and internal organs, GI tract perforation and hemorrhage, peri-*

tonitis. [Selenium] *Arrhythmias, pulmonary edema, bronchospasm, seizures, vomiting, GI bleeding.*

selenious acid [Inorganic acid] *Pulmonary edema, bronchospasm, circulatory collapse, laryngeal spasm and edema, severe chemical burns to skin, mucous membranes, and internal organs, GI tract perforation and hemorrhage, peritonitis.* [Selenium] *Arrhythmias, pulmonary edema, bronchospasm, seizures, vomiting, GI bleeding.*

selenious acid, dithallium (1+) salt [Selenium] *Arrhythmias, pulmonary edema, bronchospasm, seizures, vomiting, GI bleeding.* [Thallium] *Pulmonary edema, respiratory failure, circulatory collapse, seizures.*

selenite (n.o.s.) [Selenium] *Arrhythmias, pulmonary edema, bronchospasm, seizures, vomiting, GI bleeding.*

selenium [Selenium] *Arrhythmias, pulmonary edema, bronchospasm, seizures, vomiting, GI bleeding.*

selenium dioxide [Selenium] *Arrhythmias, pulmonary edema, bronchospasm, seizures, vomiting, GI bleeding.*

selenium disulfide [Selenium] *Arrhythmias, pulmonary edema, bronchospasm, seizures, vomiting, GI bleeding.* [Sulfur] *Respiratory tract irritation, pulmonary edema, anaphylaxis.*

selenium hexafluoride [Selenium] *Arrhythmias, pulmonary edema, bronchospasm, seizures, vomiting, GI bleeding.* [Fluorine] *CNS depression, respiratory arrest, cardiovascular collapse, shock, arrhythmias.*

selenium oxide [Selenium] *Arrhythmias, pulmonary edema, bronchospasm, seizures, vomiting, GI bleeding.*

selenium oxychloride [Selenium] *Arrhythmias, pulmonary edema, bronchospasm, seizures, vomiting, GI bleeding.*

selenium sulfide [Selenium] *Arrhythmias, pulmonary edema, bronchospasm, seizures, vomiting, GI bleeding.* [Sulfur] *Respiratory tract irritation, pulmonary edema, anaphylaxis.*

selenourea [Selenium] *Arrhythmias, pulmonary edema, bronchospasm, seizures, vomiting, GI bleeding.*

self-heating substance, corrosive (n.o.s.) [Corrosive] *Upper airway burns and edema, circulatory collapse, severe chemical burns to skin, toxic systemic effects, GI tract perforation and hemorrhage, peritonitis.*

self-heating substance, oxidizing (n.o.s.) [Oxidizer] *Pulmonary and laryngeal edema, circulatory arrest, hypovolemic shock, chemical burns of skin, mucous membranes, and internal organs.*

self-heating substance, poisonous (n.o.s.) [Poison] *Cardiovascular collapse, pulmonary edema, CNS depression, coma, seizures, nausea, vomiting, cardiopulmonary arrest.*

self-reactive substance (n.o.s.) [Poison] *Cardiovascular collapse, pulmonary edema, CNS depression, coma, seizures, nausea, vomiting, cardiopulmonary arrest.*

semicarbazide HCl [Hydrazine] *Seizures, hemolysis of red blood cells, pulmonary edema.*

shale oil [Aliphatic hydrocarbon] *Arrhythmias, asphyxiation, anesthesia.*

shellac [Hydrocarbon mixture] *CNS depression, respiratory arrest, seizures, arrhythmias, pulmonary edema.*

silane [Silane/chlorosilane] *Respiratory tract irritation, pulmonary edema.*

silicofluoric acid [Fluorine] *CNS depression, respiratory arrest, cardiovascular collapse, shock, arrhythmias.*

silicofluoride (n.o.s.) [Fluorine] *CNS depression, respiratory arrest, cardiovascular collapse, shock, arrhythmias.*

silicon [Irritant] *Severe immediate or delayed upper airway or respiratory tract irritation, pulmonary edema, glottic spasm, airway obstruction.*

silicon chloride [Chlorine] *Severe respiratory tract irritation, pulmonary edema, irritation of skin, eyes, and mucous membranes.*

silicon tetrachloride [Chlorine] *Severe respiratory tract irritation, pul-*

HazMat

monary edema, irritation of skin, eyes, and mucous membranes.

silicon tetrafluoride [Fluorine] *CNS depression, respiratory arrest, cardiovascular collapse, shock, arrhythmias.*

silver [Poison] *Cardiovascular collapse, pulmonary edema, CNS depression, coma, seizures, nausea, vomiting, cardiopulmonary arrest.*

silver arsenite [Arsenic] *Heavy metal toxicity, vomiting, GI bleeding, CNS depression, pulmonary edema, cardiac arrest.*

silver cyanide [Cyanide] *Impairment of cellular oxygenation and adenosine triphosphate production, hypoxia, death.*

silver nitrate [Nitrate/nitrite] *Methemoglobinemia, hypotension, circulatory collapse.*

silver picrate [Poison] *Cardiovascular collapse, pulmonary edema, CNS depression, coma, seizures, nausea, vomiting, cardiopulmonary arrest.*

silvex [Chlorophenoxy herbicide] *CNS depression, CNS stimulation, respiratory failure, ventricular fibrillation, seizures.*

sludge acid [Poison] *Cardiovascular collapse, pulmonary edema, CNS depression, coma, seizures, nausea, vomiting, cardiopulmonary arrest.*

smoke bomb [Irritant] *Severe immediate or delayed upper airway or respiratory tract irritation, pulmonary edema, glottic spasm, airway obstruction.* [Corrosive] *Upper airway burns and edema, circulatory collapse, severe chemical burns to skin, toxic systemic effects, GI tract perforation and hemorrhage, peritonitis.*

smokeless powder [Explosive] *Multiple trauma, highly toxic chemical exposure.*

soda lime [Inorganic base/alkaline corrosive] *Upper airway burns and edema, pulmonary edema, skin burns, circulatory collapse, GI tract perforation and hemorrhage, peritonitis.*

sodium; sodium alloy (n.o.s.) [Flammable solid] *Shock, severe chemical and thermal burns, severe respiratory tract*

irritation, pulmonary edema, respiratory arrest, ECG changes, sudden death.

sodium acid sulfate [Inorganic acid] *Pulmonary edema, bronchospasm, circulatory collapse, laryngeal spasm and edema, severe chemical burns to skin, mucous membranes, and internal organs, GI tract perforation and hemorrhage, peritonitis.*

sodium aluminate [Poison] *Cardiovascular collapse, pulmonary edema, CNS depression, coma, seizures, nausea, vomiting, cardiopulmonary arrest.*

sodium aluminum hydride [Poison] *Cardiovascular collapse, pulmonary edema, CNS depression, coma, seizures, nausea, vomiting, cardiopulmonary arrest.*

sodium amalgam [Mercury] *Circulatory collapse, arrhythmias, respiratory failure, pulmonary edema, neurotoxic effects.*

sodium amide [Inorganic base/alkaline corrosive] *Upper airway burns and edema, pulmonary edema, skin burns, circulatory collapse, GI tract perforation and hemorrhage, peritonitis.*

sodium ammonium vanadate [Poison] *Cardiovascular collapse, pulmonary edema, CNS depression, coma, seizures, nausea, vomiting, cardiopulmonary arrest.*

sodium arsanilate [Arsenic] *Heavy metal toxicity, vomiting, GI bleeding, CNS depression, pulmonary edema, cardiac arrest.*

sodium arsenate [Arsenic] *Heavy metal toxicity, vomiting, GI bleeding, CNS depression, pulmonary edema, cardiac arrest.*

sodium arsenite [Arsenic] *Heavy metal toxicity, vomiting, GI bleeding, CNS depression, pulmonary edema, cardiac arrest.*

sodium azide *Hypotension, arrhythmias, asystole, seizures, coma.*

sodium bichromate [Inorganic acid] *Pulmonary edema, bronchospasm, circulatory collapse, laryngeal spasm and edema, severe chemical burns to skin, mucous membranes, and internal* *organs, GI tract perforation and hemorrhage, peritonitis.*

sodium bifluoride [Fluorine] *CNS depression, respiratory arrest, cardiovascular collapse, shock, arrhythmias.*

sodium binoxalate [Oxalate] *Cardiovascular collapse, arrhythmias, seizures.*

sodium bisulfate [Poison] *Cardiovascular collapse, pulmonary edema, CNS depression, coma, seizures, nausea, vomiting, cardiopulmonary arrest.*

sodium bisulfite [Sulfur] *Respiratory tract irritation, pulmonary edema, anaphylaxis.*

sodium borohydride [Boron] *Respiratory tract irritation, laryngeal spasm and edema, pulmonary edema, severe chemical burns.*

sodium bromate [Bromate] *CNS and respiratory system depression, delayed-onset renal failure.*

sodium cacodylate [Arsenic] *Heavy metal toxicity, vomiting, GI bleeding, CNS depression, pulmonary edema, cardiac arrest.*

sodium carbonate [Inorganic base/alkaline corrosive] *Upper airway burns and edema, pulmonary edema, skin burns, circulatory collapse, GI tract perforation and hemorrhage, peritonitis.*

sodium chlorate [Chlorate] *Hemolysis, methemoglobinemia, hypoperfusion, CNS depression, delayed-onset renal failure.*

sodium chlorite [Hypochlorite] *Circulatory collapse, respiratory tract irritation, upper airway obstruction, pulmonary edema.*

sodium chloroacetate [Ester] *CNS depression, respiratory tract irritation, bronchitis, pneumonitis.*

sodium chromate [Poison] *Cardiovascular collapse, pulmonary edema, CNS depression, coma, seizures, nausea, vomiting, cardiopulmonary arrest.*

sodium cuprocyanide [Cyanide] *Impairment of cellular oxygenation and adenosine triphosphate production, hypoxia, death.*

sodium cyanide [Cyanide] *Impairment of cellular oxygenation and adenosine triphosphate production, hypoxia, death.*

sodium 2-diazo-1-naphthol-4-sulfonate; sodium 2-diazo-1-naphthol-5-sulfonate [Phenol] *Coma, hypotension, arrhythmias, pulmonary edema, respiratory arrest.*

sodium dichloroisocyanate [Hypochlorite] *Circulatory collapse, respiratory tract irritation, upper airway obstruction, pulmonary edema.*

sodium dichloroisocyanurate [Hypochlorite] *Circulatory collapse, respiratory tract irritation, upper airway obstruction, pulmonary edema.*

sodium dichloro-S-triazinetrione [Hypochlorite] *Circulatory collapse, respiratory tract irritation, upper airway obstruction, pulmonary edema.*

sodium dichromate [Poison] *Cardiovascular collapse, pulmonary edema, CNS depression, coma, seizures, nausea, vomiting, cardiopulmonary arrest.*

sodium dinitro-o-cresolate [Phenol] *Coma, hypotension, arrhythmias, pulmonary edema, respiratory arrest.*

sodium dithionite [Sulfur] *Respiratory tract irritation, pulmonary edema, anaphylaxis.*

sodium dodecylbenzenesulfonate [Poison] *Cardiovascular collapse, pulmonary edema, CNS depression, coma, seizures, nausea, vomiting, cardiopulmonary arrest.*

sodium fluoride [Hydrofluoric acid] *Pulmonary and laryngeal edema, circulatory collapse, severe skin burns, GI tract perforation, systemic fluoride poisoning.*

sodium fluoroacetate [Monofluoroacetate] *Ventricular arrhythmias, seizures.*

sodium fluorosilicate [Fluorine] *CNS depression, respiratory arrest, cardiovascular collapse, shock, arrhythmias.*

sodium hydrate [Inorganic base/alkaline corrosive] *Upper airway burns and edema, pulmonary edema, skin burns, circulatory collapse, GI tract perforation and hemorrhage, peritonitis.*

HazMat

sodium hydride [Inorganic base/alkaline corrosive] *Upper airway burns and edema, pulmonary edema, skin burns, circulatory collapse, GI tract perforation and hemorrhage, peritonitis.*

sodium hydrogen fluoride [Hydrofluoric acid] *Pulmonary and laryngeal edema, circulatory collapse, severe skin burns, GI tract perforation, systemic fluoride poisoning.*

sodium hydrogen sulfate [Sulfur] *Respiratory tract irritation, pulmonary edema, anaphylaxis.*

sodium hydrosulfide [Hydrogen sulfide] *Severe respiratory tract irritation, pulmonary edema, respiratory paralysis.*

sodium hydrosulfite [Sulfur] *Respiratory tract irritation, pulmonary edema, anaphylaxis.*

sodium hydroxide [Inorganic base/alkaline corrosive] *Upper airway burns and edema, pulmonary edema, skin burns, circulatory collapse, GI tract perforation and hemorrhage, peritonitis.*

sodium hypochlorite [Hypochlorite] *Circulatory collapse, respiratory tract irritation, upper airway obstruction, pulmonary edema.*

sodium metasilicate [Inorganic base/alkaline corrosive] *Upper airway burns and edema, pulmonary edema, skin burns, circulatory collapse, GI tract perforation and hemorrhage, peritonitis.*

sodium methylate [Inorganic base/alkaline corrosive] *Upper airway burns and edema, pulmonary edema, skin burns, circulatory collapse, GI tract perforation and hemorrhage, peritonitis.* [Methyl alcohol] *Respiratory failure, circulatory collapse.*

sodium monoxide [Inorganic base/alkaline corrosive] *Upper airway burns and edema, pulmonary edema, skin burns, circulatory collapse, GI tract perforation and hemorrhage, peritonitis.*

sodium nitrate [Nitrate/nitrite] *Methemoglobinemia, hypotension, circulatory collapse.*

sodium nitrate & potash mixture [Nitrate/nitrite] *Methemoglobinemia, hypotension, circulatory collapse.*

sodium nitrate & potassium nitrate mixture [Nitrate/nitrite] *Methemoglobinemia, hypotension, circulatory collapse.*

sodium nitrite [Nitrate/nitrite] *Methemoglobinemia, hypotension, circulatory collapse.*

sodium nitrite & potassium nitrate mixture [Nitrate/nitrite] *Methemoglobinemia, hypotension, circulatory collapse.*

sodium pentachlorophenate [Pentachlorophenol] *Respiratory and circulatory collapse, severe hyperthermia.*

sodium percarbonate [Oxidizer] *Pulmonary and laryngeal edema, circulatory arrest, hypovolemic shock, chemical burns of skin, mucous membranes, and internal organs.*

sodium perchlorate [Chlorate] *Hemolysis, methemoglobinemia, hypoperfusion, CNS depression, delayed-onset renal failure.*

sodium permanganate [Inorganic acid] *Pulmonary edema, bronchospasm, circulatory collapse, laryngeal spasm and edema, severe chemical burns to skin, mucous membranes, and internal organs, GI tract perforation and hemorrhage, peritonitis.*

sodium peroxide [Oxidizer] *Pulmonary and laryngeal edema, circulatory arrest, hypovolemic shock, chemical burns of skin, mucous membranes, and internal organs.*

sodium persulfate [Sulfur] *Respiratory tract irritation, pulmonary edema, anaphylaxis.*

sodium phenolate [Phenol] *Coma, hypotension, arrhythmias, pulmonary edema, respiratory arrest.*

sodium phosphate [Inorganic acid] *Pulmonary edema, bronchospasm, circulatory collapse, laryngeal spasm and edema, severe chemical burns to skin, mucous membranes, and internal* organs, GI tract perforation and hemorrhage, peritonitis.

sodium phosphide [Phosphine] *Severe pulmonary irritation, pulmonary edema.*

sodium picramate [Flammable solid] *Shock, severe chemical and thermal burns, severe respiratory tract irritation, pulmonary edema, respiratory arrest, ECG changes, sudden death.*

sodium–potassium alloy (n.o.s.) [Flammable solid] *Shock, severe chemical and thermal burns, severe respiratory tract irritation, pulmonary edema, respiratory arrest, ECG changes, sudden death.*

sodium selenate [Selenium] *Arrhythmias, pulmonary edema, bronchospasm, seizures, vomiting, GI bleeding.*

sodium selenite [Selenium] *Arrhythmias, pulmonary edema, bronchospasm, seizures, vomiting, GI bleeding.*

sodium sesquicarbonate [Organic base/amine] *Pulmonary edema, cardiac depression, seizures.*

sodium silicate [Inorganic base/alkaline corrosive] *Upper airway burns and edema, pulmonary edema, skin burns, circulatory collapse, GI tract perforation and hemorrhage, peritonitis.*

sodium silicofluoride [Fluorine] *CNS depression, respiratory arrest, cardiovascular collapse, shock, arrhythmias.*

sodium sulfate & diperoxydodecane diacid mixture [Organic peroxide] *Pulmonary and laryngeal edema, circulatory arrest, hypovolemic shock, chemical burns to skin, mucous membranes, and internal organs.* [Sulfur] *Respiratory tract irritation, pulmonary edema, anaphylaxis.*

sodium sulfide [Hydrogen sulfide] *Severe respiratory tract irritation, pulmonary edema, respiratory paralysis.*

sodium superoxide [Oxidizer] *Pulmonary and laryngeal edema, circulatory arrest, hypovolemic shock, chemical burns of skin, mucous membranes, and internal organs.*

sodium tellurite [Poison] *Cardiovascular collapse, pulmonary edema, CNS depression, coma, seizures, nausea, vomiting, cardiopulmonary arrest.*

sodium thioglycolate [Inorganic base/alkaline corrosive] *Upper airway burns and edema, pulmonary edema, skin burns, circulatory collapse, GI tract perforation and hemorrhage, peritonitis.*

solox [Higher alcohol (4+ carbons)] *CNS depression, respiratory failure, arrhythmias.* [Hydrocarbon mixture] *CNS depression, respiratory arrest, seizures, arrhythmias, pulmonary edema.*

solvent, aromatic hydrocarbon (n.o.s.) [Aromatic hydrocarbon] *Arrhythmias, respiratory failure, pulmonary edema, paralysis, brain and kidney damage.*

solvent, chlorinated (n.o.s.) [Halogenated aliphatic hydrocarbon] *CNS depression, respiratory arrest, circulatory collapse.*

soman [Organophosphate] *Pulmonary edema, respiratory muscle paralysis, respiratory failure, bradycardia, acetylcholinesterase inhibition, hypotension, pulmonary edema, overstimulation of parasympathetic nervous system, striated muscle, sympathetic ganglia, and CNS.*

spirit of nitroglycerin [Nitrate/nitrite] *Methemoglobinemia, hypotension, circulatory collapse.*

stain (n.o.s.) [Hydrocarbon mixture] *CNS depression, respiratory arrest, seizures, arrhythmias, pulmonary edema.*

stannane [Organotin] *Respiratory failure, pulmonary edema, cerebral edema.*

stannic chloride [Inorganic acid] *Pulmonary edema, bronchospasm, circulatory collapse, laryngeal spasm and edema, severe chemical burns to skin, mucous membranes, and internal organs, GI tract perforation and hemorrhage, peritonitis.*

stannic phosphide [Phosphine] *Severe pulmonary irritation, pulmonary edema.*

stannous chloride [Inorganic acid] *Pulmonary edema, bronchospasm, circulatory collapse, laryngeal spasm and edema, severe chemical burns to skin, mucous membranes, and internal*

HazMat

organs, GI tract perforation and hemorrhage, peritonitis.

stearyl alcohol [Higher alcohol (4+ carbons)] *CNS depression, respiratory failure, arrhythmias.*

steel swarf [Iron] *Hypovolemic shock.*

stibine [Poison] *Cardiovascular collapse, pulmonary edema, CNS depression, coma, seizures, nausea, vomiting, cardiopulmonary arrest.*

Stoddard solvent [Hydrocarbon mixture] *CNS depression, respiratory arrest, seizures, arrhythmias, pulmonary edema.*

straw [Flammable solid] *Shock, severe chemical and thermal burns, severe respiratory tract irritation, pulmonary edema, respiratory arrest, ECG changes, sudden death.*

Strobane [Halogenated aliphatic hydrocarbon] *CNS depression, respiratory arrest, circulatory collapse.*

strontium; strontium alloy (n.o.s.) [Poison] *Cardiovascular collapse, pulmonary edema, CNS depression, coma, seizures, nausea, vomiting, cardiopulmonary arrest.*

strontium arsenite [Arsenic] *Heavy metal toxicity, vomiting, GI bleeding, CNS depression, pulmonary edema, cardiac arrest.*

strontium chlorate [Chlorate] *Hemolysis, methemoglobinemia, hypoperfusion, CNS depression, delayed-onset renal failure.*

strontium chromate [Poison] *Cardiovascular collapse, pulmonary edema, CNS depression, coma, seizures, nausea, vomiting, cardiopulmonary arrest.*

strontium nitrate [Nitrate/nitrite] *Methemoglobinemia, hypotension, circulatory collapse.*

strontium perchlorate [Chlorate] *Hemolysis, methemoglobinemia, hypoperfusion, CNS depression, delayed-onset renal failure.*

strontium peroxide [Oxidizer] *Pulmonary and laryngeal edema, circulatory arrest, hypovolemic shock, chemical burns of skin, mucous membranes, and internal organs.*

strontium phosphide [Phosphine] *Severe pulmonary irritation, pulmonary edema.*

strontium sulfide [Chlorate] *Hemolysis, methemoglobinemia, hypoperfusion, CNS depression, delayed-onset renal failure.*

strychnine; strychnine salt (n.o.s.) [Strychnine] *Convulsions, acidosis, diaphragmatic spasms, respiratory arrest.*

styrene [Aromatic hydrocarbon] *Arrhythmias, respiratory failure, pulmonary edema, paralysis, brain and kidney damage.*

styrene oxide [Aromatic hydrocarbon] *Arrhythmias, respiratory failure, pulmonary edema, paralysis, brain and kidney damage.*

substituted nitrophenol pesticide (n.o.s.) [Dinitrophenol] *Respiratory and circulatory collapse, pulmonary edema, hyperthermia.*

succinic acid peroxide [Organic acid] *Pulmonary edema, circulatory collapse, laryngeal edema and spasm, severe chemical burns to skin, mucous membranes, and internal organs, GI tract perforation and hemorrhage, peritonitis.*

succinonitrile [Cyanide] *Impairment of cellular oxygenation and adenosine triphosphate production, hypoxia, death.*

sulfallate [Carbamate] *Acetylcholinesterase inhibition (reversible), bradycardia, hypotension, respiratory muscle paralysis, respiratory arrest, pulmonary edema.*

sulfamic acid [Inorganic acid] *Pulmonary edema, bronchospasm, circulatory collapse, laryngeal spasm and edema, severe chemical burns to skin, mucous membranes, and internal organs, GI tract perforation and hemorrhage, peritonitis.*

sulfide (n.o.s.); sulfide salt (n.o.s.) [Hydrogen sulfide] *Severe respiratory tract irritation, pulmonary edema, respiratory paralysis.*

sulfotep [Organophosphate] *Pulmonary edema, respiratory muscle paraly-*

sis, *respiratory failure, bradycardia, acetylcholinesterase inhibition, hypotension, pulmonary edema, overstimulation of parasympathetic nervous system, striated muscle, sympathetic ganglia, and CNS.*

sulfoxide [Sulfur] *Respiratory tract irritation, pulmonary edema, anaphylaxis.*

sulfur [Sulfur] *Respiratory tract irritation, pulmonary edema, anaphylaxis.*

sulfur chloride [Sulfur] *Respiratory tract irritation, pulmonary edema, anaphylaxis.*

sulfur chloride & carbon tetrachloride mixture [Carbon tetrachloride] *CNS depression, respiratory arrest, circulatory collapse.* [Sulfur] *Respiratory tract irritation, pulmonary edema, anaphylaxis.*

sulfur chloride pentafluoride [Fluorine] *CNS depression, respiratory arrest, cardiovascular collapse, shock, arrhythmias.* [Sulfur] *Respiratory tract irritation, pulmonary edema, anaphylaxis.*

sulfur dioxide [Sulfur] *Respiratory tract irritation, pulmonary edema, anaphylaxis.*

sulfur dioxide & ozone mixture [Ozone] *Pulmonary edema, airway obstruction.* [Sulfur] *Respiratory tract irritation, pulmonary edema, anaphylaxis.*

sulfur hexafluoride [Simple asphyxiant] *Asphyxiation.*

sulfur monochloride [Sulfur] *Respiratory tract irritation, pulmonary edema, anaphylaxis.*

sulfur pentafluoride [Fluorine] *CNS depression, respiratory arrest, cardiovascular collapse, shock, arrhythmias.* [Sulfur] *Respiratory tract irritation, pulmonary edema, anaphylaxis.*

sulfur phosphide [Phosphine] *Severe pulmonary irritation, pulmonary edema.*

sulfur tetrafluoride [Hydrofluoric acid] *Pulmonary and laryngeal edema, circulatory collapse, severe skin burns, GI tract perforation, systemic fluoride poisoning.* [Sulfur] *Respiratory tract irritation, pulmonary edema, anaphylaxis.*

sulfur trioxide [Inorganic acid] *Pulmonary edema, bronchospasm, circulatory collapse, laryngeal spasm and edema, severe chemical burns to skin, mucous membranes, and internal organs, GI tract perforation and hemorrhage, peritonitis.*

sulfur trioxide & chlorosulfonic acid mixture [Inorganic acid] *Pulmonary edema, bronchospasm, circulatory collapse, laryngeal spasm and edema, severe chemical burns to skin, mucous membranes, and internal organs, GI tract perforation and hemorrhage, peritonitis.* [Sulfur] *Respiratory tract irritation, pulmonary edema, anaphylaxis.*

sulfuric acid [Inorganic acid] *Pulmonary edema, bronchospasm, circulatory collapse, laryngeal spasm and edema, severe chemical burns to skin, mucous membranes, and internal organs, GI tract perforation and hemorrhage, peritonitis.*

sulfuric acid & hydrofluoric acid mixture [Inorganic acid] *Pulmonary edema, bronchospasm, circulatory collapse, laryngeal spasm and edema, severe chemical burns to skin, mucous membranes, and internal organs, GI tract perforation and hemorrhage, peritonitis.* [Hydrofluoric acid] *Pulmonary and laryngeal edema, circulatory collapse, severe skin burns, GI tract perforation, systemic fluoride poisoning.*

sulfuric anhydride [Inorganic acid] *Pulmonary edema, bronchospasm, circulatory collapse, laryngeal spasm and edema, severe chemical burns to skin, mucous membranes, and internal organs, GI tract perforation and hemorrhage, peritonitis.*

sulfuric trioxide [Inorganic acid] *Pulmonary edema, bronchospasm, circulatory collapse, laryngeal spasm and edema, severe chemical burns to skin, mucous membranes, and internal organs, GI tract perforation and hemorrhage, peritonitis.*

sulfurous acid [Inorganic acid] *Pulmonary edema, bronchospasm, circula-*

HazMat

tory collapse, laryngeal spasm and edema, severe chemical burns to skin, mucous membranes, and internal organs, GI tract perforation and hemorrhage, peritonitis.

sulfurous acid 2-(*p-tert*-butylphenoxy)-1-methylethyl-2-chloroethyl ester [Poison] *Cardiovascular collapse, pulmonary edema, CNS depression, coma, seizures, nausea, vomiting, cardiopulmonary arrest.*

sulfuryl chloride [Inorganic acid] *Pulmonary edema, bronchospasm, circulatory collapse, laryngeal spasm and edema, severe chemical burns to skin, mucous membranes, and internal organs, GI tract perforation and hemorrhage, peritonitis.*

sulfuryl fluoride [Fluorine] *CNS depression, respiratory arrest, cardiovascular collapse, shock, arrhythmias.* [Sulfur] *Respiratory tract irritation, pulmonary edema, anaphylaxis.*

superphosphate (n.o.s.) [Inorganic acid] *Pulmonary edema, bronchospasm, circulatory collapse, laryngeal spasm and edema, severe chemical burns to skin, mucous membranes, and internal organs, GI tract perforation and hemorrhage, peritonitis.*

2,4,5-T [Chlorophenoxy herbicide] *CNS depression, CNS stimulation, respiratory failure, ventricular fibrillation, seizures.*

2,4,5-T acid [Chlorophenoxy herbicide] *CNS depression, CNS stimulation, respiratory failure, ventricular fibrillation, seizures.*

2,4,5-T amine (n.o.s.); 2,4,5-T ester (n.o.s.); 2,4,5-T salt (n.o.s.) [Chlorophenoxy herbicide] *CNS depression, CNS stimulation, respiratory failure, ventricular fibrillation, seizures.*

tabun [Organophosphate] *Pulmonary edema, respiratory muscle paralysis, respiratory failure, bradycardia, acetylcholinesterase inhibition, hypotension, pulmonary edema, overstimulation of parasympathetic nervous system, striated muscle, sympathetic ganglia, and CNS.*

tannic acid [Organic acid] *Pulmonary edema, circulatory collapse, laryngeal edema and spasm, severe chemical burns to skin, mucous membranes, and internal organs, GI tract perforation and hemorrhage, peritonitis.*

tar [Aromatic hydrocarbon] *Arrhythmias, respiratory failure, pulmonary edema, paralysis, brain and kidney damage.* [Benzene] *Arrhythmias, respiratory failure, pulmonary edema, CNS depression, liver and kidney damage.*

TBZ (thiabendazole) [Thiabendazole] *Cardiovascular collapse, respiratory tract irritation.*

TCDD (2,3,7,8-tetrachlorodibenzo-*p*-dioxin) [Chlorophenoxy herbicide] *CNS depression, CNS stimulation, respiratory failure, ventricular fibrillation, seizures.*

TDE (1,1-dichloro-2,2-bis-(*p*-chlorophenyl) ethane) [DDT] *CNS disruption, respiratory control center paralysis, ventricular fibrillation, seizures, respiratory arrest.*

TDI (toluene diisocyanate) [Isocyanate/aliphatic thiocyanate] *CNS depression, respiratory arrest, respiratory paralysis, pulmonary edema, cyanide toxicity.*

tear gas [Irritant] *Severe immediate or delayed upper airway or respiratory tract irritation, pulmonary edema, glottic spasm, airway obstruction.*

tecto; tecto 60 [Thiabendazole] *Cardiovascular collapse, respiratory tract irritation.*

tellurium [Poison] *Cardiovascular collapse, pulmonary edema, CNS depression, coma, seizures, nausea, vomiting, cardiopulmonary arrest.*

tellurium hexafluoride [Poison] *Cardiovascular collapse, pulmonary edema, CNS depression, coma, seizures, nausea, vomiting, cardiopulmonary arrest.*

temephos [Organophosphate] *Pulmonary edema, respiratory muscle paralysis, respiratory failure, bradycardia, acetylcholinesterase inhibition, hypoten-*

sion, *pulmonary edema, overstimulation of parasympathetic nervous system, striated muscle, sympathetic ganglia, and CNS.*

TEPP [Organophosphate] *Pulmonary edema, respiratory muscle paralysis, respiratory failure, bradycardia, acetylcholinesterase inhibition, hypotension, pulmonary edema, overstimulation of parasympathetic nervous system, striated muscle, sympathetic ganglia, and CNS.*

terbufos [Organophosphate] *Pulmonary edema, respiratory muscle paralysis, respiratory failure, bradycardia, acetylcholinesterase inhibition, hypotension, pulmonary edema, overstimulation of parasympathetic nervous system, striated muscle, sympathetic ganglia, and CNS.*

terebene [Turpentine/terpene] *Respiratory failure, pulmonary edema, tachycardia.*

terpene; terpene hydrocarbon (n.o.s.) [Turpentine/terpene] *Respiratory failure, pulmonary edema, tachycardia.*

terphenyl [Turpentine/terpene] *Respiratory failure, pulmonary edema, tachycardia.*

terpin hydrate [Turpentine/terpene] *Respiratory failure, pulmonary edema, tachycardia.*

terpineol [Turpentine/terpene] *Respiratory failure, pulmonary edema, tachycardia.*

terpinolene [Turpentine/terpene] *Respiratory failure, pulmonary edema, tachycardia.*

tetrabromo-o-cresol [Phenol] *Coma, hypotension, arrhythmias, pulmonary edema, respiratory arrest.*

tetrabromoethane; 1,1,2,2-tetrabromoethane [Halogenated aliphatic hydrocarbon] *CNS depression, respiratory arrest, circulatory collapse.*

1,2,4,5-tetrachlorobenzene [Aromatic hydrocarbon] *Arrhythmias, respiratory failure, pulmonary edema, paralysis, brain and kidney damage.*

2,3,7,8-tetrachlorodibenzo-p-dioxin (TCDD) [Chlorophenoxy herbicide] *CNS depression, CNS stimulation, respiratory failure, ventricular fibrillation, seizures.*

tetrachlorodifluoroethane [Chlorinated fluorocarbon] *Asphyxiation, anesthesia, arrhythmias.*

tetrachloroethane; 1,1,1,2-tetrachloroethane [Halogenated aliphatic hydrocarbon] *CNS depression, respiratory arrest, circulatory collapse.*

tetrachloroethylene [Carbon tetrachloride] *CNS depression, respiratory arrest, circulatory collapse.*

2,3,4,6-tetrachlorophenol [Phenol] *Coma, hypotension, arrhythmias, pulmonary edema, respiratory arrest.*

tetrachlorvinfos; tetrachlorvinphos [Organophosphate] *Pulmonary edema, respiratory muscle paralysis, respiratory failure, bradycardia, acetylcholinesterase inhibition, hypotension, pulmonary edema, overstimulation of parasympathetic nervous system, striated muscle, sympathetic ganglia, and CNS.*

tetraethyl dithiopyrophosphate [Organophosphate] *Pulmonary edema, respiratory muscle paralysis, respiratory failure, bradycardia, acetylcholinesterase inhibition, hypotension, pulmonary edema, overstimulation of parasympathetic nervous system, striated muscle, sympathetic ganglia, and CNS.*

tetraethyl dithiopyrophosphate & compressed gas mixture [Organophosphate] *Pulmonary edema, respiratory muscle paralysis, respiratory failure, bradycardia, acetylcholinesterase inhibition, hypotension, pulmonary edema, overstimulation of parasympathetic nervous system, striated muscle, sympathetic ganglia, and CNS.*

tetraethyl lead [Lead] *Circulatory collapse, coma, rare seizures.*

tetraethyl pyrophosphate [Organophosphate] *Pulmonary edema, respiratory muscle paralysis, respiratory failure, bradycardia, acetylcholinesterase inhibition, hypotension, pulmonary*

HazMat

edema, overstimulation of parasympathetic nervous system, striated muscle, sympathetic ganglia, and CNS.

tetraethyl pyrophosphate & compressed gas mixture [Organophosphate] *Pulmonary edema, respiratory muscle paralysis, respiratory failure, bradycardia, acetylcholinesterase inhibition, hypotension, pulmonary edema, overstimulation of parasympathetic nervous system, striated muscle, sympathetic ganglia, and CNS.*

tetraethyl silicate [Silane/chlorosilane] *Respiratory tract irritation, pulmonary edema.*

tetraethyl tin [Organotin] *Respiratory failure, pulmonary edema, cerebral edema.*

tetraethylammonium perchlorate [Chlorate] *Hemolysis, methemoglobinemia, hypoperfusion, CNS depression, delayed-onset renal failure.*

tetraethylenepentamine [Organic base/amine] *Pulmonary edema, cardiac depression, seizures.*

1,1,1,2-tetrafluoroethane (R134A refrigerant) [Chlorinated fluorocarbon] *Asphyxiation, anesthesia, arrhythmias.*

tetrafluoroethylene [Halogenated aliphatic hydrocarbon] *CNS depression, respiratory arrest, circulatory collapse.*

tetrafluorohydrazine [Hydrazine] *Seizures, hemolysis of red blood cells, pulmonary edema.*

tetrafluoromethane [Chlorinated fluorocarbon] *Asphyxiation, anesthesia, arrhythmias.*

tetrahydrobenzaldehyde [Aldehyde] *Seizures, respiratory failure, pulmonary edema.*

tetrahydrofuran [Ether] *Anesthesia, respiratory arrest.*

tetrahydrofurfurylamine [Organic base/amine] *Pulmonary edema, cardiac depression, seizures.*

tetrahydronaphthalene [Naphthalene] *Delayed-onset acute intravascular hemolysis.*

tetrahydronaphthyl hydroperoxide [Organic peroxide] *Pulmonary and laryngeal edema, circulatory arrest, hypovolemic shock, chemical burns to skin, mucous membranes, and internal organs.* [Naphthalene] *Delayed-onset acute intravascular hemolysis.*

tetrahydrophthalic anhydride [Organic acid] *Pulmonary edema, circulatory collapse, laryngeal edema and spasm, severe chemical burns to skin, mucous membranes, and internal organs, GI tract perforation and hemorrhage, peritonitis.*

tetrahydropyridine [Aromatic hydrocarbon] *Arrhythmias, respiratory failure, pulmonary edema, paralysis, brain and kidney damage.*

tetrahydrothiophene [Sulfur] *Respiratory tract irritation, pulmonary edema, anaphylaxis.*

tetralin hydroperoxide [Organic peroxide] *Pulmonary and laryngeal edema, circulatory arrest, hypovolemic shock, chemical burns to skin, mucous membranes, and internal organs.* [Naphthalene] *Delayed-onset acute intravascular hemolysis.*

Tetram [Organophosphate] *Pulmonary edema, respiratory muscle paralysis, respiratory failure, bradycardia, acetylcholinesterase inhibition, hypotension, pulmonary edema, overstimulation of parasympathetic nervous system, striated muscle, sympathetic ganglia, and CNS.*

tetramethoxysilane [Silane/chlorosilane] *Respiratory tract irritation, pulmonary edema.*

tetramethrin [Pyrethrin/pyrethroid] *Respiratory paralysis, convulsions.*

tetramethyl ammonium hydroxide [Organic base/amine] *Pulmonary edema, cardiac depression, seizures.*

tetramethyl lead [Lead] *Circulatory collapse, coma, rare seizures.*

tetramethyl silane [Silane/chlorosilane] *Respiratory tract irritation, pulmonary edema.*

1,1,3,3-tetramethylbutyl hydroxide [Organic peroxide] *Pulmonary and* *laryngeal edema, circulatory arrest, hypovolemic shock, chemical burns to skin, mucous membranes, and internal organs.*

1,1,3,3-tetramethylbutylperoxy-2-ethyl hexanoate [Organic peroxide] *Pulmonary and laryngeal edema, circulatory arrest, hypovolemic shock, chemical burns to skin, mucous membranes, and internal organs.*

tetramethylmethylenediamine [Organic base/amine] *Pulmonary edema, cardiac depression, seizures.*

tetranitromethane [Nitrate/nitrite] *Methemoglobinemia, hypotension, circulatory collapse.*

tetrapropyl dithionopyrophosphate [Organophosphate] *Pulmonary edema, respiratory muscle paralysis, respiratory failure, bradycardia, acetylcholinesterase inhibition, hypotension, pulmonary edema, overstimulation of parasympathetic nervous system, striated muscle, sympathetic ganglia, and CNS.*

tetrapropyl-o-titanate [Poison] *Cardiovascular collapse, pulmonary edema, CNS depression, coma, seizures, nausea, vomiting, cardiopulmonary arrest.*

Tetryl [Naphthalene] *Delayed-onset acute intravascular hemolysis.*

textile waste (n.o.s.) [see also: animal fabric with oil; vegetable fabric with oil] [Thallium] *Pulmonary edema, respiratory failure, circulatory collapse, seizures.* [Chlorate] *Hemolysis, methemoglobinemia, hypoperfusion, CNS depression, delayed-onset renal failure.*

textile-treating compound [Poison] *Cardiovascular collapse, pulmonary edema, CNS depression, coma, seizures, nausea, vomiting, cardiopulmonary arrest.*

thallic oxide [Thallium] *Pulmonary edema, respiratory failure, circulatory collapse, seizures.*

thallium acetate [Thallium] *Pulmonary edema, respiratory failure, circulatory collapse, seizures.*

thallium carbonate; thallous carbonate [Thallium] *Pulmonary*

edema, respiratory failure, circulatory collapse, seizures.

thallium chlorate [Thallium] *Pulmonary edema, respiratory failure, circulatory collapse, seizures.* [Chlorate] *Hemolysis, methemoglobinemia, hypoperfusion, CNS depression, delayed-onset renal failure.*

thallium chloride; thallous chloride [Thallium] *Pulmonary edema, respiratory failure, circulatory collapse, seizures.*

thallium mixture (n.o.s.); thallium salt (n.o.s.) [Thallium] *Pulmonary edema, respiratory failure, circulatory collapse, seizures.*

thallium nitrate [Nitrate/nitrite] *Methemoglobinemia, hypotension, circulatory collapse.* [Thallium] *Pulmonary edema, respiratory failure, circulatory collapse, seizures.*

thallium sulfate; thallous sulfate [Thallium] *Pulmonary edema, respiratory failure, circulatory collapse, seizures.*

thallous carbonate; thallium carbonate [Thallium] *Pulmonary edema, respiratory failure, circulatory collapse, seizures.*

thallous chloride; thallium chloride [Thallium] *Pulmonary edema, respiratory failure, circulatory collapse, seizures.*

thallous malonate [Thallium] *Pulmonary edema, respiratory failure, circulatory collapse, seizures.*

thallous sulfate; thallium sulfate [Thallium] *Pulmonary edema, respiratory failure, circulatory collapse, seizures.*

thanite [Isocyanate/aliphatic thiocyanate] *CNS depression, respiratory arrest, respiratory paralysis, pulmonary edema, cyanide toxicity.*

thiabendazole [Thiabendazole] *Cardiovascular collapse, respiratory tract irritation.*

thiapentanal [Poison] *Cardiovascular collapse, pulmonary edema, CNS depression, coma, seizures, nausea, vomiting, cardiopulmonary arrest.*

2-(4-thiazolyl) benzimidazole [Thiabendazole] *Cardiovascular collapse, respiratory tract irritation.*

Thibenzole [Thiabendazole] *Cardiovascular collapse, respiratory tract irritation.*

thimerosal [Mercury] *Circulatory collapse, arrhythmias, respiratory failure, pulmonary edema, neurotoxic effects.*

thinner, paint and varnish [Hydrocarbon mixture] *CNS depression, respiratory arrest, seizures, arrhythmias, pulmonary edema.*

thioacetamide [Sulfur] *Respiratory tract irritation, pulmonary edema, anaphylaxis.*

thioacetic acid [Organic acid] *Pulmonary edema, circulatory collapse, laryngeal edema and spasm, severe chemical burns to skin, mucous membranes, and internal organs, GI tract perforation and hemorrhage, peritonitis.* [Sulfur] *Respiratory tract irritation, pulmonary edema, anaphylaxis.*

thiocarbazide [Hydrazine] *Seizures, hemolysis of red blood cells, pulmonary edema.*

thiocyanates, aliphatic (n.o.s.) [Isocyanate/aliphatic thiocyanate] *CNS depression, respiratory arrest, respiratory paralysis, pulmonary edema, cyanide toxicity.*

Thiodan [Aldrin/dieldrin/endrin] *Seizures, respiratory failure.*

4,4'-thiodianiline [Aniline] *Methemoglobinemia, hypoxia.*

thiofanox [Carbamate] *Acetylcholinesterase inhibition (reversible), bradycardia, hypotension, respiratory muscle paralysis, respiratory arrest, pulmonary edema.*

thioglycol [Sulfur] *Respiratory tract irritation, pulmonary edema, anaphylaxis.*

thioglycolate salt (n.o.s.) [Organic acid] *Pulmonary edema, circulatory collapse, laryngeal edema and spasm, severe chemical burns to skin, mucous membranes, and internal organs, GI tract perforation and hemorrhage, peritonitis.*

thioglycolic acid [Organic acid] *Pulmonary edema, circulatory collapse, laryngeal edema and spasm, severe chemical burns to skin, mucous membranes, and internal organs, GI tract perforation and hemorrhage, peritonitis.*

thiolactic acid [Organic acid] *Pulmonary edema, circulatory collapse, laryngeal edema and spasm, severe chemical burns to skin, mucous membranes, and internal organs, GI tract perforation and hemorrhage, peritonitis.*

thiomethanol [Sulfur] *Respiratory tract irritation, pulmonary edema, anaphylaxis.*

thionazin [Organophosphate] *Pulmonary edema, respiratory muscle paralysis, respiratory failure, bradycardia, acetylcholinesterase inhibition, hypotension, pulmonary edema, overstimulation of parasympathetic nervous system, striated muscle, sympathetic ganglia, and CNS.*

thionyl chloride [Sulfur] *Respiratory tract irritation, pulmonary edema, anaphylaxis.*

thiophene [Sulfur] *Respiratory tract irritation, pulmonary edema, anaphylaxis.*

thiophenol [Sulfur] *Respiratory tract irritation, pulmonary edema, anaphylaxis.*

thiophosgene [Phosgene] *Severe respiratory irritation, alveolar damage, pulmonary edema.*

thiophosphoryl chloride [Phosphorus] *Hypovolemic shock, severe tissue burns, severe respiratory irritation, pulmonary edema, respiratory arrest, arrhythmias, sudden death.*

thiosemicarbazide [Hydrazine] *Seizures, hemolysis of red blood cells, pulmonary edema.*

thiourea [Naphthalene] *Delayed-onset acute intravascular hemolysis.*

thiram [Dithiocarbamate] *Hypotension, respiratory failure.*

thorium; thorium mixture (n.o.s.) [Flammable solid] *Shock, severe chemical and thermal burns, severe respiratory tract irritation, pulmonary edema, respiratory arrest, ECG changes, sudden death.* [Poison] *Cardiovascular collapse, pulmonary edema, CNS depression, coma, seizures, nausea, vomiting, cardiopulmonary arrest.*

thorium dioxide [Poison] *Cardiovascular collapse, pulmonary edema, CNS depression, coma, seizures, nausea, vomiting, cardiopulmonary arrest.*

thorium nitrate [Nitrate/nitrite] *Methemoglobinemia, hypotension, circulatory collapse.*

thymol [Phenol] *Coma, hypotension, arrhythmias, pulmonary edema, respiratory arrest.*

tin; tin mixture (n.o.s.) [Poison] *Cardiovascular collapse, pulmonary edema, CNS depression, coma, seizures, nausea, vomiting, cardiopulmonary arrest.*

tin chloride [Poison] *Cardiovascular collapse, pulmonary edema, CNS depression, coma, seizures, nausea, vomiting, cardiopulmonary arrest.*

tin tetrachloride [Poison] *Cardiovascular collapse, pulmonary edema, CNS depression, coma, seizures, nausea, vomiting, cardiopulmonary arrest.*

tincture, medicinal (n.o.s.) [Poison] *Cardiovascular collapse, pulmonary edema, CNS depression, coma, seizures, nausea, vomiting, cardiopulmonary arrest.*

titanium [Poison] *Cardiovascular collapse, pulmonary edema, CNS depression, coma, seizures, nausea, vomiting, cardiopulmonary arrest.*

titanium hydride [Poison] *Cardiovascular collapse, pulmonary edema, CNS depression, coma, seizures, nausea, vomiting, cardiopulmonary arrest.*

titanium sulfate [Poison] *Cardiovascular collapse, pulmonary edema, CNS depression, coma, seizures, nausea, vomiting, cardiopulmonary arrest.*

titanium tetrachloride [Poison] *Cardiovascular collapse, pulmonary edema, CNS depression, coma, seizures, nausea, vomiting, cardiopulmonary arrest.*

titanium tetrachloride & vanadium oxytrichloride mixture [Poison] *Cardiovascular collapse, pulmonary edema, CNS depression, coma, sei-*
zures, nausea, vomiting, cardiopulmonary arrest.

titanium trichloride; titanium trichloride mixture (n.o.s.) [Poison] *Cardiovascular collapse, pulmonary edema, CNS depression, coma, seizures, nausea, vomiting, cardiopulmonary arrest.*

Toe Puffs, nitrocellulose-based [Flammable solid] *Shock, severe chemical and thermal burns, severe respiratory tract irritation, pulmonary edema, respiratory arrest, ECG changes, sudden death.*

o-**tolidine** [Aniline] *Methemoglobinemia, hypoxia.*

toluene [Aromatic hydrocarbon] *Arrhythmias, respiratory failure, pulmonary edema, paralysis, brain and kidney damage.*

toluene diisocyanate (TDI) [Isocyanate/aliphatic thiocyanate] *CNS depression, respiratory arrest, respiratory paralysis, pulmonary edema, cyanide toxicity.*

toluene sulfonic acid [Organic acid] *Pulmonary edema, circulatory collapse, laryngeal edema and spasm, severe chemical burns to skin, mucous membranes, and internal organs, GI tract perforation and hemorrhage, peritonitis.*

toluenediamine [Aniline] *Methemoglobinemia, hypoxia.*

m-**toluidine; *o*-toluidine; *p*-toluidine** [Aniline] *Methemoglobinemia, hypoxia.*

o-**toluidine HCl** [Aniline] *Methemoglobinemia, hypoxia.*

toluol [Aromatic hydrocarbon] *Arrhythmias, respiratory failure, pulmonary edema, paralysis, brain and kidney damage.* [Phenol] *Coma, hypotension, arrhythmias, pulmonary edema, respiratory arrest.*

toluylenediamine [Aniline] *Methemoglobinemia, hypoxia.*

N-*m*-tolylphthalamic acid [Aniline] *Methemoglobinemia, hypoxia.*

toxaphene [Toxaphene] *Respiratory failure, seizures, exhaustion, death.*

HazMat

2,4,5-TP [Chlorophenoxy herbicide] *CNS depression, CNS stimulation, respiratory failure, ventricular fibrillation, seizures.*

tree-killing compound, corrosive [Poison] *Cardiovascular collapse, pulmonary edema, CNS depression, coma, seizures, nausea, vomiting, cardiopulmonary arrest.* [Corrosive] *Upper airway burns and edema, circulatory collapse, severe chemical burns to skin, toxic systemic effects, GI tract perforation and hemorrhage, peritonitis.*

tree-killing compound, flammable [Flammable/combustible liquid] *CNS depression, respiratory arrest, convulsions, arrhythmias, pulmonary edema.* [Poison] *Cardiovascular collapse, pulmonary edema, CNS depression, coma, seizures, nausea, vomiting, cardiopulmonary arrest.*

tremolite [Asbestos] *Asbestosis, lung cancer, malignant mesothelioma.*

triallyl borate [Boron] *Respiratory tract irritation, laryngeal spasm and edema, pulmonary edema, severe chemical burns.*

triallylamine [Organic base/amine] *Pulmonary edema, cardiac depression, seizures.*

triamiphos [Organophosphate] *Pulmonary edema, respiratory muscle paralysis, respiratory failure, bradycardia, acetylcholinesterase inhibition, hypotension, pulmonary edema, overstimulation of parasympathetic nervous system, striated muscle, sympathetic ganglia, and CNS.*

triatomic oxygen [Ozone] *Pulmonary edema, airway obstruction.*

triazine pesticide (n.o.s.) [Irritant] *Severe immediate or delayed upper airway or respiratory tract irritation, pulmonary edema, glottic spasm, airway obstruction.*

triaziquone [Poison] *Cardiovascular collapse, pulmonary edema, CNS depression, coma, seizures, nausea, vomiting, cardiopulmonary arrest.*

tri(1-aziridinyl)phosphine oxide [Poison] *Cardiovascular collapse, pulmonary edema, CNS depression, coma, seizures, nausea, vomiting, cardiopulmonary arrest.*

triazofos [Organophosphate] *Pulmonary edema, respiratory muscle paralysis, respiratory failure, bradycardia, acetylcholinesterase inhibition, hypotension, pulmonary edema, overstimulation of parasympathetic nervous system, striated muscle, sympathetic ganglia, and CNS.*

tribasic copper sulfate [Copper] *Respiratory tract irritation, respiratory arrest, hemorrhagic gastritis.*

tribromomethane [Chlorinated fluorocarbon] *Asphyxiation, anesthesia, arrhythmias.*

tributyl aluminum [Poison] *Cardiovascular collapse, pulmonary edema, CNS depression, coma, seizures, nausea, vomiting, cardiopulmonary arrest.*

S,S,S-tributyl phosphorotrithiolate [Organophosphate] *Pulmonary edema, respiratory muscle paralysis, respiratory failure, bradycardia, acetylcholinesterase inhibition, hypotension, pulmonary edema, overstimulation of parasympathetic nervous system, striated muscle, sympathetic ganglia, and CNS.*

tributylamine [Organic base/amine] *Pulmonary edema, cardiac depression, seizures.*

trichlorfon [Organophosphate] *Pulmonary edema, respiratory muscle paralysis, respiratory failure, bradycardia, acetylcholinesterase inhibition, hypotension, pulmonary edema, overstimulation of parasympathetic nervous system, striated muscle, sympathetic ganglia, and CNS.*

trichloroacetic acid [Organic acid] *Pulmonary edema, circulatory collapse, laryngeal edema and spasm, severe chemical burns to skin, mucous membranes, and internal organs, GI tract perforation and hemorrhage, peritonitis.*

trichloroacetyl chloride [Halogenated aliphatic hydrocarbon] *CNS* *depression, respiratory arrest, circulatory collapse.*

trichlorobenzene; 1,2,4-trichlorobenzene [Aromatic hydrocarbon] *Arrhythmias, respiratory failure, pulmonary edema, paralysis, brain and kidney damage.*

trichlorobutene [Halogenated aliphatic hydrocarbon] *CNS depression, respiratory arrest, circulatory collapse.*

trichloro(chloromethyl)silane [Silane/chlorosilane] *Respiratory tract irritation, pulmonary edema.*

trichloro(dichlorophenyl)silane [Silane/chlorosilane] *Respiratory tract irritation, pulmonary edema.*

trichloroethane; 1,1,1-trichloroethane; 1,1,2-trichloroethane [Halogenated aliphatic hydrocarbon] *CNS depression, respiratory arrest, circulatory collapse.*

trichloroethylene [Carbon tetrachloride] *CNS depression, respiratory arrest, circulatory collapse.*

trichloroethylsilane [Silane/chlorosilane] *Respiratory tract irritation, pulmonary edema.*

trichlorofluoromethane (Freon 11) [Chlorinated fluorocarbon] *Asphyxiation, anesthesia, arrhythmias.*

trichlorofluoromethane & chlorodifluoromethane & dichlorodifluoromethane mixture [Chlorinated fluorocarbon] *Asphyxiation, anesthesia, arrhythmias.*

trichlorofluoromethane & dichlorodifluoromethane mixture [Chlorinated fluorocarbon] *Asphyxiation, anesthesia, arrhythmias.*

trichloroisocyanuric acid [Hypochlorite] *Circulatory collapse, respiratory tract irritation, upper airway obstruction, pulmonary edema.*

trichloromethanesulfenyl chloride [Sulfur] *Respiratory tract irritation, pulmonary edema, anaphylaxis.*

trichloromonofluoromethane [Chlorinated fluorocarbon] *Asphyxiation, anesthesia, arrhythmias.*

trichloronate [Organophosphate] *Pulmonary edema, respiratory muscle paralysis, respiratory failure, bradycardia, acetylcholinesterase inhibition, hypotension, pulmonary edema, overstimulation of parasympathetic nervous system, striated muscle, sympathetic ganglia, and CNS.*

trichlorophenol [Phenol] *Coma, hypotension, arrhythmias, pulmonary edema, respiratory arrest.*

trichlorophenoxy ethyl sulfate sodium salt (n.o.s.) [Chlorophenoxy herbicide] *CNS depression, CNS stimulation, respiratory failure, ventricular fibrillation, seizures.*

trichlorophenoxyacetic acid; 2,4,5-trichlorophenoxyacetic acid [Chlorophenoxy herbicide] *CNS depression, CNS stimulation, respiratory failure, ventricular fibrillation, seizures.*

2,4,5-trichlorophenoxypropionic acid [Chlorophenoxy herbicide] *CNS depression, CNS stimulation, respiratory failure, ventricular fibrillation, seizures.*

trichlorophenylsilane [Silane/chlorosilane] *Respiratory tract irritation, pulmonary edema.*

trichlorosilane [Silane/chlorosilane] *Respiratory tract irritation, pulmonary edema.*

trichloro-S-triazinetrione; trichloro-S-triazinetrione salt (n.o.s.) [Hypochlorite] *Circulatory collapse, respiratory tract irritation, upper airway obstruction, pulmonary edema.*

trichlorotrifluorethane (Freon 13) [Chlorinated fluorocarbon] *Asphyxiation, anesthesia, arrhythmias.*

trichlorotrifluoroethane & dichlorodifluoromethane mixture [Chlorinated fluorocarbon] *Asphyxiation, anesthesia, arrhythmias.*

tricresyl phosphate; tri-o-cresyl phosphate [Triorthocresyl phosphate] *Delayed-onset neurotoxicity, ascending paralysis of the extremities.*

triethanolamine dodecylbenzene sulfonate [Poison] *Cardiovascular*

HazMat

collapse, pulmonary edema, CNS depression, coma, seizures, nausea, vomiting, cardiopulmonary arrest.

triethoxysilane [Silane/chlorosilane] Respiratory tract irritation, pulmonary edema.

triethyl phosphite [Phosphorus] Hypovolemic shock, severe tissue burns, severe respiratory irritation, pulmonary edema, respiratory arrest, arrhythmias, sudden death.

O,O,O-triethyl phosphorothioate [Organophosphate] Pulmonary edema, respiratory muscle paralysis, respiratory failure, bradycardia, acetylcholinesterase inhibition, hypotension, pulmonary edema, overstimulation of parasympathetic nervous system, striated muscle, sympathetic ganglia, and CNS.

triethylamine [Organic base/amine] Pulmonary edema, cardiac depression, seizures.

triethylene glycol [Ethylene glycol] Respiratory failure, pulmonary edema, paralysis, cardiovascular collapse, severe acidosis.

triethylene tetramine [Poison] Cardiovascular collapse, pulmonary edema, CNS depression, coma, seizures, nausea, vomiting, cardiopulmonary arrest.

trifluoroacetic acid [Organic acid] Pulmonary edema, circulatory collapse, laryngeal edema and spasm, severe chemical burns to skin, mucous membranes, and internal organs, GI tract perforation and hemorrhage, peritonitis.

trifluoroacetyl chloride [Organic acid] Pulmonary edema, circulatory collapse, laryngeal edema and spasm, severe chemical burns to skin, mucous membranes, and internal organs, GI tract perforation and hemorrhage, peritonitis.

trifluoroamine oxide [Fluorine] CNS depression, respiratory arrest, cardiovascular collapse, shock, arrhythmias.

trifluorobromomethane [Chlorinated fluorocarbon] Asphyxiation, anesthesia, arrhythmias.

trifluorochloroethylene [Chlorinated fluorocarbon] Asphyxiation, anesthesia, arrhythmias.

trifluorochloromethane [Chlorinated fluorocarbon] Asphyxiation, anesthesia, arrhythmias.

trifluoroethane [Chlorinated fluorocarbon] Asphyxiation, anesthesia, arrhythmias.

trifluoromethane (gas or cryogenic liquid) [Chlorinated fluorocarbon] Asphyxiation, anesthesia, arrhythmias.

3-(trifluoromethyl) benzenamine [Aniline] Methemoglobinemia, hypoxia.

2-trifluoromethylaniline; 3-trifluoromethylaniline [Aniline] Methemoglobinemia, hypoxia.

3-trifluoromethylphenylisocyanate [Isocyanate/aliphatic thiocyanate] CNS depression, respiratory arrest, respiratory paralysis, pulmonary edema, cyanide toxicity.

trifluralin [Irritant] Severe immediate or delayed upper airway or respiratory tract irritation, pulmonary edema, glottic spasm, airway obstruction.

triisobutyl aluminum [Poison] Cardiovascular collapse, pulmonary edema, CNS depression, coma, seizures, nausea, vomiting, cardiopulmonary arrest.

triisobutylene [Aliphatic hydrocarbon] Arrhythmias, asphyxiation, anesthesia.

triisocyanatoisocyanurate of isophoronediisocyanate [Poison] Cardiovascular collapse, pulmonary edema, CNS depression, coma, seizures, nausea, vomiting, cardiopulmonary arrest.

triisopropyl borate [Boron] Respiratory tract irritation, laryngeal spasm and edema, pulmonary edema, severe chemical burns.

trimethoxysilane [Silane/chlorosilane] Respiratory tract irritation, pulmonary edema.

trimethyl aluminum [Poison] Cardiovascular collapse, pulmonary edema, CNS depression, coma, seizures, nausea, vomiting, cardiopulmonary arrest.

trimethyl norpinanyl hydroperoxide [Aromatic hydrocarbon] *Arrhythmias, respiratory failure, pulmonary edema, paralysis, brain and kidney damage.*

trimethyl phosphite [Phosphorus] *Hypovolemic shock, severe tissue burns, severe respiratory irritation, pulmonary edema, respiratory arrest, arrhythmias, sudden death.*

trimethylacetyl chloride [Organic acid] *Pulmonary edema, circulatory collapse, laryngeal edema and spasm, severe chemical burns to skin, mucous membranes, and internal organs, GI tract perforation and hemorrhage, peritonitis.*

trimethylamine [Organic base/amine] *Pulmonary edema, cardiac depression, seizures.*

trimethylbenzene [Aromatic hydrocarbon] *Arrhythmias, respiratory failure, pulmonary edema, paralysis, brain and kidney damage.*

trimethylborate [Boron] *Respiratory tract irritation, laryngeal spasm and edema, pulmonary edema, severe chemical burns.*

trimethylchlorosilane [Silane/chlorosilane] *Respiratory tract irritation, pulmonary edema.*

trimethylcyclohexylamine [Organic base/amine] *Pulmonary edema, cardiac depression, seizures.*

trimethylene chlorohydrin [Dichloropropane/dichloropropene] *Pulmonary edema, bronchospasm, alveolar hemorrhage.*

trimethylhexamethylene diisocyanate [Isocyanate/aliphatic thiocyanate] *CNS depression, respiratory arrest, respiratory paralysis, pulmonary edema, cyanide toxicity.*

trimethylhexamethylenediamine [Organic base/amine] *Pulmonary edema, cardiac depression, seizures.*

trimethylolpropane phosphite [Poison] *Cardiovascular collapse, pulmonary edema, CNS depression, coma, seizures, nausea, vomiting, cardiopulmonary arrest.*

trimethyloxysilane [Silane/chlorosilane] *Respiratory tract irritation, pulmonary edema.*

2,2,4-trimethylpentane [Aliphatic hydrocarbon] *Arrhythmias, asphyxiation, anesthesia.*

2,4,4-trimethylpentyl-2-peroxyphenoxyacetate [Ester] *CNS depression, respiratory tract irritation, bronchitis, pneumonitis.*

trimethyltin chloride [Organotin] *Respiratory failure, pulmonary edema, cerebral edema.*

trinitrobenzene [Aromatic hydrocarbon] *Arrhythmias, respiratory failure, pulmonary edema, paralysis, brain and kidney damage.* [Nitrate/nitrite] *Methemoglobinemia, hypotension, circulatory collapse.*

trinitrobenzoic acid [Organic acid] *Pulmonary edema, circulatory collapse, laryngeal edema and spasm, severe chemical burns to skin, mucous membranes, and internal organs, GI tract perforation and hemorrhage, peritonitis.* [Nitrate/nitrite] *Methemoglobinemia, hypotension, circulatory collapse.*

trinitrophenol [Dinitrophenol] *Respiratory and circulatory collapse, pulmonary edema, hyperthermia.*

trinitrotoluene; 2,4,6-trinitrotoluene [Aromatic hydrocarbon] *Arrhythmias, respiratory failure, pulmonary edema, paralysis, brain and kidney damage.* [Nitrate/nitrite] *Methemoglobinemia, hypotension, circulatory collapse.*

triphenyl phosphate [Triorthocresyl phosphate] *Delayed-onset neurotoxicity, ascending paralysis of the extremities.*

triphenyltin chloride [Organotin] *Respiratory failure, pulmonary edema, cerebral edema.*

tripropylaluminum [Poison] *Cardiovascular collapse, pulmonary edema, CNS depression, coma, seizures, nausea, vomiting, cardiopulmonary arrest.*

tripropylamine [Organic base/amine] *Pulmonary edema, cardiac depression, seizures.*

HazMat

tripropylene [Aliphatic hydrocarbon] *Arrhythmias, asphyxiation, anesthesia.*

tris(1-aziridinyl)phosphine oxide [Poison] *Cardiovascular collapse, pulmonary edema, CNS depression, coma, seizures, nausea, vomiting, cardiopulmonary arrest.*

tris(2-chloroethyl)amine [Organic base/amine] *Pulmonary edema, cardiac depression, seizures.*

tris(2,3-dibromopropyl)phosphate [Phosphorus] *Hypovolemic shock, severe tissue burns, severe respiratory irritation, pulmonary edema, respiratory arrest, arrhythmias, sudden death.*

trisodium phosphate [Inorganic base/ alkaline corrosive] *Upper airway burns and edema, pulmonary edema, skin burns, circulatory collapse, GI tract perforation and hemorrhage, peritonitis.*

trisodium phosphate, chlorinated [Inorganic base/alkaline corrosive] *Upper airway burns and edema, pulmonary edema, skin burns, circulatory collapse, GI tract perforation and hemorrhage, peritonitis.* [Hypochlorite] *Circulatory collapse, respiratory tract irritation, upper airway obstruction, pulmonary edema.*

trypan blue [Naphthalene] *Delayed-onset acute intravascular hemolysis.*

tungsten hexafluoride [Fluorine] *CNS depression, respiratory arrest, cardiovascular collapse, shock, arrhythmias.*

turpentine; turpentine substitute [Turpentine/terpene] *Respiratory failure, pulmonary edema, tachycardia.*

undecane [Aliphatic hydrocarbon] *Arrhythmias, asphyxiation, anesthesia.*

uracil mustard [Poison] *Cardiovascular collapse, pulmonary edema, CNS depression, coma, seizures, nausea, vomiting, cardiopulmonary arrest.*

uranium [Radioactive] *DNA or RNA damage, severe GI or hematologic damage, loss of bone marrow function, immunocompromise, systemic infection, carcinoma.*

uranium acetate [Radioactive] *DNA or RNA damage, severe GI or hemato-*

logic damage, loss of bone marrow function, immunocompromise, systemic infection, carcinoma. [Ester] *CNS depression, respiratory tract irritation, bronchitis, pneumonitis.*

uranium hexafluoride [Radioactive] *DNA or RNA damage, severe GI or hematologic damage, loss of bone marrow function, immunocompromise, systemic infection, carcinoma.* [Fluorine] *CNS depression, respiratory arrest, cardiovascular collapse, shock, arrhythmias.*

uranium nitrate hexahydrate [Radioactive] *DNA or RNA damage, severe GI or hematologic damage, loss of bone marrow function, immunocompromise, systemic infection, carcinoma.* [Nitrate/nitrite] *Methemoglobinemia, hypotension, circulatory collapse.*

uranyl acetate [Radioactive] *DNA or RNA damage, severe GI or hematologic damage, loss of bone marrow function, immunocompromise, systemic infection, carcinoma.* [Ester] *CNS depression, respiratory tract irritation, bronchitis, pneumonitis.*

uranyl nitrate [Radioactive] *DNA or RNA damage, severe GI or hematologic damage, loss of bone marrow function, immunocompromise, systemic infection, carcinoma.* [Nitrate/nitrite] *Methemoglobinemia, hypotension, circulatory collapse.*

urea hydrogen peroxide [Organic peroxide] *Pulmonary and laryngeal edema, circulatory arrest, hypovolemic shock, chemical burns to skin, mucous membranes, and internal organs.*

urea nitrate [Nitrate/nitrite] *Methemoglobinemia, hypotension, circulatory collapse.*

urea peroxide [Organic peroxide] *Pulmonary and laryngeal edema, circulatory arrest, hypovolemic shock, chemical burns to skin, mucous membranes, and internal organs.*

urethane [Isocyanate/aliphatic thiocyanate] *CNS depression, respiratory* *arrest, respiratory paralysis, pulmonary edema, cyanide toxicity.*

valeraldehyde [Aldehyde] *Seizures, respiratory failure, pulmonary edema.*

valeric acid (n-pentanoic acid) [Organic acid] *Pulmonary edema, circulatory collapse, laryngeal edema and spasm, severe chemical burns to skin, mucous membranes, and internal organs, GI tract perforation and hemorrhage, peritonitis.*

valeryl chloride [Organic acid] *Pulmonary edema, circulatory collapse, laryngeal edema and spasm, severe chemical burns to skin, mucous membranes, and internal organs, GI tract perforation and hemorrhage, peritonitis.*

valinomycin [Poison] *Cardiovascular collapse, pulmonary edema, CNS depression, coma, seizures, nausea, vomiting, cardiopulmonary arrest.*

Valone [Warfarin/hydroxycoumarin/indanedione] *Anticoagulation effect, internal hemorrhage.*

vanadium oxytrichloride [Poison] *Cardiovascular collapse, pulmonary edema, CNS depression, coma, seizures, nausea, vomiting, cardiopulmonary arrest.*

vanadium oxytrichloride & titanium tetrachloride mixture [Poison] *Cardiovascular collapse, pulmonary edema, CNS depression, coma, seizures, nausea, vomiting, cardiopulmonary arrest.*

vanadium pentoxide [Poison] *Cardiovascular collapse, pulmonary edema, CNS depression, coma, seizures, nausea, vomiting, cardiopulmonary arrest.*

vanadium tetrachloride [Poison] *Cardiovascular collapse, pulmonary edema, CNS depression, coma, seizures, nausea, vomiting, cardiopulmonary arrest.*

vanadium trioxide [Poison] *Cardiovascular collapse, pulmonary edema, CNS depression, coma, seizures, nausea, vomiting, cardiopulmonary arrest.*

vanadyl sulfate [Poison] *Cardiovascular collapse, pulmonary edema, CNS depression, coma, seizures, nausea, vomiting, cardiopulmonary arrest.*

vanillin [Phenol] *Coma, hypotension, arrhythmias, pulmonary edema, respiratory arrest.*

varnish [Hydrocarbon mixture] *CNS depression, respiratory arrest, seizures, arrhythmias, pulmonary edema.*

varnish drier (n.o.s.) [Poison] *Cardiovascular collapse, pulmonary edema, CNS depression, coma, seizures, nausea, vomiting, cardiopulmonary arrest.*

vegetable fabric with oil (n.o.s.) [Flammable/combustible liquid] *CNS depression, respiratory arrest, convulsions, arrhythmias, pulmonary edema.*

vegetable fiber, burnt (n.o.s.) [Irritant] *Severe immediate or delayed upper airway or respiratory tract irritation, pulmonary edema, glottic spasm, airway obstruction.*

vegetable fiber with oil (n.o.s.) [Flammable/combustible liquid] *CNS depression, respiratory arrest, convulsions, arrhythmias, pulmonary edema.*

vinyl acetate [Ester] *CNS depression, respiratory tract irritation, bronchitis, pneumonitis.*

vinyl bromide [Bromine/methyl bromide] *Severe respiratory irritation, pulmonary edema, respiratory failure, coma, convulsions, death.*

vinyl butyl ether [Ether] *Anesthesia, respiratory arrest.*

vinyl butyrate [Ester] *CNS depression, respiratory tract irritation, bronchitis, pneumonitis.*

vinyl chloride [Carbon tetrachloride] *CNS depression, respiratory arrest, circulatory collapse.*

vinyl chloroacetate [Ester] *CNS depression, respiratory tract irritation, bronchitis, pneumonitis.*

vinyl ether [Ether] *Anesthesia, respiratory arrest.*

vinyl ethyl ether [Ether] *Anesthesia, respiratory arrest.*

HazMat

vinyl fluoride [Halogenated aliphatic hydrocarbon] *CNS depression, respiratory arrest, circulatory collapse.*

vinyl isobutyl ether [Ether] *Anesthesia, respiratory arrest.*

vinyl methyl ether [Ether] *Anesthesia, respiratory arrest.*

vinyl pyridine [Aromatic hydrocarbon] *Arrhythmias, respiratory failure, pulmonary edema, paralysis, brain and kidney damage.*

vinyl toluene [Aromatic hydrocarbon] *Arrhythmias, respiratory failure, pulmonary edema, paralysis, brain and kidney damage.*

vinyl trichlorosilane [Silane/chlorosilane] *Respiratory tract irritation, pulmonary edema.*

vinylidene chloride [Halogenated aliphatic hydrocarbon] *CNS depression, respiratory arrest, circulatory collapse.*

vinylidene fluoride [Halogenated aliphatic hydrocarbon] *CNS depression, respiratory arrest, circulatory collapse.*

VM&P naphtha [Hydrocarbon mixture] *CNS depression, respiratory arrest, seizures, arrhythmias, pulmonary edema.*

warfarin; warfarin salt (n.o.s.) [Warfarin/hydroxycoumarin/indanedione] *Anticoagulation effect, internal hemorrhage.*

warfarin sodium [Warfarin/hydroxycoumarin/indanedione] *Anticoagulation effect, internal hemorrhage.*

water-reactive solid (n.o.s.) [Flammable solid] *Shock, severe chemical and thermal burns, severe respiratory tract irritation, pulmonary edema, respiratory arrest, ECG changes, sudden death.*

weed-killing compound, corrosive [Poison] *Cardiovascular collapse, pulmonary edema, CNS depression, coma, seizures, nausea, vomiting, cardiopulmonary arrest.* [Corrosive] *Upper airway burns and edema, circulatory collapse, severe chemical burns to skin, toxic systemic effects, GI tract perforation and hemorrhage, peritonitis.*

weed-killing compound, flammable [Flammable/combustible liquid] *CNS depression, respiratory arrest, convulsions, arrhythmias, pulmonary edema.* [Poison] *Cardiovascular collapse, pulmonary edema, CNS depression, coma, seizures, nausea, vomiting, cardiopulmonary arrest.*

white asbestos [Asbestos] *Asbestosis, lung cancer, malignant mesothelioma.*

white phosphorus [Phosphorus] *Hypovolemic shock, severe tissue burns, severe respiratory irritation, pulmonary edema, respiratory arrest, arrhythmias, sudden death.*

wood alcohol [Methyl alcohol] *Respiratory failure, circulatory collapse.*

wood filler [Hydrocarbon mixture] *CNS depression, respiratory arrest, seizures, arrhythmias, pulmonary edema.*

wood preservative [Hydrocarbon mixture] *CNS depression, respiratory arrest, seizures, arrhythmias, pulmonary edema.*

wool waste [Irritant] *Severe immediate or delayed upper airway or respiratory tract irritation, pulmonary edema, glottic spasm, airway obstruction.*

xenon (gas or cryogenic liquid) [Simple asphyxiant] *Asphyxiation.*

xylene (xylol) [Aromatic hydrocarbon] *Arrhythmias, respiratory failure, pulmonary edema, paralysis, brain and kidney damage.*

xylenol [Aromatic hydrocarbon] *Arrhythmias, respiratory failure, pulmonary edema, paralysis, brain and kidney damage.* [Phenol] *Coma, hypotension, arrhythmias, pulmonary edema, respiratory arrest.*

xylidine [Aromatic hydrocarbon] *Arrhythmias, respiratory failure, pulmonary edema, paralysis, brain and kidney damage.*

xylol (xylene) [Aromatic hydrocarbon] *Arrhythmias, respiratory failure, pulmonary edema, paralysis, brain and kidney damage.*

xylyl bromide [Aromatic hydrocarbon] *Arrhythmias, respiratory failure,* *pulmonary edema, paralysis, brain and kidney damage.* [Bromine/methyl bromide] *Severe respiratory irritation, pulmonary edema, respiratory failure, coma, convulsions, death.*

xylylene dichloride [Aromatic hydrocarbon] *Arrhythmias, respiratory failure, pulmonary edema, paralysis, brain and kidney damage.*

yellow phosphorus [Phosphorus] *Hypovolemic shock, severe tissue burns, severe respiratory irritation, pulmonary edema, respiratory arrest, arrhythmias, sudden death.*

zinc; zinc salt (n.o.s.) [Zinc] *Respiratory tract irritation, metal fume fever, pulmonary edema.*

zinc acetate [Zinc] *Respiratory tract irritation, metal fume fever, pulmonary edema.*

zinc ammonium chloride [Zinc] *Respiratory tract irritation, metal fume fever, pulmonary edema.*

zinc ammonium nitrate [Nitrate/nitrite] *Methemoglobinemia, hypotension, circulatory collapse.* [Zinc] *Respiratory tract irritation, metal fume fever, pulmonary edema.*

zinc arsenate [Arsenic] *Heavy metal toxicity, vomiting, GI bleeding, CNS depression, pulmonary edema, cardiac arrest.* [Zinc] *Respiratory tract irritation, metal fume fever, pulmonary edema.*

zinc arsenate & zinc arsenite mixture [Arsenic] *Heavy metal toxicity, vomiting, GI bleeding, CNS depression, pulmonary edema, cardiac arrest.* [Zinc] *Respiratory tract irritation, metal fume fever, pulmonary edema.*

zinc arsenite [Arsenic] *Heavy metal toxicity, vomiting, GI bleeding, CNS depression, pulmonary edema, cardiac arrest.* [Zinc] *Respiratory tract irritation, metal fume fever, pulmonary edema.*

zinc arsenite & zinc arsenate mixture [Arsenic] *Heavy metal toxicity, vomiting, GI bleeding, CNS depression, pulmonary edema, cardiac arrest.* [Zinc] *Respiratory tract irritation, metal fume fever, pulmonary edema.*

zinc bisulfite [Zinc] *Respiratory tract irritation, metal fume fever, pulmonary edema.* [Sulfur] *Respiratory tract irritation, pulmonary edema, anaphylaxis.*

zinc borate [Zinc] *Respiratory tract irritation, metal fume fever, pulmonary edema.* [Boron] *Respiratory tract irritation, laryngeal spasm and edema, pulmonary edema, severe chemical burns.*

zinc bromate [Zinc] *Respiratory tract irritation, metal fume fever, pulmonary edema.* [Bromate] *CNS and respiratory system depression, delayed-onset renal failure.*

zinc bromide [Zinc] *Respiratory tract irritation, metal fume fever, pulmonary edema.* [Bromine/methyl bromide] *Severe respiratory irritation, pulmonary edema, respiratory failure, coma, convulsions, death.*

zinc carbonate [Zinc] *Respiratory tract irritation, metal fume fever, pulmonary edema.*

zinc chlorate [Zinc] *Respiratory tract irritation, metal fume fever, pulmonary edema.* [Chlorate] *Hemolysis, methemoglobinemia, hypoperfusion, CNS depression, delayed-onset renal failure.*

zinc chloride [Zinc] *Respiratory tract irritation, metal fume fever, pulmonary edema.*

zinc chromate [Zinc] *Respiratory tract irritation, metal fume fever, pulmonary edema.*

zinc cyanide [Zinc] *Respiratory tract irritation, metal fume fever, pulmonary edema.* [Cyanide] *Impairment of cellular oxygenation and adenosine triphosphate production, hypoxia, death.*

zinc dithionite [Zinc] *Respiratory tract irritation, metal fume fever, pulmonary edema.*

zinc fluoride [Zinc] *Respiratory tract irritation, metal fume fever, pulmonary edema.* [Fluorine] *CNS depression, respiratory arrest, cardiovascular collapse, shock, arrhythmias.*

zinc fluorosilicate [Zinc] *Respiratory tract irritation, metal fume fever, pulmonary edema.* [Fluorine] *CNS*

depression, respiratory arrest, cardiovascular collapse, shock, arrhythmias.

zinc formate [Zinc] *Respiratory tract
irritation, metal fume fever, pulmonary
edema.*

zinc hydrosulfite [Zinc] *Respiratory tract
irritation, metal fume fever, pulmonary
edema.* [Sulfur] *Respiratory tract irritation, pulmonary edema, anaphylaxis.*

zinc nitrate [Nitrate/nitrite] *Methemoglobinemia, hypotension, circulatory collapse.* [Zinc] *Respiratory tract irritation,
metal fume fever, pulmonary edema.*

zinc permanganate [Inorganic acid]
*Pulmonary edema, bronchospasm, cir-
culatory collapse, laryngeal spasm and
edema, severe chemical burns to skin,
mucous membranes, and internal
organs, GI tract perforation and hemorrhage, peritonitis.* [Zinc] *Respiratory
tract irritation, metal fume fever, pulmonary edema.*

zinc peroxide [Zinc] *Respiratory tract
irritation, metal fume fever, pulmonary
edema.*

zinc phenolsulfonate [Zinc] *Respiratory tract irritation, metal fume fever,
pulmonary edema.* [Sulfur] *Respiratory
tract irritation, pulmonary edema, anaphylaxis.*

zinc phosphide [Zinc] *Respiratory tract
irritation, metal fume fever, pulmonary
edema.* [Phosphine] *Severe pulmonary
irritation, pulmonary edema.*

zinc resinate [Zinc] *Respiratory tract
irritation, metal fume fever, pulmonary
edema.*

zinc selenate [Selenium] *Arrhythmias,
pulmonary edema, bronchospasm, seizures, vomiting, GI bleeding.* [Zinc]
*Respiratory tract irritation, metal fume
fever, pulmonary edema.*

zinc selenite [Selenium] *Arrhythmias,
pulmonary edema, bronchospasm, seizures, vomiting, GI bleeding.* [Zinc]
*Respiratory tract irritation, metal fume
fever, pulmonary edema.*

zinc silicofluoride [Zinc] *Respiratory
tract irritation, metal fume fever, pulmonary edema.* [Fluorine] *CNS*

depression, respiratory arrest, cardiovascular collapse, shock, arrhythmias.

zinc sulfate [Zinc] *Respiratory tract
irritation, metal fume fever, pulmonary
edema.*

zineb [Dithiocarbamate] *Hypotension,
respiratory failure.*

ziram [Dithiocarbamate] *Hypotension,
respiratory failure.*

zirconium [Poison] *Cardiovascular collapse, pulmonary edema, CNS depression, coma, seizures, nausea, vomiting,
cardiopulmonary arrest.*

zirconium hydride [Poison] *Cardiovascular collapse, pulmonary edema,
CNS depression, coma, seizures, nausea, vomiting, cardiopulmonary arrest.*

zirconium nitrate [Nitrate/nitrite]
*Methemoglobinemia, hypotension, cir-
culatory collapse.*

zirconium picramate [Flammable
solid] *Shock, severe chemical and thermal burns, severe respiratory tract irritation, pulmonary edema, respiratory
arrest, ECG changes, sudden death.*
[Poison] *Cardiovascular collapse, pulmonary edema, CNS depression,
coma, seizures, nausea, vomiting, cardiopulmonary arrest.*

zirconium potassium fluoride [Fluo-
rine] *CNS depression, respiratory
arrest, cardiovascular collapse, shock,
arrhythmias.*

zirconium sulfate [Poison] *Cardiovascular collapse, pulmonary edema, CNS
depression, coma, seizures, nausea,
vomiting, cardiopulmonary arrest.*

zirconium tetrachloride [Poison]
*Cardiovascular collapse, pulmonary
edema, CNS depression, coma, seizures, nausea, vomiting, cardiopulmonary arrest.*

Zytron [Organophosphate] *Pulmonary
edema, respiratory muscle paralysis, respiratory failure, bradycardia, acetylcholinesterase inhibition, hypotension, pulmonary edema, overstimulation of
parasympathetic nervous system, striated
muscle, sympathetic ganglia, and CNS.*